Clinical Applications of SPECT-CT

Hojjat Ahmadzadehfar
Hans-Jürgen Biersack • Ken Herrmann
Editors

Clinical Applications of SPECT-CT

Second Edition

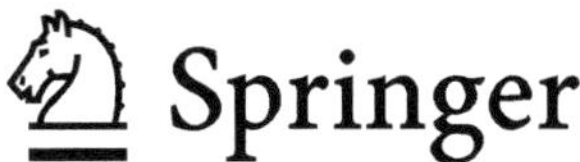

Editors
Hojjat Ahmadzadehfar
Department of Nuclear Medicine
Klinikum Westfalen
Dortmund, Germany

Hans-Jürgen Biersack
Department of Nuclear Medicine
University Hospital Bonn
Bonn, Germany

Ken Herrmann
Deptartment of Nuclear Medicine
Universitätsklinikum Essen
Essen, Germany

ISBN 978-3-030-65849-6   ISBN 978-3-030-65850-2   (eBook)
https://doi.org/10.1007/978-3-030-65850-2

This Springer imprint is published by the registered company Springer Nature Switzerland AG
The registered company address is: Gewerbestrasse 11, 6330 Cham, Switzerland

Contents

Physics and Technology of SPECT/CT

Dale L. Bailey and Kathy P. Willowson

1.1 SPECT/CT: Combining Form with Function

The introduction of combined SPECT (single photon emission computed tomography) and X-ray CT (computed tomography) scanners has changed the practice of single photon imaging in nuclear medicine forever. The original motivators to produce a combined SPECT/CT system were to provide improved anatomical localisation of the distribution of the SPECT radiopharmaceutical and to improve the capability of the SPECT scanner to produce images that can be corrected for the photon scattering and attenuation that cause degradation of the image.

The functional information contained in the SPECT images is complemented by the anatomical information (the 'form') provided by the CT scanner in numerous ways, including:

- Anatomical localisation of the SPECT radiopharmaceutical distribution.
- Correction for photon attenuation.
- Correcting for scattered radiation.

- Ability to determine the impact of the partial volume effect (PVE) due to the limited spatial resolution of the SPECT camera.
- The ability to calibrate the SPECT images in absolute units of radioactivity ($kBq\ ml^{-1}$).
- Introducing new clinical applications based on quantitative imaging in SPECT that require absolute radioactivity measures.
- The ability to convert the quantitative SPECT images into standardised uptake values (SUV).

This chapter will concentrate on the physics and technology relevant to combined SPECT and X-ray CT imaging.

1.2 The Development of Multimodality SPECT/CT Imaging

The first multimodal imaging performed with SPECT was developed to provide more accurate attenuation correction methods. In the 1980s, a number of groups were actively producing crude CT-like measurements on the gamma camera using radionuclide transmission sources such as Gadolinuiom-153 (Gd-153) [1–4]. The radionuclide sources were used to produce external photon beams with which the patient could be irradiated to produce a transmission image. The advantage of these measurements is that they could be performed on the gamma camera thus

D. L. Bailey (✉) · K. P. Willowson
Department of Nuclear Medicine, Royal North Shore Hospital, Sydney, NSW, Australia
e-mail: dale.bailey@sydney.edu.au;
kathy.willowson@sydney.edu.au

H. Ahmadzadehfar et al. (eds.), *Clinical Applications of SPECT-CT*,
https://doi.org/10.1007/978-3-030-65850-2_1

obviating the need for a separate second detector. When a transmission radionuclide of different photon energy to the emission radionuclide's γ-ray energy was used, the emission and transmission measurements could be made simultaneously [1]. An example is shown in Fig. 1.1. For further discussion about these systems, the reader is referred to the review article by Bailey [5]. This technology found extensive use in SPECT myocardial perfusion imaging for correcting photon attenuation and has been incorporated into imaging guidelines issued by professional organisations [6].

However, even while these developments were being implemented others were starting to explore the use of CT with SPECT. Moore used a CT scan as the 'true' density distribution for attenuation correction in the early 1980s [7], and Fleming showed how a CT scan could be used in an iterative algorithm to produce quantitative SPECT reconstructions [8]. Hasegawa led a group in the early 1990s that sought to integrate many of these developments by producing a single detector that could record the X-rays from a CT source as well as the γ photons emitted by an in vivo radiopharmaceutical [9]. The

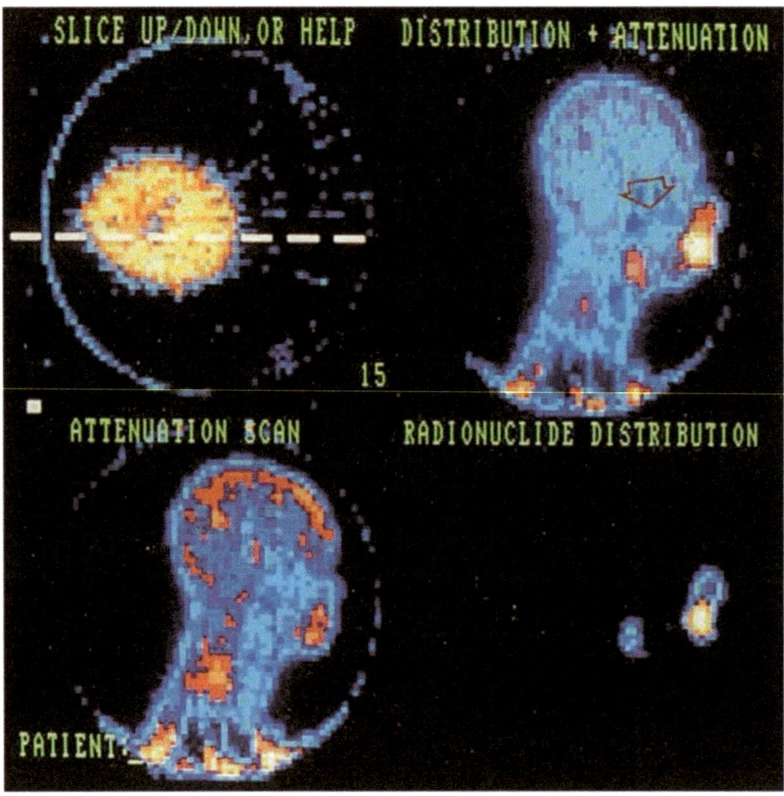

Fig. 1.1 An example from the mid-1980s of a simultaneous emission and transmission scan acquired with a gamma camera in a subject with a locally advanced cancer of the base of the tongue, intended for treatment with catheter-directed intra-arterial chemotherapy. The low resolution anatomical image is produced using a Gd-153 external radionuclide source. Gd-153 has two γ photons of energies 97 and 103 keV and thus is readily separated by pulse height discrimination from Tc-99 m (140 keV). The image shows an example of intra-arterially administered [^{99m}Tc]-MAA ("RADIONUCLIDE DISTRIBUTION" in lower right corner) and the reconstruction from the Gd-153 transmission source ("ATTENUATION SCAN" bottom left) in the sagittal plane. The fused image is shown in the top right corner and a reference image, a transaxial section, in top left corner. The red arrow on the fused image shows the approximate location of the tumour, indicating that the current location of the catheter needed to be revised for better tumour targeting. For further information, see Butler et al. [33]

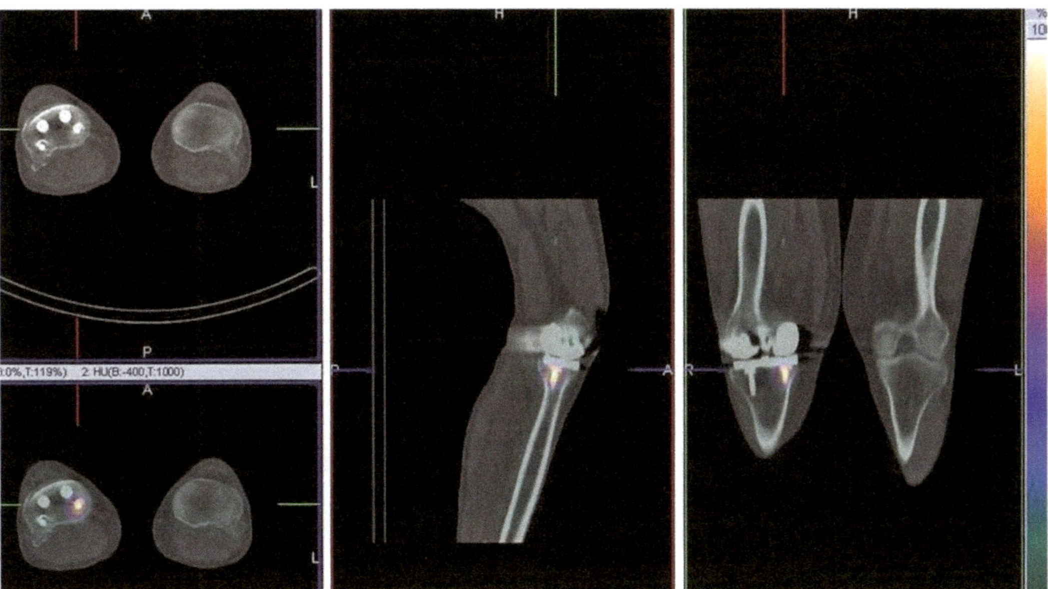

Fig. 1.2 An example from a contemporary SPECT/CT system demonstrating focally increased uptake on a ^{99m}Tc bone scan around an orthopaedic screw 3 years after knee replacement. The potential causes include infection, loosening or bony reaction to the screw

original detector was made from high-purity Germanium but they explored other detectors at a later stage [10]. In addition, the same group combined a diagnostic CT scanner with a conventional gamma camera [11] using standard detectors. The combined clinical scanners shared a common patient table for sequential SPECT and CT imaging. In the late 1990s, a combined gamma camera and X-ray CT system became commercially available based on a low beam current (1.0–2.5 mA) X-ray tube (GE Discovery VG Hawkeye) [12]. Having demonstrated the benefits of combined multi-modal SPECT/CT imaging on this platform, which was enormously successful commercially, other groups and vendors explored the added value of integrating a fully capable diagnostic CT scanner with dual-head SPECT gamma cameras (e.g., see [13]).

Today, combined SPECT and CT scanners are available in a variety of configurations with different CT scanner performance from flat panel detectors using cone-beam CT geometry, originally developed for on-board imaging on radiotherapy LINACs, to high-end conventional fast multi-detector (e.g., 2, 4, 6, 16, and 64 slice) systems. Figure 1.2 shows a recent clinical example from such a device.

1.3   Radiation and Interaction with Matter

The ability to produce cross-sectional images of the human body, whether using an external source of X-ray photons or from an internal source of γ photons, utilises radiation that can penetrate the body's tissues. Radiation can be divided into particulate radiation, such as alpha, beta and positron, or electromagnetic radiation, that is, mass-less quantised energy. Examples of different types of electromagnetic radiation that the reader would be more familiar with include radio waves, visible light, infrared radiation (heat), and microwaves as well as the high energy radiations which can cause ionisation of atoms such as X-rays, γ-rays, and cosmic (γ) radiation. Table 1.1 lists some properties of some of the ionising radiation encountered in nuclear medicine.

In general, nuclear medicine utilises γ radiation to form images with a gamma camera, annihilation radiation emitted after positron-electron

Table 1.1 Types of radiation and properties used in nuclear medicine imaging and therapy

Type of radiation	Symbol	Mass (kg)	Origin	Typical energy (MeV)
Alpha	α^{2+}	6.64×10^{-27}	Nucleus	>2
Beta	β^-	9.11×10^{-31}	Nucleus	0.2–4.0+
Positron	β^+	9.11×10^{-31}	Nucleus	0.2–4.0+
X-ray	X	0	Electron shells	0.04–0.10
Gamma	γ	0	Nucleus	0.05–0.5
Annihilation	$\gamma\pm$	0	Outside atom	0.511
Bremsstrahlung	–	0	Outside atom	0.2–4.0+
Auger	–	9.11×10^{-31}	Electron shells	<0.05

The radiations without mass are all electromagnetic

annihilation with a PET camera, X-rays to measure tissue density using a CT scanner, and alpha or beta radiation for radionuclide therapy. A further secondary form of radiation, Bremsstrahlung, is produced as an electron path deviates due to the influence of a nearby charged particle (usually the nucleus of an atom). From classical physics, we know that any force acting on a charged particle causing acceleration will result in radiation being produced. As an electron, in an X-ray tube or produced as a result of β^- decay, passes through matter, it will experience many deviations and collisions resulting in a continuous spectrum of radiation being emitted, the Bremsstrahlung, literally 'braking radiation' in German. Superimposed onto this continuous spectrum is the characteristic radiation emitted when electrons drop down from outer shells to fill the vacancies caused by ionisation, resulting in a polychromatic spectrum of energies (Fig. 1.3) as opposed to the monochromatic radiation seen with most γ-emitters used in nuclear medicine imaging.

Electromagnetic radiation interacts with matter by three principal mechanisms: the photoelectric effect, Compton scattering, and pair production. The photoelectric effect is the predominant mechanism by which X-rays interact with matter, and for the γ-ray energies used in nuclear medicine, the predominant mode of interaction is Compton scattering. This distinction has implications when using X-ray CT data in SPECT attenuation correction algorithms as the absorption profile is different.

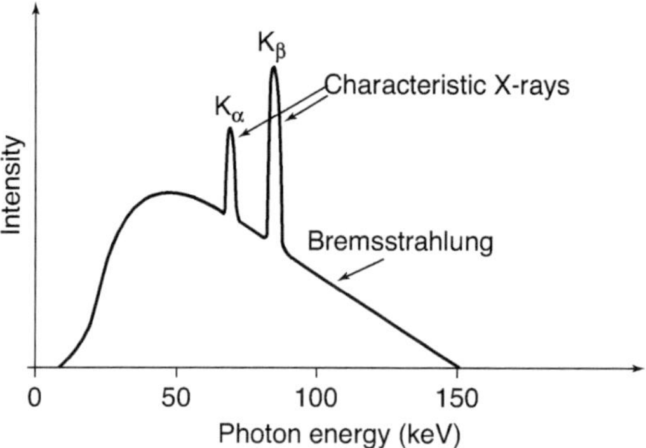

Fig. 1.3 A hypothetical X-ray spectrum is shown illustrating the polychromatic nature of the photons produced by the continuum of Bremsstrahlung radiation superimposed with the characteristic radiation corresponding to different transitions within the electron shells

X-rays, being in general of lower photon energy than γ-rays, tend to be totally absorbed by the photoelectric interaction with inner shell orbital electrons in the tissues of the body. The higher energy γ-rays are more likely to interact with a weakly bound outer shell electron in a Compton interaction whereby they lose some energy in the elastic scattering and change direction. The two effects are illustrated in Fig. 1.4.

The energy of the scattered photon can be found from the Compton equation:

$$E_\gamma' = \frac{E_\gamma}{1 + \dfrac{E_\gamma}{m_e c^2}\left[1 - \cos\left(\theta_C\right)\right]} \tag{1.1}$$

where E_γ and E_γ' are the incident and scattered photon energies, respectively, m_e is the non-

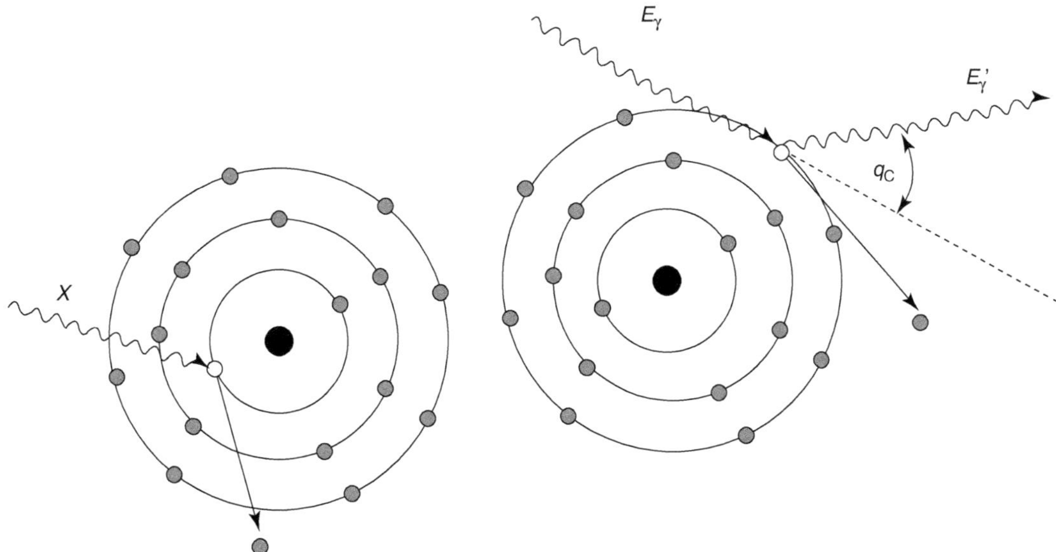

Fig. 1.4 The photoelectric effect (left) is where an incident photon (**X**) displaces an inner shell electron thereby leaving a vacancy and ionising the atom. X-rays and Auger electrons may be produced after as the vacancy is filled by an outer shell electron. Compton scattering (right) is more probable at higher photon energies. The incoming photon (**E$_\gamma$**) elastically scatters off a weakly bound outer shell electron changing direction and resulting in a photon of slightly lower energy (**E$_\gamma$'**)

relativistic rest mass of the electron, c is the speed of light ($m_e c^2 = 0.511$ MeV), and θ_C is the angle through which the photon has been scattered (the 'Compton angle').

1.3.1 Photon Attenuation

For a well-collimated source of photons and detector, attenuation takes the form of a mono-exponential function, i.e.,

$$I_x = I_0\, e^{-\mu x} \tag{1.2}$$

where I represents the photon beam intensity, the subscripts '0' and 'x' refer, respectively, to the unattenuated beam intensity and the intensity measured through a thickness of material of thickness x, and μ refers to the attenuation coefficient of the material (units:cm^{-1}). Attenuation is a function of the photon energy and the electron density (Z number) of the attenuator. The attenuation coefficient is a measure of the probability that a photon will be attenuated by a unit length of the medium. The situation of a well-collimated source and detector is referred to as narrow-beam condition.

However, when dealing with in vivo imaging, we do not have a well-collimated source, but rather a source emitting photons in all directions equally. Under these uncollimated conditions, photons whose original emission direction would have taken them out of the acceptance angle of the detector may be scattered such that they are detected. This is known as 'broad-beam' conditions indicating increased acceptance of scattered photons leading to an overall lower effective attenuation coefficient (Fig. 1.5). A table of broad- and narrow-beam attenuation coefficients for radionuclides commonly used in nuclear medicine is given in Table 1.2. This distinction between the broad and narrow-beam cases is important when it comes to applying attenuation and scatter correction in SPECT reconstruction as it will have a large impact on the reconstructed data.

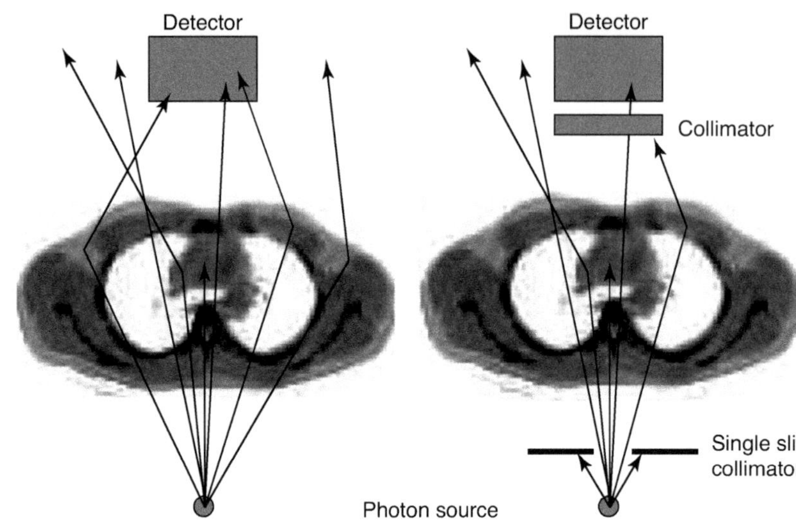

Fig. 1.5 An illustration of the difference between narrow-beam and broad-beam geometry is shown. In the broad-beam cause, more photons are detected compared to the narrow-beam situation so that the effect of attenuation appears to be lessened. When the source is internally distributed within the body and radiation is being given off in all directions, it is a broad-beam situation

Table 1.2 Attenuation Coefficients for commonly used single photon radionuclides in water

Radionuclide	Peak (keV)	NIST XCOM	Narrow beam (cm^{-1})	Broad beam (cm^{-1})
Tc-99 m	140	0.151	0.149	0.121
I-131	364	0.110	0.099	†
In-111	171	0.142	0.135	0.103
	245	0.127	0.121	0.104
Ga-67	93	0.169	0.171	0.153
	185	0.139	0.143	0.107
	300	0.118	0.123	0.099
I-123	159	0.137	0.138	0.114
Tl-201	75–80, 167	–	0.159, 0.137	0.123

These are values that we have compiled from a variety of sources. The NIST (US National Institute of Standards & Technology) XCOM values are available in an on-line resource (see: http://physics.nist.gov/PhysRefData/XrayMassCoef/ComTab/water.html accessed March 2013). The narrow and broad beam values have been measured on the gamma camera and are those used in our practice [18]. († − not measured to date)

1.4 SPECT Instrumentation

1.4.1 Gamma Camera

The workhorse imaging device for SPECT today remains the gamma camera (Fig. 1.6). New solid-state devices have been introduced clinically and will be discussed later. The gamma camera has remained virtually unchanged since its introduction by Anger in the late 1950s. It consists of an inorganic scintillator crystal, sodium iodide doped with small amounts of thallium (NaI(Tl)) to enhance light production, to which is coupled a close packed array of photomultiplier tubes (PMTs) which converts the light produced by the scintillator into an electrical signal. The electrical signal produced contains information about the location of the photons' interaction with the crystal plus pulse height spectroscopy (energy deposited in crystal) information.

The most common configuration for a SPECT camera today is a dual-detector device. This is because this configuration affords the most flexibility in general nuclear medicine imaging, permitting static planar imaging, moving bed whole-body planar scanning, and SPECT with the heads at various relative angles to each other, e.g., 90°, 120°, and 180°. While the gamma camera has retained the same basic design for over 50 years, refinements and improvements in the instrumentation, especially increased digitisation of the signals, have resulted in an extremely stable device suitable for rotation and translation without impacting on image quality.

As the γ-photons are emitted from the subject in all directions, a lead collimator is required between the scintillation crystal and the source to define the parallel lines of response that the photons have taken. The collimator has requirements such as high attenuation (lead is almost always used), thickness, hole shape, length and width to

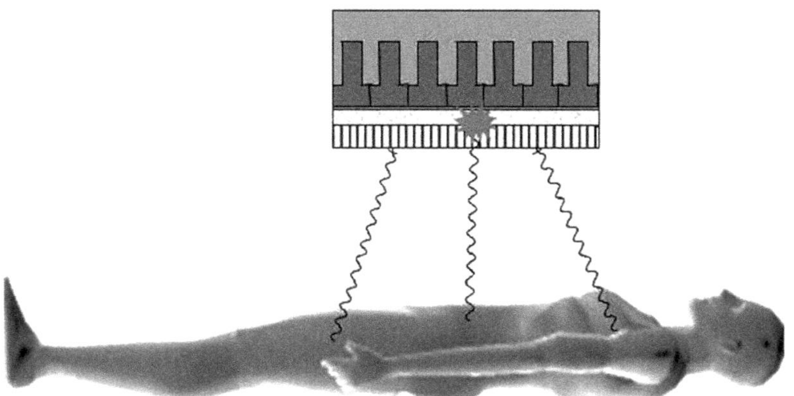

Fig. 1.6 Photons emitted from the subject travelling in a direction orthogonal to the detector pass through the holes of the collimator while the photons from other angles are attenuated. The photons emit a burst of light which is proportional in intensity to the energy absorbed in the crystal, which is then localised by the photomultiplier tube array

attenuate the photons that need to be excluded when imaging at a particular orientation to the subject. The resolution of the gamma camera is primarily limited by the geometric resolution of the collimator, which is of the order of 6–9 mm at a distance of 10 cm from the collimator. Overall resolution for the gamma camera is a function of a number of factors including the detector (intrinsic) and collimator (geometric) resolution, the distance from the emitting source to the collimator, the energy of the radionuclide, and the size and density of the object or body being imaged. The sensitivity of the gamma camera is primarily limited by the collimator. The absolute sensitivity in air for a typical gamma camera to a non-attenuating source of 140 keV γ-rays is around 100–200 detected events (counts) per second per MBq (ct.s^{-1}·MBq^{-1}), or around 0.01–0.02% of all emitted events. The collimator is the component of the imaging chain which places the greatest restriction on gamma camera performance—it has very low sensitivity given the available photon flux and its geometry imposes limits on the spatial resolution achievable. To compound this, sensitivity and spatial resolution have to be traded against each other to achieve a compromise—high sensitivity giving poor spatial resolution and higher resolution coming with decreased sensitivity.

The energy resolution of the NaI(Tl) scintillator is limited to around 10% FWHM (Full Width at Half Maximum) in the range 0.1–1.0 MeV. This precludes discriminating against photons that have undergone a scattering interaction within the body from which they originate, with a concomitant loss of energy. The net effect is that around 20–50% of all events detected by the gamma camera have been scattered within the body, accompanied by a change of direction, which gives rise to mispositioning. This degrades image quality by contributing to an increased background level and therefore decreased contrast. It also confounds attempts to quantify the radionuclide distribution. It is for this reason that scatter correction methods are required for quantitative SPECT reconstructions.

1.4.2   Solid-State Detectors

Recently, dedicated organ-specific SPECT systems with fundamentally different designs to the gamma camera have been introduced. Rather than using a conventional scintillator crystal for photon detection, these new systems use solid-state detectors which are able to convert the absorbed energy from the photon directly into an electrical signal. Due to the cost of these detectors at present, they are being developed for very specific applications such as cardiac imaging. The design for the systems includes a large number of small detectors (~10–30) which are located in a fixed position. These systems are SPECT-only devices not capable of forming planar images. Collimation is usually done using simple pinhole designs, and the reconstruction is tailored to the unique geometry of the system. Among the attractive features of these systems are high sensitivity due to the large number of detectors focused on a small field of view and improved energy resolution compared with NaI(Tl). The improved energy resolution presents the possibility of simultaneous imaging of different radionuclides with similar photon energies (e.g., ^{99m}Tc (140 keV) and ^{123}I (159 keV)). The systems can be used for more rapid image acquisition due to the improved sensitivity with reductions of 4–10-fold reported. Alternately, the improvement in sensitivity can be used to reduce the amount of radioactivity injected and hence reduce the radiation dose received by the subject.

1.5 SPECT Acquisition and Reconstruction

1.5.1 Projections and the Radon Transform

Tomographic imaging is the art of reconstructing the internal distribution of the signal of interest from external measurements. The same principles for image formation are employed in CT, SPECT, and PET as well as in other imaging modalities such as con-focal microscopy. High energy photons are used because of their ability to pass through the body with subsequent detection by an external device.

The tomographic imaging process for SPECT is shown in Fig. 1.7. Photons are emitted from the subject at all angles but the collimator on the gamma camera selects only those travelling in the required direction at a particular angle of the detector relative to the subject. As seen in the figure, each row on the detector is composed of a series of parallel projections. The projections are proportional to the sum of the intensities of the radionuclide concentration along the particular

line of sight through the subject. This can be written (ignoring photon attenuation at present) as:

$$p\left(x_r,\phi\right) = \int_{-\infty}^{+\infty} f\left(x,y\right) dy_r \qquad (1.3)$$

where $p(x_r, \phi)$ is the one-dimensional projection of the two-dimensional function $f(x,y)$ in a rotating frame of reference (indicated by the subscript 'r') at the angle ϕ. This is known as a Radon (or 'X-ray') transform—$p(x_r, \phi)$ is the Radon transform of $f(x,y)$ at angle ϕ. The reconstruction of $f(x,y)$ from the projections is known as an 'inverse problem'. Note that the dimensionality of the original function $f(x,y)$, 2D, is reduced by one in the projection to a 1D profile. However, if multiple 1D projections at different angles over 180° or 360° are acquired, rotating about the z-axis, the 2D function $f(x,y)$ can be recovered using the solution provided by the Central Slice Theorem. This relates the projections and the original distribution $f(x, y)$ as the Fourier transform of a projection $p(x_r, \phi)$ of a distribution $f(x, y)$ are equal to a section through the Fourier transform of the distribution $f(x, y)$ at the same angle (ϕ) as the projection. For a more detailed discussion of this important concept, the reader is referred to one of the following texts on the topic [14–16].

The SPECT reconstruction problem is complicated by the fact that there are extra terms which were ignored, for clarity, in Eq. (1.3). A more complete description of the projection $p(x_r, \phi)$ is shown below where there is an additional attenuation term in the integrand, and there are additive terms to account for scatter (S) and Poisson (random) noise (η).

$$p\left(x_r,\phi\right) = \int_{-\infty}^{+\infty} f\left(x,y\right) \cdot e^{\int_{-\infty}^{y} -\mu\left(x,y\right)} dy_r + S\left(x_r,\phi\right) + \eta$$

$$(1.4)$$

1.5.2 Image Reconstruction: Filtered Back-Projection (FBP)

The classical method for image reconstruction in emission tomography is the filtered back-projection algorithm (Fig. 1.8). The advantages of the filtered

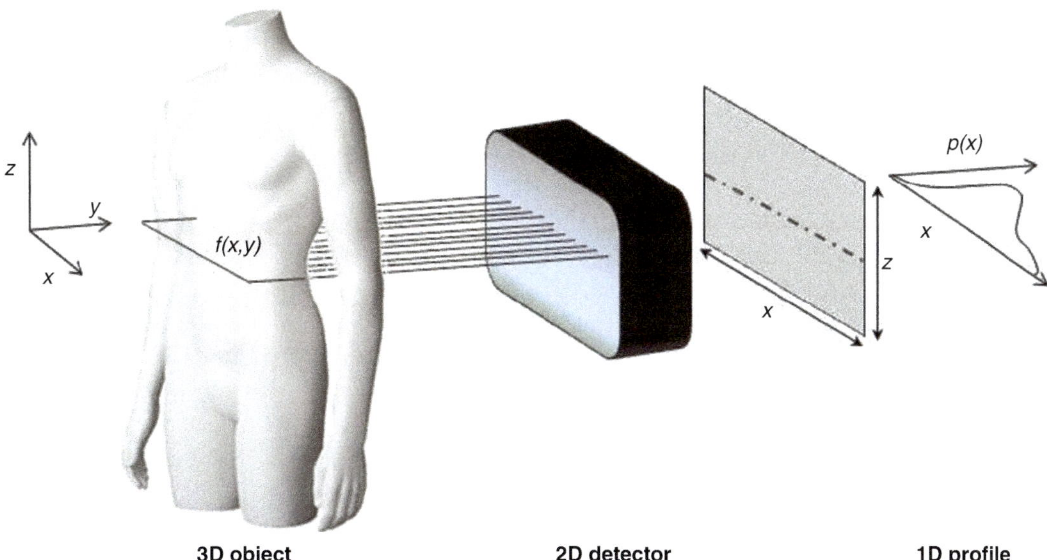

Fig. 1.7 The acquisition geometry is defined for SPECT acquisitions. The (x, y) co-ordinate system rotates about the z-axis to acquire projection $(p(x))$ at different angles. A section through the 3-dimensional radionuclide distribution in the subject $(f(x, y))$ is recorded by the detector as a 2D Radon transform. Each 1D profile in the planar image is then treated independently in the reconstruction process

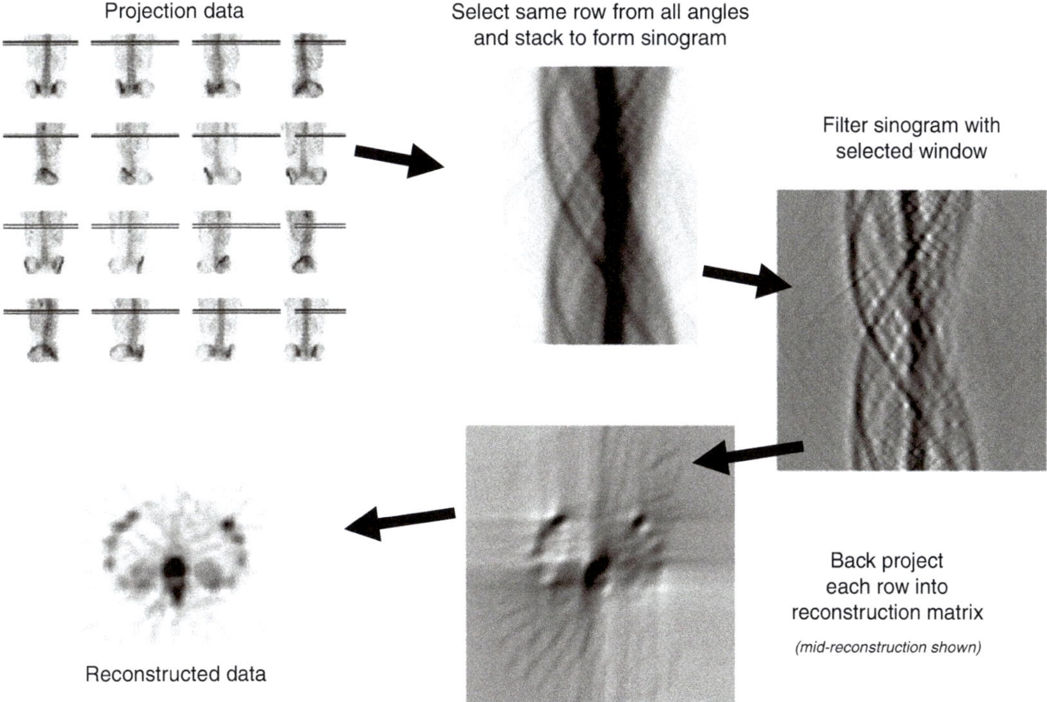

Fig. 1.8 The steps in reconstruction by filtered back-projection

back-projection approach are that it is computationally efficient and well-suited to optimisation using vector-based hardware (i.e., array processors). The alternative methods, such as iterative methods like Simultaneous Iterative Reconstruction Technique (SIRT), Algebraic Reconstruction Technique (ART), Iterative Least-Squares Techniques (ILST), or direct analytical methods (e.g., two-dimensional Fourier reconstruction), and statistical approaches (e.g., maximum-likelihood expectation-maximisation algorithm—ML-EM), are, in general, far more computationally expensive. In filtered back-projection, the projection data are firstly filtered, row by row (i.e., 1D filtering) and then back-projected. The pre-back-projection filtering is done to mitigate the blurring inherent in the back-projection operation.

Filtered back-projection was originally applied to reconstructing two-dimensional images from one-dimensional projection data recorded at many angles about the object in radioastronomy and electron microscopy. Back-projection involves projecting the acquired data back across the reconstruction matrix. At each angle, the detected events from each projection are evenly distributed between each element on the ray. After doing this from a large number of angles, the elements with the highest detected event rates will have the highest reconstructed intensity, but unfortunately elements that did not contain any signal also have an unwanted 'background' contribution from the blurring in back-projection.

In order to understand this process, we start with a simple object, a point source. The back-projected image of a point source from multiple angles has the appearance of a star. The distance between the lines of the star increases with increasing distance from the point source. If the distance from the point source is r, then the value of the final back-projected value is $1/r$. If there are a lot of projection angles, then it makes sense to say that the density of the lines in a region is proportional to $1/r$ (Fig. 1.9). All of these extra lines lead to a very blurred reconstruction. We consider that each point in the image acts independently of those around it, and so each produces a star-like pattern. The combined effect of all of these star artefacts is to produce a very blurred image of little use. However, this can be corrected by filtering the data, usually before back-projection. The filter which corrects for this blurring is called the ramp filter due to its shape (Fig. 1.10).

Conventional filtered back-projection has been the traditional choice for reconstructing the internal distribution of a radiopharmaceutical in

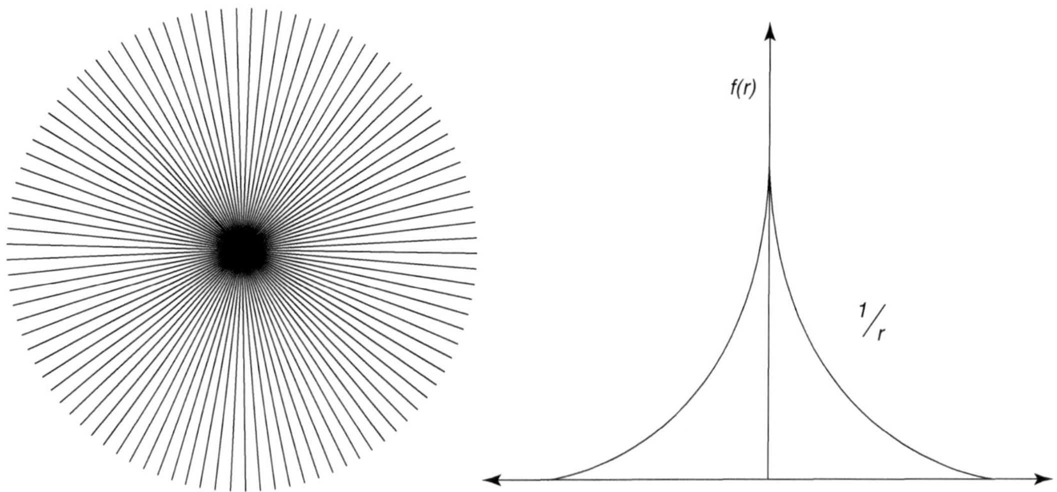

Fig. 1.9 Te 'star artefact' pattern seen on the left demonstrates the increase in density of the lines in simple back-projection that would be seen for a point source located at the centre of the matrix. The graph on the right shows diagrammatically how the density decreases rapidly at increasing radial distance from the origin

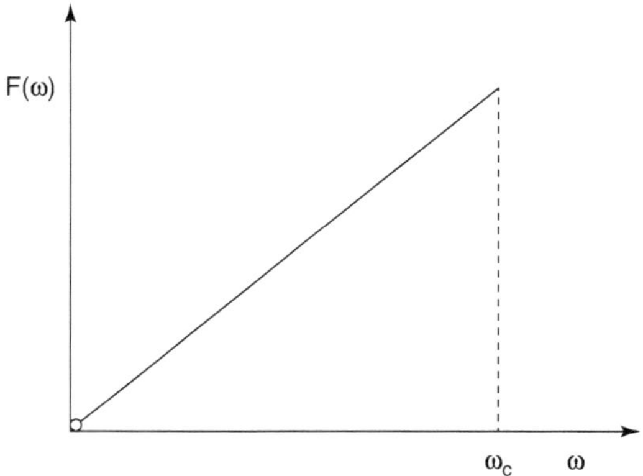

Fig. 1.10 Ramp filter in the Fourier (frequency) domain. The independent variable on the horizontal axis is the spatial frequency, ω, and the dependent variable on the vertical axis is the value that the function $F(\omega)$ takes for each value of ω. The ramp filter is truncated at a critical frequency, ω_c. The ramp filter corrects for the blurring in the back-projection process

emission tomography due to its speed. As for all radionuclide emission modalities, the recorded events for a particular line-of-response (LOR, one projection bin in a parallel acquisition geometry) consist of the integrated, *attenuated* contributions from all emission sources along the line-of-sight. Without applying any correction for attenuation, the contributions from locations deeper in the object will be relatively decreased due to attenuation compared with more peripheral emission origins. Filtered back-projection reconstruction does not handle this type of inconsistency well, as the relationship between attenuation and emission is inseparable. This is not the case in PET, where attenuation correction using measured transmission data is a simple and accurate correction. Correction for attenuation has been the major restriction on quantitative SPECT studies, to the point where SPECT was previously considered non-quantitative. Considerable progress on this topic has been made in recent years.

The disadvantages of filtered back-projection are:

- Due to the random nature of radioactive decay and the statistical uncertainties ('noise') that this introduces, plus attenuation and scattering, the projection data are *inconsistent* with respect to each other, and this causes artefacts in the reconstructed image if not corrected for prior to reconstruction.
- The filtering step before back-projection done to remove the blurring inherent in back-projection amplifies the high-frequency components of the projection data, and in doing so, greatly increases the statistical noise in the projections as this is a high frequency component of the data. Thus, filtered back-projection can be thought of as a noise-amplification process.
- It is not possible to build into the reconstruction process models of the data acquisition process which affect the final reconstruction, and which are well-understood and easily characterised, such as differences in resolution at different depths in the object, attenuation, and scattering. In this sense, filtered back-projection is a naïve approach to reconstructing an image from projection data.

1.5.3 Image Reconstruction: Iterative Techniques.

In recent years, the reconstruction algorithm of choice in emission tomography has moved from filtered back-projection to an approach based on one of the statistical iterative methods, with many applications using the block-iterative, Ordered Subset EM algorithm (OSEM) [17]. This approach has numerous attractive features including the ability to model physical characteristics of the acquisition process in the reconstruction in order to enhance image quality and accuracy and to better control the signal:noise ratio (SNR) of the final image. Most reconstruction software today includes optional scatter and attenuation correction and, increasingly, depth-dependent resolution recovery (referred to as PSF (point spread function) correction).

In an iterative reconstruction, an estimate of the original distribution $f(x,y)$ is formed based on the measured projection data. This estimate is then Radon transformed and compared with the acquired projection data, which is a Radon transform of the actual distribution $f(x, y)$.

Differences are determined, and a new estimate of $f(x, y)$ is produced. This is again Radon transformed and compared with the acquired projection data. This process is carried out a number of times with each iteration hopefully converging towards a closer match between the Radon transform of the current estimate of $f(x, y)$ and the acquired projection data. When the differences fall below a pre-determined threshold, the reconstruction is considered to have found a solution. A schematic diagram of the process is shown in Fig. 1.11.

1.5.4 Corrections for Photon Attenuation and Scattering

CT data from SPECT/CT can be used to correct for photon attenuation and scattering, usually in separate steps, after scaling the voxel values from CT (or Hounsfield) units to linear attenuation coefficients (μ) appropriate for the radionuclide that was used, as the energy of the X-ray photons and the γ photons will be different. It has been shown that the conversion from the CT numbers to the higher energy γ photon attenuation has a bi-linear relationship [18] (Fig. 1.12). The CT number is a relative number that is referenced to the attenuation of water in a calibration procedure. It is defined as:

$$CT_i = K \frac{\mu_i - \mu_{water}}{\mu_{water}} \qquad (1.5)$$

where i refers to the ith element of the data, and K is a scaling factor that accounts for the operating conditions of the CT scanner (tube voltage, etc.).

The implementation of this bi-linear scaling requires the CT image to be pre-processed into two distinct data sets—one data set containing the CT values below the pre-determined threshold value where the relationship changes, and the other above the threshold. In practice, this is easily achieved by segmenting the CT image on the basis of the CT values into two separate images, applying a different regression equation to each to scale to the appropriate values for the radionuclide being used, and then

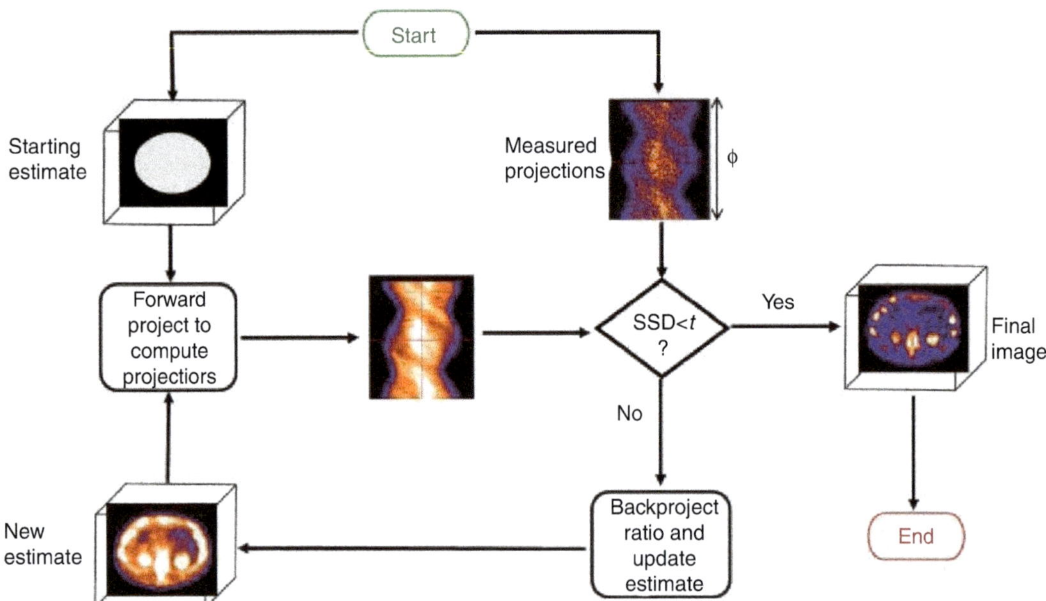

Fig. 1.11 General scheme used in iterative reconstructions is shown. Successive estimates of the reconstruction are updated until a criteria such as sum of squared differences (SSD) between acquired data and estimated reconstruction are below a threshold (t)

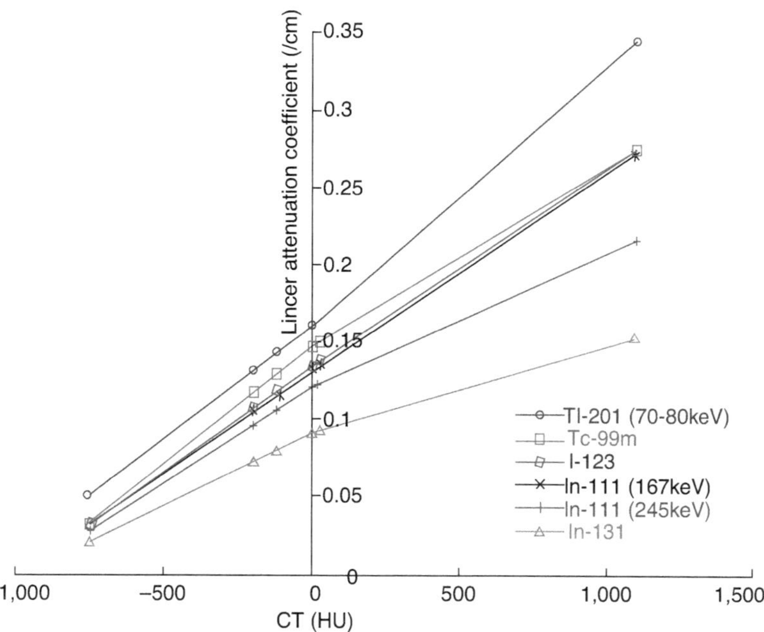

Fig. 1.12 The conversion curves for attenuation coefficients measured experimentally between commonly used radionuclides in SPECT imaging and CT (Hounsfield) numbers are shown for a variety of materials of different density. Note that the bi-linear nature increases with increasing photon energy, as the photon energies move further away from those dominated at low energy by photo-electric interaction

recombine. The majority of the pixels in the image above the threshold tend to be from bony structures only. The process for converting a CT image to an attenuation map is shown in Fig. 1.13.

If the reconstruction algorithm used for the SPECT data is filtered back-projection then CT data can be used in a post-reconstruction correction such as a modification of the Chang method [19] using measured attenuation data rather than assuming a ellipse containing a uniform attenuation coefficient [1]. The correction for photon attenuation can be included in the iterative reconstruction process as the forward-projection/back-projection steps model the image formation process.

Scatter correction can also use the CT data to improve the accuracy of the correction. The main techniques that have been validated for SPECT scatter correction are the energy window-based triple energy window (TEW) method [20], the convolution-based Transmission Dependent Scatter Correction (TDSC) [21], and the direct calculation methods based on the physics of scattering [22, 23]. The latter two methods can both use CT to improve the accuracy of the correction.

1.5.5 Corrections for Resolution

Current generation SPECT reconstruction algorithms based on iterative techniques commonly employ correction for resolution losses by implementing a PSF model at the re-projection step of the iterative algorithm. This effectively creates reconstructed data that is corrected for the effects of the system PSF; however, noise propagation can be an issue, as can artefacts introduced in the reconstructed image, particularly at boundaries of high contrast. The system PSF should ideally be modelled at varying source–to–collimator distances for each radionuclide and collimator.

The poor resolution of SPECT reconstructed data has also been addressed for the specific scenario of bone imaging in the Siemens xSPECT Bone™ algorithm, which makes use of the ordered subset conjugated gradient minimisation (OSCGM) approach. This reconstruction algorithm uses the accompanying CT data which gets segmented into five distinct zones based on HU: air, fat, soft tissue, medullary bone, and cortical bone. The zones are used to inform and enhance the resolution of the reconstructed bone SPECT data, creating SPECT images with sharp foci of uptake in anatomical bone areas (see Fig. 1.14).

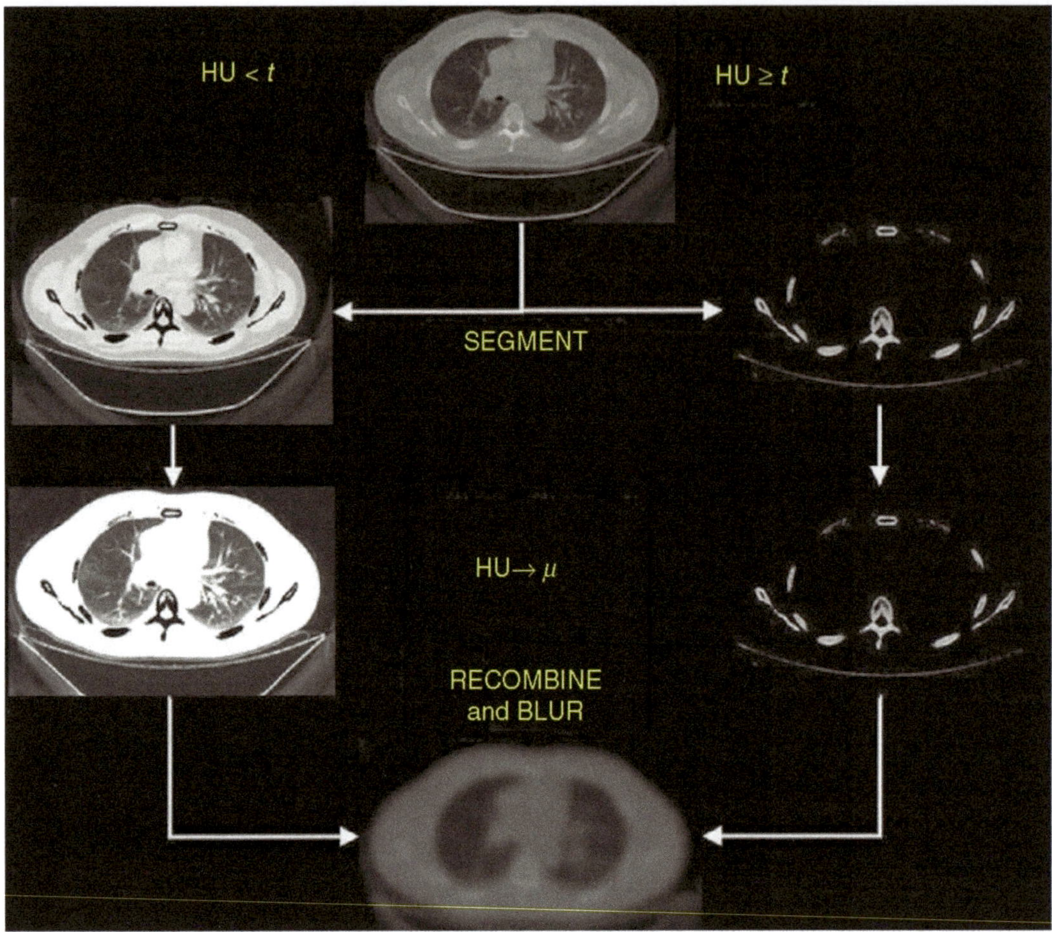

Fig. 1.13 The process to convert a CT image to an attenuation map is shown. The data are firstly classified and segmented based on the point t at which the shape of the bi-linear relationship in Fig. 1.12 between CT number (Hounsfield Unit, HU) and the attenuation coefficients change (usually around 0–50 HU). Each segmented data set is then converted using the appropriate regression equation (the 'HU → μ' step in the figure) and the data are subsequently recombined by adding together and blurred to approximately match the spatial resolution of the SPECT images, so as not to introduce any sharp boundaries or artefacts into the resultant reconstruction

1.6 CT for SPECT/CT

The use of X-rays to produce three-dimensional (3D) anatomical mapping of body density relies on technology analogous to that of SPECT, where computed tomography is performed via reconstruction of a series of one-dimensional (1D) projections acquired throughout 180°. At the most basic level, a single projection image is formed by the detection of X-rays transmitted through the patient, where the changing density or contrast across an image is representative of the differing attenuation properties within the patient due to different tissue thickness and densities that the beam must traverse. Given the loss of information in the dimension parallel to the direction of the beam (the Radon transformation), rotation of the beam and detector arrangement to acquire transmission images through many projection angles allows for the reconstruction of the 2D slice-oriented data.

Generally speaking, X-ray CT image quality is determined by a number of factors, some of which are under the operator's control, others which are governed by the hardware. Table 1.3 summarises the most common factors and their

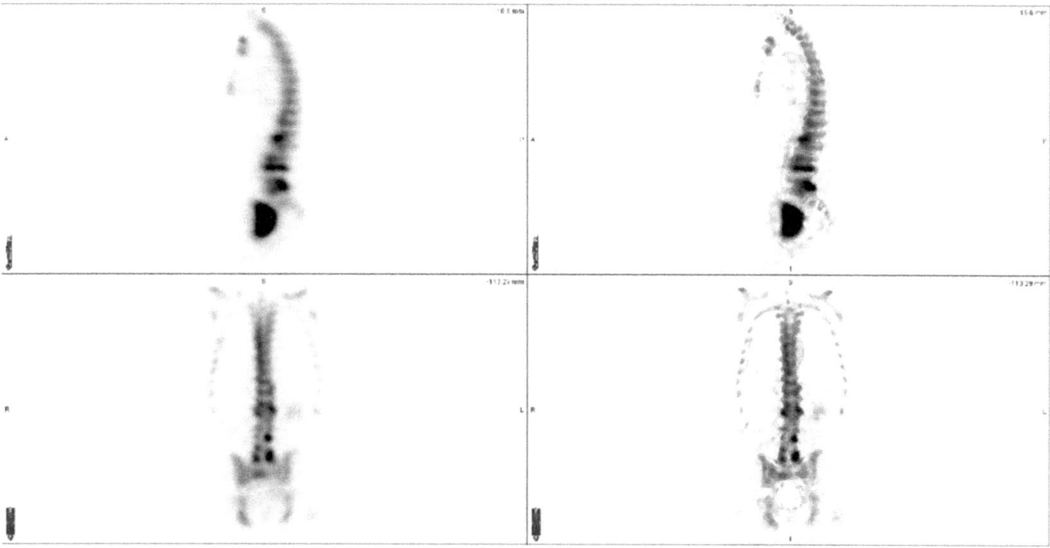

Fig. 1.14 A comparison of the Siemens standard OSEM algorithm (Flash3D) (left) and the skeletal zoning reconstruction (xSPECT Bone) (right) on a two-bed bone SPECT/CT

Table 1.3 Factors affecting CT image quality, related directly to the contrast and spatial resolution of the resulting reconstruction

Contrast resolution (CR)		Dose	Spatial resolution (SR)	
mAs	Increasing the mAs increases the number of photons contributing to the image	$D \propto \dfrac{SNR^2}{\Delta^3 T}$ Where D is dose, SNR is signal to noise ratio, Δ is the pixel dimension, and T is the slice thickness	Detector spacing and width	Influences sampling – Smaller detectors increase the cut-off (Nyquist) frequency and improve SR
Dose	Dose increases linearly with mAs		Number of projections	Increasing the number of views allows higher spatial frequencies in the image to be displayed without aliasing
Pixel and FoV size	Increasing pixel dimensions to incorporate a larger FoV will increase the photons in each pixel		Pixel and FOV size	The size of the FoV will determine the pixel dimensions for a given reconstruction matrix
Slice thickness	Increasing slice thickness increases the number of photons to produce the image		Slice thickness	Increased slice thickness reduces SR and may blur edges in the transaxial plane
Reconstruction filter	Low pass filters improve CR at the loss of spatial resolution		Reconstruction filter	Kernel shape affects SR – High pass filters give the best SR, at the expense of increasing noise
Patient size	Larger patients attenuate more x-rays, reducing the number of photons and so the signal and CR		Number of rays	Reducing the number of rays is analagous to increased spacing between detectors along an array, and deteriorates SR
Gantry rotation speed	Faster rotation reduces the mAs used to produce each image, reducing CR		Helical pitch	Increasing pitch will deteriorate the SR

impact on image quality, defined by both contrast resolution (CR) and spatial resolution (SR). Improvement of image quality requires a balance of both CR and SR, which must always be considered under the premise of keeping radiation dose as low as reasonably achievable (ALARA). The current (mA) provided to the X-ray source will determine the intensity of the photon flux which is available to contribute to the image, and the tube voltage (kV_p) will determine the energy of the flux and quality of the X-ray beam. A beam of poor quality will result in noisy projection and reconstructed data and will limit the contrast in the image. Beam current and voltage are adjustable parameters which the operator has, to some extent, control over, allowing modification depending on patient thickness and age (to limit dose). Other related factors which the operator has some control over are the size of the FoV and the matrix size or pixel dimensions. For the same FoV, if the pixel size is reduced to improve SR for a given mA and kV_p (same dose), fewer photons will be contributing to the data in each pixel of the image, resulting in a deterioration in the signal to noise ratio (SNR) and CR. As such, the SNR, pixel dimensions, slice thickness, and radiation dose are all related.

The thickness or collimation of the beam itself will depend on whether or not the system is projecting on to a single row of detectors, or a series of multiple rows of detectors, allowing for multiple slices to be acquired simultaneously (see Fig. 1.15). A thicker beam collimation results in a larger volume of the patient being scanned at one time, at the cost of decreased image resolution. Due to the fact that single-slice technology requires a beam that is highly collimated relative to the size of the detector array, a large percentage of X-rays emitted by the tube do not contribute to the image, and only a single slice is acquired for every rotation of the tube. The effective slice thickness is influenced by both the width of the fan beam and the speed of the patient table (helical or spiral CT), or the pitch (the ratio between the distance that the CT table moves during one revolution of the tube to the total collimation). Ideal image quality is reached when the distance the table travels during one revolu-

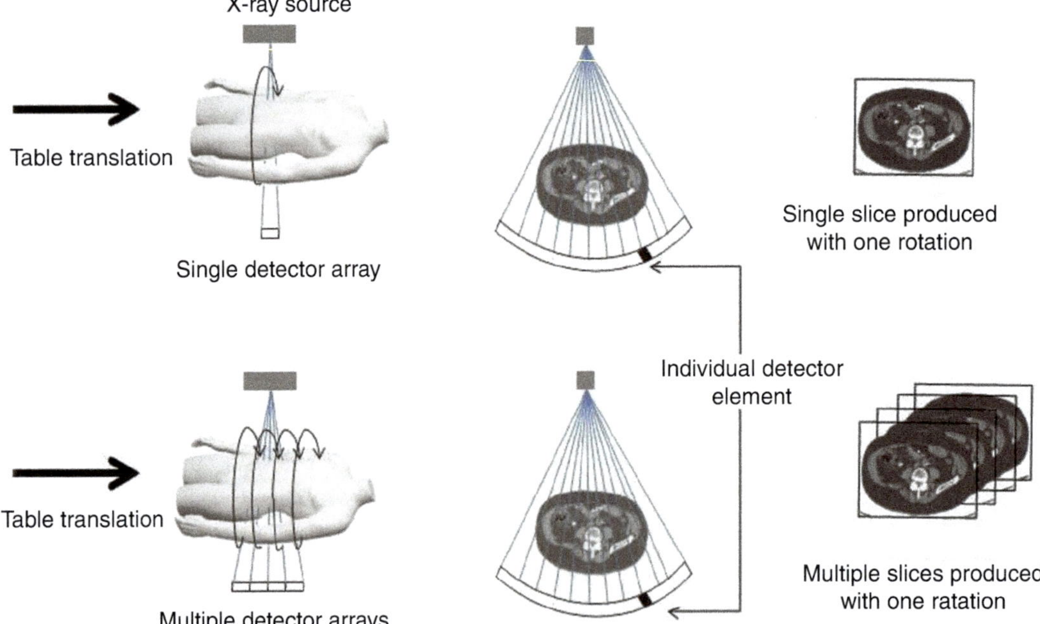

Fig. 1.15 Principles behind single slice and multi slice x-ray CT acquisition. Slice thickness is determined by the collimation of the beam, the detector width and the pitch (related to the speed at which the patient table feeds in to the scanner, and so the 'tightness' of the spiral ray traced by the rotating beam)

tion is equal to the beam collimation or slice thickness. Increasing the pitch will increase volume coverage (and reduce patient dose) but affects image quality. Image quality is also determined by reconstruction parameters, such as filtering, the interpolation algorithm used, and the reconstruction increment, or the degree of overlap between slices, which improves image quality when kept to a minimum at the cost of increased image storage space and computing time.

Alternatively, multi-slice scanners allow for faster image acquisition of the same volume with no compromise on image quality. The effective slice thickness is determined by the number of detector arrays available, the collimation of the beam, and the binning of detector elements. Since the beam is pre-collimated to fall on an entire row of detector arrays, the fan beam extends to a cone-beam geometry, which also has implications for the reconstruction algorithm and requires corrections for beam divergence.

Both the hardware and software components of CT scanners have undergone many developments since the introduction of X-ray CT scanning in the 1970s. In terms of the role of CT scanners in nuclear medicine hybrid imaging, the first commercial SPECT/CT system was introduced in 1999 (GE Discovery VG Hawkeye). This saw the combination of a dual-head SPECT system with a low-powered X-ray CT subsystem, equivalent to a dental tube, operated at 140 kV_p and 2.5 mA. The Discovery Hawkeye employed slip-ring technology for continuous CT acquisition during patient translation through the gantry, with a rotating fan beam from an X-ray tube coupled to a single-curved detector array. The X-ray CT component of the hybrid Hawkeye system was initially single-slice technology, requiring a slow 20 s rotation time and resulting in 2.5 mm in-plane resolution for non-diagnostic quality CT data, however was adequate for the purposes of attenuation correction of the SPECT data and low-resolution anatomical localisation. The Discovery Hawkeye system was updated to the Infinia Hawkeye 4 SPECT/CT with four-slice CT, each of 5 mm thickness, improving axial resolution. It also introduced spiral acquisition which improved (i.e., reduced)

total CT scanning time. Such systems offered cost-effective tools for hybrid imaging where diagnostic quality CT was not required and were also favourable in the nuclear medicine community due to their 'low-dose' status and small installation footprint.

Fully diagnostic CT scanners were integrated into commercial hybrid scanners in 2004 in the form of the Siemens Symbia T series and the Philips Precedence, which incorporate dual-head SPECT systems with diagnostic-performance multi-slice CT scanners comparable with conventional CT scanners. The Siemens Symbia T series, available with a 1-, 2-, 6-, or 16-slice CT, uses a diagnostic quality CT operating at up to 130 kVp and 345 mA (T16) with a rotation speed of as little as 0.5 seconds. Both high-end and low-end CT performance components from various generations of SPECT/CT systems can be used for attenuation correction; however, the high-end systems see an improvement in signal-to-noise characteristics in the reconstructed data, and highly detailed anatomical data are available with the multi-slice options due to improved spatial resolution and scan speeds. Current models of scanners that employ up to 64-slice CT in conjunction with SPECT allow for short scan times that are adequate for high-speed studies involving iodinated contrast and coronary angiography studies [24].

An alternative CT technology was introduced to hybrid scanners in 2008 with the launch of the Philips Brightview XCT, which saw a flat panel cone-beam CT component (CBCT) mounted on the same rotatable gantry as the SPECT component, in a co-planar geometry. This co-planar configuration offers the advantage of reduced room size requirements and reduced system weight compared to traditional hybrid systems, and the extended geometry of the flat panel detector along the longitudinal axis has the potential to reduce dose required for a given image quality and volume. The CT component was still relatively slow when compared to conventional CT scanners (minimum rotation time of 12 seconds), and of low power, operating on tube characteristics of 120 kV_p and 80 mA (maximum). The CBCT technology consists of an X-ray source and flat panel detector mounted on opposite sides of the gantry with a lateral offset such that a single projection covers slightly more than half the CT field of view (FoV). The use of flat panel detectors enables 1 mm isotropic reconstructed voxel size for the entire FoV and can be as small as 0.33 mm isotropic for high-resolution sub-volume reconstructions. The different geometry of the CBCT system requires some additional processing steps to be performed at reconstruction. As a result of the lateral offset between the X-ray source and detector, each X-ray projection corresponds to only a half-field projection of the object, resulting in truncation that must be compensated for by combining the projections from the opposite side of the gantry. The combined projections must in turn have a weighting factor applied to correct for the central overlap region. Alternatively, the cone-beam geometry can be accurately modelled in iterative reconstruction algorithms to directly account for the truncation of projection data.

Due to the fact that the primary X-ray beam for the CT component of hybrid systems can produce large amounts of X-ray scatter, significantly higher than that emitted by the radiopharmaceutical used for emission imaging, multimodality systems typically have the imaging planes of the X-ray source and the gamma camera separated by an axial distance of 50 cm or more. The future of SPECT/CT scanners lies in the possibility of truly simultaneous SPECT and CT imaging, with a common detector capable of discriminating between primary emission photons and both scattered photons and the X-ray source, which would require superior temporal and energy resolution [25].

As is the case with standard clinical CT scanning, the CT component of multimodality imaging can suffer from image artefacts. Beam hardening is a phenomenon due to the use of a polychromatic X-ray spectrum. Since X-ray attenuation coefficients are energy dependent, lower energy X-rays will be attenuated more than higher energy X-rays when passing through the same thickness of tissue. As a result, as the beam propagates through the patient, the shape of the spectrum is skewed towards higher energies, and the average energy of the beam becomes increased (or 'harder'). Artefacts are produced in reconstructed CT data due to the fact that different degrees of beam hardening occur at different projection angles, thus rendering the data inconsistent between different projections. Corrections for beam hardening are required during reconstruction of the CT data. Motion artefacts can also be a problem in CT reconstruction and may produce ghosting in the resulting image. The other primary artefact seen in CT reconstruction is partial volume averaging. CT numbers for a given voxel in the reconstructed data are proportional to the attenuation coefficient in the corresponding volume of the patient. If voxels contain only one type of tissue, then this representation is not problematic. However, if multiple tissue types are viewed within a single voxel (such as bone and soft tissue), the CT number is no longer an accurate representation of the corresponding tissue volume, but is instead an average value. Partial volume effects can be reduced with the use of thinner CT slices, and multiple reconstructions at different positions (e.g., 1.25 mm thick and 3 mm thick slices) may be useful.

In addition to CT artefacts, some information on the CT image can potentially result in further artefacts on the reconstructed SPECT data when used for attenuation correction. Attenuation correction artefacts lead to an artificial over- or under-estimate of counts in the reconstructed SPECT data. One common issue arises through the use of contrast media. High-density contrast media may result in erroneously high counts in the corresponding region on the attenuation corrected SPECT data due to the false high-density voxel values on the co-registered CT data used to derive the attenuation correction map. While contrast media exhibits high attenuation and hence signal intensity for low energy X-rays, absorbed by the photo-electric effect, at the higher energies of most γ photon energies, it has an attenuation coefficient close to water. Thus, contrast in a CT scan can lead to erroneously high attenuation coefficients for correcting in SPECT if it is not recognised and scaled separately. Attenuation correction artefacts may be accompanied by streaking in the image and can often be resolved by comparing to the non-attenuation corrected data. Truncation can also be a potential source of image artefacts. If the SPECT and CT FoV are not the same size, areas of the emission image outside that covered by the CT image will not be corrected for attenuation by the reconstruction algorithm. This often occurs in the 'arms-down' imaging position. Also, misregistration between the two modalities will lead to incorrect compensation in various parts of the reconstructed image, particularly noticeable at boundaries of variable tissue densities, for example, between liver and lung. In terms of cardiac and respiratory motion, even when diagnostic quality CT is used in hybrid systems, SPECT acquisition is of the order of minutes, as opposed to the CT acquisition in seconds or sub-seconds. As such, using the CT data for attenuation correction requires blurring to match the resolution of the SPECT data so as to avoid attenuation correction artefacts.

The radiation dose from the X-ray CT component of hybrid imaging is often seen as a limiting factor in multimodality imaging. Vendors have been continuously striving to reduce radiation dose to patients through improvements in both hardware and software. Certainly, the power of the beam is a big factor when considering patient dose, yet beam intensity and quality must always be balanced against patient size to achieve adequate image quality and signal-to-noise. Faster patient scanning is desirable, yet reducing slice overlap too much can introduce image artefacts. Furthermore, in terms of avoiding respiratory and cardiac motion, if the primary goal of the CT acquisition is for attenuation correction and anatomical localisation, such scan speeds may not be necessary. The major vendors have introduced X-ray CT systems which use automated tube current modulation, such that the beam current is varied during the scan depending on the thickness of the patient at a given slice, as determined by the scout or topogram. Furthermore, the recent introduction of statistical iterative reconstruction of X-ray CT data, as opposed to conventional filtered back-projection, has resulted in a new meaning of the phrase 'low-dose CT'. Iterative algorithms are based on the principle that, unlike FBP, it is not assumed that noise is evenly distributed across the entire image, and it is instead selectively identified and minimised during reconstruction based on a mathematical model. The ability to selectively reduce image noise allows higher quality image data at lower radiation dose compared to FBP to be generated. Dose reductions of the order of 60% are typical, at no cost to temporal or spatial resolution in the reconstructed image [24]. Statistical modelling of the reconstruction process is ideal for incorporating non-standard geometries and corrections; however, it does in turn result in increased computation time due to complex modelling in software. In terms of hybrid scanners in nuclear medicine clinics, this may not be an issue, given that the CT data can be acquired prior to the SPECT study, and reconstruction can take place during the acquisition of emission data.

1.7 Quantitative SPECT/CT

The requirements for producing quantitative data in emission tomography, in general, are: (i) a reconstruction algorithm that behaves in a linear fashion in terms of the reconstructed radioactivity concentration, (ii) an algorithm to compensate for photon absorption within the body, (iii) an algorithm to remove scattered radiation from the data, and (iv) the ability to calibrate the reconstructed data in $kBq.cc^{-1}$. There are several other factors that may influence the quantitative accuracy of reconstructed SPECT data including decreased apparent radioactivity concentration in objects less than approximately three times the spatial resolution of the system and therefore affected by the partial volume effect, count rate losses due to dead time within the instrumentation, radioactive decay during the acquisition process, and corrections and normalisations for spatial and temporal variations in detector response.

Historically, quantification in SPECT has been challenging due to the source-depth dependent nature of attenuation, and the fact that the requirements listed above must be individually determined for each different radionuclide (gamma energy) and can be affected by window width, detector crystal thickness, and collimator choice. For these reasons, much of the quantitative SPECT techniques were first developed in-house by specialised groups around the world. A number of clinical studies demonstrating in vivo validation of the accuracy of reconstruction in quantitative SPECT using [99mTc]-labelled radiopharmaceuticals have recently appeared [26–28]. The data are presented as radioactivity concentrations (in $kBq.cm^{-3}$). From this it is straightforward to display the data as SUV units, as is done in PET. Increasingly, other radionuclides are being investigated for quantitative SPECT reconstruction, including ^{111}In, ^{123}I, ^{131}I, ^{177}Lu, [186]Re, and [201]Tl.

In 2013, quantitative SPECT became available through vendor-based software, initially by Siemens (xSPECT and Broad Quant algorithms) and followed shortly by GE (Q.Metrix software). The current vendor release software can allow for SPECT quantification and the display of data in SUVs, equivalent to that which we see in PET. A range of radionuclide reconstructions are available; however, [99mTc] bone imaging and theranostics applications such as ^{177}Lu-DOTATATE and [177]Lu -PSMA imaging for dosimetry estimates have featured prominently in the literature.

For further reading on the clinical applications of SPECT and the potential for quantitative SPECT/CT, the reader is referred to some recent review articles [29–31].

1.8 Radiation Dose from SPECT/ CT

The addition of a CT scan to a conventional SPECT study will increase the total radiation dose to the subject from the procedure. Any increase in the radiation dose must be balanced against the perceived benefit to the subject. However, it is useful to view this increase in dose relative to the dose from the radiopharmaceutical. It is worth remembering that previously in nuclear medicine attempts to better localise foci of uptake of the radiopharmaceutical were often done by augmenting the original scan with a second radiotracer to aid in localisation. For example, adrenal imaging was often augmented with a [99mTc] renal scan to ascertain the likelihood of the focal uptake being intraadrenal or in a separate mass anatomically separated from the kidney [32]. In this case, very

little extra information may be achieved with the second scan, but there is a not insignificant radiation dose associated with the extra procedure. We would argue that an additional CT scan in this example provides a lot more information about the anatomy of the subject for a comparable or lower effective dose of radiation, especially when using Automated Exposure Reduction (AER) on the CT scanner.

Table 1.4 contains estimates of effective dose (ED) from a variety of radiopharmaceutical and CT procedures as they are used routinely in nuclear medicine.

1.9 QC for SPECT/CT

In addition to the quality control (QC) required for performing optimal SPECT studies, SPECT/CT introduces a number of extra procedures necessary to maintain high-quality clinical studies. Principal among these is testing the accuracy of the co-registration between the SPECT and CT data. As the systems are physically distinct, the physical offset between the systems needs to be determined for application when combining the data. The different manufacturers have different approaches to this adjustment, but all systems require validation of the accuracy of the co-registration which should be performed at regular intervals including after any service or maintenance procedure which has the potential to modify the offset.

The QC requirements for quantitative SPECT are still to be developed. These will need to include a regular check of the agreement between the measured dose calibrator readings and reconstructed SPECT values of radioactivity. As there will potentially be a variety of different SPECT radionuclides used, with different photon energies necessitating different collimators, adjustable PHA energy windows, *etc.*, separate calibrations and checking will be required for each. With the co-operation and implementation by the manufacturer of the SPECT/CT systems, many of the required parameters (such as required for scatter correction) could be pre-defined and fixed for a particular radionuclide/collimator/PHA setting. Strict adherence to the predetermined operating conditions and regular vali-

Table 1.4 A comparison of effective dose from CT procedures used in association with SPECT/CT and conventional radiation dose from a variety of radiopharmaceuticals

Procedure	ED (mSv)	Comment and reference
CT head Hawkeye Infinia 4	0.1	Not diagnostic quality – for AC and anatomical localisation only [34]
CT chest Hawkeye Infinia 4	0.9	
CT abdo/pelvis Hawkeye Infinia 4	1.5	
CT head Symbia T6	0.7	Diagnostic quality. Operating at a 130 kV_p with variable tube current 20–345 mAs [35]
CT chest Symbia T6	7.4	
CT abdo/pelvis Symbia T6	6.1–8.6	
Ventilation lung scan with [^{99m}Tc]-DTPA	0.3	Assumes normal clearance from lung [36]
V/Q lung scan	2.5	40 MBq Technegas (no clearance), 200 MBq [^{99m}Tc]-MAA [36]
[^{99m}Tc]-MAG3 for renal localisation (300 MBq)	3.7	Assumes normal renal function [36]
[^{123}I]-mIBG (4 MBq·kg^{-1})	5.8	Assumed 80 kg person [36]
[^{99m}Tc]-MDP bone scan (800 MBq)	4.6	Assumes normal renal clearance [37]
[^{18}F]-FDG PET scan (370 MBq)	7.0	Without CT [37]
[^{99m}Tc]-SestaMIBI (1100 MBq)	9.0	[36]
'Low-dose' FDG PET/CT scan (250–300 MBq and 130 kVp/80 mA with AER^a)	~15	[38]
^{201}Tl brain SPECT (120 MBq)	26.4	[36]
^{67}Ga (400 MBq)	48.0	[36]

^{a}AER – Automated Exposure Reduction

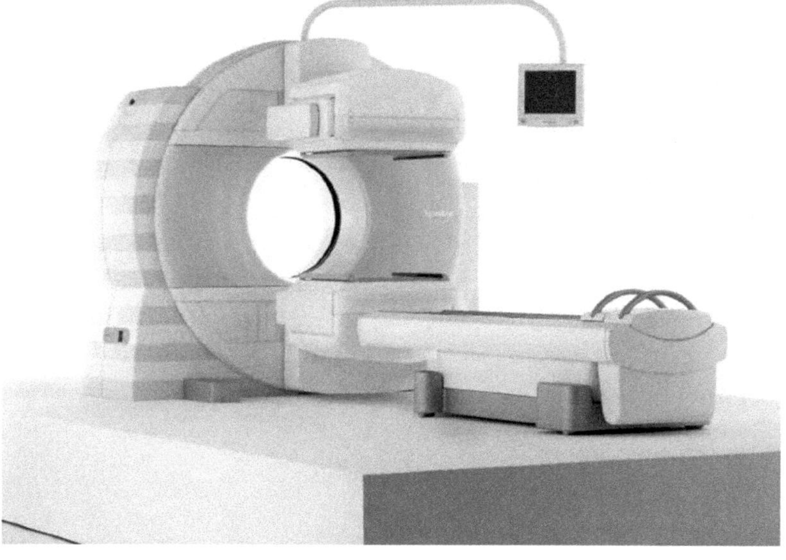

Fig. 1.16 A contemporary SPECT/CT system. The diagnostic quality CT is contained in the large "doughnut" gantry with the two variable angle gamma camera detectors fixed to the front of this (image courtesy of Siemens Healthcare)

dation will be an essential feature when deploying quantitative SPECT.

1.10 Combined SPECT and CT

It is our view that combined SPECT/CT multimodality imaging is a game-changer in terms of the evolution of SPECT for clinical applications. As listed at the beginning of this chapter, there are numerous benefits that the CT data provide both for image interpretation and for improving the quality and accuracy of SPECT images. The near-simultaneous acquisition, in a single imaging session on the same scanning bed, of the emission and transmission (CT) measurements creates the possibility to routinely provide quantitative SPECT data, that is, images reconstructed in units of kBq.cm^{-3}. Clinical applications of this are now being developed. An example of a dual-head SPECT/CT is shown in Fig. 1.16.

References

1. Bailey DL, Hutton BF, Walker PJ. Improved SPECT using simultaneous emission and transmission tomography. J Nucl Med. 1987;28:844–51.
2. Greer KL, Harris CC, Jaszczak RJ, Coleman RE, Hedland LW, Floyd CE, Manglos SH. Transmission computed tomography data acqusiition with a SPECT system. J Nucl Med Tech. 1987;15:53–6.
3. Malko JA, Gullberg GT, Kowalsky WP, Van Heertum RL. A count-based algorithm for attenuation-corrected volume determination using data from an external flood source. J Nucl Med. 1985;26:194–200.
4. Morozumi T, Nakajima M, Ogawa K, Yuta S. Attenuation correction methods using the information of attenuation distribution for single photon emission CT. Med Imag Tech. 1984;2:20–8.
5. Bailey DL. Transmission scanning in emission tomography. Eur J Nucl Med. 1998;25:774–87.
6. Heller G, Links J, Bateman T, Ziffer J, Ficaro E, Cohen M, Hendel R. American Society of Nuclear Cardiology and Society of nuclear medicine joint position statement: attenuation correction of myocardial perfusion SPECT scintigraphy. J Nucl Cardiol. 2004;11:229–30.
7. Moore SC. Attenuation compensation. In: Ell PJ, Holman BL, editors. Computed emission tomography. London: Oxford University Press; 1982.
8. Fleming JS. A technique for using CT images in attenuation correction and quantification in SPECT. Nucl Med Commun. 1989;10:83–97.
9. Hasegawa BH, Gingold EL, Reilly SM, Liew SC, Cann C. Description of a simultaneous emission-transmission CT system. Proc SPIE. 1990:1231.
10. Iwata K, Kwon S-I, Hasegawa BH, Bennett PR, Cirignano L, Shah KS. Description of a prototype combined CT-SPECT system with a single CdZnTe detector. In: IEEE Nuclear science symposium 2000. IEEE; 2000. p. 16/1–5.
11. Tang HR, Brown JK, Da Silva AJ, Matthay KK, Price DC, Huberty JP, Hawkins RA, Hasegawa BH. Implementation of a combined X-ray CT-scintillation camera imaging system for localizing and measuring radionuclide uptake: experiments in phantoms and patients. IEEE Trans Nucl Sci. 1999;46:551–7.
12. Patton JA, Debelke D, Sandler MP. Image fusion using an integrated, dual-head coincidence cameras with X-ray tube-based attenuation maps. J Nucl Med. 2000;41:1364–8.
13. Bailey DL, Roach PJ, Bailey EA, Hewlett J, Keijzers R. Development of a cost-effective modular SPECT/CT scanner. Eur J Nucl Med Mol Imaging. 2007;34:1415–26.
14. Defrise M, Kinahan P, Michel C. Chapter 4. Image reconstruction algorithms in PET. In: Bailey DL, Townsend DW, Valk PE, Maisey MN, editors. Positron emission tomography: basic sciences. London: Springer; 2005.
15. Defrise M, Kinahan PE. Chapter 2. Data acquisition and image reconstruction for 3D PET. In: Bendriem B, Townsend DW, editors. The theory and practice of 3D PET. Dordecht, The Netherlands: Kluwer Academic; 1998.
16. Kinahan P, Defrise M, Clackdoyle R. Chapter 20. Analytical Iimage reconstruction methods. In: Wernick MN, Aarsvold JN, editors. Emission tomography. London: Elsevier Academic Press; 2004.
17. Hudson HM, Larkin RS. Accelerated image reconstruction using ordered subsets of projection data. IEEE Trans Med Imag. 1994;MI-13:601–9.
18. Brown S, Bailey DL, Willowson K, Baldock CA. Investigation of the relationship between linear attenuation coefficients and CT Hounsfield units using radionuclides for SPECT. App Radiat Isot. 2008;66:1206–12.
19. Chang LT. A method for attenuation correction in radionuclide computed tomography. IEEE Trans Nucl Sci. 1978;NS-25:638–43.
20. Ichihara T, Ogawa K, Motomura N, Kubo A, Hashimoto S. Compton scatter compensation using the triple-energy window method for single- and dual-isotope SPECT. J Nucl Med. 1993;34:2216–21.
21. Meikle SR, Hutton BF, Bailey DL. A transmission dependent method for scatter correction in SPECT. J Nucl Med. 1994;35:360–7.
22. Beekman FJ, Kamphuis C, Frey EC. Scatter compensation methods in 3D iterative SPECT reconstruction: a simulation study. Phys Med Biol. 1997;42:1619–32.
23. Kadrmas DJ, Frey EC, Karimi SS, Tsui BM. Fast implementations of reconstruction-based scatter compensation in fully 3D SPECT image reconstruction. Phys Med Biol. 1998;43:857–73.
24. ABADI S, Brook OR, Rispler S, Frenkel A, Engel A, Keidar Z. Hybrid cardiac SPECT/64-slice CTA-derived LV function parameters: correlation and reproducibility assessment. Eur J Radiol. 2010;75:154–8.
25. Seo Y, Mari C, Hasegawa BH. Technological development and advances in single-photon emission computed tomography/computed tomography. Semin Nucl Med. 2008;38:177–98.
26. Willowson K, Bailey DL, Baldock C. Quantitative SPECT using CT-derived corrections. Phys Med Biol. 2008;53:3099–112.
27. Willowson K, Bailey DL, Baldock C. Quantifying lung shunting during planning for radio-embolization. Phys Med Biol. 2011;56:N145–52.
28. Zeintl J, Vija AH, Yahil A, Hornegger J, Kuwert T. Quantitative accuracy of clinical 99mTc SPECT/CT using ordered-subset expectation maximization with 3-dimensional resolution recovery, attenuation, and scatter correction. J Nucl Med. 2010;51:921–8.
29. Bailey DL, Willowson KP. An evidence-based review of quantitative SPECT imaging and potential clinical applications. J Nucl Med. 2013;54:83–9.
30. Mariani G, Bruselli L, Kuwert T, Kim EE, Flotats A, Israel O, Dondi M, Watanabe N. A review on the clin-

ical uses of SPECT/CT. Eur J Nucl Med Mol Imaging. 2010;37:1959–85.

31. Seret A, Nguyen D, Bernard C. Quantitative capabilities of four state-of-the-art SPECT-CT cameras. EJNMMI Res. 2012;2:45.

32. Ong Y-Y, Cohn D, Wijaya J, Roach PJ. The importance of renal localization with MIBG scintigraphy. Clin Nucl Med. 2002;27:479–82.

33. Butler SP, Bailey DL, McLaughlin AF, Khafagi FA, Stephens FO. SPECT evaluation of arterial perfusion in regional chemotherapy. J Nucl Med. 1988;29:593–8.

34. Sawyer LJ, Starritt HC, Hiscock SC, Evans MJ. Effective doses to patients from CT acquisitions on the Ge Infinia Hawkeye: a comparison of calculation methods. Nucl Med Commun. 2008;29:144–9.

35. Larkin AM, Serulle Y, Wagner S, Noz ME, Friedman K. Quantifying the increase in radiation exposure associated with SPECT/CT compared to SPECT alone for routine nuclear medicine examinations. Int J Mol Imaging. 2011;2011:897202.

36. ICRP. ICRP publication 53: radiation dose to patients from radiopharmaceuticals. Ann ICRP. 1988;18

37. Towson JEC. Radiation dosimetry and protection in pet. In: Valk P, Bailey DL, Townsend DW, Maisey MN, editors. Positron emission tomography: basic science and clinical practice. London: Springer-Verlag; 2003.

38. Willowson KP, Bailey EA, Bailey DL. A retrospective evaluation of radiation dose associated with low dose FDG protocols in whole-body PET/CT. Australas Phys Eng Sci Med. 2012;35:49–53.

Faiq Shaikh and Francisca Mulero

2.1 Introduction

Radiomics as a medical image analysis technology is coming of age in the realms of clinical practice and clinical development. Quantitative image analysis has been used as a methodology to evaluate disease processes using medical images for a few decades now; radiomics is a newer approach that involves intricate feature extraction and classification techniques and leverage sophisticated statistical approaches, such as machine learning (ML). Standard structural imaging modalities, such as computed tomography (CT) and magnetic resonance imaging (MRI), were first to be used for radiomic analysis efforts and still comprise the majority of scientific work being done in this space. More recently, a significant body of scientific literature has been accumulating for radiomics performed on positron emission tomography (PET) images. Meta-analysis of these early PET studies has shown that radiomic analysis lacked in reproducibility given its high sensitivity to variations in voxel size, segmentation and reconstruction algorithms used, which is why standardized uptake value (SUV) still remains the gold standard for

PET signal measurement [1]. Single photon emission computed tomography (SPECT) is another functional imaging modality where radiomics can play a role in extracting more information than what meets the eye. However, there are concerns with the reproducibility and reliability of SPECT-based radiomic analysis similar to those seen with PET. This is both a challenge and an opportunity. And while AI-driven approaches, of which radiomics is one, can be very promising for all imaging, including SPECT, the challenges related to data availability, annotation, and medicolegal considerations thereof need to be addressed for the application of radiomics to become mainstream [2]. In this chapter, we review the landscape of the recent efforts in SPECT radiomics and discuss the challenges and opportunities that abound its applications in clinical practice and development.

2.2 Radiomics as a Methodology

Conceptually, radiomics is an analytical process of using medical images to extract microstructural or "microfuncitional" information by extracting data from each boxes, which may then be useful for disease classification, stratification, therapy response assessment, and prognostication. In that sense, it is a non-invasive alternative to molecular and other histopathology-based disease assessments. Developing imaging-based biomarkers for these purposes is a sophisticated process that

F. Shaikh (✉)
Advanced Imaging, Image Analysis Group,
Philadelphia, PA, USA

F. Mulero
Molecular Imaging, Centro Nacional de
Investigaciones Oncologicas (CNIO), Madrid, Spain
e-mail: fmulero@cnio.es

involves choosing the right medical images and employing adequate ML approaches that deliver useful radiomic signatures of clinical significance. Typically, these radiomic signatures are based on the morphology and tissue heterogeneity, but when using functional modalities, such as PET and SPECT, these signatures provide insights into the physiologic or biochemical processes and perturbations there of [3]. AI/ML models developed for radiomic analysis are improving in their accuracy and predictive power when compared to conventional interpretive approaches. Radiomics is being considered as a potential quantitative analysis methodology to be applied to SPECT imaging in the realm of neurologic, cardiac, oncologic, and immunologic diseases [4].

The basic steps involved in the radiomics methodology (see Fig. 2.1) are as follows:

- *Image acquisition*: This is the first step in this process. In most settings, radiomic analysis can be performed on medical images acquired as per standard clinical protocols. However, modified protocols that render higher spatial resolution or "richer" raw data can be useful. The main concern is to have a standardized acquisition protocol across the cohort in order to minimize variations in the feature extraction process [1]. Furthermore, post-acquisition processing, including filtering techniques and iterative reconstruction, should also be standardized in order to minimize inter- and even intra-centre variability. Filtering techniques are used to improve results [1].

- *Lesion detection and segmentation*: This is a key requisite step in this methodology. It is critical to identify the right lesion(s) and segment them in a way to include the whole lesion while removing the surrounding or background tissue [5]. The process of segmentation may be manual, whereby a radiologist identifies the lesion and drawing a region/volume of interest (ROI/VOI). Alternatively, it may be semiautomated, whereby the lesion is manually selected and the algorithm identifies its boundaries and draws a VOI. There are also fully automated segmentation software programs that can identify the lesion and draw an ROI/VOI. All these

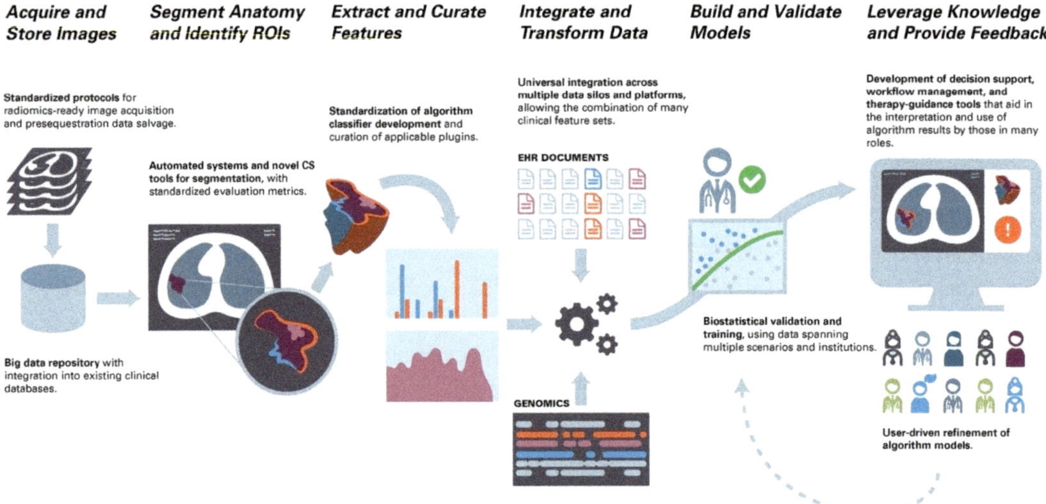

Fig. 2.1 Typical radiomics workflow. The basic steps include image sequestration and preacquisition data salvage, data transfer and repository maintenance, image segmentation, feature extraction and classification, covariance matrices and data modelling, integration into clinical decision support systems, and biostatistic and outcome analysis. ROI, region of interest. (Used under CC license from Technical Challenges in the Clinical Application of Radiomics. Faiq A. Shaikh, Brian J. Kolowitz, Omer Awan, Hugo J. Aerts, Anna von Reden, Safwan Halabi, Sohaib A. Mohiuddin, Sana Malik, Rasu B. Shrestha, Christopher Deible. JCO Clinical Cancer Informatics. 2017;1:1–8.)

methods allow for manual readjustment to ensure correct lesion demarcation with human oversight. Whichever method adopted, precise, consistent, and accurate segmentation of all lesions is critical for a reliable and reproducible delta radiomics assessment.

- *Feature extraction*: This is the core step of the radiomics technique in which a large set of features (which are mathematically determined based on the values within a voxel) are extracted from these images. The size of the feature set depends on the modality, and there are a variety of libraries available for each. The radiomic signatures can be created using features extracted in a "pre-engineered" or "hand-crafted" fashion or through a "black-box" approach that depends on ML [6–8]. Radiomic features are based on the morphology, histogram, or texture analysis. These features may be semantic (providing description about shape, size, tissue relation to surrounding material, surface area and volume) or agnostic (providing histograms and texture-based features). These extracted features are highly variable, and feature reduction is applied to reduce redundancy. LASSO (least absolute shrinkage and selection operator) is a regression analysis technique that performs variable selection and regularization to improve prediction and accuracy and can be employed in this step to extract a smaller subset of features that is more likely to yield the radiomic signature of interest [8]. Second-order radiomic analysis has been most commonly applied across all modalities as it provides valuable information regarding the local spatial distribution of voxel values, calculating local features at each voxel within the in-plane image and deriving parameters from the distributions of the local features. A number of texture features can be derived that provide a measure of intralesional heterogeneity.

- *Feature classification and model development*: The extracted radiomic features are "raw data" that needs to be classified into signatures of statistical value. These signatures are critical in the development of non-invasive biomarkers that can quantify tissue-level changes otherwise not visualized in the medical image. Correlation heat maps of the extracted radiomic features are created and those with high variance are used (see Fig. 2.2). Feature classification is performed

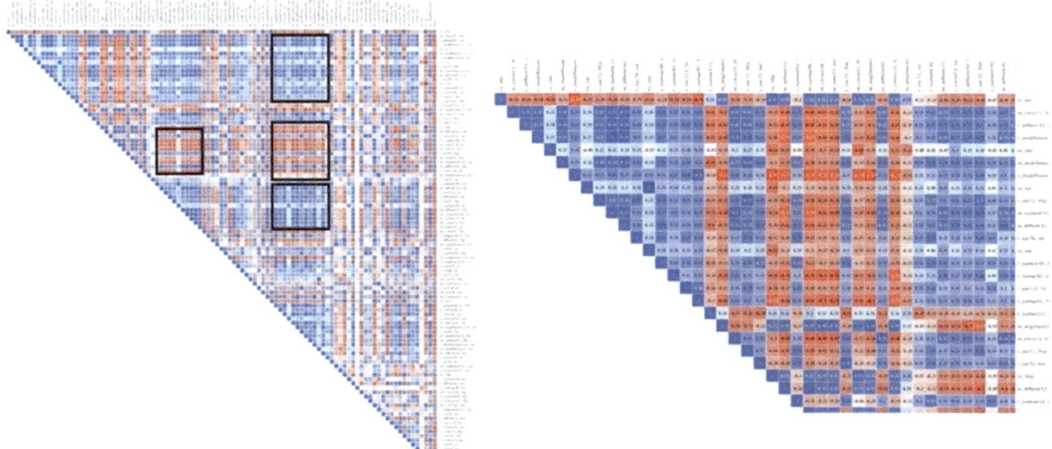

Fig. 2.2 Correlation analysis heatmap showing blocks of highly correlated radiomic features (black frames on the left and positive with red color or negative correlation with blue color on the right). When identifying such groups of highly correlated features, all but the one with the highest variance are removed from further analysis. In this case, the correlation coefficient was set to 95%. (Used under the creative commons license from Papanikolaou N, Matos C, Koh DM. How to develop a meaningful radiomic signature for clinical use in oncologic patients. Cancer Imaging. 2020;20:33.)

using computational techniques that can involve machine learning approaches, such as random forest (RF) or support vector machine (SVM). In scenarios with complex data (from radiomics and other non-radiological sources), more complex techniques, such as convolutional neural network (CNN) or deep learning neural network (DLNN), may be employed to derive insights for important go/no-go decisions or predict/assess therapy response [9]. These algorithms need to have high accuracy rates when tested using a test set. The true "test" of a radiomic model is the assessment of its performance across various centers in a clinical trial or practice. While radiomic models cannot be fully transferable to all types of populations and disease subtypes, it should have reasonable applicability in similar clinical settings, using similar equipment and protocols, and in relatable cohorts.

2.3 Clinical Application of Radiomics Using SPECT

2.3.1 Oncologic SPECT Radiomics

While still niche, the most salient application of SPECT radiomics has been in the field of oncology. This trend follows the momentum seen in the realm of PET radiomics. As SPECT plays an important role in the clinical management of a number of malignant diseases, radiomics-based studies have been performed with encouraging results in this space. The main areas of potential application of SPECT radiomics in oncology would be:

- Disease detection and classification.
- Clinical course prediction and prognostication.
- Therapy response prediction/assessment.
- Complimenting or as an alternative to nonimaging biomarkers.
- Pharmacokinetic and pharmacodynamic assessment for the clinical development of novel therapeutics.

Technetium-99 m albumin nanoparticle studies are performed for the evaluation of primary and secondary hepatic malignancies in clinical practice. Radiomic analysis of these scans has been performed that yielded signatures consisting of skewness, kurtosis, and distribution histograms to study the intra-tumoral tissue heterogeneity [10] (see Fig. 2.3). This enables qualitative and quantitative assessment of pathophysiologic processes, such as fibrosis, necrosis, metaplasia, and vasculogenesis. This, in turn, allows for quantification of the extent of cirrhosis, metastatic potential, or response to therapy. The hepatic tissue density changes detected through radiomic analysis can prove to be a harbinger of liver tumors that would be otherwise detected at a later stage through conventional imaging methods. In small animal studies, radiomic approaches have been used to study the varying patterns of radiotracer distribution, which can help distinguish between healthy and tumoral livers, which can be helpful to assess the extent of invisible tumor burden in a patient [10]. Other related approaches in this domain include the radiomic analysis of Tc-99 m sulfur colloid SPECT to predict the Child-Pugh class in hepatocellular carcinoma (HCC) patients [11, 12].

These approaches have yielded promising results in animal models and can be potentially translated for clinical use eventually. In humans, a biomarker that quantifies hidden tumor burden in the liver can be a tremendously useful endpoint for patients with HCC as well as metastatic liver disease. Skewness is a direct imaging-based parameter that correlates with the inhomogeneous distribution of macrophage cells and can be quantified to show the altered tissue function even before the visual manifestation of liver tumor foci on standard imaging. This can be developed as a prognostic biomarker of malignant disease progression in HCC patients [10, 11].

Novel AI approaches have been introduced that use SPECT data in oncologic imaging interpretation. One such example is that of PSMA-AI that uses DLNN to anaylze and interpret PSMA-targeted Tc99m-MIP-1404 SPECT/CT images [13]. The results shows that PSMA-AI generated reproducible results and could compliment

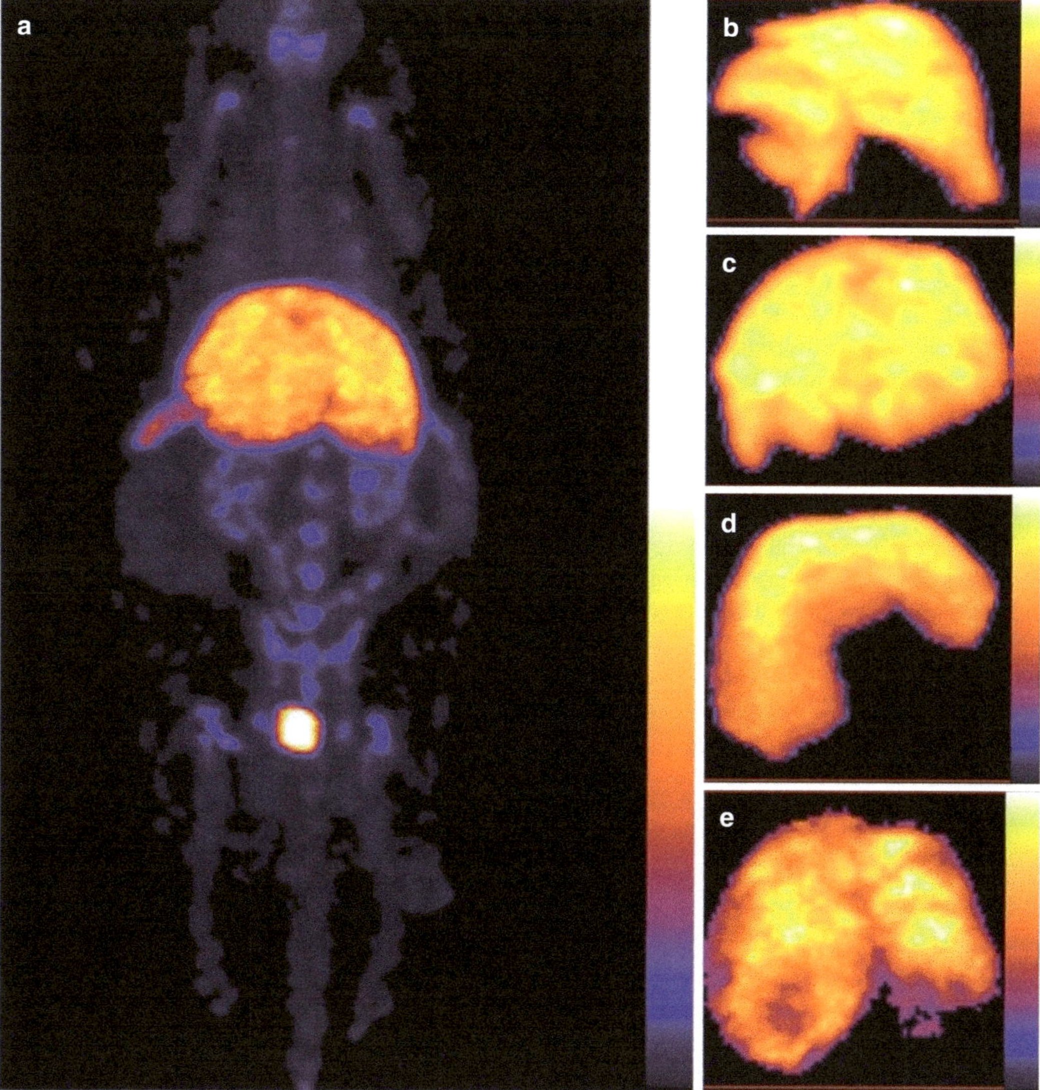

Fig. 2.3 The result of 99mTc-protein nanoparticle whole-body SPECT scan. b–e Selected projections of the segmented liver in control, obese, metastatic, and primary tumor groups, respectively, from top to bot (Used under Creative Commons license from Veres DS, Máthé D, Hegedűs N. et al. Radiomic detection of microscopic tumorous lesions in small animal liver SPECT imaging. EJNMMI Res. 2019;9:67.)

human interpretation. Radiomic analysis can be added in this approach as an additional layer of rich data generation that the PSMA-AI can use to improve its predictive values as compared to human interpretation.

Tc99m-Sestamibi SPECT/CT has been used to differentiate between oncocytomas (hot lesions) and renal cell carcinoma (cold lesions). Radiomic analysis of these cold spots has been performed in an attempt to differentiate between various subtypes of RCC [14]. While there were challenges related to mis-segmentation and high variation, this approach highlights the potential of radiomics for clinically performed SPECT studies.

SPECT imaging plays a critical role in the successful planning and monitoring of antibody-targeted radionuclide imaging and therapy (radio-immunotherapy). ^{111}In-ibritumomab tiuxetan is a SPECT agent that is used prior to the administration of ^{90}Y-ibritumomab tiuxetan radioimmunotherapy to determine eligibility for its treatment by determining whether there is sufficient and uniform antibody retention within the tumor. Features extracted using radiomic texture analysis that describe the relationships between gray-level intensity and position of pixels from these images can help assess the underlying biological complexity and tissue heterogeneity.

Longitudinal SPECT imaging is also used to monitor antibody biodistribution and dosimetry in patients. This has been performed in patients receiving anti-carcinoembryonic antigen (CEA) ^{131}I-A5B7 antibody in combination with the vascular disrupting agent (VDA), combretastatin A4-phosphate for gastrointestinal carcinoma [15]. Performing texture analysis on these SPECT images would allow the quantification of the heterogeneity of antigen distribution noninvasively, before and after therapy. This strategy can be useful in the clinical trials as it can speak to the resistance of some tumors to antigen-targeted therapy. It has been demonstrated in animal studies that texture analysis (using gray-level co-occurrence matrix feature extraction) of ^{125}I-A5B7 SPECT can show spatial heterogeneity variations of antibody distribution between well- and poorly differentiated liver metastases before antivascular treatment [16].

For radionuclide therapies of cancer, the concept of intra-tumoral heterogeneity is important as it can determine the treatment response to radionuclide therapy, especially when the bystander effect is required to kill neighboring cells that do not express the target. In a study using preclinical colon tumor models that express carcinoembryonic antigen (CEA), treatment response to ^{131}I-labeled anti-CEA antibody has been shown to depend on the vascular supply and CEA distribution [17].

2.3.2 Neurologic SPECT Radiomics

SPECT imaging has a number of applications in the management of neurologic diseases. For the radiomic analysis of neurologic SPECT images, the lesion identification and segmentation are performed on the MR images co-registered with the SPECT images.

Imaging of the dopaminergic system with ^{123}I-ioflupane-dopamine transporter (DAT) is a widely used SPECT study in the clinical workup for Parkinson's disease. DAT SPECT images are typically assessed visually; however, adding radiomics can provide a new set of information that can help predict clinical outcomes (see Fig. 2.4) [18]. Such a noninvasive biomarker could be useful for the purposes of prognostic assessment and would be crucial in designing clinical trials [19]. Radiomic models can provide a more accurate and objective alternative to the clinical metrics, such as (i) the UPDRS (part III—motor) score, disease duration as measured from (ii) time of diagnosis (DD-diag.) and (iii) time of appearance of symptoms (DD-sympt.), or (iv) the Montreal Cognitive Assessment (MoCA) score [19]. However, in order to do that, the radiomic models will require reference regions for normalization.

The radiomic features extracted from the caudate, putamen, and ventral striatum of DaTscan images at different timepoints of disease evolution could serve to quantify heterogeneity and texture in radiotracer uptake [20]. Quantifying feature eccentricity from the more affected ventral striatum may provide a useful predictor [20]. Thus, a combined approach involving standard SPECT interpretation and radiomic analysis performed on DAT SPECT imaging can improve the overall prediction of clinical outcomes.

Radiomics-based Haralick texture metrics extracted from striatal DAT SPECT have been shown to have a greater sensitivity to PD symptoms as compared to the routine mean uptake analysis [21]. These metrics may serve as a noninvasive imaging biomarker for disease progression.

These efforts in DAT SPECT radiomics are consistent with the aims of the Parkinson's Progressive Marker Initiative (PPMI), which emphasizes on the promotion of quantitative measurement and analysis of imaging used in the management of Parkinson's disease.

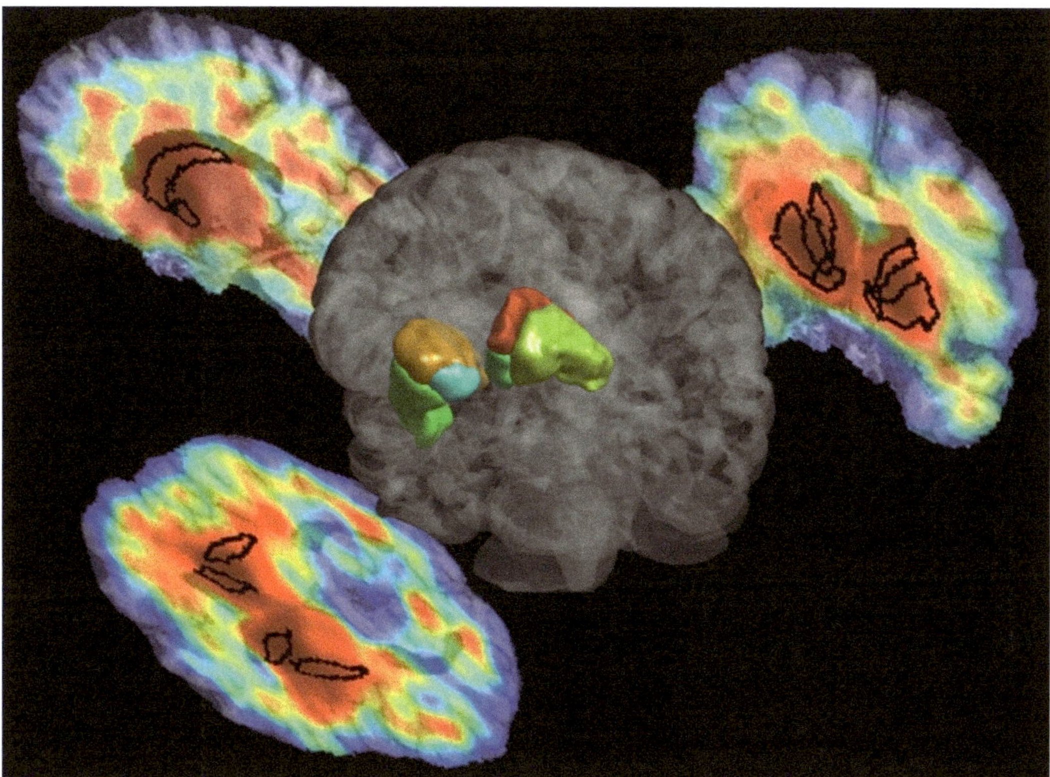

Fig. 2.4 3D volume rendering of six segmentations (caudate, putamen and VS; both right and left) for a typical study, as well as trans axial, coronal, and sagittal slices through the DAT SPECT image with superimposed segmentations. (Used under the Creative commons license from Rahmim A, Huang P, Shenkov N, Fotouhi S, Davoodi-Bojd E, Lu L, Mari Z, Soltanian-Zadeh, H, Sossi V. Improved prediction of outcome in Parkinson's disease using radiomics analysis of longitudinal DAT SPECT images. NeuroImage: Clinical. 2017 Jan 1;16:539–44.)

2.3.3 Cardiac SPECT Radiomics

Myocardial perfusion imaging (MPI) using SPECT is an established diagnostic test for patients suspected with coronary artery disease (CAD). 99mTc-Sestamibi is one of the preferred radiotracers used for this indication. Clinically, these studies are analyzed and interpreted manually with some support from a computer-aided diagnosis (CAD) program. Radiomics has the potential to improve the diagnostic and prognostic yield of MPI SPECT by way of providing biomarkers that correlate with perfusion heterogeneity [22].

In a standard MPI SPECT study, most features are not reproducible due to the low resolution. In studies where radiomic analysis was performed on MPI SPECT, it was observed that the most significant features were the intensity skewness and GLCM cluster shade for the right coronary artery (RCA), and intensity at 90% volume histogram for left circumflex artery (LCX). It has also been shown that left anterior descending artery (LAD) and RCA extracted from the vascular plot had more significant correlation than bull's eye plot, while LCX from the latter plot was noted to be more significant [23].

Radiomic analysis, regardless of the modality and indication, is highly sensitive to these factors, which impact the results even more profoundly in case of MPI SPECT. It is critically important to assess the robustness of cardiac SPECT radiomics features against variations in image acquisition and reconstruction parameters. For this purpose, the coefficient of variation (COV), which is a widely adopted metric, needs to be measured for each of the radiomic features for all imaging settings. It has been noted that the repeatability and reproducibility of SPECT/CT cardiac radiomic features under different imaging settings are feature-dependent. The radiomic features that exhibited low COV against changes in all imaging settings included the Inverse Difference Moment Normalized (IDMN) and Inverse Difference Normalized (IDN) features from the Gray Level Co-occurrence Matrix (GLCM), Run Percentage (RP) from the Gray Level Co-occurrence Matrix (GLRLM), Zone Entropy (ZE) from the Gray Level Size Zone Matrix (GLSZM), and Dependence Entropy (DE) from the Gray Level Dependence Matrix (GLDM) [24]. Of these image acquisition parameters, matrix size has been found to have the largest impact on feature variability [24].

123-iodine meta-iodobenzylguanidine (^{123}I-mMIBG) SPECT imaging is a study performed clinically in the management of cardiomyopathy, and its interpretation is largely manual. However, texture analysis performed to study regional washout from non-infarcted tissue can improve the predictive capability of cardiac events using multivariate analysis of regional washout associated with territories adjacent to myocardial infarction [25]. In a study by Currie et al., artificial neural network (ANN)-based analysis was performed on the ^{123}I-MIBG images, and the calculated planar global washout of >30% was shown to be the best indicator for risk of cardiac event when accompanied by a decline in left ventricular ejection fraction of >10% [25]. This is encouraging for new ML-driven efforts (such as radiomics) for automated feature extraction from raw image datasets in nuclear cardiology.

2.3.4 Other Applications of SPECT Radiomics

Preclinical studies have demonstrated that changes in opacity in SPECT/CT with Tc-99 m-MDP can be used for the assessment of bone remodeling. One such study compared the increase of bone opacity and decrease of

Tc-99 m-MDP activity variables [26]. Radiomics can be applied here to study bone healing, bone grafting, and bone replacement, which can improve the prognostic value of these studies (see Fig. 2.5).

Theranostics is a molecular imaging technique that involves specific molecular targeting for the purposes of diagnostics and therapy [27]. One example of a theranostic approach using ^{111}In/^{90}Y-ibritumomab tiuxetan has been described above (in the oncologic SPECT radiomics section). Visualization of the potential target for a specific therapeutic is a tremendously powerful tool that minimizes untoward effects and improves therapeutic efficacy. Radiomics approaches can increase the range of information revealing the tissue processes that can guide treatment and those that reflect changes secondary to treatment. This way, radiomics can impact both the diagnostic and therapeutic arms of theranostics, respectively. Texture analysis-based radiomic features can identify and target activity of the theranostic agents and study the cellular- and tissue-level changes induced by their action. Quantification of involved processes such as T-cell recruitment and resulting apoptosis/necrosis as features extracted from the SPECT study performed as a part of the theranostics can be highly useful in patient selection and therapy response assessment in clinical studies [28]. When using radiomics for such sophisticated approaches, which may involve multimodal imaging, it is important to implement image-quality harmonization and perform optimal integrative analysis (by choosing the right ML methods) [29].

2.4 Challenges and Opportunities of SPECT Radiomics

While reviewing the current landscape of radiomics-related work using SPECT, it becomes quite apparent that the field of SPECT radiomics is still in its infancy. Most of the studies are preclinical, using animal models. Furthermore, only a few indications within each specialty have been

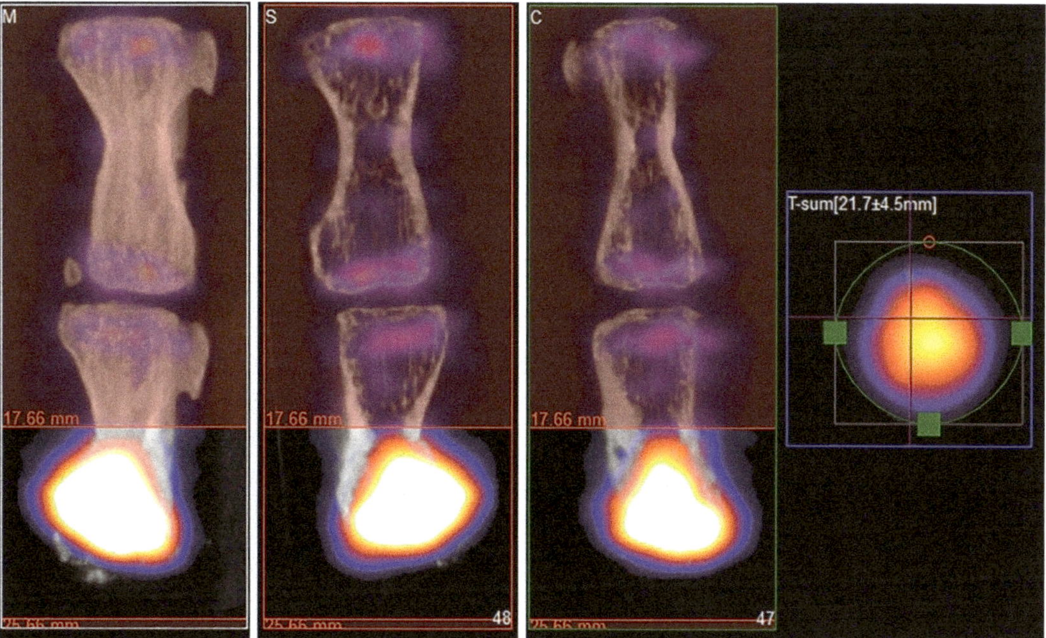

Fig. 2.5 Tc-99m-MDP activity in *caudal vertebrae* of treated rats after 8 weeks. The C5 *vertebrae* (down) were treated and filled with a bone graft which was selected as VOI in SPECT at 8 weeks after surgery. The color intensity shows the activity of Tc-99 m-MDP in the last region of *vertebra*. The upper bones are C4 control *vertebrae*. (Used under the creative commons license from Budán F, Szigeti K, Weszl M, et al. Novel radiomics evaluation of bone formation utilizing multimodal (SPECT/X-ray CT) in vivo imaging. PLoS One. 2018;13(9):e0204423. Published 2018 Sep 25. doi: https://doi.org/10.1371/journal.pone.0204423.)

the focus of such efforts. Having said that, the initial results are encouraging. Learning from the experience with PET radiomics, one can expect an expansion of the breadth and scope of such studies, both in terms of indications and technical advancements that will make SPECT radiomics ready for prime time in human studies and eventual clinical practice.

The main challenges in this path include the availability of high-quality data to develop such models. SPECT is not as ubiquitous in clinical use the way CT or even PET is. This poses a limitation in the development of ML-based radiomic models that require large training and validation sets. Another major challenge, which has been alluded to above, is that of the robustness of SPECT models being affected by the variations in the imaging parameters (related to acquisition protocol, scanner types, patient preparation, and other factors). This limits the way radiomics could be applied as a reproducible and reliable

methodology across multiple centers with reasonably similar imaging parameters and patient populations. One way to address this problem is to design large-scale studies in which all variables are represented. This goes back to our initial challenge of data paucity for SPECT studies. However, smarter trial designs, multicenter collaborations, improved data liquidity and availability, and leveraging the power of AI can help overcome this challenge. Furthermore, designing radiomic models that address multimodal imaging (SPECT/CT, SPECT/MR) and other -omics (genomics, transcriptomics, metabolomics, pathomics, etc.) will improve the specificity and predictive values of these methods.

Having a well-articulated clinical question based on a real-world need and designing a radiomic methodology that attempts to answer thst question by using a rich data set is critical to the success of a radiomics-based application. Optimizing each step of the workflow, including

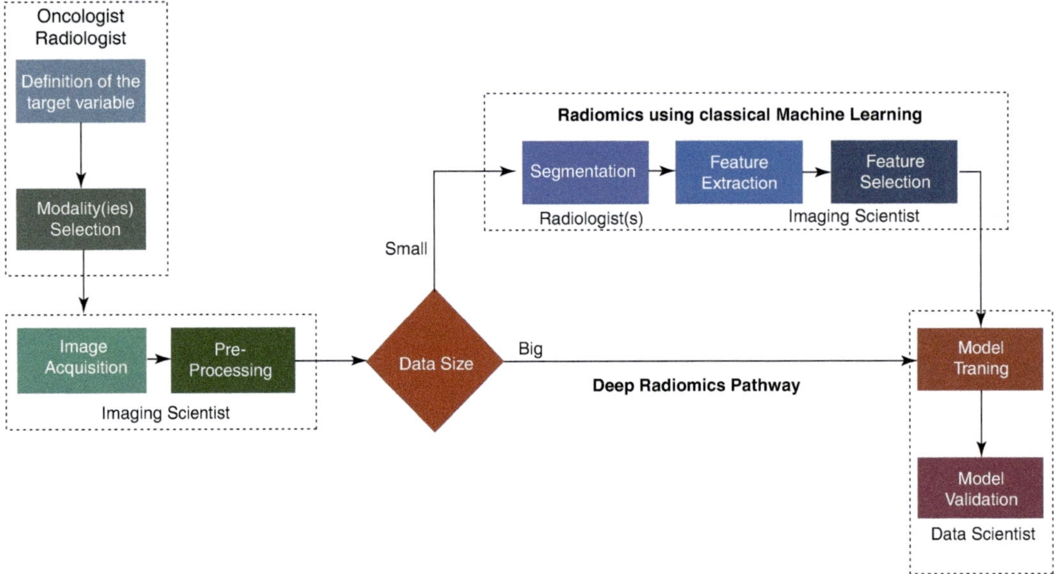

Fig. 2.6 A multidisciplinary radiomics workflow. Initially a group of clinicians should define the clinical problem that the proposed model should deal with and make decisions on what kind of imaging modalities should be recruited. Imaging scientists need to make sure that acquisition protocols are optimally designed producing high-quality images, as well as for the preprocessing of the images. Then depending on the size of the available imaging studies, we need to decide which pipeline to use. In case of big data (in the order of thousands), a deep radiomics approach can be suggested avoiding tedious and time-consuming processes like tumor segmentation by multiple radiologists. In addition, deep convolutional neural networks have been proven more efficient to model complex problems compared with traditional machine learning algorithms, as long as data availability requirement is satisfied. Finally, the data sets are allocated for training, validation, and testing purposes. (Used under the creative commons license from Papanikolaou N, Matos C, Koh DM. How to develop a meaningful radiomic signature for clinical use in oncologic patients. Cancer Imaging. 2020;20:33.)

preprocessing the data prior to analysis and applying the most suitable statistical/ML strategies, will render high accuracy rates (see Fig. 2.6) [30]. Testing these models in real-world is another key step that ensures that a radiomic model is ready for clinical use.

This is an exciting time to be involved in the fields of functional/molecular imaging and informatics, as recent and ongoing advancements have enabled us to merge these fields to devise advanced quantitative image analysis approaches that make help revive and promote modalities, such as SPECT in the era of precision medicine.

References

1. Zwanenburg A. Radiomics in nuclear medicine: robustness, reproducibility, standardization, and how to avoid data analysis traps and replication crisis. Eur J Nucl Med Mol Imaging. 2019;46(13):2638–55.

2. Aktolun C. Artificial intelligence and radiomics in nuclear medicine: potentials and challenges. Eur J Nucl Med Mol Imaging. 2019;46:2731–6.

3. Larue RT, Defraene G, De Ruysscher D, Lambin P, Van Elmpt W. Quantitative radiomics studies for tissue characterization: a review of technology and methodological procedures. Br J Radiol. 2017;90(1070):20160665.

4. Ibrahim A, Vallieres M, Woodruff H, Primakov S, Beheshti M, Keek S, Sanduleanu S, Walsh S, Morin O, Lambin P, Hustinx R. Radiomics analysis for clinical decision support in nuclear medicine. In: Seminars in nuclear medicine. WB Saunders; 2019.

5. Parmar C, Velazquez ER, Leijenaar R, Jermoumi M, Carvalho S, Mak RH, Mitra S, Shankar BU, Kikinis R, Haibe-Kains B, Lambin P. Robust radiomics feature quantification using semiautomatic volumetric segmentation. PLoS One. 2014;9(7):e102107.

6. Gillies RJ, Kinahan PE, Hricak H. Radiomics: images are more than pictures, they are data. Radiology. 2016;278(2):563–77.

7. Kumar V, Gu Y, Basu S, Berglund A, Eschrich SA, Schabath MB, Forster K, Aerts HJ, Dekker A, Fenstermacher D, Goldgof DB. Radiomics: the process and the challenges. Magn Resonance Imaging. 2012;30(9):1234–48.

8. Zheng B, Liu L, Zhang Z, et al. Radiomics score: a potential prognostic imaging feature for postoperative survival of solitary HCC patients. BMC Cancer. 2018;18:1148.

9. Parmar C, Grossmann P, Bussink J, Lambin P, Aerts HJ. Machine learning methods for quantitative radiomic biomarkers. Sci Rep. 2015;5:13087.

10. Veres DS, Máthé D, Hegedűs N, Horváth I, Kiss FJ, Taba G, Tóth-Bodrogi E, Kovács T, Szigeti K. Radiomic detection of microscopic tumorous lesions in small animal liver SPECT imaging. EJNMMI Res. 2019;9(1):67.

11. Schaub S, Hippe D, Bowen S, Wootton L, Chaovalitwongse W, Kinahan P, Apisarnthanarax S, Nyflot M. Radiomics of sulfur colloid SPECT/CT to predict child-pugh class in hepatocellular carcinoma patients. Med Phys. 2019;46(6):E174.

12. Bell M, Turkbey EB, Escorcia FE. Radiomics, radiogenomics, and next-generation molecular imaging to augment diagnosis of hepatocellular carcinoma. Cancer J. 2020;26(2):108–15.

13. Pouliot F, Sjöstrand K, Stambler N, Richter J, Gjertsson K, Johnsson K, Wong V, Jensen J, Edenbrandt L, Anand A. Prospective evaluation of a novel deep learning algorithm (PSMA-AI) in the assessment of 99mTc-MIP-1404 SPECT/CT in patients with low or intermediate risk prostate cancer, 2019.

14. Ashrafinia S, Jones K, Gorin MA, Rowe SP, Javadi MS, Pomper MG, Allaf ME, Rahmim A. Reproducibility of cold uptake radiomics in 99m Tc-Sestamibi SPECT imaging of renal cell carcinoma. In: 2017 IEEE Nuclear Science Symposium and Medical Imaging Conference (NSS/MIC). IEEE; 2017. p. 1–4.

15. Meyer T, Gaya AM, Dancey G, Stratford MR, Othman S, Sharma SK, Wellsted D, Taylor NJ, Stirling JJ, Poupard L, Folkes LK, Chan PS, Pedley RB, Chester KA, Owen K, Violet JA, Malaroda A, Green AJ, Buscombe J, Padhani AR, Rustin GJ, Begent RH. A phase I trial of radioimmunotherapy with 131I-A5B7 anti-CEA antibody in combination with combretastatin-A4-phosphate in advanced gastrointestinal carcinomas. Clin Cancer Res. 2009;15:4484–92.

16. Rajkumar V, Goh V, Siddique M, et al. Texture analysis of (125)I-A5B7 anti-CEA antibody SPECT differentiates metastatic colorectal cancer model phenotypes and anti-vascular therapy response. Br J Cancer. 2015;112(12):1882–7. https://doi.org/10.1038/bjc.2015.166.

17. El Emir E, Qureshi U, Dearling JL, Boxer GM, Clatworthy I, Folarin AA, et al. Predicting response to radioimmunotherapy from the tumor microenvironment of colorectal carcinomas. Cancer Res. 2007;67:11896–905.

18. Rahmim A, Huang P, Shenkov N, Fotouhi S, Davoodi-Bojd E, Lu L, Mari Z, Soltanian-Zadeh H, Sossi V. Improved prediction of outcome in Parkinson's disease using radiomics analysis of longitudinal DAT SPECT images. NeuroImage: Clin. 2017;16:539–44.

19. Adams M, Tang J. Convolutional neural network based motor score prediction using DAT SPECT imaging of Parkinson's disease. J Nucl Med. 2019;60(Suppl. 1):405.

20. Huang P, Shenkov N, Fotouhi S, Davoodi-Bojd E, Lu L, Mari Z, Soltanian-Zadeh H, Sossi V, Rahmim A. Radiomics analysis of longitudinal DaTscan images for improved progression tracking in Parkinson's disease. J Nucl Med. 2017;58(Suppl. 1):412.

21. Rahmim A, Salimpour Y, Blinder S, Klyuzhin I, Sossi V. Optimized haralick texture quantification to track Parkinson's disease progression from DAT SPECT images. J Nucl Med. 2016;57(Suppl. 2):428.

22. Ashrafinia S, Dalaie P, Yan R, Ghazi P, Marcus C, Taghipour M, Huang P, Pomper M, Schindler T, Rahmim A. Radiomics analysis of clinical myocardial perfusion SPECT to predict coronary artery calcification. J Nucl Med. 2018;59(Suppl. 1):512.

23. Ashrafinia S, Dalaie P, Yan R, Huang P, Pomper M, Schindler T, Rahmim A. Application of texture and radiomics analysis to clinical myocardial perfusion SPECT imaging. J Nucl Med. 2018;59(Suppl. 1):94.

24. Ashrafinia S, Ghazi P, Marcus CV, Taghipour M, Yan R, Valenta I, Pomper M, Schindler TH, Rahmim A. Robustness and reproducibility of radiomic features in 99mTc-Sestamibi SPECT imaging of myocardial perfusion. Med Phys. 2017;44(6)

25. Currie G, Iqbal B, Kiat H. Intelligent imaging: radiomics and artificial neural networks in heart failure. J Med Imaging Radiat Sci. 2019;50(4):571–4. https://doi.org/10.1016/j.jmir.2019.08.006.

26. Budán F, Szigeti K, Weszl M, et al. Novel radiomics evaluation of bone formation utilizing multimodal (SPECT/X-ray CT) in vivo imaging. PLoS One. 2018;13(9):e0204423. Published 2018 Sep 25. https://doi.org/10.1371/journal.pone.0204423.

27. Yordanova A, Eppard E, Kürpig S, Bundschuh RA, Schönberger S, Gonzalez-Carmona M, Feldmann G, Ahmadzadehfar H, Essler M. Theranostics in nuclear medicine practice. OncoTargets Ther. 2017;10:4821.

28. Keek SA, Leijenaar RT, Jochems A, Woodruff HC. A review on radiomics and the future of theranostics for patient selection in precision medicine. Br J Radiol. 2018;91(1091):20170926.

29. Ha S. Perspectives in radiomics for personalized medicine and theranostics. Nucl Med Mol Imaging. 2019;53:164–6. https://doi.org/10.1007/s13139-019-00578-x.

30. Papanikolaou N, Matos C, Koh DM. How to develop a meaningful radiomic signature for clinical use in oncologic patients. Cancer Imaging. 2020;20:33.

Stephan Walrand and Michel Hesse

3.1   Introduction

Likely, most nuclear clinicians will naturally acknowledge that SPECT/CT is the best tool beside PET/CT to get an accurate individual dosimetry in internal radiotherapy. But is it really needed? Often, internal radiotherapies are performed without any real individual dosimetry assessment. So why should we use the state-of-the-art SPECT/CT system?

This practice is linked with two wrong beliefs commonly spread in the nuclear medicine community: increasing the tumours absorbed dose a little bit can just improve a little bit the patient outcome, and the efficacy of external photon beam radiotherapy improved because the irradiation devices improved, so our only option is also to improve our tumour tracers.

The first belief comes from the way we are used to assess the efficacy of internal radiothera-

pies, i.e. by measuring the change in tumour size or in metabolism a few months after the therapy. And indeed, in this case, increasing a little bit the absorbed dose just increases a little bit the response, as early tissue (organ or tumour) toxicity is a smooth function of the absorbed dose [1–5]; killing a fraction of the tissue cells reduces the tissue metabolism by a similar fraction.

However, late tissue toxicity owns an absorbed dose threshold [6–8]; above a critical fraction of cells killed, the tissue will not be able to recover, and will 'die'. Decay, production of free radicals by ionisation, hits of the radicals to the DNA are all random process. The recovering capacity of a tissue depends on its state. As a result, the normal tissue complication probability (NTCP) and the tumour control probability (TCP) are not step functions, but are quite steeply S-shape functions, i.e. going from 0 to 1 within a few Gy. In addition, the dosimetry of critical organs is highly patient dependent [1]. It is thus of paramount importance to give the maximal activity to the patient that is still safe for him. Indeed, for some patients, the resulting increase in the tumour absorbed dose, even small, could be sufficient to shift from a cancer relapse to a controlled disease. In external beam radiotherapy (EBRT), this feature is called the therapeutic window. Figure 3.1 illustrates this concept applied to ^{90}Y-DOTATOC used in peptide receptor radiotherapy (PRRT). Even if dosimetry assessments are not accurate enough to ensure being in narrow therapeutic windows, the maximal chance

---

Preamble
Versus the previous 2013 version, recent breakthroughs in the field lead to add 6 new subsections to the "SPECT/CT based dosimetry studies" section, while two new sections have been added to the chapter. The conclusion has thus been fully re-written.

S. Walrand (✉) · M. Hesse
Nuclear Medicine, Université Catholique de Louvain, Brussels, Belgium
e-mail: stephan.walrand@uclouvain.be;
michel.hesse@uclouvain.be

© The Author(s), under exclusive license to Springer Nature Switzerland AG 2022
H. Ahmadzadehfar et al. (eds.), *Clinical Applications of SPECT-CT*,
https://doi.org/10.1007/978-3-030-65850-2_3

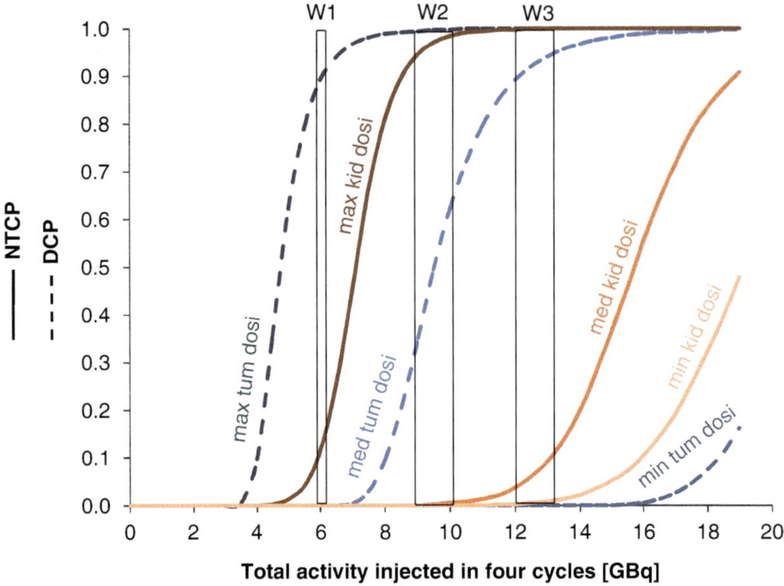

Fig. 3.1 Illustration of the therapeutic windows (TW) concept applied to ^{90}Y-DOTATOC PRRT. The disease control probability (DCP) and kidney NTCP were computed for their respective minimum, median, and maximum dosimetry measured by ^{86}Y-DOTATOC PET in the phase 1 clinical study using amino acid infusion [1, 9]. The curves were computed for a disease owning five tumours, and the tissue radiation tolerance parameters were extracted from [6, 10]. For a patient owning both the median tumour and median kidney dosimetry, W3 is a good TW choice giving a probability of 90% to be curative and of 10% to get a late renal failure. If his tumour dosimetry is the maximal one observed, then W2 is a better choice avoiding any risk of late renal failure. A patient with the maximal kidney dosimetry observed can be cured only if he also owns the maximal tumour dosimetry observed (W1)

for the patient outcome is to be as close as possible to his individual therapeutic window.

During the last decades, the efficacy of EBRT and the sophistication of the devices used have increased together. From these points of view, the recent CyberKnife system is really impressive [11]. In reality, there is no real innovation regarding the CyberKnife hardware (the knife part); it is the combination of a linear accelerator and of a standard industrial 6-axis robot used in car manufacturing, both existing since three decades. So why did this system appear only recently? The major benefit of the CyberKnife is to allow decreasing the absorbed dose to the critical tissues by increasing the number of different beam paths crossing the patient body to target the tumour. This (the cyber part) required motion tracking and an accurate individual treatment planning that uses state-of-the-art multimodality imaging [12–14] including elaborated Monte Carlo simulations of the absorbed dose spreading along the beam paths. This feasibility results from the continuous development of such treatment planning assessment in EBRT during the last decades [15].

Internal radiotherapy had the good fortune to begin with two pathologies owning a large therapeutic window: the radio-synovectomy and the thyroid cancer ^{131}I radio-ablation. These two therapies were used with success by simply injecting a standard activity. Sometimes, an early success durably formats the behaviours, and despite a lot of efforts spent during two decades, no such ideal radio-compound was found for the other cancers. For the patient benefit and also for the long-term future of nuclear medicine, we have to push the available internal radiotherapies to their optimal efficiency by performing an individual treatment planning at the same quality level than that routinely performed in EBRT. This was formalized by the European Union Council in its 2013/59/ Euratom directive [16]. That directive equates radionuclide therapies with EBRT regarding the necessity to get dosimetry as precise as possible to treat patient lesions in an optimized way while preserving healthy tissues. Let emphasize that a dosimetry method displaying a good dose–toxicity correlation on a patient's sample is not sufficient; as the goal is to inject to the patient the maximal activity that he can safely receive, the dosimetry has to be accurate on a patient per patient basis.

3.2 SPECT Versus Planar

There are four effects which definitely disqualify the use of planar-based dosimetry in most of internal radiotherapies: (1) γ-rays attenuation-scatter, (2) tissues overlapping, (3) multi-compartment organ and (4) heterogeneous organ uptake.

1. There is no way to accurately correct gamma-ray attenuation in planar acquisition; use of conjugated planar views, even jointly with a planar transmission scan, is a crude approximation. This method is only valid for an infinitely thin organ without any other activity overlapping. Use of a point scatter kernel to correct for the organs cross-contamination is hampered by the lack of information about the activity depth distribution. This cross-contamination is very cumbersome regarding that biological half-life of the organs is different and that the critical organs can be located close to tissue owning higher activity, such as liver, spleen, tumour, bowels close to the kidneys in PRRT.
2. The critical organs can partially or fully be overlapped by higher taking up tissues. Often, this problem is casually considered and several papers proposed patient dosimetry assessment based on planar views using correction method for the overlapping issues. But to our knowledge, only one [17] presented a validation on phantoms, which should be done for all proposed methods. However, these phantoms were simple: no full overlap, identical effective half-life for the different tissues and no appearing and disappearing activities (bowel in PRRT). Let emphasize that such overlap correction methods have to accurately

work for the worst patient case to whom it is not ethically defendable to tell that we cannot do an accurate treatment planning, because we chose to not use the best tool.

Sandström et al. [18] compared the absorbed dose assessed from conjugate planar views and SPECT/CT in 24 patients imaged 1, 24, 96 and 168 h post ^{177}Lu-DOTATATE therapy. Both modalities were corrected for attenuation; a ^{57}Co transmission scan was performed with the planar modality for this purpose. The planar view to SPECT total kidney absorbed dose ratio ranged from 0.8 to 5.4. Six patients out of 24 had a relative deviation higher than 40%. This clearly disqualifies planar imaging in PRRT pre-therapy planning. Garkavij et al. [19] observed the same problem, in 16 patients also treated with ^{177}Lu-DOTATATE, although with a lower maximal planar view to SPECT total kidney absorbed dose ratio of 1.8. The reason explaining this huge discrepancy between planar and SPECT based dosimetry, in both studies, originated from significant radioactivity overlap as illustrated in Fig. 3.2. In an older ^{90}Y-DOTATOC study, Valkema et al. reported that organs overlapping prevent accurate planar dosimetry assessment underwent in 6 out of 43 patients [20].

3. Some critical organs own several compartments displaying different uptakes, biological washouts, and radiosensitivities. For example, in PRRT, the renal cortex and medulla represent about 70% and 30% of the kidney activity, respectively [21]. The critical tissue, i.e. the glomerular, is located into the cortex. The medulla to cortex S-factor is about one-fourth of that from the cortex to the cortex [22]. The volume, uptake, and biological washout of these compartments are also patient-dependent [1, 23]. These three points require separately assessing the number of decays occurring in the medulla and in the renal cortex, which cannot be done in planar view.
4. Even if the organ has a homogeneous radiosensitivity, i.e. the spatial variations of the radiosensitivity are smaller than the ionizing particle range, such as the liver in ^{90}Y-radioembolization, assessing the intra-

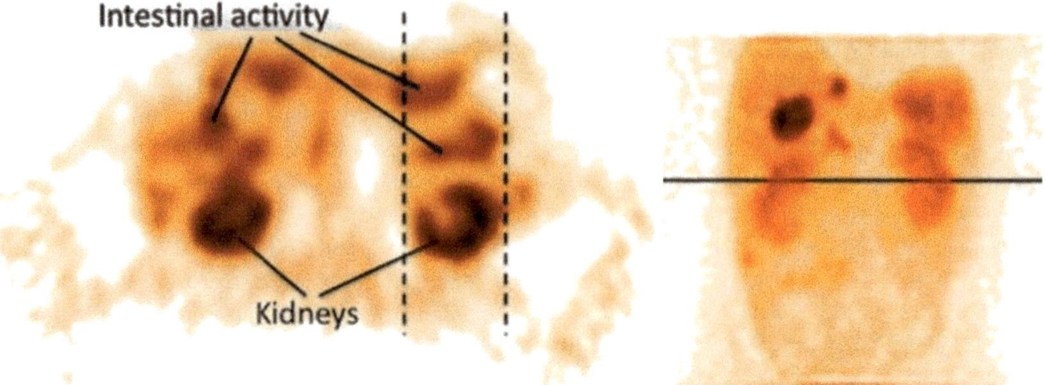

Fig. 3.2 Two images illustrating an imaging situation that results in an overestimated absorbed dose to the kidneys. The activity uptake in the contents of the intestine that overlaps the kidney in the planar image (as indicated by dashed lines) contributes to the absorbed dose, which is not the case in the single-photon emission computed tomography image. Note that the overlapping activity is difficult to detect in the planar images. Reprinted from [19] with permission of John Willey and Sons

organ absorbed dose distribution is still needed. Indeed, studies have shown that the NTCP does not depend only on the mean organ absorbed dose but also on its distribution [24, 25]. NTCP can be calculated using the equivalent uniform dose (EUD) formalism that account for the absorbed dose distribution [10]. For homogeneous density organs, the EUD can be computed based on a fast convolution of the SPECT image by a dose deposition kernel, preferably deconvolved by the SPECT system spatial resolution [26].

Lastly, the argument, which is still sometimes advanced nowadays [17], that planar views have to be used because SPECT is too much time consuming, is not relevant. Irradiating a patient from the inside is a medical act as serious as irradiating him from the outside and should be done in the same sophisticated way.

3.3 SPECT/CT Versus SPECT

Hybrid SPECT/CT system allows a better co-registration accuracy of the two modalities than that obtain by trying to acquire the patient with exactly the same geometry in two different systems or than to use delicate non-rigid fusion. This favourably impacts the activity quantification. Regarding dosimetry assessment, this also helps to link the activity observed to the tissue owning it.

Activity quantification requires the knowledge of the patient attenuation map. SPECT systems equipped with a gamma-ray transmission source are rare. The attenuation map can be derived from the CT Hounsfield values using appropriate rescaling [27]. The issue regarding the additional irradiation received by the patient from the CT performed at the different SPECT time points needed to assess the pharmacokinetics is purely philosophical regarding the four higher order of magnitude of the absorbed dose received during the therapy.

Recent literature review showed that SPECT/CT performed better in absolute quantification than conventional SPECT system [28]. On acquisitions of a torso phantom, Shcherbinin et al. [29] reported errors between 3% and 5% for the isotopes ^{99m}Tc, ^{123}I, ^{131}I, and ^{111}In. The phantom contained two sources centrally and peripherally placed with no surrounding activity. For ^{99m}Tc in a cardiac torso phantom, Vandervoort et al. [30] reported an error of 8% in simulation and within 4% for the acquisition. Both studies included attenuation, scatter and collimator PSF in the iterative reconstruction.

Willowson et al. [31] evaluated SPECT/CT quantification for ^{99m}Tc in phantoms and in patients. The acquisitions were first corrected for scattering using a transmission-dependent scatter correction (TDSC) method developed on site, and afterwards reconstructed with a commercial OSEM software. The scatter-corrected data, the associated reconstructed data and the co-registered attenuation map were then passed to an iterative Chang attenuation correction algorithm using the CT-derived attenuation correction map. Last, a dead-time correction was performed. In the torso phantom, the relative deviation of the total liver-specific activity assessment was 2%. Clinical evaluation in 12 lung ventilation/perfusion studies after injection of calibrated ^{99m}Tc-MAA activity gave a relative deviation ranging from −7.4 to 3.7% (mean absolute relative deviation of 2.6%).

Beauregard et al. [32] evaluated a commercially available SPECT/CT system in quantitative ^{177}Lu imaging using the manufactory iterative reconstruction algorithm that included CT-based attenuation correction, scatter correction using a triple energy acquisition window and collimator PSF. In addition, they added a camera sensitivity calibration function of the count rate in order to correct for the dead time. They performed seven acquisitions of a 20 cm-diameter phantom with background activity ranging from 0 to 1 GBq including two cylindrical active sources independently ranging from 0 to 0.7 GBq. The deviation activity ranged from −9.5% to 4.1% and from −14.9% to 4.3%, for the whole phantom and for the sources, respectively. The total body activity deviation on five treated patients versus the injected activity (mean ± std. activity = 8.9 ± 0.9 GBq) ranged from −4.9% to 0.0% with dead time correction (from −15.2% to −10.2% without).

Those studies show that SPECT/CT can be used for individualized dosimetry treatment planning. The maximal safe activity found to be injected can be reduce by 10% in order to account for the current quantification accuracy.

Ahmadzadehfar et al. [33] evaluated the impact of ^{99m}Tc-MAA SPECT/CT on SIRT treatment planning and its added value to angiography in 90 studies performed on 76 patients. The accurate co-registration of the two modalities obtained with a hybrid SPECT/CT system allows determining in a robust way which tissue corresponds to the activity observed (Fig. 3.3). Extrahepatic accumulation was detected by planar imaging, SPECT and SPECT/CT in 12%, 17% and 42% of examinations, respectively. The sensitivity for detecting extrahepatic shunting with planar imaging, SPECT and SPECT/CT was 32%, 41% and 100%, respectively, all with a specificity higher than 93%. They concluded that ^{99m}Tc-MAA SPECT/CT is valuable for identifying extrahepatic visceral sites at risk for postradioembolization complications.

3.4 Choice of a Surrogate

^{90}Y is the majorly used radionuclide in internal radiotherapy which does not own any isotope having an appropriated half-life and emitting γ-rays that can be imaged by SPECT. The choice of the good SPECT surrogate is a crucial point which has not yet been sufficiently investigated. ^{90}Y is mainly used in PRRT, radioimmunotherapy and liver radioembolization.

When introducing PRRT, the community thought that tissues uptake should mainly depend on the peptide, perhaps a little bit on the chelator and marginally on the radionuclide which is confined in the chelator cage. Later, Reubi et al. showed that receptor affinity for a same chelator-peptide also strongly depends on the labelled radionuclide [34], e.g. by a factor 2 when replacing Y by Ga in DOTATATE labelling. However, contrary to tumours, organ uptakes are not always only receptor-dependent. For example, an important part of the ^{90}Y-DOTATOC kidney uptake is not receptor-dependent, and ^{111}In-DOTATOC-based dosimetry has shown a good correlation with kidney toxicity post therapy [6].

However, this shows that the choice of a radionuclide surrogate for individualized treatment planning in PRRT requires an initial validation proving identical pharmacokinetics along a patient-per-patient basis. Such studies in PRRT are still lacking. This validation can be performed by imaging the ^{90}Y therapy by bremsstrahlung SPECT or by PET imaging of the compound

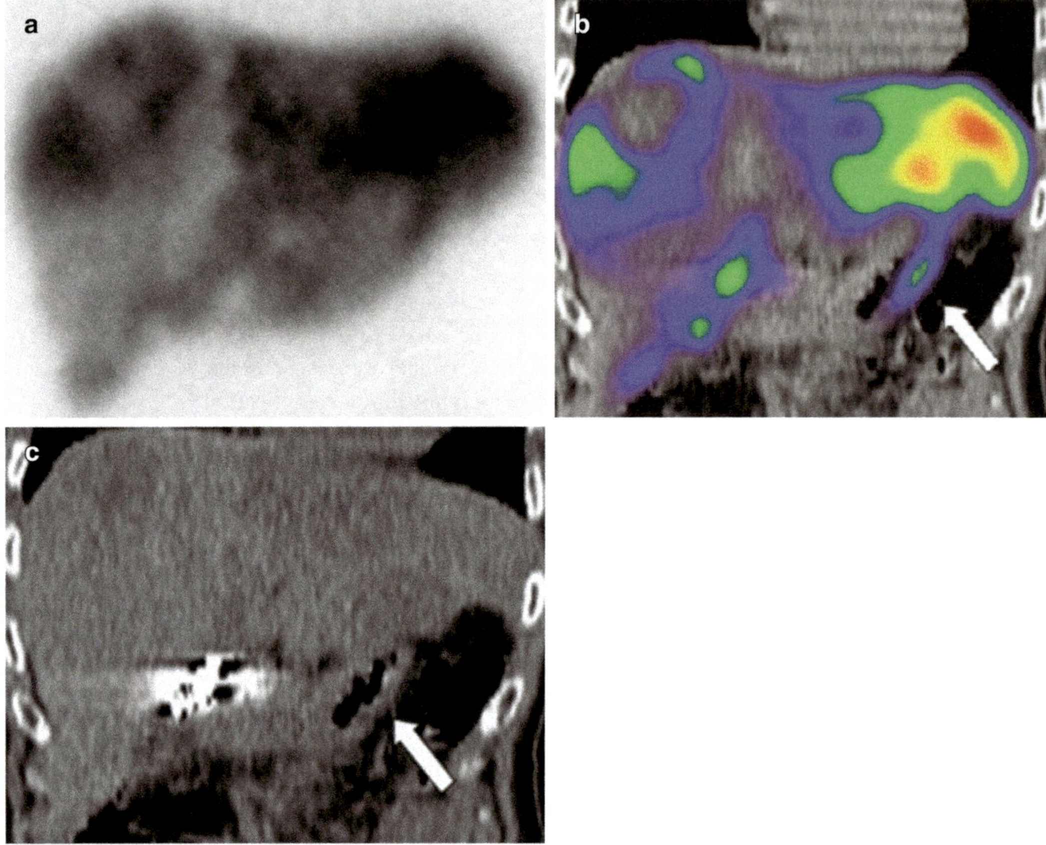

Fig. 3.3 Duodenal accumulation (arrows) in a patient with colorectal cancer, not definable on planar images: planar scan (**a**), SPECT/CT coronal view (**b**), and CT coronal view (**c**). Reprinted from [33] with permission of the Society of Nuclear Medicine

labelled with [86]Y [35]; however, both modalities require state-of-the-art correction methods.

In radioimmunotherapy, Minarik et al. [36] compared in three patients the absorbed doses obtained from a pretherapeutic 300 MBq ^{111}In-ibritumomab SPECT/CT to those obtained post ^{90}Y-ibritumomab therapy by bremsstrahlung SPECT/CT using corrections developed on site (see Bremsstrahlung SPECT/CT chapter). The absolute relative differences between absorbed dose computed from ^{111}In and ^{90}Y SPECT/CT were 8.8 ± 13.7 and 8.9 ± 4.0 (mean ± std. in %), for the liver and kidneys, respectively. This supports considering ^{111}In as a surrogate of ^{90}Y in radioimmunotherapy. Compared to peptides, the active site in antibodies is located farther from the radionuclide which likely reduces its impact.

However, a validation on a larger patient series is still needed.

For ^{90}Y-loaded glass spheres, Chiesa et al. [25] performed in 35 patients a co-registering of the ^{99m}Tc-MAA SPECT with the ^{90}Y bremsstrahlung SPECT. In the 29 patients treated with the same intentional catheter positioning that in the pretherapeutic study, the biodistribution was markedly different between the two modalities in two patients (7%) and seems only attributable to the different physical properties of spheres and MAA.

For ^{90}Y resin spheres, Jiang et al. [37] conducted an interesting study in 81 paired ^{99m}Tc-MAA and ^{90}Y bremsstrahlung SPECT performed in 75 patients, the catheter being intended to be set in the same position in the two radioemboliza-

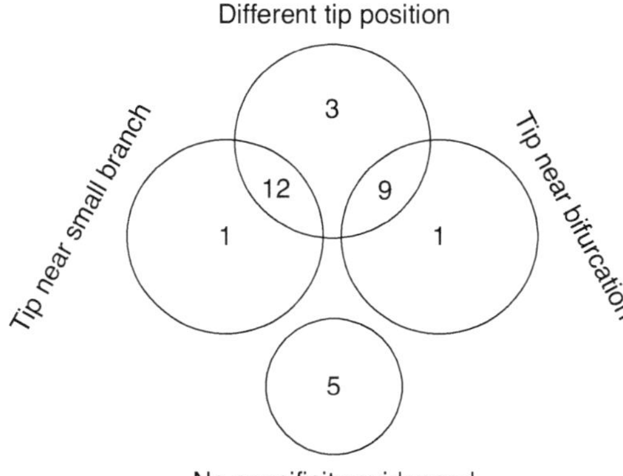

Fig. 3.4 Summary of results from [37] that analyzed in the angiograms the catheter tip position in paired studies showing a segmental perfusion difference (SPD) between ^{99m}Tc-MAA and ^{90}Y SPECT, i.e. 31 out of 81 resin spheres radioembolizations

tions using angiography. They observed a segmental perfusion difference (SPD) between the two SPECT modalities in 31 patients. Analyzing the position of the catheter tip on the two angiograms performed, they noted that 24 SPDs correspond to a different tip position between the two radioembolizations, 2 SPDs occurred with the same tip position, but close to an arterial bifurcation or close to a small branch (Fig. 3.4). However, in 5 SPDs, no particular specificity was evidenced besides the physical properties of the particles.

The correlation dependence on the distance between the catheter tip and the first arterial branch was recently confirmed for ^{90}Y-loaded glass spheres radioembolization in 23 patients [38]. A better correlation was also observed for non-tumoral tissue versus tumours [39, 40].

In a recent study, Smits et al. [41] showed that a ^{166}Ho-scout SPECT/CT performed in the morning of the therapeutic ^{166}Ho radioembolization, itself performed in the afternoon, provided better tumour dose estimation than a ^{99m}Tc-MAA SPECT/CT preformed 4 days earlier. However, it is not clear whether this improvement is attributable to the use of the same device or to the shorter delay with the therapeutic procedure. Good agreement was obtained for both procedures for the non-tumoral dose prediction.

The same team also observed a good agreement for the LSF [42], while ^{99m}Tc MAA systematically exhibited an LSF overestimation likely related to the physical differences between the two devices. Similar overestimation is observed in ^{90}Y-loaded glass spheres radioembolization using ^{99m}Tc-MAA SPECT/CT [43], with the overestimation still being larger using planar imaging [44, 45]. In a phantom study, Kunnen et al. [46] proved dosimetry feasible using a safe 100 MBq ^{90}Y scout activity.

The readers can find a detailed discussion about the challenges of individualized radioembolization therapy using ^{99m}TC-MAA SPECT/CT [47].

3.5 SPECT/CT-Based Dosimetry Studies

3.5.1 Yttrium-90 Spheres Dose–Response

Garin et al. [7] performed a dose–response retrospective study in 36 patients for HCC treated with ^{90}Y-loaded glass spheres. The absorbed doses to liver and tumours were assessed using the ^{99m}Tc-MAA SPECT/CT performed within 1–2 weeks before the therapy and iteratively reconstructed with attenuation and with dual-energy windows scatter correction. The catheter line was counted after therapy in order to estimate the actual injected activity. The planned absorbed dose to the targeted liver volume was 120 Gy based on the MAA, without exceeding 30 Gy for the lungs. Compared to the planning only using the lung shunt and the targeted liver volume, this dose assessment allowed increasing the injected activity in four patients owning large lesions. Mean absorbed doses for non-responding and responding tumours were 124 ± 63 Gy and 328 ± 107 Gy, respectively. The 30 months overall survival evidenced a 205 Gy tumour absorbed dose responding threshold.

Chiesa et al. [48, 49] retrospectively analyzed treatment with ^{90}Y-loaded glass spheres in 52 patients (36, 7 and 9 Child Pugh A5, A6 and B7, respectively). Voxel dosimetry was computed from the ^{99m}Tc-MAA SPECT performed within 3–4 weeks before the therapy and corrected for attenuation using CT co-registration. All the administrations were lobar, aiming to deliver a mean absorbed dose of 120 Gy to the target lobe including tumour based on the lobe mass measured on CT. There was an overlap in the absorbed doses of the non-responding tumours (0 → 500 Gy) and of the responding tumours (250 → 1500 Gy). Kappadath et al. [50] using ^{90}Y-bremssthralung SPECT/CT-based dosimetry for glass spheres HCC radioembolization in 34 patients also observed such large doses overlap between non-responding and responding tumours.

Strigari et al. [8] retrospectively analyzed HCC treatment with ^{90}Y-resin spheres in 73 patients. The administered activity was determined using the BSA method. Entire liver was treated in 35 patients, a right and left lobar approach was used in 35 and 3 patients, respectively. The liver and tumour dosimetry was assessed on the fusion of the pre-therapeutic ^{99m}Tc-MAA SPECT with a CT using a dedicated software. An elliptical constant attenuation map was used in the SPECT reconstruction with an effective attenuation coefficient of 0.11 cm^{-1} to account for the scatter. The TCP fit, based on RECIST or EASL criteria, showed that two different radio-resistant tumour populations coexisted: 60 and 40% of the tumours had a TD$_{50}$ around a BED of 50 and 130 Gy, respectively. Complete response was observed in all tumours above BED = 200 Gy (AD = 145).

This much higher threshold for tumour response observed in liver-radioembolization studies compared to the traditional 40 Gy observed in EBRT is partly explained by the fact that in internal therapy due to the beta range, the outer shell of the tumour receives about half of the mean absorbed dose.

3.5.2 Yttrium-90 Spheres Dose–Toxicity

In the study [8] summarised here above, Strigari et al. measured a median liver dose of 36 Gy ranging from 6 to 78 Gy. 58, 13 and 2 patients were classified Child-Pugh A, B and C, respectively. The liver was considered as a purely parallel organ ($n = 1$ in the Lyman–Burman Kutcher model). Liver BED was computed with $\alpha/\beta = 2.5$ Gy and using 2.5 h for the sublethal damage repair half-time. The common terminology criteria for adverse events (version 4 National Cancer Institute, Cancer Therapy Evaluation Program) was used to qualify late liver toxicity (4.5 months follow-up). Figure 3.5 shows the liver toxicity–dose relationship considering grades ≥ 2 as liver toxicity threshold, i.e. at least severe or medically significant.

In the study [48, 49] summarised in the previous section, Chiesa et al. assessed the liver toxicity as the occurrence, during the first 6 months after therapy, of any of: clinically detectable ascites, hepatic encephalopathy, bleeding from oesophageal varices, total bilirubin >3 mg/dL and prothrombin time INR (international normalized ratio) >2.2. Figure 3.6a shows that the NCTP strongly depend on the Child Pugh status. Figure 3.6b shows that for Child Pugh A, the NCTP$_{50}$ occurred around AD = 100 Gy, twofold higher than the AD = 50 Gy observed by Strigari et al. (Fig. 3.5).

Compared to resin spheres, the lower toxicity and efficacy per Gy of the glass one result from a much higher dose distribution heterogeneity as proved by Monte Carlo simulations of spheres transport in hepatic arterial tree [51–53]. d'Abadie et al. [54] taking this heterogeneity into account, using ^{90}Y TOF-PET-based EUD, reunified observed dose–responses between glass spheres, resin spheres and EBRT together.

3.5.3 Yttrium-90 PRRT

Pretherapy dosimetry with ^{86}Y-DOTATOC PET gave impressive renal and bone marrow dose–toxicity correlation in ^{90}Y-DOTATOC therapy [1, 2]. However, its cost, and also the need to infuse amino acids to mimic the therapy, prevent its use in clinical therapy. Fortunately, ^{90}Y-DOTATOC therapy is performed in several cycles in order to reduce the organs toxicity, and thus dosimetry

Fig. 3.5 Normal-tissue complication probability of liver toxicity (solid line) vs. liver BED. Dashed-line represents 95% confidence interval. Vertical bars represent SD (caused by number of data in each group that created each point). Exp = experimental data. Reprinted from [8] with authorization of the Society of Nuclear Medicine Liver absorbed dose (AD) was added by the author of the present chapter

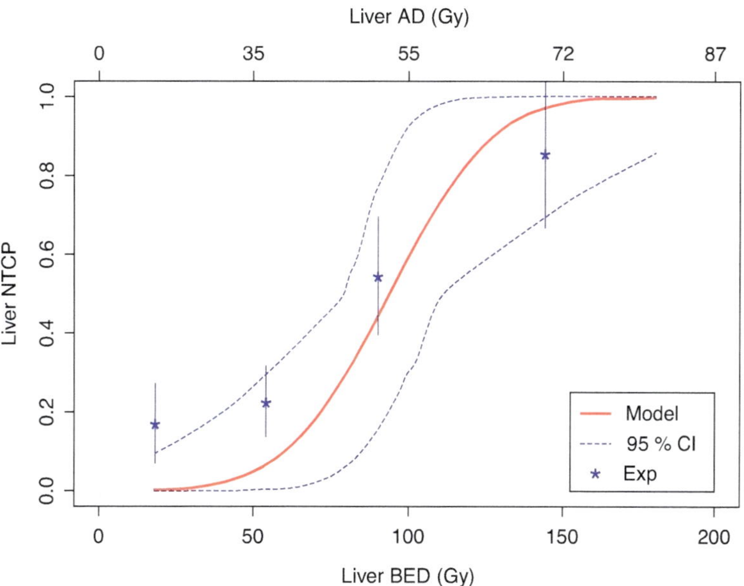

Fig. 3.6 NTCP histogram in function of mean absorbed dose to the lobe excluding tumour for the different Child Pugh populations. Reprinted from [48] with permission of Minerva Medica

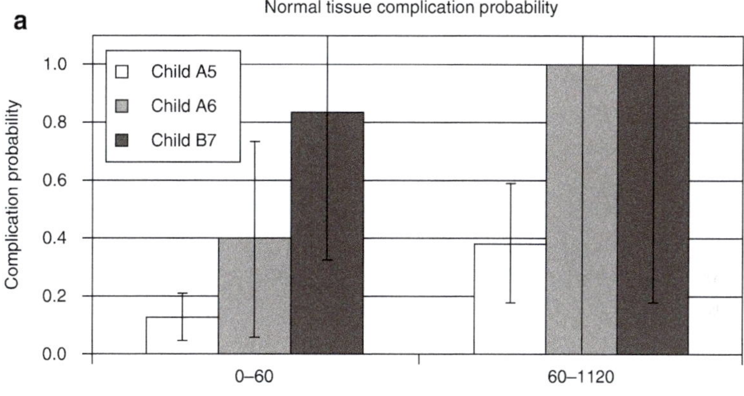

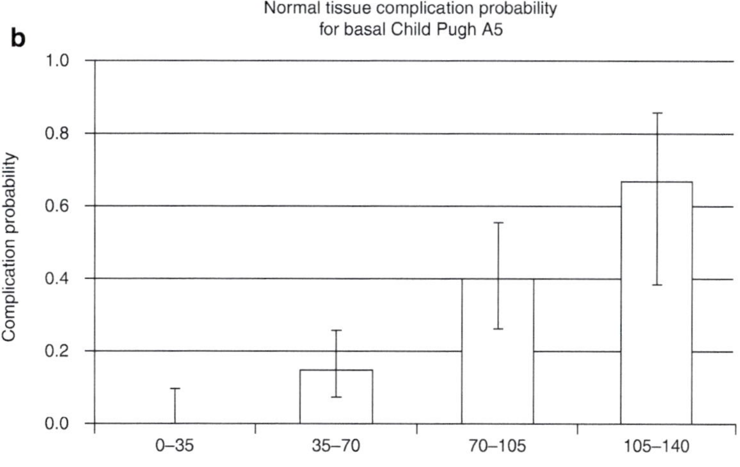

performed after one cycle can be used to optimize the activity to be injected in the next one.

Menda et al. [55] conducted a prospective post cycle renal dosimetry using ^{90}Y-bremss. SPECT/CT in 25 patients having neuroendocrine tumours. A ^{90}Y TOF-PET/CT [56] was used at the first time for BREMSS for SPECT/CT calibration purpose. The study confirmed the very high variability of inter-patient renal dosimetry as already observed using ^{86}Y-DOTATOC PET [1], advocating the interest to individually optimize the injected ^{90}Y activity.

3.5.4 Holmium-166

Smits et al. [57] conducted a phase 1 dose-escalation study in ^{166}Ho liver radioembolization with a state-of-the-art design. 6, 3, 3 and 3 patients received activities in order to get a whole-liver absorbed dose of 20, 40, 60 and 80 Gy, respectively, calculated assuming a homogeneous distribution of the activity in the whole liver, i.e. neglecting the tumour liver burden. After coil embolization of undesirable artery branch, ^{99m}Tc-MAA was injected and followed by a SPECT or SPECT/CT imaging. Within 2 weeks, a second angiography was performed with injection of a 250 MBq scout activity of ^{166}Ho spheres followed by a SPECT or SPECT/CT imaging. The same day, a third angiography was performed with injection of the therapeutic ^{166}Ho spheres activity. Both ^{166}Ho radioembolizations intended with the same catheter positioning than that in the ^{99m}Tc-MAA one. SPECT or SPECT/CT and MRI imaging were performed 3–5 post therapy. In all patients, the three SPECT modalities showed similar patterns of the presence or absence of extrahepatic deposition of activity. Regarding the adverse events, the authors concluded that ^{166}Ho radioembolization with a whole-liver dose of 60 Gy is feasible.

In a recent study, the same team showed that it is advocated to use ^{166}Ho-scout SPECT/CT to select patients and to personalize the administered activity in order to target a mean tumour-absorbed dose >90 Gy and a parenchymal dose <55 Gy [58]. In this 40 patients study, only one CTCAE grade 5 related to the radioembolization was observed within the 3 months follow-up, while 90 Gy was the tumour threshold giving a significantly better patients outcome.

Identifying on ^{99m}Tc-MAA SPECT/CT whether the uptake is located in normal liver or tumoral tissue can be highly challenging. Stella et al. [59] conducted a prospective study on 65 ^{166}Ho liver radioembolizations for neuroendocrine metastases. Patients were radioembolized with a scout ($n = 29$) or a therapeutic ($n = 36$) ^{166}Ho activity. After the ^{166}Ho SPECT/CT, the patients remained on the camera table and were immediately injected with 50 MBq ^{99m}Tc-stannous phytate which accumulates in Kupffer cells, present in healthy liver tissue, but not in tumorous tissue. Ten minutes after the injection, a triple-energy window SPECT/CT was performed. Dosimetry performed on the ^{166}Ho window SPECT/CT, corrected for ^{99m}Tc cross scattering, was proven sufficiently accurate in VOIs >25 mL for clinical purpose.

3.5.5 Lutetium-177 Antibody

Woliner-van der Weg et al. [60] calculated the bone marrow dosimetry for 13 colorectal cancer patients in ^{177}Lu-labeled di-HSG-peptide therapy. 3D dosimetry was performed on lumbar vertebrae imaged by SPECT/CT at 3, 24 and 72 h after ^{177}Lu administration. 3D dosimetry proved superior in identifying patients at risk of developing any grade of bone marrow toxicity compared to blood- or 2D image-based methods.

In a more recent trial, Blakkisrud et al. [61] studied the bone marrow absorbed dose for 8 non-Hodgkin lymphoma patients treated with ^{177}Lu-lilotomab satetraxetan, with or without additional cold lilotomab. Using SPECT/CT imaging of the L2–L4 vertebrae, they observed that cold lilotomab administration reduced the red-marrow absorbed dose. They also obtained a clear correlation between red-marrow absorbed dose and hematologic toxicity. They concluded that, contrary to some non-imaging method, estimations of bone marrow absorbed dose by

SPECT/CT imaging could be predictive of hematologic adverse events.

3.5.6 Lutetium-177 PRRT

Santoro et al. [62] evaluated the organs at risk in 12 patients treated with ^{177}Lu-DOTATATE using 4 SPECT/CT performed after the first and second cycles. The mean dosimetry for kidney and red marrow was 0.43 ± 0.13 mGy/MBq and 0.04 ± 0.02 mGy/MBq, respectively. As the maximal tolerated dose for red marrow is about tenfold lower than that of kidney [2], this explains why haematological toxicity is the limiting factor in 26% of individually optimized ^{177}Lu PRRT [63].

Hagmarker et al. [64] using the thoracic vertebra activity in ^{177}Lu-DOTATATE SPECT/CT-planar hybrid method found similar red-marrow dosimetry, i.e. 0.06 (0.02–0.12) mGy/MBq in 22 patients without skeletal metastasizes. They observed a dose–toxicity relation (Fig. 3.7) in line with that observed in ^{90}Y-DOTATOC trial using ^{86}Y-DOTATOC PET-based red-marrow dosimetry [2]. In 200 patients, Garsk et al. [63] observed fourfold lower mean blood-based red-marrow dosimetry, i.e. 0.016 mGy/MBq, which was unable to predict the haematological toxicity observed in 40 patients.

Transferrin transchelation [4, 65] is likely the origin of this difference. Indeed, in this binding competition, human transferrin benefits from two major assets versus inorganic chelators:

– Transferring is an active protein: it has two domains, each one containing an anion and a metal binding site. The anion sites act as padlocks: when the metal enter into the metal binding site, the protein geometry changes to enclose the metal which can be released only if a synergic anion binds the appropriate anion binding site [66]. This mechanism ensures that the metal will only be released at an appropriate cell target, e.g. in the red marrow.
– Inorganic chelators have to wait the release of a metal ion by another chelator in order to bind it, which is rare from a good competitor. In contrary, kinetics and spectrometry studies evidenced that transferrin is able to make a ternary (or mixed) complex with the initial metal–chelator complex [67]. During the life of this ternary complex, the metal ion is transferred from the chelator to the transferrin metal binding site.

A recent study in human [68] showed that only 23% and 2% of ^{177}Lu-DOTATATE remain intact after 24 h and 96 h post injection, respectively.

The results of these five studies [60–64] urge for using SPECT/CT in red-marrow dosimetry for all ^{177}Lu therapies and clearly discard the unsuitable blood-based estimation which was although recently used to advocate the useless of dosimetry therapy planning [69].

Ilan et al. [70] observed in ^{177}Lu-DOTATATE therapy of 24 patients, a correlation between tumour volume reduction and three time points

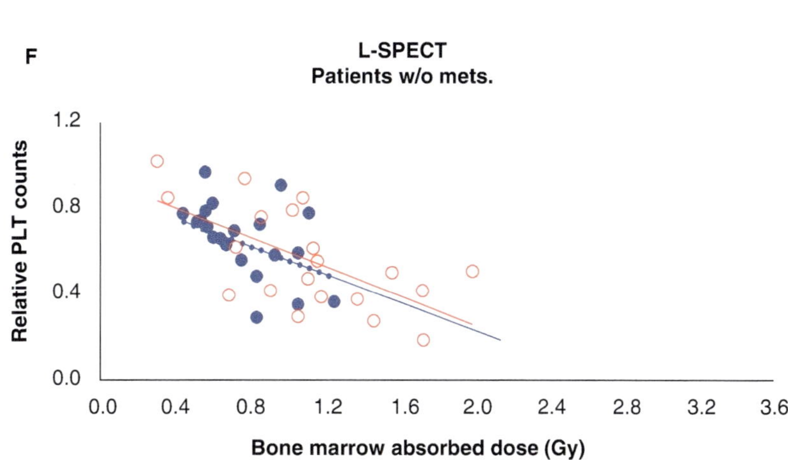

Fig. 3.7 Blue solid circles: relative platelet counts decrease as a function of the hybrid SPECT/CT-planar-based red-marrow dose in ^{177}Lu-DOTATATE therapy (reprinted from [64] with courtesy of Dr. P Bernhardt). Red empty circles: decrease observed in the ^{90}Y-DOTATOC trial using ^{86}Y-DOTATOC PET-based dosimetry added by the authors [2]

SPECT/CT-based absorbed dose. The correlation was remarkably impressive when excluding tumours smaller than 4 cm.

Advances in computational techniques open the way to improved corrections methods for ^{177}Lu SPECT/CT: analytical [71] or MC code [72] to correct for attenuation-scattering and collimator penetration; deep learning algorithm in order to reduce the acquisition time [73].

3.5.7 Iodine-131

Gregory et al. [74] studied the quantitative imaging of ^{123}I and ^{131}I with different SPECT/CT systems. Cylindrical phantoms were used for calibration factors, and 3D-printed phantom mimicking patient's activity distributions were then used to analyze SPECT/CT quantitative imaging. Their results showed that dead-time and calibration factors varied between systems, but that global calibration factors might be used for SPECT/CT from the same manufacturer and with the same crystal size.

Dewaraja et al. [75] in 39 patients with relapsed or refractory non-Hodgkin lymphoma treated with ^{131}I-tositumomab observed a clear separation of progression-free survival for a tumour dose threshold of 2 Gy. Doses were estimated on three time points SPECT/CT using a dose planning MC code. This low-dose threshold is explained by the high radiosensitivity of follicular lymphoma.

3.5.8 Alpha Emitters

Benabdallah et al. [76] evaluated the absolute quantification of [223]Ra in bone metastasis therapy. To evaluate the calibration factors, they used the NEMA IEC body phantom with the spheres filled with [223]Ra activity concentration ranging from 1.8 to 22.8 kBq/mL. SPECT/CT was performed with a camera equipped with a 5/8″ crystal and triple-energy windows around 85, 154 and 270 keV together with three additional windows for scatter corrections. A TORSO phantom was then used to simulate tumours with tumour to

normal tissue ratio close to clinical conditions. They so achieved a quantification of the [223]Ra activity with an error smaller than 19%.

3.5.9 SPECT/CT-Based Individualized Therapy Planning

Obsolete medical dogmas are often extremely hard to clear, the most sad stories being the numerous decades needed to implement asepsis in surgery [77] or to treat helicobacter infection in peptic ulcers [78]. Even Louis Pasteur, showing with his microscope the bacteria's present on the lancets, was not able in his lifetime to convince the surgeons to wash their hands and tools between each patient surgery. Nowadays, despite clear evidences [79–81] and in infringement of international authorities recommendations (ICRP 140: first main point, [82]) and rules (Directive 2013/59 Euratom: art. 56, [16]), EANM continue to claim that radionuclide therapy is just similar to chemotherapy, avoiding to mention SPECT/CT in its argumentation [83].

In spite of the abundant literature evidencing strong dose–response and toxicity relationships joined to highly patient-dependent pharmacokinetics here above discussed, this persistent dogma prevented up to recently any randomized trial of individualized therapy planning in molecular radiotherapy. Hopefully, the dynamic and proactive radioembolization community has seriously considered SPECT/CT and, by using it in individualized therapy planning, has evidenced impressive patient outcome improvements [84, 85].

Levillain et al. [84] performed a multicentre retrospective analysis on 58 patients with intrahepatic cholangiocarcinoma treated with ^{90}Y-loaded resin spheres, 47% of them using the empirical BSA methods and 53% using the ^{99m}Tc-MAA SPECT/CT-based partition model. Median overall survival was 14.9 months using the partition model, while was only 5.5 months using the BSA method (Fig. 3.8a). They concluded that SPECT/CT-based personalized activity prescription should be performed.

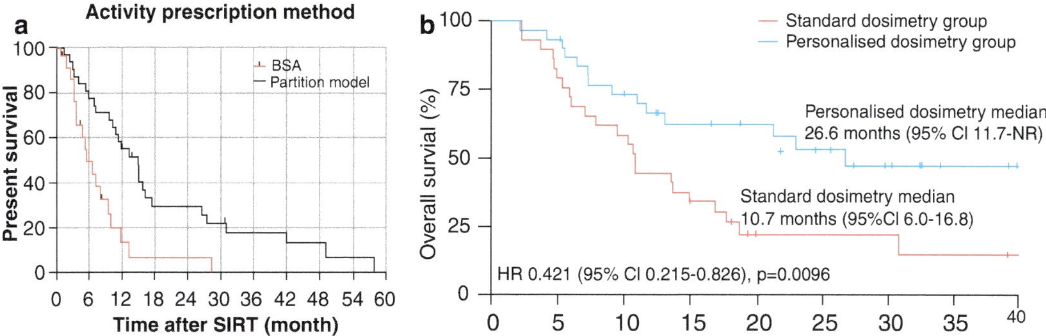

Fig. 3.8 Patients' survival after different liver radioembolization planning. (**a**) Comparison between empirical BSA planning and ^{99m}Tc-MAA SPECT/CT-based partition model (reprinted from [84] with authorization of Springer). (**b**) Comparison between standard dosimetry aiming 120 Gy to the perfused lobe and personalized dosimetry aiming at least 205 Gy in the largest treated tumour, both using ^{99m}Tc-MAA SPECT/CT. (reprinted from [85] with permission of Elsevier)

Garin et al. [85] went one step further in conducting a prospective randomized multicentre phase 2 trial using ^{90}Y-loaded glass spheres in patients with HCC. Outcomes were compared between standard dosimetry aiming 120 Gy to the perfused lobe and personalised dosimetry aiming to deliver at least 205 Gy to the largest treated lesion, both using ^{99m}Tc-MAA SPECT/CT-based dosimetry. The prespecified statistical criterion for stopping early for efficacy occurred after 29 and 31 patients being treated with standard and personalized dosimetry, respectively. Median overall survival was 26.6 months in the personalised dosimetry group, while was only 10.7 months in the standard dosimetry group (Fig. 3.8b).

In parallel to these comparison studies, Del Petre et al. [86], Sundlov et al. [87] and Garske-Roman et al. [63] performed SPECT/CT-based individualized planning ^{177}Lu-DOTATATE therapy in 52, 51 and 200 patients aiming a renal BED = 27Gy, D = 23Gy and D = 23Gy, respectively. They evidenced that applying the standard recommendation of four 7.4GBq-cycles results in undertreating 85, 73 and 49% of the patients.

Garske-Roman et al. [63] observed an impressive progression-free survival (PFS) and overall survival (OS) improvement of patients who were able to reach the 23Gy renal dose limit ($n = 114$) versus those who cannot due to haematological toxicities ($n = 40$) (Fig. 3.9).

The patient outcome improvement observed in these individualized therapy planning studies clearly proves the inadequacy of the EANM position on radionuclide therapy [83, 88].

3.5.10 Perspectives: Compton Cameras

Electronic collimation of dual photons emitted in opposite directions makes PET sensitivity and spatial resolution better than those of SPECT by a factor of about 100 and 3, respectively. Early in 1974, such electronics collimation was also proposed for single photon by using a two layers detector [89]. The first layer is optimized to favour Compton scattering while the second is a conventional γ camera that records the scattered gamma-ray. The Compton relation allows deriving information about the incoming direction and energy of the primary gamma-ray (see [90] for a detailed description of camera principles and recent developments).

Compared to SPECT using conventional γ camera, Compton camera has the benefit of a usable wide range of gamma energies from 100 keV to several MeV, of a very large FOV and of allowing SPECT using a few camera positions, and in theory even from a single camera position.

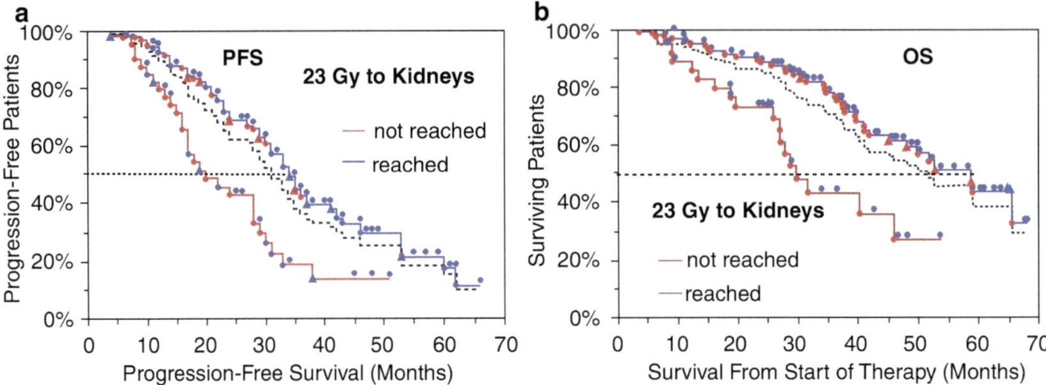

Fig. 3.9 Progression-free survival (**a**) and overall survival (**b**) in ^{177}Lu-DOTA-octreotate therapy in relation to absorbed dose to the kidneys, best morphological response according to RECIST 1.1, and proliferation rate (Ki-67 index) (reprinted from [9] with courtesy of Dr. Sundin)

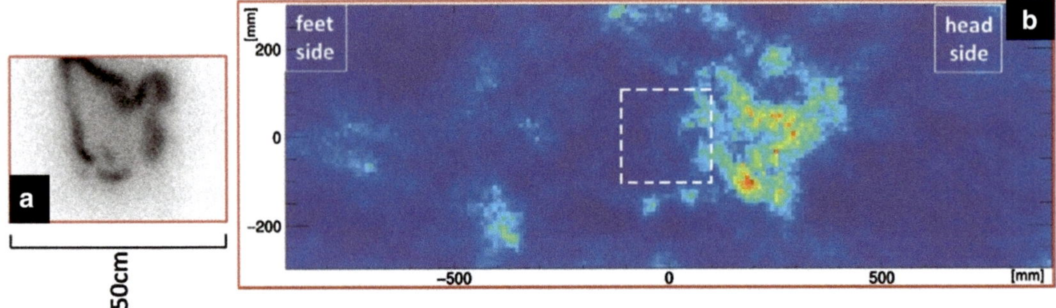

Fig. 3.10 Image of a patient injected with 2.9 MBq of ^{223}Ra (reprinted from [92] with permission of Elsevier). (**a**): 30 min planar acquisition with a MGEP Anger camera. b: whole-body reconstructed slice from a 10 min acquisition using a 22 × 22 cm² handheld Compton camera (the left image (**a**) was rotated to respect orientation, and dashed square was added to (**b**) by the authors to visualize the size and position of the camera)

However, during three decades, Compton camera development was hampered by the lack of electronics readout sufficiently transparent to gamma rays in order to use efficient crystals in the first detector layer. This bottle neck was broken in 2002 by the development of thin multipixel photo counter (MPPC) [91]. Due to their capability to image a very large FOV in once, compact and mobile Compton cameras development was boosted after 2011 for the Fukushima plan survey using helicopters or drones.

Figure 3.10 shows a whole-body SPECT slice performed post ^{223}Ra therapy using a 22 × 22 cm² handheld Compton camera developed for the Fukushima plan survey [92]. A single central camera position of 10 min and 20 cm below the patient table was used. Simultaneous use of several cameras will significantly increase the imaging quality by increasing the sensitivity and the range of sampled gamma-ray directions. As most therapeutic α-emitters, such as ^{223}Ra, ^{225}Ac and ^{211}As, have high energy gamma-ray emitters in their daughters cascade, Compton camera will be the detector of choice in order to perform whole-body 3D dosimetry post α-therapy cycle [93, 94], allowing activity optimization for the next cycles. Obviously, Compton cameras will also be useful for whole-body 3D dosimetry using conventional β-emitters.

3.6 Conclusions

These last 3 years, several dynamics teams implemented SPECT/CT-based individualized planning in ^{90}Y radioembolizations [84, 85] and in

[177]Lu therapies [63, 86, 87]. Their results clearly proved the high-interpatient dosimetry variations. Impressive patient outcome improvements were also observed. It is extraordinary to notice that all these teams are European, while the EANM persists in claiming that radionuclides therapy is similar to chemotherapy [83], even claiming in infringement of international rules that these therapies can be performed by *'just giving a net activity according to the package insert'* [84], i.e. as such as for conventional drug therapies.

Other recent SPECT/CT studies [62, 64] also cleared the persistent assumption that ^{177}Lu cannot be taken up by the bone marrow in ^{177}Lu-DOTATATE therapy. Indeed, these studies evidenced that the bone marrow dosimetry is about fourfold higher than that estimated using the blood-based method. Such difference was already observed 10 years ago in ^{90}Y-DOTATOC therapy using [86]Y-DOTATOC PET-based dosimetry [2, 4]. However, this observation was completely overlooked in the Erasmus phase I/II or in NETTER-1 phase III study, which both considered to only use the inappropriate blood-based method.

No doubt that these breakthroughs in radionuclide therapies will stimulate other teams to move to state-of-the-art dosimetry planning, a strategy which made the success of the external beam radiotherapy.

References

1. Barone R, Borson-Chazot F, Valkema R, Walrand S, Chauvin F, Gogou L, Kvols LK, Krenning EP, Jamar F, Pauwels S. Patient-specific dosimetry in predicting renal toxicity with (90)Y-DOTATOC: relevance of kidney volume and dose rate in finding a dose-effect relationship. J Nucl Med. 2005;46:99S–106S.
2. Pauwels S, Barone R, Walrand S, Borson-Chazot F, Valkema R, Kvols LK, Krenning EP, Jamar F. Practical dosimetry of peptide receptor radionuclide therapy with (90)Y-labeled somatostatin analogs. J Nucl Med. 2005;46:92S–8S.
3. Walrand S, Lhommel R, Goffette P, Van den Eynde M, Pauwels S, Jamar F. Hemoglobin level significantly impacts the tumor cell survival fraction in humans after internal radiotherapy. EJNMMI Res. 2012;2:20.
4. Walrand S, Barone R, Pauwels S, Jamar F. Experimental facts supporting a red marrow uptake due to radiometal transchelation in 90Y-DOTATOC therapy and relationship to the decrease of platelet counts. Eur J Nucl Med Mol Imaging. 2011;38(7):1270–80.
5. Flamen P, Vanderlinden B, Delatte P, Ghanem G, Ameye L, Van Den Eynde M, Hendlisz A. Multimodality imaging can predict the metabolic response of unresectable colorectal liver metastases to radioembolization therapy with Yttrium-90 labeled resin spheres. Phys Med Biol. 2008;53(22):6591–603.
6. Wessels BW, Konijnenberg MW, Dale RG, Breitz HB, Cremonesi M, Meredith RF, Green AJ, Bouchet LG, Brill AB, Bolch WE, Sgouros G, Thomas SR. MIRD pamphlet no. 20: the effect of model assumptions on kidney dosimetry and response—implications for radionuclide therapy. J Nucl Med. 2008;49(11):1884–99.
7. Garin E, Lenoir L, Rolland Y, Edeline J, Mesbah H, Laffont S, Porée P, Clément B, Raoul JL, Boucher E. Dosimetry based on 99mTc-macroaggregated albumin SPECT/CT accurately predicts tumor response and survival in hepatocellular carcinoma patients treated with 90Y-loaded glass spheres: preliminary results. J Nucl Med. 2012;53(2):255–63.
8. Strigari L, Sciuto R, Rea S, Carpanese L, Pizzi G, Soriani A, Iaccarino G, Benassi M, Ettorre GM, Maini CL. Efficacy and toxicity related to treatment of hepatocellular carcinoma with 90Y-SIR spheres: radiobiologic considerations. J Nucl Med. 2010;51(9):1377–85.
9. Jamar F, Barone R, Mathieu I, Walrand S, Labar D, Carlier P, de Camps J, Schran H, Chen T, Smith MC, Bouterfa H, Valkema R, Krenning EP, Kvols LK, Pauwels S. 86Y-DOTA0-D-Phe1-Tyr3-octreotide (SMT487)—a phase 1 clinical study: pharmacokinetics, biodistribution and renal protective effect of different regimens of amino acid co-infusion. Eur J Nucl Med Mol Imaging 2003;30(4): 510–518.
10. Gay HA, Niemierko A. A free program for calculating EUD-based NTCP and TCP in external beam radiotherapy. Phys Med. 2007;23:115–25.
11. Adler JR, Chang SD, Murphy MJ, Doty J, Geis P, Hancock SL. The Cyberknife: a frameless robotic system for radiosurgery. In: Stereotactic and functional neurosurgery. 1997;69:124–8.
12. Devic S. MRI simulation for radiotherapy treatment planning. Med Phys. 2012;39(11):6701–11.
13. Scripes PG, Yaparpalvi R. Technical aspects of positron emission tomography/computed tomography in radiotherapy treatment planning. Semin Nucl Med. 2012;42(5):283–8.
14. Götz L, Spehl TS, Weber WA, Grosu AL. PET and SPECT for radiation treatment planning. Q J Nucl Med Mol Imaging. 2012;56(2):163–72.
15. Taylor ML, Kron T, Franich RD. A contemporary review of stereotactic radiotherapy: inherent dosimetric complexities and the potential for detriment. Acta Oncol. 2011;50(4):483–508.
16. https://eur-lex.europa.eu/legal-content/EN/TXT/?uri =CELEX%3A32013L0059

17. Berker Y, Goedicke A, Kemerink GJ, Aach T, Schweizer B. Activity quantification combining conjugate-view planar scintigraphies and SPECT/CT data for patient-specific 3-D dosimetry in radionuclide therapy. Eur J Nucl Med Mol Imaging. 2011;38(12):2173–85.

18. Sandström M, Garske U, Granberg D, Sundin A, Lundqvist H. Individualized dosimetry in patients undergoing therapy with (177)Lu-DOTA-D-Phe (1)-Tyr (3)-octreotate. Eur J Nucl Med Mol Imaging. 2010;37(2):212–25.

19. Garkavij M, Nickel M, Sjögreen-Gleisner K, Ljungberg M, Ohlsson T, Wingårdh K, Strand SE, Tennvall J. 177Lu-[DOTA0,Tyr3] octreotate therapy in patients with disseminated neuroendocrine tumors: Analysis of dosimetry with impact on future therapeutic strategy. Cancer. 2010;116(4): 1084–92.

20. Valkema R, Pauwels S, Kvols LK, Kwekkeboom DJ, Jamar F, de Jong M, et al. Long-term follow-up of renal function after peptide receptor radiation therapy with 90Y-DOTA0, Tyr3-octreotide and 177Lu-DOTA0, Tyr3-octreotate. J Nucl Med. 2005;46:83S–91.

21. Konijnenberg M, Melis M, Valkema R, Krenning E, de Jong M. Radiation dose distribution in human kidneys by octreotides in peptide receptor radionuclide therapy. J Nucl Med. 2007;48(1):134–42.

22. Bouchet LG, Bolch WE, Blanco HP, Wessels BW, Siegel JA, Rajon DA, Clairand I, Sgouros G. MIRD pamphlet no 19: absorbed fractions and radionuclide S values for six age-dependent multiregion models of the kidney. J Nucl Med. 2003;44(7):1113–47.

23. De Jong M, Valkema R, Van Gameren A, et al. Inhomogeneous localization of radioactivity in the human kidney after injection of [111In-DTPA]octreotide. J Nucl Med. 2004;45:1168–71.

24. Cremonesi M, Ferrari M, Bartolomei M, Orsi F, Bonomo G, Aricò D, Mallia A, De Cicco C, Pedroli G, Paganelli G. Radioembolisation with 90Y-spheres: dosimetric and radiobiological investigation for multi-cycle treatment. Eur J Nucl Med Mol Imaging. 2008;35(11):2088–96.

25. Chiesa C, Maccauro M, Romito R, Spreafico C, Pellizzari S, Negri A, Sposito C, Morosi C, Civelli E, Lanocita R, Camerini T, Bampo C, Bhoori S, Seregni E, Marchianò A, Mazzaferro V, Bombardieri E. Need, feasibility and convenience of dosimetric treatment planning in liver selective internal radiation therapy with (90)Y spheres: the experience of the National Tumor Institute of Milan. Q J Nucl Med Mol Imaging. 2011;55(2):168–97.

26. Lhommel R, van Elmbt L, Goffette P, Van den Eynde M, Jamar F, Pauwels S, Walrand S. Feasibility of 90Y TOF PET-based dosimetry in liver metastasis therapy using SIR-spheres. Eur J Nucl Med Mol Imaging. 2010;37(9):1654–62.

27. Brown S, Bailey DL, Willowson K, Baldock C. Investigation of the relationship between linear attenuation coefficients and CT Hounsfield units using radionuclides for SPECT. Appl Radiat Isot. 2008;66(9):1206–12.

28. Ritt P, Vija H, Hornegger J, Kuwert T. Absolute quantification in SPECT. Eur J Nucl Med Mol Imaging. 2011;38:S69–77.

29. Shcherbinin S, Celler A, Belhocine T, Vanderwerf R, Driedger A. Accuracy of quantitative reconstructions in SPECT/CT imaging. Phys Med Biol. 2008;53:4595–604.

30. Vandervoort E, Celler A, Harrop R. Implementation of an iterative scatter correction, the influence of attenuation map quality and their effect on absolute quantitation in SPECT. Phys Med Biol. 2007;52:1527–45.

31. Willowson K, Bailey DL, Baldock C. Quantitative SPECT reconstruction using CT-derived corrections. Phys Med Biol. 2008;53(12):3099–112.

32. Beauregard JM, Hofman MS, Pereira JM, Eu P, Hicks RJ. Quantitative (177)Lu SPECT (QSPECT) imaging using a commercially available SPECT/CT system. Cancer Imaging. 2011;11:56–66.

33. Ahmadzadehfar H, Sabet A, Biermann K, Muckle M, Brockmann H, Kuhl C, Wilhelm K, Biersack HJ, Ezziddin S. The significance of 99mTc-MAA SPECT/CT liver perfusion imaging in treatment planning for 90Y-sphere selective internal radiation treatment. Nucl Med. 2010;51(8):1206–12.

34. Reubi JC, Schär JC, Waser B, Wenger S, Heppeler A, Schmitt JS, Mäcke HR. Affinity profiles for human somatostatin receptor subtypes SST1-SST5 of somatostatin radiotracers selected for scintigraphic and radiotherapeutic use. Eur J Nucl Med. 2000;27(3):273–82.

35. Walrand S, Flux GD, Konijnenberg MW, Valkema R, Krenning EP, Lhommel R, Pauwels S, Jamar F. Dosimetry of yttrium-labelled radiopharmaceuticals for internal therapy: 86Y or 90Y imaging? Eur J Nucl Med Mol Imaging. 2011;38:S57–68.

36. Minarik D, Sjögreen-Gleisner K, Linden O, Wingårdh K, Tennvall J, Strand SE, Ljungberg M. 90Y bremsstrahlung imaging for absorbed-dose assessment in high-dose Radioimmunotherapy. J Nucl Med. 2010;51:1974–8.

37. Jiang M, Fischman A, Nowakowski FS, Heiba S, Zhang Z, Knesaurek K, Weintraub J, Josef MJ. Segmental perfusion differences on paired Tc-99m macroaggregated albumin (MAA) hepatic perfusion imaging and Yttrium-90 (Y-90) bremsstrahlung imaging studies in SIR-sphere Radioembolization: associations with angiography. J Nucl Med Radiat Ther. 2012;3:1.

38. Kafrouni M, Allimant C, Fourcade M, Vauclin S, Guiu B, Mariano-Goulart D, Bouallègue FB. Analysis of differences between 99m Tc-MAA SPECT-and 90 Y-microsphere PET-based dosimetry for hepatocellular carcinoma selective internal radiation therapy. EJNMMI Res. 2019;9:62.

39. Gnesin S, Canetti L, Adib S, Cherbuin N, Monteiro MS, Bize P, Denys A, Prior JO, Baechler S, Boubaker A. Partition model–based 99mTc-MAA SPECT/CT predictive dosimetry compared with 90Y TOF PET/CT posttreatment dosimetry in Radioembolization of hepatocellular carcinoma: a quantitative agreement comparison. J Nucl Med. 2016;57:1672–8.

40. Jadoul A, Bernard C, Lovinfosse P, Gérard L, Lilet H, Cornet O, Hustinx R. Comparative dosimetry

between 99m Tc-MAA SPECT/CT and 90 Y PET/CT in primary and metastatic liver tumors. Eur J Nucl Med Mol Imag. 2020;47(4):828–37.

41. Smits ML, Dassen MG, Prince JF, Braat AJ, Beijst C, Bruijnen RC, de Jong HW, Lam MG. The superior predictive value of 166 ho-scout compared with 99m Tc-macroaggregated albumin prior to 166 ho-microspheres radioembolization in patients with liver metastases. Eur J Nucl Med Mol Imag. 2019;9:1–9.

42. Elschot M, Nijsen JF, Lam MG, Smits ML, Prince JF, Viergever MA, van den Bosch MA, Zonnenberg BA, de Jong HW. 99m Tc-MAA overestimates the absorbed dose to the lungs in radioembolization: a quantitative evaluation in patients treated with 166 ho-microspheres. Eur J Nucl Med Mol Imaging. 2014;41:1965–75.

43. Song YS, Paeng JC, Kim HC, Chung JW, Cheon GJ, Chung JK, Lee DS, Kang KW. PET/CT-based dosimetry in 90Y-microsphere selective internal radiation therapy: single cohort comparison with pretreatment planning on 99mTc-MAA imaging and correlation with treatment efficacy. Medicine. 2015;94(23):e945.

44. Mauxion T, Hobbs R, Herman J, Lodge M, Yue J, Du Y, Wahl R, Geschwind JF, Frey E. Comparison of lung shunt fraction (LSF) from pre-therapy 99mTc MAA and post-therapy quantitative 90Y imaging in microsphere (MS) radioembolization. J Nucl Med. 2015;56:104.

45. Allred JD, Niedbala J, Mikell JK, Owen D, Frey KA, Dewaraja YK. The value of 99m Tc-MAA SPECT/CT for lung shunt estimation in 90 Y radioembolization: a phantom and patient study. Eur J Nucl Med Mol Imaging Res. 2018;8:50.

46. Kunnen B, Dietze MM, Braat AJ, Lam MG, Viergever MA, de Jong HW. Feasibility of imaging 90Y microspheres at diagnostic activity levels for hepatic radioembolization treatment planning. Med Phys. 2020;47:1105–14.

47. Chiesa C, Maccauro M. 166 ho microsphere scout dose for more accurate radioembolization treatment planning. Eur J Nucl Med Mol Imag. 2020;47:744–7.

48. Chiesa C, Mira M, Maccauro M, Romito R, Spreafico C, Sposito C, Bhoori S, Morosi C, Pellizzari S, Negri A, Civelli E, Lanocita R, Camerini T, Bampo C, Carrara M, Seregni E, Marchianò A, Mazzaferro V, Bombardieri E. A dosimetric treatment planning strategy in radioembolization of hepatocarcinoma with 90Y glass spheres. Q J Nucl Med Mol Imaging. 2012;56(6):503–8.

49. Mazzaferro V, Sposito C, Bhoori S, Romito R, Chiesa C, Morosi C, Maccauro M, Marchianò A, Bongini M, Lanocita R, Civelli E, Bombardieri E, Camerini T, Spreafico C. Yttrium-90 radioembolization for intermediate-advanced hepatocellular carcinoma: a phase 2 study. Hepatology. 2012; https://doi.org/10.1002/hep.26014.

50. Kappadath SC, Mikell J, Balagopal A, Baladandayuthapani V, Kaseb A, Mahvash A. Hepatocellular carcinoma tumor dose response after 90Y-radioembolization with glass microspheres using 90Y-SPECT/CT-based voxel dosimetry. Int J Rad Oncol Biol Phys. 2018;102:451–61.

51. Walrand S, Hesse M, Chiesa C, Lhommel R, Jamar F. The low hepatic toxicity per gray of 90Y glass microspheres is linked to their transport in the arterial tree favoring a nonuniform trapping as observed in posttherapy PET imaging. J Nucl Med. 2014;55:135–40.

52. Walrand S, Hesse M, Jamar F, Lhommel R. A hepatic dose-toxicity model opening the way toward individualized radioembolization planning. J Nucl Med. 2014;55:1317–22.

53. Crookston NR, Fung GS, Frey EC. Development of a customizable hepatic arterial tree and particle transport model for use in treatment planning. IEEE Trans Radiat Plasma Med Sci. 2018;3:31–7.

54. d'Abadie P, Hesse M, Jamar F, Lhommel R, Walrand S. ^{90}Y TOF-PET based EUD reunifies patient survival prediction in resin and glass microspheres radioembolization of HCC tumours. Phys Med Biol 2018;63:245010.

55. Menda Y, Madsen MT, O'Dorisio TM, Sunderland JJ, Watkins GL, Dillon JS, Mott SL, Schultz MK, Zamba GK, Bushnell DL, O'Dorisio MS. 90Y-DOTATOC dosimetry–based personalized peptide receptor radionuclide therapy. J Nucl Med. 2018;59:1692–8.

56. Walrand S, Jamar F, van Elmbt L, Lhommel R, Bekonde EB, Pauwels S. 4-step renal dosimetry dependent on cortex geometry applied to 90Y peptide receptor radiotherapy: evaluation using a fillable kidney phantom imaged by 90Y PET. J Nucl Med. 2010;51:1969–73.

57. Smits ML, Nijsen JF, van den Bosch MA, Lam MG, Vente MA, Mali WP, van Het Schip AD, Zonnenberg BA. Holmium-166 radioembolisation in patients with unresectable, chemorefractory liver metastases (HEPAR trial): a phase 1, dose-escalation study. Lancet Oncol. 2012;13(10):1025–34.

58. van Roekel C, Bastiaannet R, Smits ML, Bruijnen RC, Braat AJ, de Jong HW, Elias SG, Lam MG. Dose-effect relationships of holmium-166 radioembolization in colorectal cancer. J Nucl Med. 2020;26:120.

59. Stella M, Braat AJ, Lam MG, de Jong HW, van Rooij R. Quantitative 166Ho-microspheres SPECT derived from a dual-isotope acquisition with 99mTc-colloid is clinically feasible. EJNMMI Phys. 2020;7:48.

60. Woliner-van der Weg W, Schoffelen R, Hobbs RF, Gotthardt M, Goldenberg DM, Sharkey RM, Slump CH, van der Graaf WTA, Oyen WJG, Boerman OC, Sgouros G, Visser EP. Tumor and red bone marrow dosimetry: comparison of methods for prospective treatment planning in pretargeted radioimmunotherapy. Eur J Nucl Med Mol Imaging Phys. 2014;1:104.

61. Blakkisrud J, Løndalen A, Dahle J, Turner S, Holte H, Kolstad A, Stokke C. Red marrow–absorbed dose for non-hodgkin lymphoma patients treated with 177lu-lilotomab satetraxetan, a novel anti-cd37 antibody–radionuclide conjugate. J Nucl Med. 2017;58:55–61.

62. Santoro L, Mora-Ramirez E, Trauchessec D, Chouaf S, Eustache P, Pouget JP, Kotzki PO, Bardiès M, Deshayes E. Implementation of patient dosimetry in the clinical practice after targeted radiotherapy using [177 Lu-[DOTA0, Tyr3]-octreotate]. Eur J Nucl Med Mol Imaging Research. 2018;8:103.

63. Garske-Roman U, Sandström M, Fröss Baron K, Lundin L, Hellman P, Welin S, Johansson S, Khan T, Lundqvist H, Eriksson B, Sundin A, Granberg D. Prospective observational study of 177Lu-DOTA-octreotate therapy in 200 patients with advanced metastasized neuroendocrine tumours (NETs): feasibility and impact of a dosimetry-guided study protocol on outcome and toxicity. Eur J Nucl Med Mol Imaging. 2018;45:970–88.

64. Hagmarker L, Svensson J, Rydén T, van Essen M, Sundlöv A, Gleisner KS, Gjertsson P, Bernhardt P. Bone marrow absorbed doses and correlations with hematologic response during 177Lu-DOTATATE treatments are influenced by image-based dosimetry method and presence of skeletal metastases. J Nucl Med. 2019;60:1406–13.

65. EW price. Synthesis, evaluation, and application of new ligands for radiometal based radiopharmaceuticals. 2014. Thesis. University British Columbia. https://open.library.ubc.ca/cIRcle/collections/ubctheses/24/items/1.0103411

66. Hamilton DH, Turcot I, Stintzi A, Raymond KN. Large cooperativity in the removal of iron from transferrin at physiological temperature and chloride ion concentration. JBIC J Biol Inorg Chem. 2004;9:936–44.

67. Bates GW, Billups C, Saltman P. THE kinetics and mechanism of iron (III) exchange between chelates and transferrin II. THE PRESENTATION AND REMOVAL WITH ETHYLENEDIAMINETETRAACETATE. J Biol Chem. 1967;242:2816–21.

68. Lubberink M, Wilking H, Öst A, Ilan E, Sandström M, Andersson C, Fröss-Baron K, Velikyan I, Sundin A. In vivo instability of 177Lu-DOTATATE during peptide receptor radionuclide therapy. J Nucl Med. 2020;61:1337–40.

69. https://www.ema.europa.eu/en/documents/product-information/lutathera-epar-product-information_en.pdf

70. Ilan E, Sandström M, Wassberg C, Sundin A, Garske-Román U, Eriksson B, Granberg D, Lubberink M. Dose response of pancreatic neuroendocrine tumors treated with peptide receptor radionuclide therapy using 177Lu-DOTATATE. J Nucl Med. 2015;56:177–82.

71. D'Arienzo M, Cozzella ML, Fazio A, De Felice P, Iaccarino G, D'Andrea M, Ungania S, Cazzato M, Schmidt K, Kimiaei S, Strigari L. Quantitative 177Lu SPECT imaging using advanced correction algorithms in non-reference geometry. Phys Med. 2016;32:1745–52.

72. Rydén T, Heydom Lagerlöf J, Hemmingsson J, Marin I, Svensson J, Bath M, Gjertsson P, Bernhardt P. Fast GPU-based Monte Carlo code for SPECT/CT reconstructions generates improved 177Lu images. Eur J Nul Med Mol Imaging Phys. 2018;5:1.

73. Ryden T, van Essen M, Marin I, Svensson J, Bernhardt P. Deep learning generation of synthetic intermediate projections improves 177Lu SPECT images reconstructed with sparsely acquired projections. J Nucl Med. 2021;62(4):528–35.

74. Gregory RA, Murray I, Gear J, Leek F, Chittenden S, Fenwick A, Wevertt J, Scuffham J, Tipping J, Murby B, Jeans S, Stuffins M, Michopoulou S, Guy M, Morgan D, Hallam A, Hall D, Polydor H, Brown C, Gillen G, Dickinson N, Brown S, Wadsley J, Flux G. Standardized quantitative radioiodine SPECT/CT imaging for multicenter dosimetry trials in molecular radiotherapy. Phys Med Biol. 2019;64:245013.

75. Dewaraja YK, Schipper MJ, Shen J, Smith LB, Murgic J, Savas H, Youssef E, Regan D, Wilderman SJ, Roberson PL, Kaminski MS. Tumor-absorbed dose predicts progression-free survival following 131I-tositumomab radioimmunotherapy. J Nucl Med. 2014;55:1047–53.

76. Benabdallah N, Bernardini M, Biancardi M, de Labriolle-Vaylet C, Franck D, Desbrée A. 223Ra-dichloride therapy of bone metastasis: optimization of SPECT images for quantification. Eur J Nucl Med Mol Imaging Res 2019;9:20.

77. https://en.wikipedia.org/wiki/Asepsis

78. https://en.wikipedia.org/wiki/Timeline_of_peptic_ulcer_disease_and_Helicobacter_pylori

79. Cremonesi M, Ferrari ME, Bodei L, Chiesa C, Sarnelli A, Garibaldi C, Pacilio M, Strigari L, Summers PE, Orecchia R, Grana CM. Correlation of dose with toxicity and tumour response to 90 Y-and 177 Lu-PRRT provides the basis for optimization through individualized treatment planning. Eur J Nucl Med Mol Imag. 2018;45:2426–41.

80. Sundlöv A, Sjögreen-Gleisner K. Peptide receptor radionuclide therapy–prospects for personalised treatment. Clin Oncol. 2021;33(2):92–7.

81. Cremonesi M, Ferrari M, Botta F. Dosimetry in PRRT. In: Clinical applications of nuclear medicine targeted therapy. Springer International Publishing; 2018. p. 297–313.

82. https://www.icrp.org/page.asp?id=10

83. Giammarile F, Muylle K, Bolton RD, Kunikowska J, Haberkorn U, Oyen W. Dosimetry in clinical radionuclide therapy: the devil is in the detail. Eur J Nucl Med Mol Imag. 2017;44:1–3.

84. Levillain H, Derijckere ID, Ameye L, Guiot T, Braat A, Meyer C, Vanderlinden B, Reynaert N, Hendlisz A, Lam M, Deroose CM. Personalised radioembolization improves outcomes in refractory intra-hepatic cholangiocarcinoma: a multicenter study. Eur J Nucl Med Mol Imag. 2019;46:2270–9.

85. Garin E, Tselikas L, Guiu B, Chalaye J, Edeline J, de Baere T, Assenat E, Tacher V, Robert C, Terroir-Cassou-Mounat M, Mariano-Goulart D. Personalised versus standard dosimetry approach of selective internal radiation therapy in patients with locally advanced hepatocellular carcinoma (DOSISPHERE-01): a randomised, multicentre, open-label phase 2 trial. Lancet Gastroenterol Hepatol. 2021;6(1):17–29.

86. Del Prete M, Buteau FA, Arsenault F, Saighi N, Bouchard LO, Beaulieu A, Beauregard JM. Personalized 177 Lu-octreotate peptide receptor radionuclide therapy of neuroendocrine tumours: initial results from the P-PRRT trial. Eur J Nucl Med Mol Imag. 2019;46:728–42.

87. Sundlöv A, Sjögreen-Gleisner K, Svensson J, Ljungberg M, Olsson T, Bernhardt P, Tennvall J. Individualised 177 Lu-DOTATATE treatment of neuroendocrine tumours based on kidney dosimetry. Eur J Nucl Med Mol Imag. 2017;44:1480–9.

88. Konijnenberg M, Herrmann K, Kobe C, Verburg F, Hindorf C, Hustinx R, Lassmann M. EANM position paper on article 56 of the council directive 2013/59/ Euratom (basic safety standards) for nuclear medicine therapy. Eur J Nucl Med Mol Imaging. 2020;15:1–6.

89. Todd RW, Nightingale JM, Everett DB. A proposed γ camera. Nature. 1974;251:132–4.

90. Zaidi H, Sgouros G, editors. Therapeutic applications of Monte Carlo calculations in nuclear medicine. 2nd ed. CRC Press; 2002.

91. Buzhan P, Dolgoshein B, Ilyin A, Kantserov V, Kaplin V, Karakash A, Pleshko A, Popova E, Smirnov S, Volkov Y, Filatov L. The advanced study of silicon photomultiplier. In: Advanced technology and particle physics; 2002. p. 717–28.

92. Fujieda K, Kataoka J, Mochizuki S, Tagawa L, Sato S, Tanaka R, Matsunaga K, Kamiya T, Watabe T, Kato H, Shimosegawa E. First demonstration of portable Compton camera to visualize 223-Ra concentration for radionuclide therapy. Nucl Instrum Methods Phys Res Sect A: Accel Spectrom Detect Assoc Equip. 2020;958:162802.

93. Lee T, Kim M, Lee W, Kim B, Lim I, Song K, Kim J. Performance evaluation of a Compton SPECT imager for determining the position and distribution of 225Ac in targeted alpha therapy: a Monte Carlo simulation based phantom study. Appl Radiat Isot. 2019;154:108893.

94. Nagao Y, Yamaguchi M, Watanabe S, Ishioka NS, Kawachi N, Watabe H. Astatine-211 imaging by a Compton camera for targeted radiotherapy. Appl Radiat Isot. 2018;139:238–43.

SPECT/CT Imaging in Hyperparathyroidism and Benign Thyroid Disorders

Nicolas Aide, Elif Hindié, Stéphane Bardet, and David Taïeb

4.1 Hyperparathyroidism

4.1.1 Embryology

The superior parathyroid glands (also called PIV) are derived from the fourth branchial pouch. The third branchial pouches give rise to the inferior parathyroid glands (also called PIII) and the thymus. The superior parathyroid glands are most commonly found at the upper and middle third of the thyroid lobes. The inferior parathyroid glands are more varied in location and are usually found near the lower pole of the thyroid lobe below the lobe in the thyrothymic ligament. In some cases, the migration patterns are aberrant (insufficient or excessive), with clinical implications.

Depending on the underlying causal mechanism, ectopic pathological parathyroid glands can be found in various situations and locations. The detection of ectopic glands by nuclear physi-cians, radiologists, and surgeons requires a thorough knowledge of anatomy and a comprehensive understanding of the embryological evolution.

(a) **Glands located in aberrant situations due to congenital ectopia:** This is typically observed in PIII glands that can be located in upper (undescended thyrothymic complex) or lower positions. Undescended PIII glands can be located on the lateral and cranial side of the upper thyroid lobe pole, adjacent to the carotid sheath on its anteromedial side, and are associated with a rudimentary thymus. PIII glands can also be pulled down with the thymus, into the anterior mediastinum near the great vessels. Congenital ectopias of PIV are rarely major ectopias that can be found on the posterior aspect of the superior thyroid lobe pole in a latero-cricoid, latero-pharyngeal, or inter-cricothyroid position.

(b) **Acquired gland ectopias:** This mechanism of migration is more commonly observed with PIV glands and is most likely related to displacement by gravity of large adenomas against the prevertebral plane into the posterior mediastinum. During this course, the glands remain in very close contact with the oesophagus and can even pass behind the oesophagus, with exceptional crossing of the midline.

(c) **Supranumerary parathyroid glands:** These are mainly located in the thymus due to fragmentation of PIII glands during embryogenesis. They can also be located

N. Aide
Department of Nuclear Medicine, University Hospital, Caen, France

E. Hindié
Department of Nuclear Medicine, Haut-Lévêque Hospital, University of Bordeaux, Bordeaux, France

S. Bardet
Department of Nuclear Medicine, François Baclesse Cancer Centre, Caen, France

D. Taïeb (✉)
Department of Nuclear Medicine, la Timone university hospital, Aix-marseille university, Marseille, France
e-mail: david.taieb@ap-hm.fr

© The Author(s), under exclusive license to Springer Nature Switzerland AG 2022
H. Ahmadzadehfar et al. (eds.), *Clinical Applications of SPECT-CT*,
https://doi.org/10.1007/978-3-030-65850-2_4

alongside the vagus nerve in the carotid sheath of the neck or at lower limit sites where the inferior laryngeal nerves recur (i.e. subclavian artery on right side and in aorto-pulmonary window on left side). Parathyroid lesions can be found in close contact with the vagus nerve or within its fibres (para or intravagal).

(d) **Intrathyroidal:** Ectopic glands may be found in the thyroid gland, parathyroid tissue that originated from PIV (due to excess of migration of the gland with ultimobranchial body), or less frequently, from a supranumerary gland or a PIII gland.

(e) **Parathyroid ectopia due to autotransplant or cell dispersal:** This occurs when there is an autotransplant into the forearm (as part of a parathyroidectomy procedure for secondary HPT or MEN1 syndrome) or accidental cell grafting with subsequent parathyromatosis (e.g. rupture of the parathyroid capsule, with spillage of parathyroid cells in the surgical field).

(f) **Metastasis from a parathyroid carcinoma.** This is usually to the lung.

4.1.2 Pathophysiology, Treatment Goals, and Strategies

4.1.2.1 Primary Hyperparathyroidism

Sporadic primary hyperparathyroidism (pHPT) is only rarely diagnosed before the age of 50 and is mostly caused by solitary parathyroid adenomas. Parathyroid adenomas are monoclonal tumours which are probably related to defects in a set of specific genes that control parathyroid cell growth. Double adenomas are seen in about 5% of cases. Diffuse parathyroid hyperplasia may occur in up to 10% of sporadic cases and in all patients with MEN1 disease or with familial hypocalciuric hypercalcaemia. Carcinomas are rare and frequently related to mutations in HRPT2 gene.

In sporadic cases, a clear indication for surgery is most obviously for symptomatic patient. The controversy arises with the asymptomatic patient, and criteria have been defined by International Workshops by the NIH taking into account patient's age, renal function, and bone mineral density.

4.1.2.2 Secondary Hyperparathyroidism

Secondary hyperparathyroidism (sHPT) is a frequent and major complication for patients on long-term haemodialysis or peritoneal dialysis. With the decline of kidney function, sHPT develops due to a cascade of metabolic abnormalities: (1) phosphate retention, (2) increased FGF23 (fibroblast growth factor-23) which inhibits 1α-hydroxylase and calcitriol synthesis [1], (3) the negative net calcium balance stimulates PTH release, and (4) chronically stimulated parathyroid cells lose their expression of VDR (vitamin D receptor), CaR (calcium-sensing receptor), klotho, and FGFR1–3 and become resistant to the inhibitory effect of vitamin D, calcium, and FGF23 [1]. In patients on long-standing dialysis, parathyroid growth progressively shifts from diffuse hyperplasia of all parathyroid glands to asymmetrical nodular and tumour-like monoclonal growth.

The arsenal of medical treatment includes dietary phosphorus restriction, phosphate binders, vitamin D sterols and analogues, and calcimimetics. Patients with intact parathyroid hormone (iPTH), calcium and phosphate levels within the targets set by the National Kidney Foundation's Kidney Disease Outcomes Quality Initiative (NKF-K/DOQI™), have a lower risk of mortality [2]. When medical treatment fails to control the disease, patients with severe sHPT are typically referred for parathyroidectomy (PTx), which usually improves biological parameters, as well as clinical signs and symptoms [3]. The success of PTx depends strongly on the skill and experience of the surgeon, whose goals include suppressing HPT for as long as possible while avoiding hypoparathyroidism. The two most widely accepted surgical techniques are subtotal PTx and total PTx with autotransplantation. Neither technique has established superiority over the other in terms of surgical complications, or disease persistence or recurrence [4].

4.1.2.3 Tertiary Hyperparathyroidism

The hypercalcaemia that develops after renal transplantation is usually transient and gradually resolves with the involution of parathyroid hyperplasia. However, in about 10% of patients, HPT persists and is also called tertiary hyperparathyroidism. PTx may also be necessary in a small subset of kidney transplant patients in whom tertiary hyperparathyroidism (tHPT) did not resolve spontaneously [5].

4.1.3 Role of Parathyroid Scintigraphy

4.1.3.1 Primary Hyperparathyroidism

Initial Surgery for pHPT

For many years, bilateral cervical exploration with identification of the four parathyroid glands remained the gold standard for parathyroid surgery with a 95–98% long-term success rate [6]. In experienced hands, immediate failures are mainly due to ectopic glands located inferiorly in the mediastinum (<2% of cases) where they are virtually inaccessible from the neck [7] or some other major ectopy (undescended glands, within the sheath of carotid artery, and intrathyroidal).

In the recent years, surgical management of patients with sporadic pHPT has moved towards the development of focused minimally invasive approaches, and the use of preoperative imaging has become essential for selecting best candidates [8–11]. Parathyroid ultrasonography and scintigraphy are the imaging modalities commonly used for this purpose [12]. In MEN1 patients, the role of imaging is more limited since all glands are affected by parathyroid hyperplasia, and bilateral surgery is the rule. Nevertheless, the possibility that one of the affected glands be ectopic should not be underestimated.

Persistent or Recurrent HPT

Preoperative imaging is mandatory in the management of patients with persistent or recurrent HPT and may include noninvasive and invasive investigations [13–16].

4.1.3.2 Renal Hyperparathyroidism

Initial Surgery for rHPT

Unfortunately, the rate of persistent or recurrent disease after PTx in patients with renal hyperparathyroidism (rHPT) is far from negligible [4, 17, 18]. Parathyroid reoperation is challenging in this population because the rate of associated morbidities is particularly high [17]. Some early reports showed that parathyroid scintigraphy could be useful before initial PTx, providing both anatomic and functional information on individual parathyroid glands [19–21]. However, the use of parathyroid scintigraphy prior to the initial surgery is still debated [22, 23].

The use of parathyroid scintigraphy offers several potential advantages:

1. Identification of the four orthotopic glands: Identifying all four parathyroid glands in patients with rHPT can be difficult due to the high prevalence of nodular goitre in this patient population and the gross appearance of hyperplastic glands that may mimic thyroid tissue. Failure to identify all parathyroid glands usually results in persistent HPT [18]. Missing a parathyroid gland in the neck might further entail a difficult and extensive reoperation.

2. Localisation of ectopic and supernumerary glands: When PTx is performed by an experienced surgeon, the inability to identify an ectopic or supernumerary parathyroid is the main cause of persistence or early recurrence [17]. The high sensitivity to visualise ectopic parathyroid glands is considered the main advantage of scintigraphy over ultrasound [24].

3. Choice of the gland to be preserved: The choice of the gland depends on its gross appearance (the gland should be less likely to have severe nodular hyperplasia) as well as its anatomical situation. It is important to note that the functional information provided by parathyroid scintigraphy may guide surgeons towards the most suitable gland for preservation (least active/autonomous) [19, 20, 24, 25]. However, this requires further studies.

Persistent or Recurrent rHPT

Persistent rHPT diagnosed in the early postoperative period, or during the first 6 months, results from missed orthotopic glands, too large remnant/grafts or ectopic or supernumerary macroscopic parathyroid glands. In patients who undergo PTx + AT, the diagnosis of surgical failure is easy because parathyroid grafts are not immediately functional. Delayed recurrences due to growth of the remaining parathyroid tissue (from remnant/grafts) or supernumerary glands are sometimes observed after an appropriate initial PTx; this rate can reach 30% after 10 years of continuing dialysis [4]. Recurrence may also rarely develop from parathyromatosis, which is caused by inadvertent rupture of the parathyroid capsule, with spilling of parathyroid cells in the surgical field.

Preoperative imaging is considered mandatory before reoperation for persistent or recurrent disease [17, 26].

4.1.4 Planar Parathyroid Scintigraphy

Whatever the functional imaging protocol, the imaged field should be from the angle of the mandible to the heart, because ectopic glands may be widely distributed along the parathyroid cell migration routes. In patients with recurrent sHPT treated by PTx + AT in a muscle of the forearm, imaging protocol should also include acquisition over the parathyroid graft at the forearm.

4.1.5 Dual-Phase Protocol

This approach is based on differential sestaMIBI retention between parathyroid and thyroid tissue [19]. SestaMIBI retention is prolonged in parathyroid lesions, whereas the tracer washes out more rapidly from normal thyroid tissue.

4.1.6 Subtraction Protocol

In this protocol, ^{99m}Tc-MIBI is used in conjunction with another tracer specific to the thyroid. Either technetium-99 m-pertechnetate (^{99m}TcO$_4^-$) or iodine123 (^{123}I) can be used for thyroid scintigraphy. When using ^{99m}TcO$_4^-$, the thyroid image is acquired either before or after the ^{99m}Tc-MIBI acquisition. Patient motion may lead to artefacts on subtraction images. The main advantage of using ^{123}I is that thyroid and parathyroid images can be acquired simultaneously in a dual-energy window set-up (such as 140 ± 7 keV for ^{99m}TcO$_4^-$ and 164 ± 7 keV for ^{123}I). A typical protocol includes a magnified view of the thyroid/parathyroid area with a pinhole collimator [20] followed by a parallel-hole collimator large field of view over the neck and the mediastinum. After normalisation, ^{123}I (or ^{99m}TcO$_4^-$) thyroid images are digitally subtracted from ^{99m}Tc-MIBI images. The residual image corresponds to the parathyroid image.

4.1.7 Sensitivity and Specificity

In pHPT, overall sensitivity of parathyroid scintigraphy ranges from 68 to 86% [27–31], mainly depending on gland weights and serum PTH levels [31–38]. Subtraction method offers at least 20% higher sensitivity than single-tracer "dual-phase" imaging in studies with intra-patient analysis [39–42]. Based on published literature, the superiority of subtraction technique is especially true as regards detection of multiple parathyroid gland disease. It has been also suggested that secondary hyperplastic parathyroid glands were better detected by dual-tracer "subtraction" techniques with sensitivities ranging between 65 and 90% (Fig. 4.1) [13]. Studies that compared single-tracer and dual-tracer techniques in the setting of reoperation also found higher sensitivity for

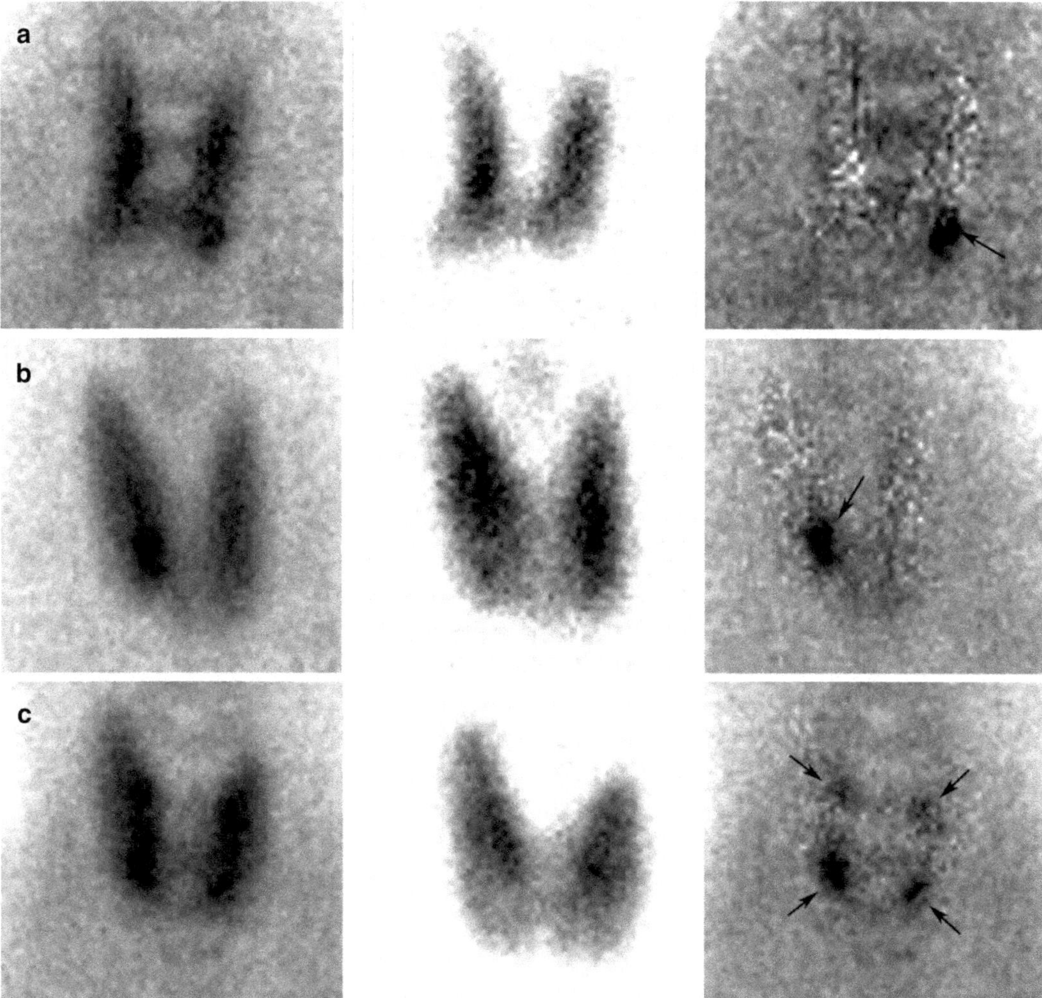

Fig. 4.1 Subtraction protocol. Injection of 12 MBq of ^{123}I at $T = -2$ h, injection of 740 of ^{99m}Tc-MIBI at T0, dual-tracer planar pinhole acquisition (20 min acquisition). ^{99m}Tc-MIBI pinhole planar image (*left*), ^{123}I pinhole planar image (*middle*), and subtraction image (^{99m}Tc-MIBI-^{123}I) (*right*). (**a**) Parathyroid adenoma located at the tip of the inferior pole of the left thyroid lobe (*arrow*). (**b**) Parathyroid adenoma located at the inner part of the right thyroid lobe (*arrow*). (**c**) Typical diffuse hyperplasia related to chronic renal failure (*arrows*)

dual-tracer techniques [43]. False-negative results are mainly attributed to small parathyroid lesions (limit of detection about 100–200 mg) and cystic adenomas (after necrosis or cystic degeneration). Thymoma, metastatic or inflammatory lymph nodes, and skeletal brown tumours may represent rare potential false-positive lesions.

4.1.8 SPECT/CT

4.1.8.1 Primary Hyperparathyroidism

SPECT/CT may provide improvement in sensitivity in comparison to single-tracer planar imaging, especially for posterior adenomas. In our opinion, the use of subtraction method using ^{123}I and ^{99m}Tc-MIBI with pinhole planar acquisition

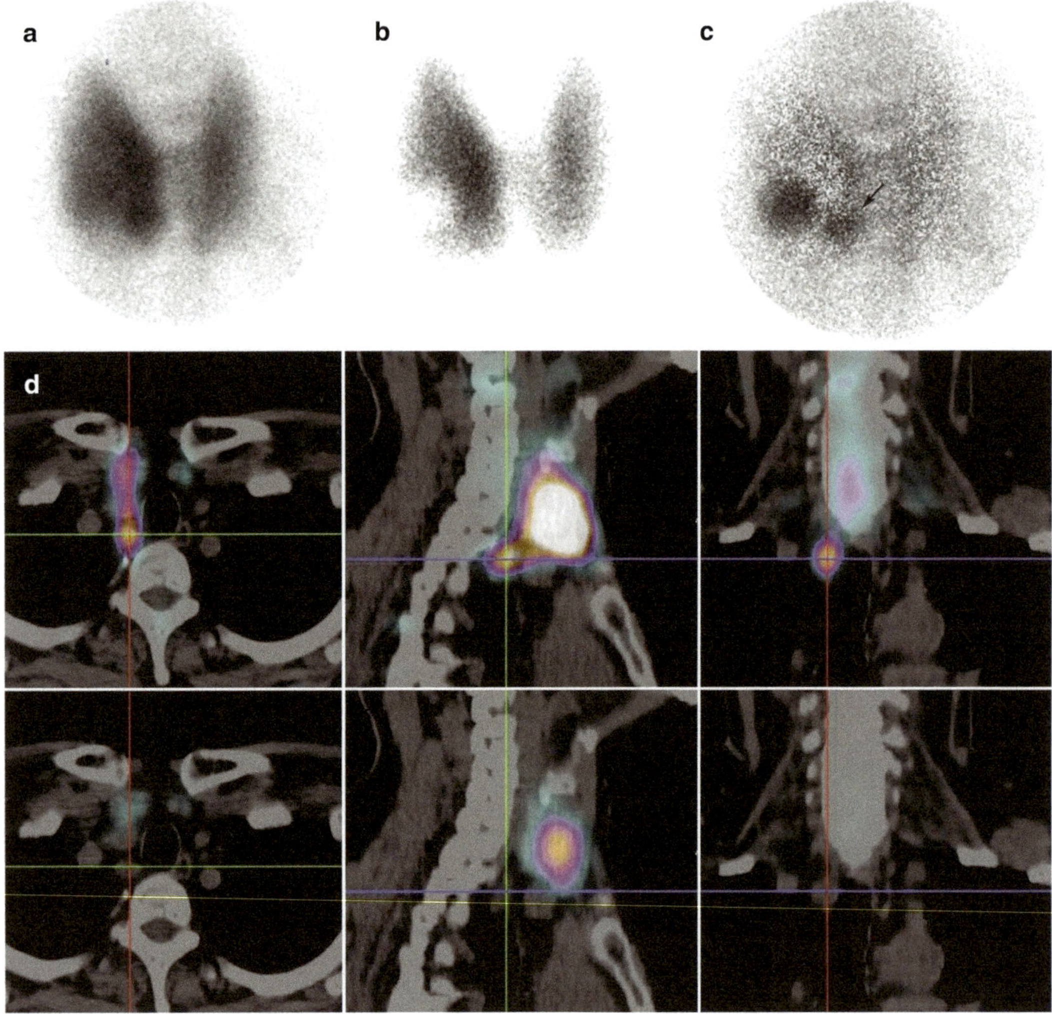

Fig. 4.2 PIV adenoma. (**a**) ^{99m}Tc-MIBI pinhole image, (**b**) ^{123}I pinhole image, (**c**) subtraction, (**d**) Dual-isotope SPECT/CT images (^{99m}Tc-MIBI *upper row*; ^{123}I *lower row*). Planar pinhole subtraction images reveal a focal accumulation of ^{99m}Tc-MIBI located in the inner and lower pole of the right thyroid lobe. Note a right thyroid nodule on ^{123}I scintigraphy. SPECT/CT demonstrates that the parathyroid gland is prolapsed behind the thyroid gland and is extended posteriorly (*black arrows*). This is a typical feature of PIV adenoma. Please note absence of ^{123}I uptake in the parathyroid adenoma (*lower row image*)

(neck) followed by SPECT/CT (neck and mediastinum) is the most sensitive approach to detect and localise hyperfunctioning glands. SPECT can be performed as single-tracer imaging or as a dual-tracer technique with simultaneous acquisition (Figs. 4.2, 4.3 and 4.4). The energy windows for acquisition are the same as for planar and pinhole images [13, 40].

SPECT/CT provides the advantage over planar techniques to localise adenomas in the anterior-posterior plane [44, 45], offering critical information for surgeons. SPECT may reclassify apparently inferior adenomas (on planar images) to superior, PIV-derived, adenomas prolapsed behind the lower pole of the thyroid gland. These adenomas can be located

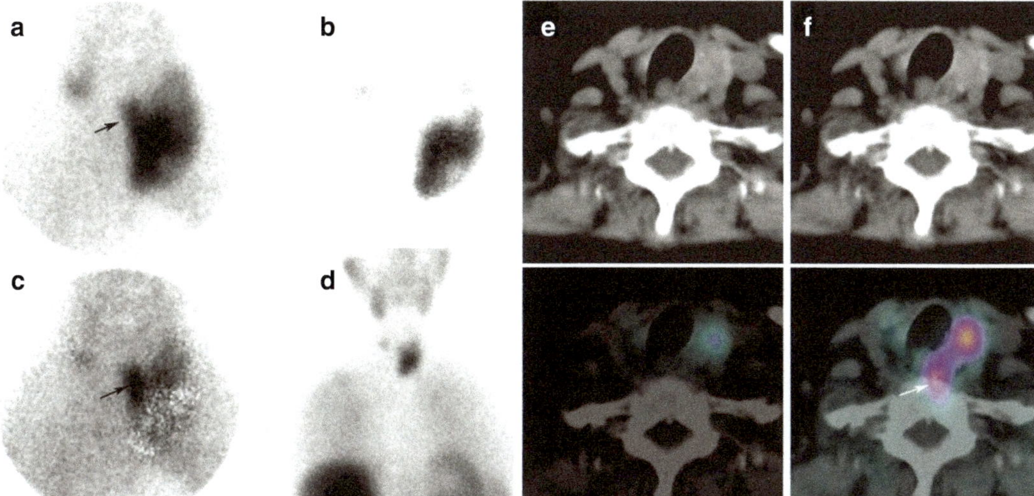

Fig. 4.3 PIV adenoma. (**a**) ^{99m}Tc-sestaMIBI, (**b**) ^{123}I, (**c**) subtraction, (**d**) cervico-mediastinal acquisition, (**e**) CT and ^{123}I SPECT/CT images, (**f**) CT and ^{99m}Tc- SPECT/CT images. Planar pinhole subtraction images reveal a focal accumulation of ^{99m}Tc-MIBI located in the inner part of the left thyroid lobe (*arrows*). SPECT/CT demonstrates that the gland is prolapsed behind the thyroid gland and is extended posteriorly as almost all large PIV adenomas (*white arrow*). This patient had nodular thyroid disease with previous right thyroid lobectomy

very deeply in the neck, in paraesophageal or in retroesophageal locations and may be missed by neck ultrasound (Figs. 4.2 and 4.3) [46]. By contrast, inferior glands are mostly located at the tip of the inferior pole of the thyroid lobe, in the thyrothymic tract or in the upper thymic horn, and remain anterior on SPECT imaging (Fig. 4.4) [45]. These 3D information may also influence the surgical strategy such as resection via an endoscopic lateral approach for posterior adenomas (most often PIV-derived) or a small cervical incision (mini-open approach) cervicotomy for PIII-derived adenomas [47]. SPECT also enables a better localisation of ectopic glands (Fig. 4.3). The precise anatomic localisation of mediastinal adenomas provided by SPECT/CT may also influence the surgical strategy (mediastinoscopy/anterior mediastinotomy vs left thoracotomy) (Fig. 4.5).

Using a single-isotope protocol, SPECT/CT acquisitions are usually performed from 10–60 min after injection of ^{99m}Tc-MIBI [48–50]. Some teams acquire both early and late SPECT images. Iterative reconstruction methods are well suited to improve image quality. There is some evidence that early-phase SPECT or SPECT/CT imaging performs better than delayed imaging, presumably because of a rapid tracer wash-out in some hyperfunctioning glands [50–52] (Table 4.1). The use of SPECT/CT also provides an advantage over SPECT alone in patients with nodular goitre [54]. To minimise radiation exposure, the CT part of the SPECT/CT acquisition should probably be limited to the neck area in cases of absence of mediastinal foci on planar images [43].

4.1.8.2 Renal Hyperparathyroidism
SPECT/CT may increase sensitivity of single-tracer planar imaging [43] but probably have little impact on sensitivity in comparison to highly sensitive subtraction protocols using pinhole collimators [13] (Fig. 4.6). SPECT/CT is particularly helpful as a complement to planar imaging to pinpoint the position of mediastinal foci and other ectopic parathyroid glands [13].

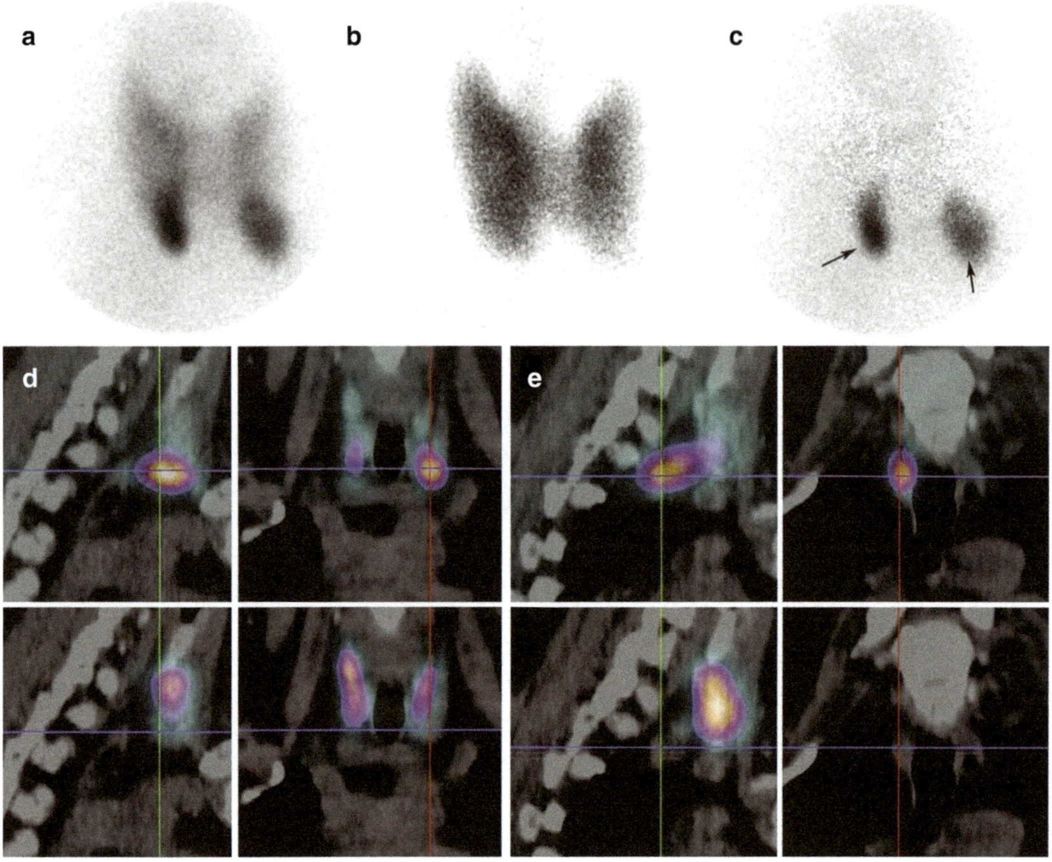

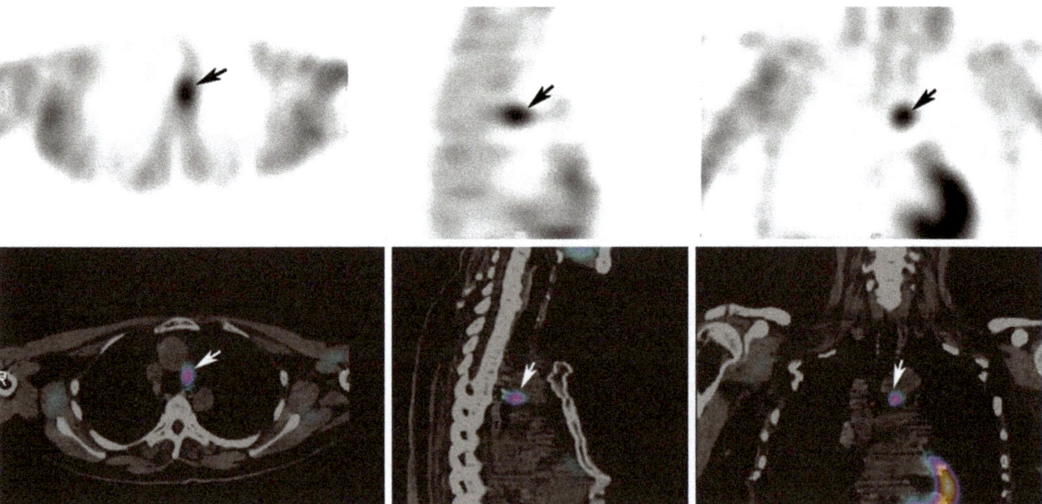

Fig. 4.4 MEN1-related HPT. (**a**) ^{99m}Tc-MIBI, (**b**) ^{123}I, (**c**) subtraction, (**d** and **e**) Dual-isotope SPECT/CT images. Planar pinhole subtraction images reveal two focal accumulation of ^{99m}Tc-MIBI located in the inferior poles of right and left thyroid lobes. SPECT/CT demonstrates a left PIII hyperfunctioning lesion (*left arrow*) (**d**) and a right PIV hyperfunctioning lesion prolapsed behind the thyroid gland (*right arrow*) (**e**). Please note absence of ^{123}I uptake in the parathyroid lesions (*lower row*)

Fig. 4.5 Parathyroid adenoma in the aortopulmonary window (*arrows*). SPECT and SPECT/CT fusion images

Table 4.1 Performance of SPECT/CT in hyperparathyroidism

Authors	Disease	Number of patients	SPECT/CT device	SPECT/CT protocol	Diagnostic performance		
					Type of analysis	Sensitivity	Specificity
Lavely et al. [50]	pHPT	98	Low-power CT	Early SPECT/CT	Per lesion	62	99
–	–	–	–	Delayed SPECT/CT	–	53	98
–	–	–	–	Early planar/delayed SPECT/CT	–	61	98
–	–	–	–	Early SPECT/CT/delayed planar	–	72	99
Patel et al. [53]	pHPT	59	Low-power CT	Early planar/delayed SPECT/CT	Per lesion	90	Na
Pata et al. [54]	pHPT + nodular goitre	18	SPECT alone	Early planar/delayed SPECT	Per neck quadrant	56	62
–	–	15	Low-power CT	Early planar/delayed SPECT/CT	–	87	87
Pata et al. [55]	pHPT	27	SPECT alone	Early planar/delayed SPECT	Per neck quadrant	87	90
–	–	28	Low-power CT	Early planar/delayed SPECT/CT	–	61	97
Ciappuccini et al. [56]	pHPT	59	Spiral CT	Early pinhole/delayed SPECT/CT	Per lesion	92	83
Shafiei et al. [57]	pHPT + nodular goitre	48	Spiral CT	Early planar + SPECT/delayed planar	Per lesion	67	87
–	–	–	–	Early planar + SPECT/CT/delayed planar	–	78	97
Zhen et al. [43]	sHPT	90	Spiral CT	Early planar/delayed planar + SPECT/CT	Per patient	79	100

pHPT primary hyperparathyroidism, *sHPT* secondary hyperparathyroidism

a

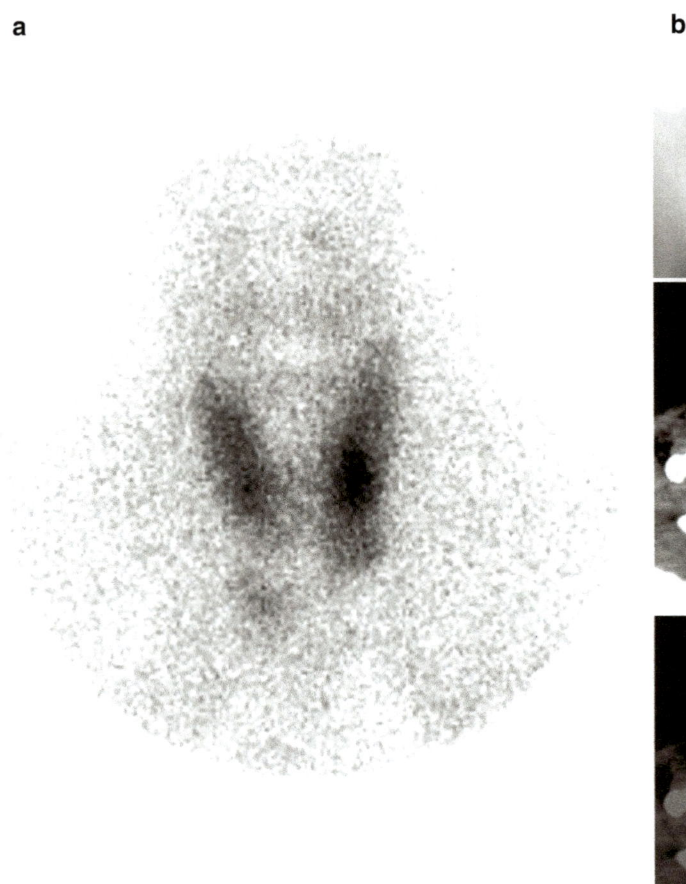

b

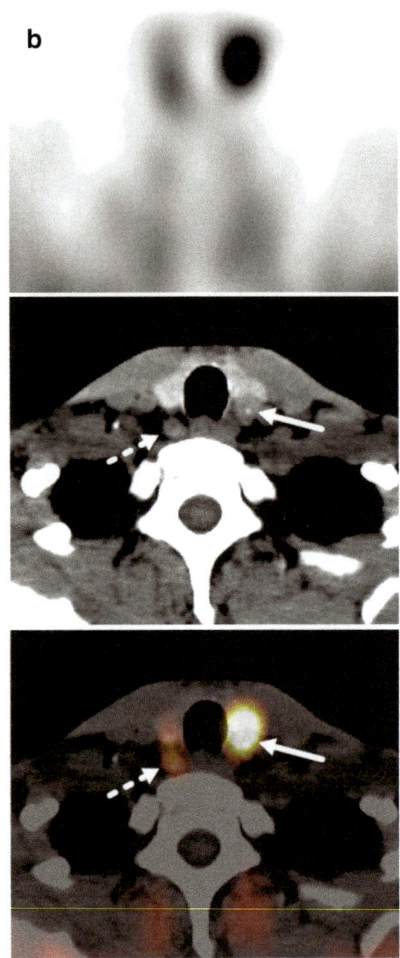

Fig. 4.6 Secondary hyperparathyroidism. (**a**) Early pinhole images and trans-axial slices (**b**, from top to bottom: SPECT, CT, and fused SPECT/CT slices) are shown. Whereas pinhole images show an intense focus on the left side, delayed SPECT/CT acquisition clearly shows a left parathyroid adenoma (*arrow*) and a second contralateral lesion at the same level, which harbours a low MIBI uptake (*dotted arrow*)

4.1.9 Conclusion Remarks

Nuclear physicians should possess thorough knowledge of the anatomy and embryology of parathyroid glands as well as the pathophysiology and management of parathyroid disorders. Refinement of parathyroid imaging studies has led to a reassessment of their role in the management of patients with primary and renal HPT. The optimal parathyroid scintigraphy protocol relies on ^{123}I/^{99m}Tc-MIBI planar pinhole acquisition centred over the thyroid area followed by cervico-mediastinal SPECT/CT acquisition. In hyperparathyroidism with negative or unconclusive findings on parathyroid scintigraphy, ^{18}F-fluorocholine PET/CT has proven successful as a second-line modality. There is currently a considerable excitement for promoting ^{18}F-fluorocholine PET/CT at the fore-font modality before initial PTx. This would however need to further establish the positive medical impact of performing this modality compared to parathyroid scintigraphy in this setting with integration of medico-economic issues.

4.2 Benign Thyroid Disorders

4.2.1 Ectopic Thyroid Tissue

Ectopic thyroid tissue is the result of abnormal migration of the gland as it travels from the floor of the primitive foregut to its destined pre-tracheal position. Patients with ectopic thyroid tissue are usually euthyroid and asymptomatic but can present with signs and symptoms of upper aerodigestive tract obstruction. One of the most frequent locations of ectopic thyroid tissue is at the base of the tongue, in particular at the region of the foramen cecum. Most patients with lingual thyroid present with hypothyroidism, usually in the absence of orthotopic thyroid. They may also be euthyroid (even when no orthotopic thyroid exists) or even hyperthyroid in patients with Graves' disease and often revealed as recurrent hyperthyroidism several years after total thyroidectomy. Ectopic tissue may also be located in the mediastinum and give rise to primary intrathoracic goitre (ectopic thyroid tissue detached from a cervical thyroid mass). Finally, ectopic thyroid can also be detected in the lateral cervical region (also called lateral aberrant thyroid) and is usually regarded as metastatic lymph node from thyroid carcinoma. Multiple ectopia of the thyroid is extremely rare.

Scintigraphy using $^{99m}TcO_4$ or ^{123}I is the most important diagnostic tool to detect ectopic thyroid tissue. SPECT/CT increases diagnostic accuracy (Fig. 4.7).

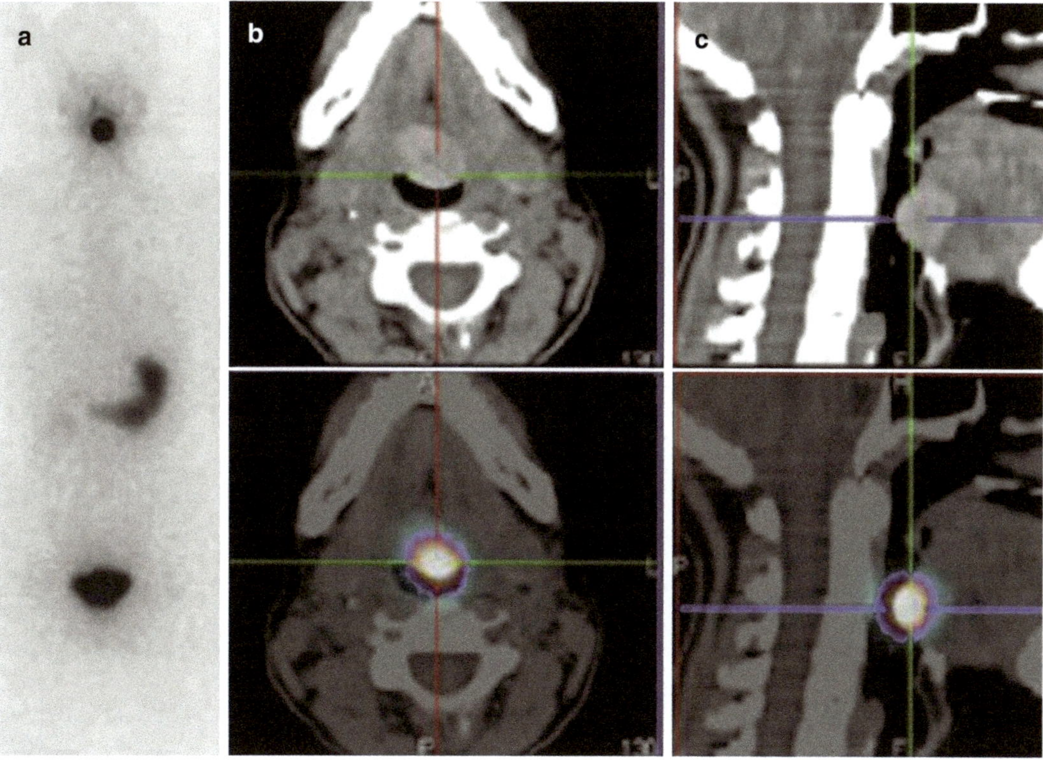

Fig. 4.7 Lingual thyroid. (**a**) Whole-body planar image, (**b**) trans-axial, and (**c**) sagittal CT and SPECT/CT images centred over the ectopic thyroid tissue. Images were acquired 2 h after injection of 37 MBq of ^{123}I in a patient presenting with a lump of the tongue. Scintigraphy was performed under LT4 treatment and after injections of recombinant human thyroid-stimulating hormone (Adapted with permission from Vercellino et al. [58])

4.2.2 Intrathoracic Goitre

Intrathoracic (substernal) goitre is usually secondary, related to a retrosternal extension of a portion of the cervical goitre. The therapy of choice is total/near-total thyroidectomy and subsequent levothyroxine substitution. SPECT/CT improved the image contrast and quantification due to attenuation and scatter corrections and enables precise localisation into the mediastinum (Fig. 4.8). It may also select potential candidates to radioiodine therapy.

4.2.3 Ovarian Teratoma

Thyroid tissue is occasionally present in ovarian teratomas (also called ovarian goitre or struma ovarii) with potential neoplastic transformation into thyroid carcinoma. It can be revealed by signs and symptoms of an adnexal mass and may be occasionally revealed by hyperthyroidism or post-therapy whole-body scan performed after adjuvant ^{131}I therapy for thyroid cancer [59]. SPECT/CT imaging may be useful to achieve a better localisation and to limit false-positive findings related to urinary elimination [60–64].

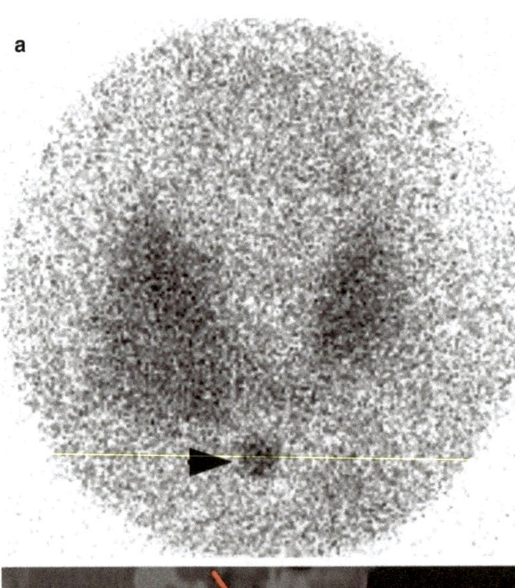

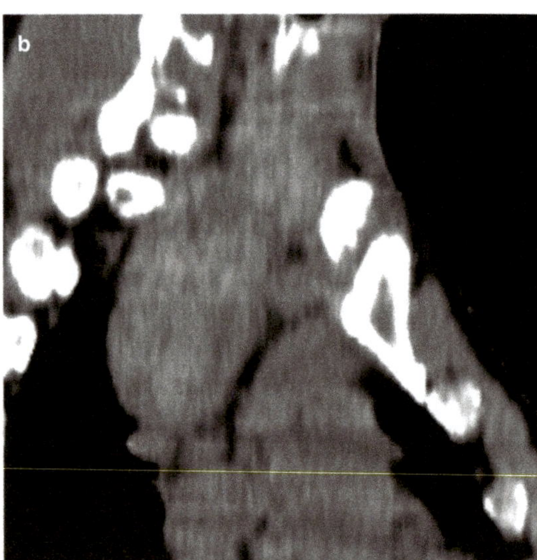

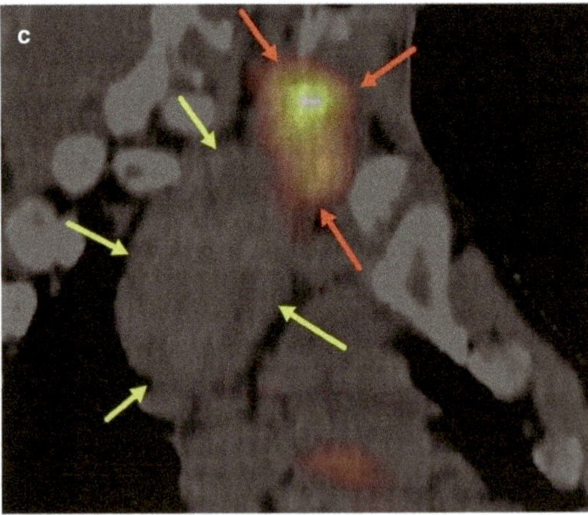

Fig. 4.8 Retrosternal goitre. (**a**) Pinhole image (*head arrow*: sternal notch landmark) and sagittal CT (**b**) and SPECT/CT (**c**) images. SPECT/CT acquisition shows that the retrosternal component of the goitre (*yellow arrows*) does not take up the tracer, as opposed to the remaining right thyroid lobe (*red arrows*), and provides useful details regarding the inferior limit of the goitre as well as its limits with surrounding organs and great vessels

References

1. Quarles LD. Role of FGF23 in vitamin D and phosphate metabolism: implications in chronic kidney disease. Exp Cell Res. 2012;318:1040–8. https://doi.org/10.1016/j.yexcr.2012.02.027.
2. Floege J, Kim J, Ireland E, Chazot C, Drueke T, de Francisco A, et al. Serum iPTH, calcium and phosphate, and the risk of mortality in a European haemodialysis population. Nephrol Dial Transplant. 2011;26:1948–55. https://doi.org/10.1093/ndt/gfq219.
3. Sharma J, Raggi P, Kutner N, Bailey J, Zhang R, Huang Y, et al. Improved long-term survival of dialysis patients after near-total parathyroidectomy. J Am Coll Surg. 2012;214:400–7. https://doi.org/10.1016/j.jamcollsurg.2011.12.046. discussion 7–8
4. Gagne ER, Urena P, Leite-Silva S, Zingraff J, Chevalier A, Sarfati E, et al. Short- and long-term efficacy of total parathyroidectomy with immediate autografting compared with subtotal parathyroidectomy in hemodialysis patients. J Am Soc Nephrol. 1992;3:1008–17.
5. Triponez F, Clark OH, Vanrenthergem Y, Evenepoel P. Surgical treatment of persistent hyperparathyroidism after renal transplantation. Ann Surg. 2008;248:18–30. https://doi.org/10.1097/SLA.0b013e3181728a2d.
6. van Heerden JA, Grant CS. Surgical treatment of primary hyperparathyroidism: an institutional perspective. World J Surg. 1991;15:688–92.
7. Henry JF, Taieb D, Van Slycke S. Parathyroid localization and imaging. In: Endocrine surgery (Springer Specialist Surgery Series). London: Springer; 2009. p. 235–52. https://doi.org/10.1007/978-1-84628-881-4_17.
8. Mihai R, Simon D, Hellman P. Imaging for primary hyperparathyroidism–an evidence-based analysis. Langenbeck's Arch Surg. 2009;394:765–84. https://doi.org/10.1007/s00423-009-0534-4.
9. Mihai R, Barczynski M, Iacobone M, Sitges-Serra A. Surgical strategy for sporadic primary hyperparathyroidism an evidence-based approach to surgical strategy, patient selection, surgical access, and reoperations. Langenbeck's Arch Surg. 2009;394:785–98. https://doi.org/10.1007/s00423-009-0529-1.
10. Taieb D, Hindie E, Grassetto G, Colletti PM, Rubello D. Parathyroid scintigraphy: when, how, and why? A concise systematic review. Clin Nucl Med. 2012;37:568–74. https://doi.org/10.1097/RLU.0b013e318251e408.
11. Kunstman JW, Kirsch JD, Mahajan A, Udelsman R. Clinical review: parathyroid localization and implications for clinical management. J Clin Endocrinol Metab. 2013;98:902–12. https://doi.org/10.1210/jc.2012-3168.
12. Ruda JM, Hollenbeak CS, Stack BC Jr. A systematic review of the diagnosis and treatment of primary hyperparathyroidism from 1995 to 2003. Otolaryngol Head Neck Surg. 2005;132:359–72. https://doi.org/10.1016/j.otohns.2004.10.005.
13. Hindie E, Ugur O, Fuster D, O'Doherty M, Grassetto G, Urena P, et al. 2009 EANM parathyroid guidelines. Eur J Nucl Med Mol Imaging. 2009;36:1201–16. https://doi.org/10.1007/s00259-009-1131-z.
14. Bergenfelz AO, Hellman P, Harrison B, Sitges-Serra A, Dralle H. Positional statement of the European Society of Endocrine Surgeons (ESES) on modern techniques in pHPT surgery. Langenbeck's Arch Surg. 2009;394:761–4. https://doi.org/10.1007/s00423-009-0533-5.
15. Bilezikian JP, Khan AA, Potts JT Jr. Guidelines for the management of asymptomatic primary hyperparathyroidism: summary statement from the third international workshop. J Clin Endocrinol Metab. 2009;94:335–9. https://doi.org/10.1210/jc.2008-1763.
16. Calzada-Nocaudie M, Chanson P, Conte-Devolx B, Delemer B, Estour B, Henry JF, et al. Management of asymptomatic primary hyperparathyroidism: French Society of Endocrinology expert consensus. Ann Endocrinol (Paris). 2006;67:7–12.
17. Dotzenrath C, Cupisti K, Goretzki E, Mondry A, Vossough A, Grabensee B, et al. Operative treatment of renal autonomous hyperparathyroidism: cause of persistent or recurrent disease in 304 patients. Langenbeck's Arch Surg. 2003;387:348–54. https://doi.org/10.1007/s00423-002-0322-x.
18. Kovacevic B, Ignjatovic M, Zivaljevic V, Cuk V, Scepanovic M, Petrovic Z, et al. Parathyroidectomy for the attainment of NKF-K/DOQI and KDIGO recommended values for bone and mineral metabolism in dialysis patients with uncontrollable secondary hyperparathyroidism. Langenbeck's Arch Surg. 2012;397(3):413–20. https://doi.org/10.1007/s00423-011-0901-9.
19. Piga M, Bolasco P, Satta L, Altieri P, Loi G, Nicolosi A, et al. Double phase parathyroid technetium-99m-MIBI scintigraphy to identify functional autonomy in secondary hyperparathyroidism. J Nucl Med. 1996;37:565–9.
20. Hindie E, Urena P, Jeanguillaume C, Melliere D, Berthelot JM, Menoyo-Calonge V, et al. Preoperative imaging of parathyroid glands with technetium-99m-labelled sestamibi and iodine-123 subtraction scanning in secondary hyperparathyroidism. Lancet. 1999;353:2200–4. https://doi.org/10.1016/S0140-6736(98)09089-8.
21. Torregrosa JV, Fernandez-Cruz L, Canalejo A, Vidal S, Astudillo E, Almaden Y, et al. (99m)Tc-sestamibi scintigraphy and cell cycle in parathyroid glands of secondary hyperparathyroidism. World J Surg. 2000;24:1386–90.
22. Taieb D, Urena-Torres P, Zanotti-Fregonara P, Rubello D, Ferretti A, Henter I, et al. Parathyroid scintigraphy in renal hyperparathyroidism: the added diagnostic value of SPECT and SPECT/CT. Clin Nucl Med. 2013;38(8):630. https://doi.org/10.1097/RLU.0b013e31829af5bf.

23. Caldarella C, Treglia G, Pontecorvi A, Giordano A. Diagnostic performance of planar scintigraphy using (9)(9)mTc-MIBI in patients with secondary hyperparathyroidism: a meta-analysis. Ann Nucl Med. 2012;26:794–803. https://doi.org/10.1007/s12149-012-0643-y.

24. Vulpio C, Bossola M, De Gaetano A, Maresca G, Bruno I, Fadda G, et al. Usefulness of the combination of ultrasonography and 99mTc-sestamibi scintigraphy in the preoperative evaluation of uremic secondary hyperparathyroidism. Head Neck. 2010;32:1226–35. https://doi.org/10.1002/hed.21320.

25. Fuster D, Ybarra J, Ortin J, Torregrosa JV, Gilabert R, Setoain X, et al. Role of pre-operative imaging using 99mTc-MIBI and neck ultrasound in patients with secondary hyperparathyroidism who are candidates for subtotal parathyroidectomy. Eur J Nucl Med Mol Imaging. 2006;33:467–73. https://doi.org/10.1007/s00259-005-0021-2.

26. Gasparri G, Camandona M, Bertoldo U, Sargiotto A, Papotti M, Raggio E, et al. The usefulness of preoperative dual-phase 99mTc MIBI-scintigraphy and IO-PTH assay in the treatment of secondary and tertiary hyperparathyroidism. Ann Surg. 2009;250:868–71. https://doi.org/10.1097/SLA.0b013e3181b0c7f4.

27. Lumachi F, Ermani M, Basso S, Zucchetta P, Borsato N, Favia G. Localization of parathyroid tumours in the minimally invasive era: which technique should be chosen? Population-based analysis of 253 patients undergoing parathyroidectomy and factors affecting parathyroid gland detection. Endocr Relat Cancer. 2001;8:63–9.

28. Siperstein A, Berber E, Barbosa GF, Tsinberg M, Greene AB, Mitchell J, et al. Predicting the success of limited exploration for primary hyperparathyroidism using ultrasound, sestamibi, and intraoperative parathyroid hormone: analysis of 1158 cases. Ann Surg. 2008;248:420–8. https://doi.org/10.1097/SLA.0b013e3181859f71.

29. Tublin ME, Pryma DA, Yim JH, Ogilvie JB, Mountz JM, Bencherif B, et al. Localization of parathyroid adenomas by sonography and technetium tc 99m sestamibi single-photon emission computed tomography before minimally invasive parathyroidectomy: are both studies really needed? J Ultrasound Med. 2009;28:183–90.

30. Lumachi F, Tregnaghi A, Zucchetta P, Marzola MC, Cecchin D, Marchesi P, et al. Technetium-99m sestamibi scintigraphy and helical CT together in patients with primary hyperparathyroidism: a prospective clinical study. Br J Radiol. 2004;77:100–3.

31. Mihai R, Gleeson F, Buley ID, Roskell DE, Sadler GP. Negative imaging studies for primary hyperparathyroidism are unavoidable: correlation of sestamibi and high-resolution ultrasound scanning with histological analysis in 150 patients. World J Surg. 2006;30:697–704. https://doi.org/10.1007/s00268-005-0338-9.

32. Kebebew E, Hwang J, Reiff E, Duh QY, Clark OH. Predictors of single-gland vs multigland parathyroid disease in primary hyperparathyroidism: a simple and accurate scoring model. Arch Surg. 2006;141:777–82. https://doi.org/10.1001/archsurg.141.8.777. discussion 82

33. Stephen AE, Roth SI, Fardo DW, Finkelstein DM, Randolph GW, Gaz RD, et al. Predictors of an accurate preoperative sestamibi scan for single-gland parathyroid adenomas. Arch Surg. 2007;142:381–6.

34. Erbil Y, Barbaros U, Yanik BT, Salmaslioglu A, Tunaci M, Adalet I, et al. Impact of gland morphology and concomitant thyroid nodules on preoperative localization of parathyroid adenomas. Laryngoscope. 2006;116:580–5. https://doi.org/10.1097/01.MLG.0000203411.53666.AD.

35. Lo CY, Lang BH, Chan WF, Kung AW, Lam KS. A prospective evaluation of preoperative localization by technetium-99m sestamibi scintigraphy and ultrasonography in primary hyperparathyroidism. Am J Surg. 2007;193:155–9. https://doi.org/10.1016/j.amjsurg.2006.04.020.

36. Siegel A, Alvarado M, Barth RJ Jr, Brady M, Lewis J. Parameters in the prediction of the sensitivity of parathyroid scanning. Clin Nucl Med. 2006;31:679–82. https://doi.org/10.1097/01.rlu.0000242212.23936.a7.

37. Berber E, Parikh RT, Ballem N, Garner CN, Milas M, Siperstein AE. Factors contributing to negative parathyroid localization: an analysis of 1000 patients. Surgery. 2008;144:74–9. https://doi.org/10.1016/j.surg.2008.03.019.

38. Swanson TW, Chan SK, Jones SJ, Bugis S, Irvine R, Belzberg A, et al. Determinants of Tc-99m sestamibi SPECT scan sensitivity in primary hyperparathyroidism. Am J Surg. 2010;199:614–20. https://doi.org/10.1016/j.amjsurg.2010.02.001.

39. Neumann DR, Esselstyn CB Jr, Go RT, Wong CO, Rice TW, Obuchowski NA. Comparison of double-phase 99mTc-sestamibi with 123I-99mTc-sestamibi subtraction SPECT in hyperparathyroidism. AJR Am J Roentgenol. 1997;169:1671–4.

40. Hindie E, Melliere D, Jeanguillaume C, Perlemuter L, Chehade F, Galle P. Parathyroid imaging using simultaneous double-window recording of technetium-99m-sestamibi and iodine-123. J Nucl Med. 1998;39:1100–5.

41. Chen CC, Holder LE, Scovill WA, Tehan AM, Gann DS. Comparison of parathyroid imaging with technetium-99m-pertechnetate/sestamibi subtraction, double-phase technetium-99m-sestamibi and technetium-99m-sestamibi SPECT. J Nucl Med. 1997;38:834–9.

42. Caveny SA, Klingensmith WC 3rd, Martin WE, Sage-El A, McIntyre RC Jr, Raeburn C, et al. Parathyroid imaging: the importance of dual-radiopharmaceutical simultaneous acquisition with 99mTc-sestamibi and 123I. J Nucl Med Technol. 2012;40:104–10. https://doi.org/10.2967/jnmt.111.098400.

43. Schalin-Jantti C, Ryhanen E, Heiskanen I, Seppanen M, Arola J, Schildt J, et al. Planar scintigraphy with 123I/99mTc-sestamibi, 99mTc-sestamibi SPECT/CT, 11C-methionine PET/CT, or selective venous sampling before reoperation of primary hyperparathyroidism? J Nucl Med. 2013;54:739–47. https://doi.org/10.2967/jnumed.112.109561.

44. Rubello D, Massaro A, Cittadin S, Rampin L, Al-Nahhas A, Boni G, et al. Role of 99mTc-sestamibi SPECT in accurate selection of primary hyperparathyroid patients for minimally invasive radio-guided surgery. Eur J Nucl Med Mol Imaging. 2006;33:1091–4. https://doi.org/10.1007/s00259-006-0162-y.

45. Taieb D, Hassad R, Sebag F, Colavolpe C, Guedj E, Hindie E, et al. Tomoscintigraphy improves the determination of the embryologic origin of parathyroid adenomas, especially in apparently inferior glands: imaging features and surgical implications. J Nucl Med Technol. 2007;35:135–9. https://doi.org/10.2967/jnmt.107.039743.

46. Harari A, Mitmaker E, Grogan RH, Lee J, Shen W, Gosnell J, et al. Primary hyperparathyroidism patients with positive preoperative sestamibi scan and negative ultrasound are more likely to have posteriorly located upper gland adenomas (PLUGs). Ann Surg Oncol. 2011;18:1717–22. https://doi.org/10.1245/s10434-010-1493-2.

47. Henry JF, Sebag F, Cherenko M, Ippolito G, Taieb D, Vaillant J. Endoscopic parathyroidectomy: why and when? World J Surg. 2008;32:2509–15. https://doi.org/10.1007/s00268-008-9709-3.

48. Martinez-Rodriguez I, Banzo I, Quirce R, Jimenez-Bonilla J, Portilla-Quattrociocchi H, Medina-Quiroz P, et al. Early planar and early SPECT Tc-99m sestamibi imaging: can it replace the dual-phase technique for the localization of parathyroid adenomas by omitting the delayed phase? Clin Nucl Med. 2011;36:749–53. https://doi.org/10.1097/RLU.0b013e318217568a.

49. Lindqvist V, Jacobsson H, Chandanos E, Backdahl M, Kjellman M, Wallin G. Preoperative 99Tc(m)-sestamibi scintigraphy with SPECT localizes most pathologic parathyroid glands. Langenbeck's Arch Surg. 2009;394:811–5. https://doi.org/10.1007/s00423-009-0536-2.

50. Lavely WC, Goetze S, Friedman KP, Leal JP, Zhang Z, Garret-Mayer E, et al. Comparison of SPECT/CT, SPECT, and planar imaging with single- and dual-phase (99m)Tc-sestamibi parathyroid scintigraphy. J Nucl Med. 2007;48:1084–9. https://doi.org/10.2967/jnumed.107.040428. jnumed.107.040428 [pii]

51. Perez-Monte JE, Brown ML, Shah AN, Ranger NT, Watson CG, Carty SE, et al. Parathyroid adenomas: accurate detection and localization with Tc-99m sestamibi SPECT. Radiology. 1996;201:85–91.

52. Burke JF, Naraharisetty K, Schneider DF, Sippel RS, Chen H. Early-phase technetium-99m sestamibi scintigraphy can improve preoperative localization in primary hyperparathyroidism. Am J Surg. 2013;205:269–73. https://doi.org/10.1016/j.amjsurg.2013.01.001. discussion 73

53. Patel CN, Salahudeen HM, Lansdown M, Scarsbrook AF. Clinical utility of ultrasound and 99mTc sestamibi SPECT/CT for preoperative localization of parathyroid adenoma in patients with primary hyperparathyroidism. Clin Radiol. 2010;65:278–87. https://doi.org/10.1016/j.crad.2009.12.005. S0009-9260(10)00024-3 [pii]

54. Pata G, Casella C, Besuzio S, Mittempergher F, Salerni B. Clinical appraisal of 99m technetium-sestamibi SPECT/CT compared to conventional SPECT in patients with primary hyperparathyroidism and concomitant nodular goiter. Thyroid. 2010;20:1121–7. https://doi.org/10.1089/thy.2010.0035.

55. Pata G, Casella C, Magri GC, Lucchini S, Panarotto MB, Crea N, et al. Financial and clinical implications of low-energy CT combined with 99m technetium-sestamibi SPECT for primary hyperparathyroidism. Ann Surg Oncol. 2011;18:2555–63. https://doi.org/10.1245/s10434-011-1641-3.

56. Ciappuccini R, Morera J, Pascal P, Rame JP, Heutte N, Aide N, et al. Dual-phase 99mTc sestamibi scintigraphy with neck and thorax SPECT/CT in primary hyperparathyroidism: a single-institution experience. Clin Nucl Med. 2012;37:223–8. https://doi.org/10.1097/RLU.0b013e31823362e5. 00003072-201203000-00001 [pii]

57. Shafiei B, Hoseinzadeh S, Fotouhi F, Malek H, Azizi F, Jahed A, et al. Preoperative (9)(9)mTc-sestamibi scintigraphy in patients with primary hyperparathyroidism and concomitant nodular goiter: comparison of SPECT-CT, SPECT, and planar imaging. Nucl Med Commun. 2012;33:1070–6. https://doi.org/10.1097/MNM.0b013e32835710b6.

58. Vercellino L, Alaoui NI, Faugeron I, Berenger N, de Labriolle-Vaylet C, Hindie E, et al. Lingual thyroid imaging with (1)(2)(3)I SPECT/CT. Eur J Nucl Med Mol Imaging. 2011;38:1173. https://doi.org/10.1007/s00259-011-1747-7.

59. Macdonald W, Armstrong J. Benign struma ovarii in a patient with invasive papillary thyroid cancer: detection with I-131 SPECT-CT. Clin Nucl Med. 2007;32:380–2. https://doi.org/10.1097/01.rlu.0000259642.36291.0d.

60. Zhen L, Li H, Liu X, Ge BH, Yan J, Yang J. The application of SPECT/CT for preoperative planning in patients with secondary hyperparathyroidism. Nucl Med Commun. 2013;34:439–44. https://doi.org/10.1097/MNM.0b013e32835f9447.

61. Tunninen V, Varjo P, Schildt J, Ahonen A, Kauppinen T, Lisinen I, et al. Comparison of five parathyroid scintigraphic protocols. Int J Mol Imaging. 2013;2013:921260.

62. Klingensmith WC 3rd, Koo PJ, Summerlin A, Fehrenbach BW, Karki R, Shulman BC, et al. Parathyroid imaging: the importance of pinhole collimation with both single- and dual-tracer acquisition. J Nucl Med Technol. Jun 2013;41(2):99–104.

63. Guerin C, Lowery A, Gabriel S, Castinetti F, Philippon M, Vaillant-Lombard J, et al. Preoperative imaging for focused parathyroidectomy: making a good strategy even better. Eur J Endocrinol. 2015;172(5):519–26.

64. Krakauer M, Wieslander B, Myschetzky PS, Lundstrom A, Bacher T, Sorensen CH, et al. A prospective comparative study of parathyroid dual-phase scintigraphy, dual-isotope subtraction scintigraphy, 4D-CT, and ultrasonography in primary hyperparathyroidism. Clin Nucl Med. Feb 2016;41(2):93–100.

SPECT/CT for Thyroid Cancer Imaging

5

Anca M. Avram and Hatice Savas

5.1 Introduction

Thyroid cancer is the most common endocrine malignancy in adults, with 52,890 estimated new cases (12,720 M:F 40,170) and 2180 deaths reported in the United States for 2020 [1]. The incidence of thyroid cancer continues to rise, with a 2.4-fold increase in incidence since 1975, based largely upon detection of small ($\leq$2 cm) tumors, which represents 87% of newly diagnosed cases [2, 3]. Based on histology, thyroid cancers are characterized as 80.2% papillary, 11.4% follicular, 3.1% Hurthle cell (or oxyphil), 3.5% medullary, and 1.7% anaplastic [4]. The 5-year survival rates for well-differentiated thyroid cancer (WDTC), which includes papillary thyroid cancer, follicular, and Hurthle cell histologies, are 99.8% for localized tumors, 97.0% with regional metastases, and 57.3% with distant metastases [5]. In general, stage for stage, the prognosis for papillary thyroid cancer and follicular thyroid cancer is similar; however, certain histologic subtypes of papillary thyroid cancer (such as tall cell variant, columnar cell variant, and diffuse sclerosing variant) and highly invasive follicular thyroid cancer have a worse prognosis [6].

Initial therapy for thyroid cancer includes near-total or total thyroidectomy with or without prophylactic or therapeutic central compartment neck dissection to remove the primary tumor and involved cervical lymph nodes [7]. New ATA guidelines permit withholding surgery or performing only lobectomy for selective patient population as well [7]. Therapeutic lateral neck compartmental dissection is performed for patients with metastatic lateral cervical lymphadenopathy [8–11]. Cervical nodal metastases are present in 20–50% of patients at initial diagnosis, even with small <1.0 cm intra-thyroidal tumors (microcarcinomas) [12–15]. The completeness of surgical resection is an important determinant of outcome, because residual metastatic lymph nodes represent the most common site of disease persistence or recurrence [16, 17]. After initial diagnosis, staging and risk stratification are used to individualize treatment decisions, inform on prognosis for an individual patient, decide on the use of postoperative 131-I therapy, and determine the frequency and intensity of follow-up [7].

The most commonly used staging system in thyroid cancer is the TNM staging of the American Joint Committee on Cancer/

A. M. Avram (✉)
Division of Nuclear Medicine, Department of
Radiology, University of Michigan Medical Center,
Ann Arbor, MI, USA
e-mail: ancaa@med.umich.edu

H. Savas
Nuclear Medicine/Radiology Department, Feinberg
School of Medicine, Northwestern Memorial
Hospital, Northwestern University, Chicago, IL, USA
e-mail: hatice.savas@nm.org

International Union against Cancer, currently in its eighth edition [7, 18]. Because this staging schema was developed to predict risk for death—not for recurrence—and does not take into account several independent prognostic variables, the American Thyroid Association (ATA) has developed a three-level risk stratification model for thyroid cancer [7]. Radioiodine (131-I) ablation is recommended for distant metastases, a primary tumor that is grossly invasive or larger than 4 cm, and selected patients with 1–4-cm tumors confined to the thyroid, with documented nodal metastases or other high-risk features. The ATA guidelines recommend against 131-I ablation for unifocal or multifocal microcarcinomas without high-risk features [7, 19, 20]. Surveillance of WDTC is usually performed using a combination of radioiodine scintigraphy, neck ultrasound, biochemical thyroglobulin (Tg) levels, and 18-F fluorodeoxyglucose (FDG) PET imaging.

5.2 Radioiodine SPECT/CT

Radionuclide imaging as traditionally performed with planar imaging using 131-I has suboptimal spatial resolution, and image quality is further degraded by septal penetration by energetic 364 keV gamma emissions. The paucity of anatomical information on radioiodine scans makes interpretation challenging; similarly, lesion localization with SPECT is also difficult and not used routinely. Furthermore, diagnostic CT has had a limited role in evaluation of WDTC due to the necessity to avoid iodinated contrast and the frequency of nodal metastases in non-enlarged cervical lymph nodes (<10 mm). Despite these individual limitations, the synergistic combination of functional and anatomical information provided by integrated SPECT/CT has been found to have many advantages over traditional planar imaging in various clinical settings. Optimal co-registration of tomographic volumes of data obtained by *gamma*-cameras with inline CT, with the patient in the same bed position, allows precise anatomic localization of radioactive foci. Additional benefits include CT-based attenuation correction and morphologic information from unenhanced CT with reduced milliampere seconds (mAs) and kilovoltage (kV) settings.

A growing number of studies confirm that radioiodine 131-I SPECT/CT is a powerful diagnostic tool, overcoming many limitations encountered with planar imaging interpretation [21–47]. Several excellent reviews of the clinical applications of hybrid 131-I/123-I SPECT/CT for imaging thyroid cancer provide context and outline the advantages of SPECT/CT imaging [41, 48–52]. 131-I SPECT/CT has been performed both at the time of first radioablation after total thyroidectomy and during long-term imaging surveillance, using either diagnostic activities between 37 and 450 MBq or post-therapy activities ranging from 1.1 to 8.1+ GBq. Advantages of SPECT/CT applied either selectively or routinely to planar scintigraphy studies have been consistently reported, with precise anatomic localization of foci of radioactivity allowing more accurate assignment of the findings as benign (thyroid remnants or normal physiologic distribution), or metastases in cervical nodes or at distant sites. One of the strengths of 131-I SPECT/CT is to substantially reduce the equivocal findings frequently reported on planar imaging. When unusual radioiodine biodistributions are encountered and a physiologic mimic of disease is suspected, SPECT/CT clarifies the interpretation of planar images, thereby avoiding false-positive diagnoses. SPECT/CT can solve difficult diagnostic interpretations and reveal metastatic lesions to unexpected sites or tissues. Due to CT-based attenuation correction, occasionally SPECT/CT can reveal more foci of pathologic activity as compared to planar studies. An integrated assessment of the size and iodine avidity of metastatic lesions based on the analysis of CT and SPECT components of the hybrid SPECT/CT study provides information about the likelihood of response to 131-I therapy and guides management decisions on alternative therapeutic options such as surgical excision for large metastases or external-beam radiation therapy for non-resectable and non–iodine-avid metastatic deposits.

5.3 Early Use of Radioiodine SPECT/CT

The use of radioiodine SPECT/CT in thyroid cancer was first reported by Even-Sapir et al. in a subgroup of 4 of 27 patients in whom SPECT/CT imaging was performed to evaluate endocrine neoplasms [53]. Subsequently, multiple studies have reported the incremental diagnostic value of SPECT/CT in patients with WDTC. The initial reports described the advantages of SPECT/CT applied to post-therapy 131-I scintigraphy: in a study evaluating co-registration of separately acquired SPECT and CT data with the aid of external fiducial markers, combined SPECT/CT improved diagnostic evaluation compared with SPECT alone in 15 of 17 patients (88%) [42]. Similarly, in a series of 25 patients with post-therapy 131-I scans, SPECT/CT improved diagnostic interpretation compared with planar images in 44% of radioactive foci, resulting in a change in management in 25% of patients [32]. In a study of 71 patients, of whom 54 had post-therapy imaging and 17 had diagnostic 131-I imaging, Tharp et al. described the incremental diagnostic value for SPECT/CT over planar imaging in 57% of patients [36]. One clear advantage of SPECT/CT reported by early investigators and confirmed in subsequent studies is its ability to substantially reduce the number of equivocal foci seen on planar imaging alone. Chen et al. reported that SPECT/CT accurately characterized 85% of foci considered inconclusive on planar imaging, resulting in altered management for 47% patients [25]. Aide et al. analyzed 55 patients studied with post-therapy 131-I scans, finding 29% indeterminate results on planar imaging and only 7% with SPECT/CT. Of the 16 patients with indeterminate planar scans, reclassification with SPECT/CT as positive or negative for disease correlated with the success or failure of radioiodine treatment at follow-up [22]. Our own experience has been primarily with diagnostic pre-ablation 131-I SPECT/CT performed after total thyroidectomy and prior to the first radioablation. In this setting, pre-ablation 131-I scans with SPECT/CT are used to complete postsurgical staging and guide subsequent 131-I therapy. In the neck region, we found incremental value of SPECT/CT over planar imaging in 53/130 (41%) of neck foci and described the typical appearances of thyroglossal duct remnant and thyroid bed remnant, which have long been recognized on planar imaging but are often difficult to distinguish from neck nodal metastases with confidence in the absence of SPECT/CT data [40, 41] (Fig. 5.1).

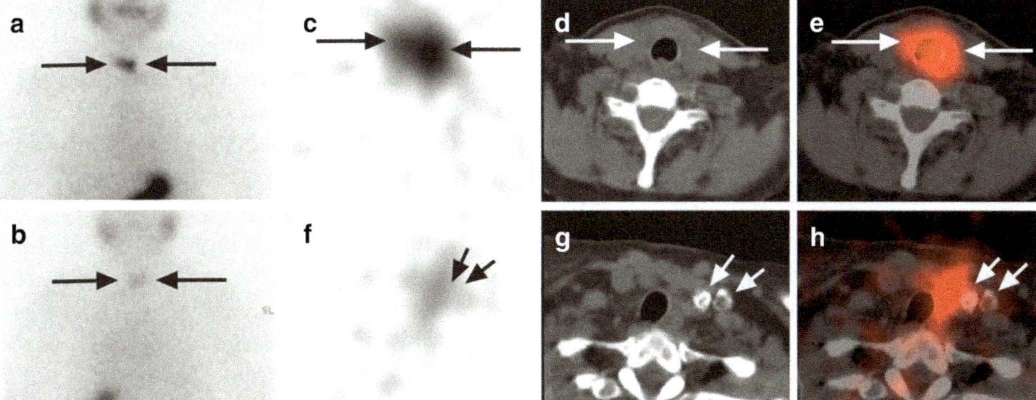

Fig. 5.1 Pre-ablation 131-I SPECT/CT imaging in a 65-year-old-woman with a 1.2 cm papillary thyroid cancer with capsular and vascular invasion, no extra-thyroidal extension, and positive surgical margins; no pathologic evidence for nodal disease (0/3 central nodes submitted); pT1b N0 Mx Stage I. Planar anterior (**a**) and posterior (**b**) images depict two foci of neck activity (arrows) corresponding on SPECT/CT (**c–e**) to soft tissue in bilateral thyroid bed (arrows) compatible with remnant thyroid tissue. However, more inferiorly, the SPECT/CT demonstrates two enlarged, partially calcified lymph nodes in the left lower neck (**g**, **h**, arrows), consistent with partially calcified metastatic cervical level IV lymph nodes, restaging: T1b N1b M0, Stage IV A disease. SPECT/CT is able to detect residual non–iodine-avid metastatic disease in patients with elevated thyroglobulin levels out of proportion to the focal activity seen on radioiodine scan. The patient was referred for surgical resection of non-iodine cervical nodal metastases. SPECT/CT can distinguish remnant thyroid tissue from nodal metastases

5.4 Utility of Post-therapy Radioiodine SPECT/CT

The majority of published reports on the utility of SPECT/CT are based on hybrid imaging performed on post-therapy scans following administration of therapeutic 131-I dosages. Maruoka et al. studied 147 patients with post-therapy 131-I SPECT/CT imaging. Compared to planar whole-body scans, SPECT/CT clarified all 25 equivocal interpretations in the neck region as either regional lymph nodes or thyroid remnant. For distant foci, SPECT/CT corrected the interpretation in 21/52 (40%) foci, identifying both metastases and benign physiological mimics, including 20 foci that were equivocal on planar imaging [28].

Kohlfuerst et al. reported on the impact of post-therapy SPECT/CT in a group of 41 patients: in 33 patients with neck lesions, SPECT/CT changed the N status in 12 (36.4%) and led to a treatment change in 8 (24.2%); in 19 patients with lesions distant from the neck, SPECT/CT changed the M status in 4 (21.1%) and led to a treatment change in 2 (10.5%); and for the entire group of 41 patients, SPECT/CT led to a treatment change in 10 (24.4%) [27]. Schmidt et al. published a study on nodal staging in 57 patients who underwent planar imaging and SPECT/CT after the first radioablation and concluded that SPECT/CT determines lymph nodal status more accurately than planar imaging: 6 of 11 lesions previously considered nodal metastases on planar imaging were reclassified as benign, and 11 of 15 lesions considered indeterminate on planar imaging were reclassified as nodal metastases; SPECT/CT provided information that clarified nodal status in 20 of 57 patients (35%), which resulted in a change in risk stratification in 25% [34]. Furthermore, the same group determined that the information obtained with 131-I SPECT/CT performed at the first radioablation can predict the occurrence or persistence of iodine-avid cervical nodal metastases in subsequent follow-up: 94% of nodal metastatic deposits smaller than 0.9 mL were eliminated after radioablation, whereas nodal metastases exceeding this size were less likely to completely resolve with 131-I

therapy [33]. Consequently, the size information obtained on CT data from the SPECT/CT study can be used to guide patient selection for excision of larger metastatic deposits. SPECT/CT improved anatomic localization of radioactive foci seen on planar post-therapy scans in 21% of cases, as demonstrated by Wang et al. in a study of 94 patients; in addition, SPECT/CT identified new metastatic foci unsuspected on planar imaging in 7% of patients. Most importantly, the additional information obtained with SPECT/CT resulted in reconsideration of the therapeutic approach in 22 of 94 patients (23%) [37].

The use of post-therapy SPECT/CT at the first radioablation has provided information on the incidence of nodal metastases in patients with T1 tumors ($\leq$2 cm, limited to the thyroid). The most commonly occurring papillary thyroid cancer in the United States is now microcarcinoma (T1a tumors, $\leq$1.0 cm); 45% of tumors in older patients (age $\geq$45 years) and 34% of tumors in younger patients (age <45 years) are microcarcinomas [54]. Although the long-term outcome of papillary microcarcinoma is excellent, it frequently spreads to cervical lymph nodes, as documented in 40.9% of cases in a series of 445 patients [14], and may occasionally metastasize to distant sites [55–58]. In a large, bicentric study of 151 patients, using a combination of nodal staging based on histopathology (pN1) (in 46% patients who underwent surgical neck dissection) and SPECT/CT imaging information (in 54% patients who did not undergo neck dissection), Mustafa et al. reported that nodal metastases occurred in 26% of T1 tumors and in 22% of microcarcinomas [30].

The effect of post-therapy 131-I SPECT/CT on American Thyroid Association (ATA) risk classification was assessed by Grewal et al. in a group of 148 intermediate- and high-risk patients (as initially determined based on clinical and histopathology criteria); 74% of patients underwent a first radioablation after total thyroidectomy, while 26% exhibited a rising trend in thyroglobulin levels and received 131-I therapy for treatment of presumed recurrent or metastatic disease. SPECT/CT changed nodal status in 15% of the postsurgical patients and in 21%

of patients suspected of recurrent tumor. Based on the SPECT/CT findings, the ATA risk classification changed due to upstaging in 7 of 109 patients (6.4%). Importantly, review of the CT images of the SPECT/CT study identified non–iodine-avid metastases in 32 of 148 patients (22%) and permitted lesion size determination. Additional imaging studies were avoided in 48% of patients [43]. Ciappucinni et al. demonstrated that post-ablation scintigraphy (planar and SPECT/CT) has prognostic value for predicting the therapeutic outcome of patients with thyroid cancer after total thyroidectomy and first radioablation. In 170 patients followed for a median of 29 months (range, 1.5–4.5 years) after initial 131-I ablative therapy, 32 (19%) patients presented with persistent or recurrent disease in subsequent follow-up: 18 with nodal metastases, 8 with distant metastases, and 6 with both nodal and distant metastases. In all patients free of disease at follow-up evaluations, initial post-ablative SPECT/CT was negative or equivocal for disease [26]. However, SPECT/CT was positive for disease in 78% of patients identified with persistent or recurrent disease at follow-up; post-therapy 131-I whole body scan (WBS) was negative in 22% with persistent or recurrent disease due to the presence of non–iodine-avid metastases, also reported by other groups in 20–30% of patients [43, 59]. The authors conclude that post-ablation scintigraphy (planar WBS and SPECT/CT) has 78% sensitivity and 100% specificity for predicting recurrent or persistent disease and is the sole independent prognostic variable for disease-free survival [26]. In a group of 42 patients studied with dual-phase post-therapy scans (performed at 3 and 7 days after therapeutic 131-I administration), SPECT/CT improved the interpretation of planar images regarding characterization of focal radioiodine accumulations as benign or malignant [44].

In a recent study with 323 patients, Szujo et al. evaluated the role of post-radioiodine therapy SPECT/CT of patients with WDTC in early-risk classification and in prediction of late prognosis. They performed both whole-body planar and neck/chest/abdomen SPECT/CT 3–6 days after the first radioactive iodine treatment. The patients were reevaluated 9–12 months later as well as at the end of follow-up (median 37 months). On the post-radioiodine therapy SPECT/CT, lymph node, lung, and bone involvement were detected in 22% of the patients including 61, 13, and 5 patients, respectively, resulting in early reclassification of 115 cases (36%). No evidence of disease was found in 251 cases at 9–12 months after radioiodine treatment and 269 patients at the end of follow-up. To predict residual disease at the end of follow-up, the sensitivities, specificities, and diagnostic accuracies of the current risk classification systems and SPECT/CT were: ATA: 77%, 47%, and 53%; ETA: 70%, 62%, and 64%; SPECT/CT: 61%, 88%, and 83%, respectively. Based on the study, the accuracy of post-radioiodine SPECT/CT outweighs that of the currently used ATA and ETA risk classification systems in the prediction of long-term outcome of DTC [60].

On a recent prospective study done in Greece, Malamitsi et al. aim to evaluate diagnostic accuracy of post-ablation SPECT/CT as compared to whole-body planar scan in N and M staging. The group also compared SPECT/CT to planar WBS to predict relapse of papillary thyroid cancer by following up the patients for 5 years. On the total number of abnormal uptake, WBS gave 27 false-positive (7.76%) and 23 false-negative (6.61%) results. On cross tabulation of NM stage through WBS and SPECT/CT, the study showed only 24 patients with N0M0 stage and 6 patients with N1M0 stage were classified correctly in the same stage by both methods. Considering N stage, there were 8 cases of upstaging from N0 to N1 and 14 cases of downstaging on SPECT/CT from N1 to N0. Considering M stage, there were 5 cases of upstaging from M0 to M1 and 2 cases of downstaging from M1 to M0. The agreement between the two methods was very low. The accuracy in determining NM stage was low on WBS (51.72%), while that of SPECT/CT 100%, respectively. There was a statistically significant difference in relapse by NM stage when assessed with SPECT/CT ($p = 0.033$), while with WBS this difference was not significant ($p = 0.209$) [46] (Table 5.1).

Table 5.1 Studies reporting utility of post-therapy 131-I SPECT/CT for evaluation of well-differentiated thyroid cancer

First author Year	#Pts/#Scans Design	Setting Indication	Isotope Activity	Camera CT settings	Site of radioactivity foci Findings/comments
Sjuzo 2017	323 Retro	Post-ablation Routine	131-I 1.1–3.7 GBq	DHV SPECT/CT 120 kV, 50 mAs	Predict residual disease at the end of follow-up Statistical comparison of residual disease detection Accuracy of post radio-iodine SPECT/CT outweighs ATA and ETA risk classification
Malamitsi 2019	58 Pros	Post-ablation Routine	131-I 2.8–5.6 GBq	Philips BrightView Not specified	On focus-based analysis, on the total number of findings, WBS gave 27 false positive (7.76%) and 23 false negative (6.61%) results The accuracy of WBS in determining NM stage was low (51.72%), while that of SPECT/CT 100%
Maruoka 2012	147/147 Retro	Post-ablation Routine	131-I 3.8–6.7 GBq	Symbia T6 130 kV, 30 mAs	Neck: SPECT/CT clarified all 25 equivocals as remnant or regional mets Distant: SPECT/CT clarified all 20 equivocal distant foci SPECT/CT improved interpretation in 21 of 52 (40%) distant foci
Qiu 2012	80/80 Retro	Suspected bone mets Routine	131-I 7.4 GBq	Not specified 120 kV	131-I SPECT/CT sensitivity 93%, specificity 97% FDG PET/CT sensitivity 86%, specificity 94% MDP bone scan sensitivity 73%, specificity 74%
Ciappuccini 2011	170/170 Pros	Post-ablation Routine	131-I 0.9–4.8 GBq	Symbia T2 ?kV, 60 mAs	Neck/distant; follow-up: median, 29 months, range 1.5–4.5 years Prognostic value SPECT/CT for recurrence in follow-up evaluation 32 (19%) pts had disease: 18 nodal mets, 8 distant mets and 6 both SPECT/CT negative or equivocal in all patients free of disease SPECT/CT positive in 78% and negative in 22% pts disease Post-ablation scintigraphy 78% sensitivity, 100% specificity for predicting recurrent disease
Oh 2011	140/140 Retro	Post-ablation Routine	131-I 3.6–9.3 GBq	Infinia Hawkeye 140 kV, 5 mAs	131-I SPECT/CT sensitivity 65%, specificity 95% 131-I planar sensitivity 65%, specificity 55% FDG PET/CT sensitivity 61%, specificity 94%
Wakabayashi 2011	42/42 Retro	Post-ablation Selected	131-I 3.7–7.4 GBq	Software registration 130 kV, 40 mAs	Interobserver agreement and reader confidence improved with SPECT/CT and delayed-phase (7 day) post-therapy imaging
Qiu 2010	561/ Pros	Post-ablation Repeat Rx Selected	131-I 3.7–7.4 GBq	Millenium Hawkeye 140 kV, 2.5 mAs	Neck SPECT/CT identified parapharyngeal metastases in 14/561 (2.5%) pts Parapharyngeal mets were associated with regional and/or distant mets

Grewal 2010	148/148 Retro	74% Post-ablation 26% Repeat Rx Routine	131-I 1.7–8 GBq	Philips Precedence 120 kV, adjusted mAs/ kg	Neck/distant SPECT/CT changed N in 15% postsurgical pts and in 21% recurrence pts SPECT/CT changed ATA risk classification in 7/109 (6.4%) pts SPECT/CT identified non-iodine avid metastases in 32/148 (22%) pts Size of nodal mets was measured on CT component of SPECT/CT SPECT/CT avoided additional imaging in 48% pts
Mustafa 2010	151/151 Pros	Post-ablation Routine	131-I 1.8–5.3 GBq	Symbia T2, T6 140 kV, 20–40 mAs	Neck Accuracy SPECT/CT > planar in 24.5% pts SPECT/CT revised N score in 24.5% pts LNM occurs in 26% pts with T1 and 22% pts with microcarcinoma (≤1 cm)
Schmidt 2010	81/81 Retro	Post-ablation Routine	131-I 1.5–5.3 GBq	Symbia T2, T6 140 kV, 40 mAs	Neck 60/61 pts with negative SPECT/CT were disease free at 5 months 17/20 pts with positive SPECT/CT were disease free at 5 months Metastasis size <0.9 mL predicted treatment success
Aide 2009	55/55 Pros	Post-ablation Routine	131-I 2.9–4.0 GBq	Symbia T2 ?kV, 60 mAs	Neck SPECT/CT clarified diagnosis in 16 pts with indeterminate planar scans: 9/9 pts without disease had negative SPECT/CT 4/5 pts with disease had positive SPECT/CT
Kohlfuerst 2009	41/53 Pros	56% Post-ablation 44% Repeat Rx Selected	131-I 2.9–7.5 GBq	Symbia T 130 kV, 25 mAs	Neck/distant SPECT/CT impact 21/33 (63.6%) pts, changed N score 12/33 (36.4%) SPECT/CT impact 14/19 (73.7%) pts, change M score 4/19 (21.1%) Changed treatment in 10/41 (24.4%) pts 8/33 (24.2%) changed treatment due to N score 2/19 (10.5%) changed treatment due to M score
Wang 2009	94/94 Retro	Post-ablation Routine	131-I 3.7–7.4 GBq	Infinia Hawkeye 140 kV, 2.5 mAs	Neck/distant Accuracy SPECT/CT > planar in 20/94 (21%) pts Changed treatment in 22/94 (23%) pts SPECT/CT identified unsuspected metastases in 7/94 (7%) pts
Schmidt 2009	57/57 Retro	Post-ablation Routine	131-I 1.5–5.3 GBq	Symbia T2, T6 140 kV, 40 mAs	Neck SPECT/CT completes N staging SPECT/CT changed N score in 20/57 (35%) pts SPECT/CT changed risk stratification in 14/57 (25%) pts

(continued)

Table 5.1 (continued)

First author Year	#Pts/#Scans Design	Setting Indication	Isotope Activity	Camera CT settings	Site of radioactivity foci Findings/comments
Chen 2008	23/37 Pros	Post-ablation Selected	131-I 3.7–7.4 GBq	Millenium Hawkeye 140 kV, 2.5 mAs	Neck/distant Incremental diagnostic value SPECT/CT > planar in 17/23 (74%) pts SPECT/CT clarified 69/81 (85%) inconclusive planar foci Changed treatment in 8/17 (47%) pts
Tharp 2004	71/71 Retro	39% Post-ablation 37% Repeat Rx 24% Dx Scan	131-I Rx: 1.4–9.7 GBq Dx: 143–187 MBq	Millenium Hawkeye 140 kV, 2.5 mAs	Neck/distant Incremental value SPECT/CT > planar in 41/71 (57%) pts Dx SPECT/CT changed treatment in 7/17 (41%) pts
Ruf 2004	25/25 Pros	Post-ablation Selected	131-I 3.7 GBq	Millenium Hawkeye 140 kV, 2.5 mAs	Neck/distant · SPECT/CT impact in 17/39 (44%) foci Changed treatment in 6/24 (25%) pts
Yamamoto 2003	17/17 Retro	Post-ablation Routine	131-I 3.7–7.4 GBq	Aquilon CT Picker Prism	Neck/distant Accuracy SPECT/CT > SPECT 15/17 (88%) pts Co-registration with external fiducial markers feasible

#Pts = number of patients; #Scans = number of scans; ds. = disease; Retro = retrospective study; Pros = prospective study; Rx = therapy; Post-ablation = post-therapy scan after first radioablation; FU Diagn. = diagnostic scan performed in follow-up after first radioablation; Routine = SPECT/CT performed on consecutive pts; Selected = SPECT/CT performed on selected pt group; LNM = lymph node metastases; Sen = sensitivity; Spec = specificity

Table 5.1 summarizes the results of studies reporting on the use of post-therapy 131-I scintigraphy with SPECT/CT.

5.5 Utility of Diagnostic and Pre-ablation Radioiodine SPECT/ CT

As emphasized on Martinique Principles, diagnostic radioactive iodine imaging has been shown to contribute to staging and risk stratification, especially by detection of unsuspected lymph node and distant metastases [20]. Surveillance diagnostic 131-I planar imaging is considered to have sensitivity for disease detection ranging between 45% and 75% (depending on the activity dose administered) and a high specificity of 96% and 100% [35, 36, 61–64]. Another radioiodine isotope, iodine-123 (123-I), may also be used for diagnostic imaging, with the advantages of a lower energy gamma emission and less likelihood for thyroidal tissue stunning. 123-I photon energy of 159 keV is better suited to modern gamma camera equipment; using low-energy, high-resolution collimators permit acquisition of high-quality images. Drawbacks of the use of 123-I are higher costs and a short half-life of 13 h, precluding multiday imaging and increasing the complexity of dosimetry calculations. Barwick et al. demonstrated in a group of 79 consecutive patients studied with surveillance 123-I planar imaging, SPECT, and SPECT/CT that SPECT/CT provided additional diagnostic information in 42% patients and provided further characterization in 70% foci seen on planar images. The authors calculated the diagnostic performance of SPECT/CT compared with planar scans and SPECT alone: planar studies demonstrated a sensitivity of 41%, specificity of 68%, and accuracy of 61%; SPECT studies demonstrated a sensitivity of 45%, specificity of 89%, and accuracy of 78%; SPECT/CT provided significant improvement in specificity, with a calculated sensitivity of 50%, specificity of 100%, and accuracy of 87% (the study group included 11 patients with non–iodine-avid disease demonstrated on anatomic imaging and elevated thyroglobulin levels) [23].

As with post-therapy 131-I scans, the incremental value of SPECT/CT as compared with planar WBS in the diagnostic or pre-ablative setting, results from improved identification and interpretation of focal uptake, correct anatomic localization and characterization of radioactive foci, and precise differentiation between metastatic lesions versus benign uptake in thyroid remnant tissue or physiologic radioiodine distribution in normal organs. Menges et al. reported on the results of 139 scans with SPECT/CT performed in 123 patients: 82 studies were performed for diagnostic follow up evaluation (follow-up diagnostic scans) after radioablation and 57 studies were performed after 131-I therapy (post-therapy scans). The sensitivity of planar and SPECT/CT images were both 62%, with no additional detection of iodine-avid lesions on SPECT/CT compared to planar [29]. However, when non-iodine-avid disease in 27 patients was included in the analysis, SPECT/CT improved sensitivity from 61% to 74%. The main benefit of SPECT/CT was significantly higher specificity than the planar images, 94% versus 74%. We have observed that occasionally SPECT/CT reveals new foci of activity as compared to planar images, particularly when additional anatomic information based on CT dataset increases diagnostic certainty for identification of a new lesion (Fig. 5.2). In a group of 117 patients studied with surveillance planar WBS and SPECT/CT (of whom 108 patients underwent diagnostic 123-I and 9 patients underwent post-therapy 131-I scans), Spanu et al. demonstrated that SPECT/CT has incremental value over planar scanning in 67.8% of patients. SPECT/CT identified more foci of pathologic activity (158 foci on SPECT/CT compared with only 116 foci on planar imaging), changed the treatment approach in 35.6% of patients with disease, and led to avoidance of unnecessary 131-I therapy in 20% of patients without disease [35]. The use of SPECT/CT technology permitted identification of parapharyngeal metastases in 14 of 561 patients (2.5%); in this group, the presence of parapharyngeal metas-

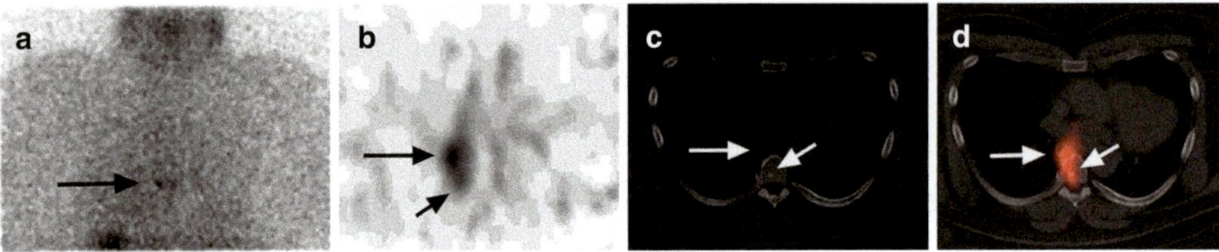

Fig. 5.2 Pre-ablation 131-I SPECT/CT imaging in a 56-year-old-man with a 7.5 cm minimally invasive follicular thyroid cancer in the left lobe with vascular and capsular invasion, extra-thyroidal extension, and negative surgical margins; with central compartment nodal disease (3+/3 central nodes submitted); pT3 N1a Mx, Stage III disease. Planar posterior chest image (**a**) depicts faint midline activity in the thorax (arrows) with an appearance suggestive of retained secretions in the esophagus. Correlative axial SPECT (**b**), axial CT (**c**), and fused SPECT/CT (**d**) demonstrate two adjacent foci in the thorax, the first is more intense and localizes to the esophagus compatible with retained secretions (long arrow); however, the second mild focus localizes to a sclerotic focus in the thoracic vertebra compatible with bone metastasis (short arrow). Restaging: T3 N1a M1, Stage IVC disease, leading to administration of 131-I therapy based on dosimetry calculations. Subsequent 131-I scan obtained at 6 months after 230 mCi (8.5 GBq) 131-I therapy documented interval resolution of bone metastasis (not shown)

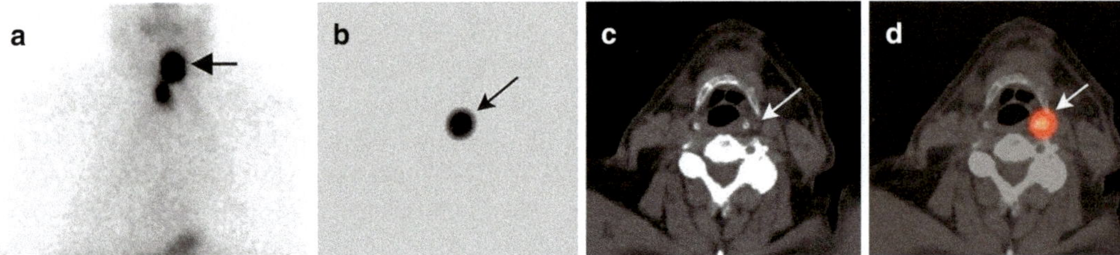

Fig. 5.3 Pre-ablation 131-I SPECT/CT scan in a 71-year-old-man with multifocal papillary thyroid cancer, the largest lesion measuring 3.0 cm in the left lobe, with extra-thyroidal extension, and negative surgical margins; 8+/21 central and 4+/8 left lateral metastatic lymph nodes were resected; pT3 N1b Mx, Stage IV A disease. Planar scan (**a**) depicts two foci of neck activity with the superior focus (arrow) corresponding on SPECT/CT (**b–d**) to a small iodine-avid cervical level IIA lymph node adjacent to the horn of the hyoid bone (arrows). Although pre-ablation I-131 scan did not alter the TNM Stage, the demonstration of an iodine-avid target in the left neck allowed selection of a medium 131-I activity for treatment, instead of low-dose 131-I remnant ablation. The more inferior neck focus was localized to the thyroid bed compatible with remnant thyroid tissue. SPECT/CT allows accurate identification of the epicenter of uptake for precise anatomic lesion localization

tases was associated with regional or distant metastases [31]. Identification of parapharyngeal lymph node metastases on SPECT/CT is particularly relevant, as these metastatic nodal deposits may remain undetected on routine neck ultrasound (Fig. 5.3).

In a group of 53 postsurgical patients studied with SPECT/CT at the first radioablation (47 with pre-ablation scans, and 6 with post-therapy scans), Wong et al. demonstrated incremental diagnostic value for SPECT/CT over planar imaging for interpretation of 47.6% of foci, as follows: in 53 of 130 neck activity foci (41%) and 17 of 17 distant foci (100%),

SPECT/CT provided clear anatomic lesion localization and lesion size measurement for predicting the likelihood of response to 131-I therapy. Rapid exclusion of physiologic activity or contamination resulted in elimination of equivocal interpretations on planar scans. Reader confidence increased for interpretation of 104 of 147 foci (71%) seen on planar images after the review of SPECT/CT [40]. This study also demonstrated that SPECT/CT imaging using low diagnostic 131-I activity (37 MBq, 1 mCi) is feasible and produces images of excellent diagnostic quality. The same investigators used pre-ablation 131-I scans with

SPECT/CT to complement clinical and histopathological data in order to complete staging and risk stratification before radioablation [39]. The patients were staged according to the TNM system using three levels of sequential information: histopathology and chest radiography, planar WBS, and SPECT/CT. The patients were restaged according to the findings on 131-I scintigraphy (planar alone, followed by combined planar and SPECT/CT information). Compared with histopathologic analysis, planar imaging and SPECT/CT changed the postsurgical thyroid cancer stage for 21% of patients. Identification of unsuspected nodal and distant metastases resulted in prescription of appropriately higher therapeutic activities whereas demonstration of residual thyroid tissue (i.e., thyroid remnant) in the absence of high-risk histopathologic features reduced the 131-I ablative dose or eliminated the need for ablation. Information obtained from the diagnostic pre-ablation planar WBS and SPECT/CT scans changed the prescribed radioactivity in 58% patients, as compared with the initially proposed therapy based on histopathologic risk stratification alone.

In a larger cohort of 320 patients studied with pre-ablation 131-I scans, the impact of diagnostic pre-ablation 131-I planar and SPECT/CT scintigraphy on N and M scores, and TNM stage was assessed in younger age <45 years, $n = 138$ (43%) and older age ≥45 years, $n = 182$ (57%) patients [65]. Subgroup analysis regarding the detection of regional and distant metastases for small tumors was also performed in 49 patients (15%) with T1a (size ≤1.0 cm) and 67 patients (21%) with T1b (size >1.0 and ≤2.0 cm).The study demonstrated that in younger patients pre-ablation 131-I scans with SPECT/CT detected distant metastases in 5/138 patients (4%), and nodal metastases in 61/138 patients (44%), including unsuspected nodal metastases in 24 of 63 (38%) patients initially assigned pN0 or pNx. In older patients, distant metastases were detected in 18/182 patients (10%), and nodal metastases in 51/182 patients (28%), including unsuspected nodal metastases in 26 of 108 (24%) patients initially assigned pN0 or pNx. Pre-ablation scans with SPECT/CT detected distant metastases in 2/49 (4%) T1a and 3/67 (4.5%) T1b patients.

For the entire group of 320 patients, pre-ablation 131-I scans with SPECT/CT detected regional metastases in 35%, and distant metastases in 8% of patients. Information acquired with pre-ablation scans changed staging in 4% of younger, and 25% of older patients. In summary, pre-ablation planar and SPECT/CT imaging contributed to staging in thyroid cancer and facilitated the selective use of 131-I therapy for targeting regional and distant metastases identified with radioiodine scintigraphy.

Diagnostic pre-ablation 131-I scans are unlikely to underestimate the extent of metastatic disease, as demonstrated by the high concordance rate (94%) between pre-ablation and post-therapy scans. In only 2% of patients did post-therapy scans reveal metastatic lesions which upstaged disease status as compared to diagnostic 131-I scan. When SPECT/CT technology is applied to pre-ablation WBS scans, the information obtained completes postsurgical staging before management decisions regarding 131-I therapy are made. Performing diagnostic radioiodine scans with planar and SPECT/CT imaging provides the opportunity to identify patients with unsuspected regional and distant metastases, defines the target of 131-I therapy, and permits adjustment of prescribed therapeutic radioactivity and dosimetry calculations, when high-dose 131-I therapy is considered [39, 66]. Avoidance of unnecessary 131-I therapy is equally important for patients in whom residual and/or metastatic disease has been excluded. SPECT/CT improves characterization of focal central neck activity as benign thyroid remnant when pathology review demonstrates no evidence of extra-thyroidal tumor extension and negative surgical excision margins, justifying omission of radioiodine administration in such patients [49] (Table 5.2).

Table 5.2 summarizes the results of studies reporting on the use of diagnostic radioiodine scintigraphy with SPECT/CT.

Table 5.2 Studies reporting utility of diagnostic SPECT/CT for evaluation of differentiated thyroid cancer

First author Year	#Pts/#Scans Design	Setting Indication	Isotope Activity	Camera CT settings	Site of radioactivity foci Findings/comments
Avram 2013	320/320 Pros	Pre-ablation Routine	131-I 37 MBq	Symbia T6 140 kV, 100 mAs	SPECT/CT change staging in 4% of younger and 35% older pts Identified regional disease in 35% and unsuspected distant disease in 8%
Menges 2012	123/139 Retro	59% FU Diagn. 41% Post-ablation Routine	131-I 407 MBq	Symbia T2, T6 140 kV, 40 mAs	SPECT/CT sensitivity 62%, specificity 98% for iodine-avid ds SPECT/CT sensitivity 78%, specificity 98% for non-iodine-avid ds Planar sensitivity 62%, specificity 78% for iodine-avid ds
Kim 2011	13/20 Retro	35% Pre-ablation 55% FU Diagn. 10% Post-ablation Selected	131-I 59–85 MBq 123-I 17–81 MBq	Symbia T2 Millenium Hawkeye CT dose 0.33 mSv	All foci were localized with SPECT/CT distinguishing benign uptake SPECT/CT supported decision not to treat with 131-I in 2 patients SPECT/CT did not contribute in 3 of 13 patients
Blum 2011	40/40 Retro	38% Pre-ablation 62% Post-ablation Selected	131-I 74 MBq	Symbia T6 Caredose 4D	SPECT/CT confirmed cryptic findings of thyroid origin ($n = 10$) SPECT/CT confirmed cryptic findings of non-thyroid origin ($n = 39$) This led to 32 cases whereby radioiodine treatment was avoided
Wong 2010	48/48 Retro	Pre-ablation Selected	131-I 37 MBq	Symbia T6 140 kV, 100 mAs	Neck/distant SPECT/CT changed TNM stage in 10/48 (21%) pts SPECT/CT changed proposed 131-I dose selection in 28/48 (58%) pts SPECT/CT identified unsuspected metastases in 4/8 pts with M1
Barwick 2010	79/85 Retro	FU Diagn. Routine	123-I 350– 400 MBq	Millenium Hawkeye 140 kV, 2.5 mAs	Neck/distant Planar: Sen 41% Spec 68% Accuracy 61% SPECT: Sen 45% Spec 89% Accuracy 78% SPECT/CT: Sen 50% Spec 100% Accuracy 87% SPECT/CT provided additional information in 42% pts and 70% foci
Spanu 2009	117/117 Pros	92% FU Diagn. 8% Post-ablation Routine	123-I 185 MBq	Millenium Hawkeye Infinia Hawkeye 4 140 kV, 2.5 mAs	Neck/distant SPECT/CT has incremental value over planar scan in 67.8% pts SPECT/CT changed treatment in 35.6% pts with disease SPECT/CT led to avoidance of 131-I therapy in 20% pts without disease SPECT/CT identified 158 foci compared to only 116 foci on planar
Wong 2008	53/56 Retro	89% Pre-ablation 11% FU Diagn. Selected	131-I 37–150 MBq	Symbia T6 140 kV, 100 mAs	Neck/distant Diagnostic value SPECT/CT > planar in 53/130 (41%) neck foci Diagnostic value SPECT/CT > planar in 17/17 (100%) distant foci SPECT/CT using diagnostic 131-I activities feasible Allows adjustment of prescribed radioiodine activity

#Pts = number of patients; # Scans = number of scans; Retro = retrospective study; Pros = prospective study; Pre-ablation = diagnostic scan before first radioablation; Post-ablation = post-therapy scan after first radioablation; FU Diagn. = diagnostic scan performed in follow-up after first radioablation; Routine = SPECT/CT performed on consecutive pts; Selected = SPECT/CT performed on selected pt group; LNM = lymph node metastases, Sen = sensitivity, Spec = specificity

5.6 SPECT/CT Evaluation of Unusual Radioactive Distributions

Unusual patterns of radioiodine biodistribution which mimic metastatic disease are well recognized and may raise a diagnostic dilemma for interpretation of planar radioiodine scintigraphy [67, 68]. Physiological radioiodine activity is seen in salivary glands, mucosa, breast, thymus, stomach, bowel, kidneys, and bladder. Salivary and urinary contamination should also be considered when unexpected focal activity distribution occurs. SPECT/CT is an excellent diagnostic tool for rapid evaluation of suspected physiologic mimics and can accurately localize radioiodine distribution to salivary glands, dental fillings, nasolacrimal secretions, retrosternal goiter, esophageal or airway secretions, hiatal hernias, bowel diverticula, breast, skin contamination, and benign uptake related to radioiodine retention in cysts, bronchiectasis, esophageal diverticulum, thymus, spermatocele, functional ovarian cyst, benign struma ovarii, teratoma, or menstruating uterus [38, 40, 69–78]. Several authors have demonstrated the utility of SPECT/CT for the evaluation of cryptic findings on radioiodine scintigraphy [24] including a wide range of physiological mimics of disease [79]. In a pictorial review of radioiodine scintigraphy for thyroid cancer evaluation, we have demonstrated the utility of SPECT/CT imaging for problem-solving in difficult interpretation cases, including salient examples of focal radioiodine uptake in the neck, thorax, and body, where benign and pathological etiologies are virtually indistinguishable on planar imaging, yet easily characterized with SPECT/CT [80].

Several reports outline the usefulness of SPECT/CT for revealing unusual metastatic lesions in the liver, kidney, central nervous system, erector spinae muscle, and rectus abdominis muscle [81–85]. SPECT/CT is useful for evaluation of distant metastatic disease [25, 27, 35, 37, 40, 86, 87]. SPECT/CT can confirm osseous and pulmonary sites of metastases, providing additional anatomical diagnostic information to guide management decisions. In the thorax, SPECT/CT can precisely localize malignancy to bone (ribs or spine), lung, or mediastinal lymph nodes (Fig. 5.4).

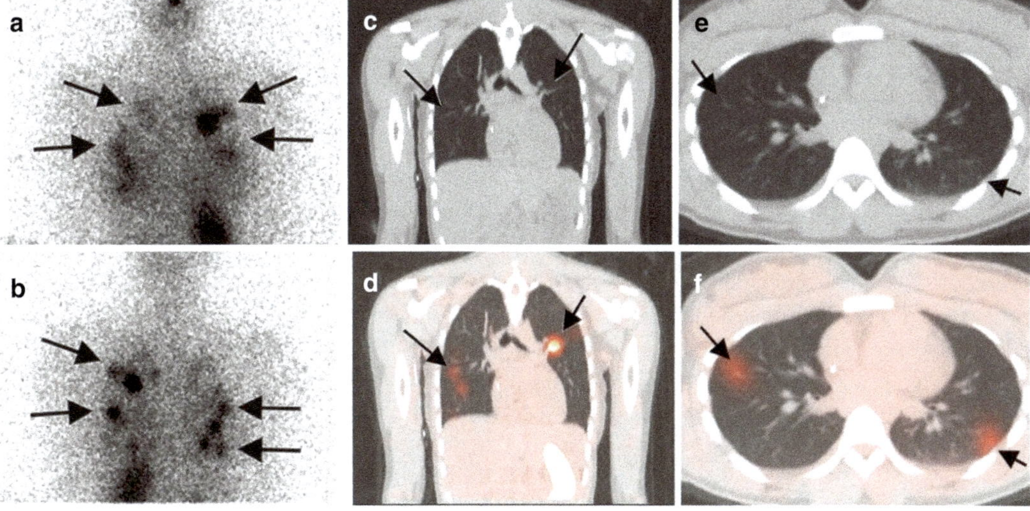

Fig. 5.4 Pre-ablation 131-I scan in a 19-year-old-woman with unifocal papillary thyroid cancer (2 cm tumor in the left lobe with focal lymphovascular invasion and extrathyroidal extension) associated with lymph nodal metastases in the left neck at presentation: 3+/17 lymph nodes resected in the surgical specimen of total thyroidectomy; T3 N1b Mx, Stage I disease. Planar anterior (**a**) and posterior (**b**) images demonstrate the presence of pulmonary metastatic disease. T1b N1b M1, Stage II disease. Correlative coronal, axial CT (**c** and **e**), and fused SPECT/CT (**d** and **f**) images reveal multifocal chest activity corresponding to multiple bilateral pulmonary nodules, the largest of which measures 5 mm. Identification of unsuspected pulmonary metastases on pre-ablation scan permitted administration of high-dose 131-I therapy based on dosimetry calculations

5.7 Changes to Clinical Management

Most of the changes in the new eighth edition of the American Joint Committee on Cancer/International Union against Cancer will be to downstage a significant number of patients into lower stages and aim to reflect their low risk of dying from thyroid cancer more accurately. It is important to remember that the risk of death from thyroid cancer does not match the risk of recurrence in many patients. Therefore, more individualized and accurate assessments of the risk of recurrence and dying from the disease should have a substantial impact on both initial therapeutic decision-making (e.g., extent of thyroid surgery, need for radioactive iodine treatment, and/or need for TSH suppressive therapy) and on follow-up management strategies [18]. In conjunction with pre-ablation or post-therapy scans, SPECT/CT has been used for completion of thyroid cancer staging, impacting clinical management, and providing important prognostic information. It is a powerful diagnostic tool which allows precise localization of radioactivity and improved characterization of benign and malignant radioactivity distributions compared to planar imaging. Routine implementation of SPECT/CT imaging with radioiodine scintigraphy may lead to reassessment of current management protocols in thyroid cancer. The use of radioiodine SPECT/CT has been reported to change clinical management in a significant numbers of patients, both when used routinely on all consecutive patients and when used on selected patients with inconclusive planar images. Potential changes in management include decisions such as administration or withholding radioiodine treatment, referral for surgical reintervention and guiding the extent of surgery, patient selection for external-beam radiation therapy, and the use of alternative imaging strategies such as 18F-FDG PET/CT when non–iodine-avid metastatic disease is suspected. Depending on the clinical context, the timing of the radioiodine scan (pre-ablation or post-therapy), and the therapeutic protocols at each institution, a change in management has

been reported in 11–58% patients in various studies [24, 26, 28, 33, 36, 37, 40, 51].

Radioiodine SPECT/CT also provides prognostic information regarding success of radioiodine treatment as determined by clinical follow-up and surveillance diagnostic 131-I whole-body imaging. Schmidt et al. using short-term follow-up reported that almost all patients with negative post-therapy SPECT/CT (60/61 patients) had a negative 5-month diagnostic 131-I scan, and even the majority with positive post-therapy SPECT-CT (17/20 patients) still had negative diagnostic scan [33]. The authors identified a neck nodal volume of <0.9 mL on SPECT/CT to be highly likely to respond to 131-I therapy and commented that surgical reintervention for resection of lymph nodal metastases of this size would be excessive. The positivity or negativity for disease as determined by post-therapy SPECT/CT correlated more closely to success or failure of radioiodine treatment than the planar imaging findings [22]. Identification of unsuspected distant metastases in 4% of younger patients and 10% of older patients was associated with an upstage in disease status and led to prescription of therapeutic 131-I activity based on dosimetric calculations. In patients for whom 131-I therapy is considered based on histopathologic prognostic factors, pre-ablation 131-I scintigraphy can detect metastases in normal-size cervical lymph nodes (which may not appear suspicious on postoperative neck ultrasonography), can identify pulmonary micrometastases (which are too small to be detected on routine chest X-ray and may remain undetected on computed tomography), and can diagnose bone metastases at an early stage before cortical disruption is identified on bone X-rays. The information obtained with diagnostic radioiodine studies has the potential to impact management decisions, e.g., whether to proceed or omit therapeutic 131-I administration, refer for surgical debulking prior to 131-I therapy, or perform additional imaging studies when non–iodine-avid disease is demonstrated by negative radioiodine scans but elevated thyroglobulin levels. The benefits of obtaining this information at an early postoperative time point in the disease process are not negligible, because

131-I therapy is most effective for smaller metastatic deposits, and early identification of regional and distant metastases is important for successful therapy [33, 88] (Fig. 5.5).

To determine the effectiveness of a management strategy based on radiotheragnostics principles, Avram et al. analyzed their routine evaluation with postoperative diagnostic 131-I

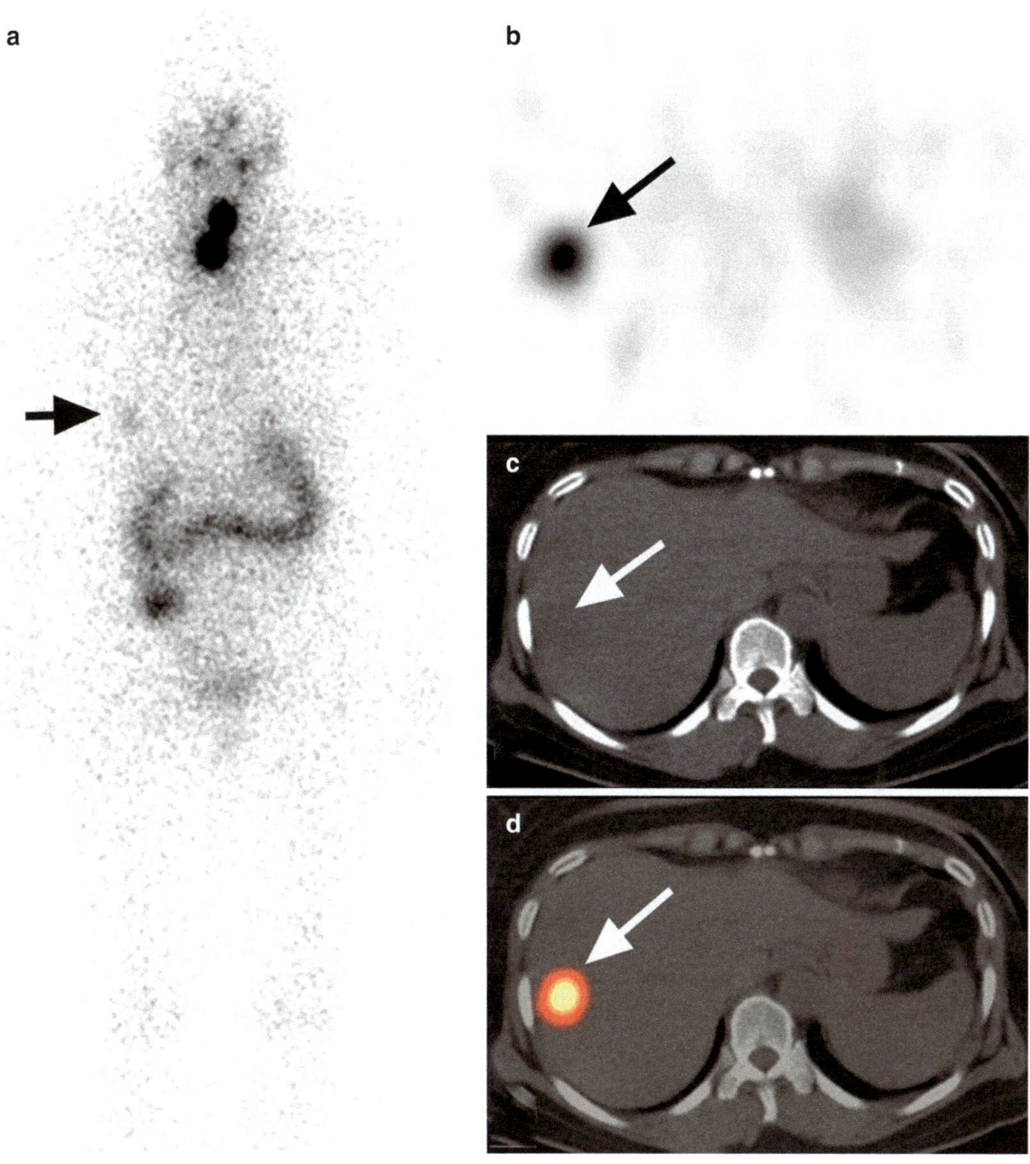

Fig. 5.5 Diagnostic 131-I SPECT/CT imaging in a 56-year-old-woman with 1.2 cm papillary thyroid cancer without capsular invasion, no extra-thyroidal extension, and negative surgical margins; no pathologic evidence for nodal disease (0/3 central nodes submitted); pT1b N0 M0, Stage I disease. Planar scan (**a**) depicts focal neck activity characterized on SPECT/CT as remnant thyroid tissue. There is a faint focus of uptake in the right lower thorax on planar anterior whole-body image (arrow) Correlative axial SPECT (**b**), CT (**c**), and fused SPECT/CT (**d**) reveal focal activity in the liver corresponding to a 0.8 cm hypodense lesion (arrows) also confirmed on liver US and MRI, consistent with hepatic metastasis. Restaging: T1b N0 M1, Stage IVC disease. Identification of unsuspected hepatic metastasis on pre-ablation scan permitted administration of high-dose 131-I therapy instead of low-dose 131-I remnant ablation. Subsequent 131-I scan obtained at 6 months after 200 mCi (7.4 GBq) 131-I therapy confirmed interval resolution of liver metastasis (not shown)

SPECT/CT scans for completion of staging and risk stratification and individualized 131-I therapy guided by diagnostic scan findings in addition to surgical pathology and postoperative stimulated thyroglobulin (Tg) levels on 320 patients. The study showed that the patient-individualized therapeutic strategy is associated with good clinical outcomes with complete response after a single postoperative 131-I treatment in 88% of patients presenting with histopathology risk factors and regional metastases and in 42% patients with distant metastatic disease [89].

tomy for differentiated thyroid cancer They found 341 positive foci in 150 patients (97.4%) by SPECT/CT and 213 corresponding positive finding in 118 patients (76.6%) by US. Ultrasound detected 30–46% of iodine uptake foci in superior lateral regions, 49% in pyramidal lobe/thyroglossal duct area (both $p < 0.05$), 74–77% in inferior lateral regions, and 22% in isthmus (both $p > 0.05$). They concluded that US is less sensitive than post-therapy 131-I SPECT/CT scans for remnant detection in patients after thyroidectomy, especially for remnants located above the lower margin of thyroid cartilage [92].

5.8 Comparison to Other Imaging Modalities

Qiu et al. studied patients with suspected bone metastases and compared the test performance of 99mTc-methylene diphosphonate (MDP) bone scan, 131-I SPECT/CT, and FDG PET. They found that 131-I SPECT/CT sensitivity 93% and specificity 97% were higher than FDG PET sensitivity 86% and specificity 94%, and both were higher than bone scintigraphy sensitivity 79% and specificity 84%. FDG PET positivity was associated with poor prognostic features, survival rate of 69% compared to 93% in FDG PET negative patients [90].

Oh et al. studied the performance of WBS, SPECT/CT, and FDG PET. The 131-I SPECT/CT sensitivity of 65% and specificity of 95% were similar to FDG PET sensitivity of 61% and specificity of 98%, and both were higher than planar whole-body scan sensitivity 65% and specificity 55%. Subgroup analysis found that 131-I-SPECT/CT sensitivity was better in patients with a single 131-I treatment, whereas FDG PET had higher sensitivity patients with multiple 131-I challenges [91]. On a recent study performed with Bulzacka and Macarawicz, they evaluated the utility of neck US for detection of thyroid remnants and compared the diagnostic capability of identification of lymph node metastases in neck with post-therapy 131-I SPEC/CT and neck ultrasound in patients after thyroidec-

5.9 Utility of Radioiodine SPECT/CT for Lesional Dosimetry

Future directions for the use of hybrid radioiodine imaging involve the use of SPECT/CT to perform lesion-specific dosimetry. Lesion radioiodine uptake and retention can be quantified on SPECT, and tumor volume can be measured on the CT component of the SPECT/CT study, permitting calculation of radiation absorbed dose to tumor. Follow-up with SPECT/CT can be used to determine therapeutic responses and assess tumor shrinkage. An example of this approach has been reported in a patient with a large skull metastasis causing infringement on the brain [93]. Other authors have demonstrated the feasibility of patient-specific three-dimensional dosimetry using multiple SPECT/CT images, in which the patient's own anatomy and spatial distribution of radioactivity over time are factored into the calculation of radiation absorbed dose to tumor (lesion dosimetry) or to an organ of interest (organ dosimetry) [94]. The CT images of SPECT/CT studies are used to provide the density and composition of each voxel for use in a Monte Carlo calculation and to define organs or regions of interest for computing spatially averaged doses. The longitudinal series of SPECT images is used to perform time integration of activity in each voxel and to obtain the cumulated activity per voxel [94]. The goal of patient-specific voxel-based absorbed dose calculations is to improve prediction of the biologic effects of radionuclide therapy.

5.10 Disadvantages and Limitations of SPECT/CT

Disadvantages of SPECT/CT include additional imaging time and possible patient discomfort and claustrophobia from lying in a confined position for approximately 20 min in the tightly enclosed space of the SPECT/CT gantry, and additional radiation exposure from the CT component of the study (1–4 mSv with each acquisition) [95]. SPECT/CT has an axial field of view limited to 40 cm in the current imaging systems; therefore, evaluation of both neck and distant radioactive foci may require two separate SPECT/CT acquisitions [95]. Analysis of benefit and potential risk should be performed on an individual basis in the young female and particularly in the pediatric population [96]. Kim studied 13 children with 131-I/123-I diagnostic SPECT/CT reporting that the SPECT/CT helped clarify equivocal foci in the neck, helping to inform decisions including not to proceed to 131-I treatment [97].

Recognizing the limitations of SPECT/CT is important: the spatial resolution of SPECT is limited by the partial-volume effect in small lesions; although metastases in normal-sized neck lymph nodes are frequently diagnosed, micro-metastatic lesions cannot be detected with SPECT/CT. Similarly, SPECT/CT is insensitive for the detection of residual locally invasive thyroid cancer after surgery, unless there is gross residual tumor volume or anatomic findings of invasion. Therefore, SPECT/CT radioiodine studies must always be interpreted in the context of the surgical pathology report, which clarifies the presence or absence of tumor invasion into local structures and completion of surgical resection. These elements are of critical importance when one is interpreting the significance of para-tracheal central neck activity as benign thyroid remnant versus residual disease. When patho-logic review of the surgical resection specimen of total thyroidectomy demonstrates no evidence of tumor extrathyroidal extension and surgical exci-sion margins are negative, focal paratracheal cen-tral neck activity can be characterized as a benign thyroid remnant. Non–iodine-avid disease, which occurs in 20–30% of differentiated thyroid can-cer [59, 98], may remain undetected on SPECT/CT and lead to false-negative interpretations (Fig. 5.1). The possibility of non–iodine-avid dis-ease needs to be considered in the context of Hurthle cell thyroid cancer, papillary thyroid cancer with unfavorable histology (e.g., tall cell, columnar, or cribriform variants), and poorly dif-ferentiated thyroid cancer (such as trabecular, insular, or solid variants). Therefore, the review of histopathology and biochemical data—thyro-globulin, thyrotropin, free thyroxine—remains essential for accurate interpretation of the find-ings on radioiodine planar and SPECT/CT scintigraphy.

5.11 Conclusion

Considerable progress in the interpretation of radioiodine scintigraphy in thyroid cancer has been achieved by the introduction of SPECT/CT. SPECT/CT is a powerful diagnostic tool that allows accurate anatomic localization and charac-terization of radioiodine foci and has substantially improved the interpretation of classic radioiodine scintigraphy. SPECT/CT reduces the number of equivocal radioiodine foci encountered in the neck and body and allows more precise characterization of the etiology (benign vs. malignant) of focal radioiodine uptake seen on WBS, contributing to completion of staging in thyroid cancer by improved characterization of N and M scores. Accurate staging and risk stratification are impor-tant for thyroid cancer management as they deter-mine the prognosis for survival and risk of recurrence and guide therapeutic decisions and intensity of surveillance. The additional informa-tion obtained with SPECT/CT impacts manage-ment in a significant number of patients. The new technology of SPECT/CT has changed the field and may lead to reassessment of current manage-ment protocols and guidelines in thyroid cancer.

Acknowledgments None.

Disclosure Statement: The authors have nothing to disclose.

References

1. Siegel RL, Miller KD, Jemal A. Cancer statistics, 2020. CA Cancer J Clin. 2020;70(1):7–30.
2. Davies L, Welch HG. Increasing incidence of thyroid cancer in the United States, 1973–2002. JAMA. 2006;295(18):2164–7.
3. Vaccarella S, Dal Maso L, Laversanne M, Bray F, Plummer M, Franceschi S. The impact of diagnostic changes on the rise in thyroid cancer incidence: a population-based study in selected high-resource countries. Thyroid. 2015;25(10):1127–36.
4. Hundahl SA, Fleming ID, Fremgen AM, Menck HR. A National Cancer Data Base report on 53,856 cases of thyroid carcinoma treated in the U.S., 1985–1995 [see comments]. Cancer. 1998;83(12):2638–48.
5. Simard EP, Ward EM, Siegel R, Jemal A. Cancers with increasing incidence trends in the United States: 1999 through 2008. CA Cancer J Clin. 2012;62(2):118–28.
6. Volante M, Landolfi S, Chiusa L, Palestini N, Motta M, Codegone A, et al. Poorly differentiated carcinomas of the thyroid with trabecular, insular, and solid patterns: a clinicopathologic study of 183 patients. Cancer. 2004;100(5):950–7.
7. Haugen BR, Alexander EK, Bible KC, Doherty GM, Mandel SJ, Nikiforov YE, et al. 2015 American Thyroid Association management guidelines for adult patients with thyroid nodules and differentiated thyroid cancer: the American Thyroid Association guidelines task force on thyroid nodules and differentiated thyroid cancer. Thyroid. 2016;26(1):1–133.
8. Gemsenjager E, Perren A, Seifert B, Schuler G, Schweizer I, Heitz PU. Lymph node surgery in papillary thyroid carcinoma. J Am Coll Surg. 2003;197(2):182–90.
9. Goropoulos A, Karamoshos K, Christodoulou A, Ntitsias T, Paulou K, Samaras A, et al. Value of the cervical compartments in the surgical treatment of papillary thyroid carcinoma. World J Surg. 2004;28(12):1275–81.
10. Kupferman ME, Patterson M, Mandel SJ, LiVolsi V, Weber RS. Patterns of lateral neck metastasis in papillary thyroid carcinoma. Arch Otolaryngol Head Neck Surg. 2004;130(7):857–60.
11. Asimakopoulos P, Nixon IJ, Shaha AR. Differentiated and medullary thyroid cancer: surgical management of cervical lymph nodes. Clin Oncol (R Coll Radiol). 2017;29(5):283–9.
12. Chow SM, Law SC, Chan JK, Au SK, Yau S, Lau WH. Papillary microcarcinoma of the thyroid-prognostic significance of lymph node metastasis and multifocality. Cancer. 2003;98(1):31–40.
13. Grebe SK, Hay ID. Thyroid cancer nodal metastases: biologic significance and therapeutic considerations. Surg Oncol Clin N Am. 1996;5(1):43–63.
14. Mercante G, Frasoldati A, Pedroni C, Formisano D, Renna L, Piana S, et al. Prognostic factors affecting neck lymph node recurrence and distant metastasis in papillary microcarcinoma of the thyroid: results of a study in 445 patients. Thyroid. 2009;19(7):707–16.
15. Scheumann GF, Gimm O, Wegener G, Hundeshagen H, Dralle H. Prognostic significance and surgical management of locoregional lymph node metastases in papillary thyroid cancer. World J Surg. 1994;18(4):559–67; discussion 67–8.
16. Shah MD, Hall FT, Eski SJ, Witterick IJ, Walfish PG, Freeman JL. Clinical course of thyroid carcinoma after neck dissection. Laryngoscope. 2003;113(12):2102–7.
17. Wang TS, Dubner S, Sznyter LA, Heller KS. Incidence of metastatic well-differentiated thyroid cancer in cervical lymph nodes. Arch Otolaryngol Head Neck Surg. 2004;130(1):110–3.
18. Tuttle RM, Haugen B, Perrier ND. Updated American Joint Committee on Cancer/Tumor-Node-Metastasis Staging System for Differentiated and Anaplastic Thyroid Cancer (eighth edition): what changed and why? Thyroid. 2017;27(6):751–6.
19. Perrier ND, Brierley JD, Tuttle RM. Differentiated and anaplastic thyroid carcinoma: major changes in the American Joint Committee on Cancer eighth edition cancer staging manual. CA Cancer J Clin. 2018;68(1):55–63.
20. Tuttle RM, Ahuja S, Avram AM, Bernet VJ, Bourguet P, Daniels GH, et al. Controversies, consensus, and collaboration in the use of (131)I therapy in differentiated thyroid cancer: a joint statement from the American Thyroid Association, the European Association of Nuclear Medicine, the Society of Nuclear Medicine and Molecular Imaging, and the European Thyroid Association. Thyroid. 2019;29(4):461–70.
21. Lee SW. SPECT/CT in the treatment of differentiated thyroid cancer. Nucl Med Mol Imaging. 2017;51(4):297–303.
22. Aide N, Heutte N, Rame JP, Rousseau E, Loiseau C, Henry-Amar M, et al. Clinical relevance of single-photon emission computed tomography/computed tomography of the neck and thorax in postablation (131)I scintigraphy for thyroid cancer. J Clin Endocrinol Metab. 2009;94(6):2075–84.
23. Barwick T, Murray I, Megadmi H, Drake WM, Plowman PN, Akker SA, et al. Single photon emission computed tomography (SPECT)/computed tomography using Iodine-123 in patients with differentiated thyroid cancer: additional value over whole body planar imaging and SPECT. Eur J Endocrinol. 2010;162(6):1131–9.
24. Blum M, Tiu S, Chu M, Goel S, Friedman K. I-131 SPECT/CT elucidates cryptic findings on planar whole-body scans and can reduce needless therapy with I-131 in post-thyroidectomy thyroid cancer patients. Thyroid. 2011;21(11):1235–47.
25. Chen L, Luo Q, Shen Y, Yu Y, Yuan Z, Lu H, et al. Incremental value of 131I SPECT/CT in the management of patients with differentiated thyroid carcinoma. J Nucl Med. 2008;49(12):1952–7.

26. Ciappuccini R, Heutte N, Trzepla G, Rame JP, Vaur D, Aide N, et al. Postablation (131)I scintigraphy with neck and thorax SPECT-CT and stimulated serum thyroglobulin level predict the outcome of patients with differentiated thyroid cancer. Eur J Endocrinol. 2011;164(6):961–9.
27. Kohlfuerst S, Igerc I, Lobnig M, Gallowitsch HJ, Gomez-Segovia I, Matschnig S, et al. Posttherapeutic (131)I SPECT-CT offers high diagnostic accuracy when the findings on conventional planar imaging are inconclusive and allows a tailored patient treatment regimen. Eur J Nucl Med Mol Imaging. 2009;36(6):886–93.
28. Maruoka Y, Abe K, Baba S, Isoda T, Sawamoto H, Tanabe Y, et al. Incremental diagnostic value of SPECT/CT with 131I scintigraphy after radioiodine therapy in patients with well-differentiated thyroid carcinoma. Radiology. 2012;265(3):902–9.
29. Menges M, Uder M, Kuwert T, Schmidt D. 131I SPECT/CT in the follow-up of patients with differentiated thyroid carcinoma. Clin Nucl Med. 2012;37(6):555–60.
30. Mustafa M, Kuwert T, Weber K, Knesewitsch P, Negele T, Haug A, et al. Regional lymph node involvement in T1 papillary thyroid carcinoma: a bicentric prospective SPECT/CT study. Eur J Nucl Med Mol Imaging. 2010;37(8):1462–6.
31. Qiu ZL, Xu YH, Song HJ, Luo QY. Localization and identification of parapharyngeal metastases from differentiated thyroid carcinoma by 131I-SPECT/CT. Head Neck. 2011;33(2):171–7.
32. Ruf J, Lehmkuhl L, Bertram H, Sandrock D, Amthauer H, Humplik B, et al. Impact of SPECT and integrated low-dose CT after radioiodine therapy on the management of patients with thyroid carcinoma. Nucl Med Commun. 2004;25(12):1177–82.
33. Schmidt D, Linke R, Uder M, Kuwert T. Five months' follow-up of patients with and without iodine-positive lymph node metastases of thyroid carcinoma as disclosed by (131)I-SPECT/CT at the first radioablation. Eur J Nucl Med Mol Imaging. 2010;37(4):699–705.
34. Schmidt D, Szikszai A, Linke R, Bautz W, Kuwert T. Impact of 131I SPECT/spiral CT on nodal staging of differentiated thyroid carcinoma at the first radioablation. J Nucl Med. 2009;50(1):18–23.
35. Spanu A, Solinas ME, Chessa F, Sanna D, Nuvoli S, Madeddu G. 131I SPECT/CT in the follow-up of differentiated thyroid carcinoma: incremental value versus planar imaging. J Nucl Med. 2009;50(2):184–90.
36. Tharp K, Israel O, Hausmann J, Bettman L, Martin WH, Daitzchman M, et al. Impact of 131I-SPECT/CT images obtained with an integrated system in the follow-up of patients with thyroid carcinoma. Eur J Nucl Med Mol Imaging. 2004;31(10):1435–42.
37. Wang H, Fu HL, Li JN, Zou RJ, Gu ZH, Wu JC. The role of single-photon emission computed tomography/computed tomography for precise localization of metastases in patients with differentiated thyroid cancer. Clin Imaging. 2009;33(1):49–54.
38. Wong KK, Avram AM. Posttherapy I-131 thymic uptake demonstrated with SPECT/CT in a young girl with papillary thyroid carcinoma. Thyroid. 2008;18(8):919–20.
39. Wong KK, Sisson JC, Koral KF, Frey KA, Avram AM. Staging of differentiated thyroid carcinoma using diagnostic 131I SPECT/CT. AJR Am J Roentgenol. 2010;195(3):730–6.
40. Wong KK, Zarzhevsky N, Cahill JM, Frey KA, Avram AM. Incremental value of diagnostic 131I SPECT/CT fusion imaging in the evaluation of differentiated thyroid carcinoma. AJR Am J Roentgenol. 2008;191(6):1785–94.
41. Wong KK, Zarzhevsky N, Cahill JM, Frey KA, Avram AM. Hybrid SPECT-CT and PET-CT imaging of differentiated thyroid carcinoma. Br J Radiol. 2009;82(982):860–76.
42. Yamamoto Y, Nishiyama Y, Monden T, Matsumura Y, Satoh K, Ohkawa M. Clinical usefulness of fusion of 131I SPECT and CT images in patients with differentiated thyroid carcinoma. J Nucl Med. 2003;44(12):1905–10.
43. Grewal RK, Tuttle RM, Fox J, Borkar S, Chou JF, Gonen M, et al. The effect of posttherapy 131I SPECT/CT on risk classification and management of patients with differentiated thyroid cancer. J Nucl Med. 2010;51(9):1361–7.
44. Wakabayashi H, Nakajima K, Fukuoka M, Inaki A, Nakamura A, Kayano D, et al. Double-phase (131)I whole body scan and (131)I SPECT-CT images in patients with differentiated thyroid cancer: their effectiveness for accurate identification. Ann Nucl Med. 2011;25(9):609–15.
45. Spanu A, Nuvoli S, Gelo I, Mele L, Piras B, Madeddu G. Role of diagnostic (131)I SPECT/CT in long-term follow-up of patients with papillary thyroid microcarcinoma. J Nucl Med. 2018;59(10):1510–5.
46. Malamitsi JV, Koutsikos JT, Giourgouli SI, Zachaki SF, Pipikos TA, Vlachou FJ, et al. I-131 postablation SPECT/CT predicts relapse of papillary thyroid carcinoma more accurately than whole body scan. In Vivo. 2019;33(6):2255–63.
47. Lee CH, Jung JH, Son SH, Hong CM, Jeong JH, Jeong SY, et al. Risk factors for radioactive iodine-avid metastatic lymph nodes on post I-131 ablation SPECT/CT in low- or intermediate-risk groups of papillary thyroid cancer. PLoS One. 2018;13(8):e0202644.
48. Avram AM. Role of SPECT/CT, versus traditional practices, in individualizing treatment of thyroid carcinoma: reply. J Nucl Med. 2012;53(11):1819.
49. Avram AM. Radioiodine scintigraphy with SPECT/CT: an important diagnostic tool for thyroid cancer staging and risk stratification. J Nucl Med. 2012;53(5):754–64.
50. Barwick TD, Dhawan RT, Lewington V. Role of SPECT/CT in differentiated thyroid cancer. Nucl Med Commun. 2012;33(8):787–98.
51. Toubert ME, Vija L, Vercellino L, Banayan S, Faugeron I, Berenger N, et al. Additional diagnostic value of hybrid SPECT-CT systems imaging in patients with differentiated thyroid cancer. Am J Clin Oncol. 2014;37(3):305–13.

52. Xue YL, Qiu ZL, Song HJ, Luo QY. Value of (131) I SPECT/CT for the evaluation of differentiated thyroid cancer: a systematic review of the literature. Eur J Nucl Med Mol Imaging. 2013;40(5):768–78.

53. Even-Sapir E, Keidar Z, Sachs J, Engel A, Bettman L, Gaitini D, et al. The new technology of combined transmission and emission tomography in evaluation of endocrine neoplasms. J Nucl Med. 2001;42(7):998–1004.

54. Hughes DT, Haymart MR, Miller BS, Gauger PG, Doherty GM. The most commonly occurring papillary thyroid cancer in the United States is now a microcarcinoma in a patient older than 45 years. Thyroid. 2011;21(3):231–6.

55. Hay ID, Grant CS, van Heerden JA, Goellner JR, Ebersold JR, Bergstralh EJ. Papillary thyroid microcarcinoma: a study of 535 cases observed in a 50-year period. Surgery. 1992;112(6):1139–46; discussion 46–7.

56. Hay ID, Hutchinson ME, Gonzalez-Losada T, McIver B, Reinalda ME, Grant CS, et al. Papillary thyroid microcarcinoma: a study of 900 cases observed in a 60-year period. Surgery. 2008;144(6):980–7; discussion 7–8.

57. Ross DS, Litofsky D, Ain KB, Bigos T, Brierley JD, Cooper DS, et al. Recurrence after treatment of micropapillary thyroid cancer. Thyroid. 2009;19(10):1043–8.

58. Strate SM, Lee EL, Childers JH. Occult papillary carcinoma of the thyroid with distant metastases. Cancer. 1984;54(6):1093–100.

59. Mian C, Barollo S, Pennelli G, Pavan N, Rugge M, Pelizzo MR, et al. Molecular characteristics in papillary thyroid cancers (PTCs) with no 131I uptake. Clin Endocrinol. 2008;68(1):108–16.

60. Szujo S, Sira L, Bajnok L, Bodis B, Gyory F, Nemes O, et al. The impact of post-radioiodine therapy SPECT/CT on early risk stratification in differentiated thyroid cancer; a bi-institutional study. Oncotarget. 2017;8(45):79825–34.

61. Delbeke D, Schoder H, Martin WH, Wahl RL. Hybrid imaging (SPECT/CT and PET/CT): improving therapeutic decisions. Semin Nucl Med. 2009;39(5):308–40.

62. Filesi M, Signore A, Ventroni G, Melacrinis FF, Ronga G. Role of initial iodine-131 whole-body scan and serum thyroglobulin in differentiated thyroid carcinoma metastases. J Nucl Med. 1998;39(9):1542–6.

63. Lind P, Kohlfurst S. Respective roles of thyroglobulin, radioiodine imaging, and positron emission tomography in the assessment of thyroid cancer. Semin Nucl Med. 2006;36(3):194–205.

64. van Sorge-van Boxtel RA, van Eck-Smit BL, Goslings BM. Comparison of serum thyroglobulin, 131I and 201Tl scintigraphy in the postoperative follow-up of differentiated thyroid cancer. Nucl Med Commun. 1993;14(5):365–72.

65. Avram AM, Fig LM, Frey KA, Gross MD, Wong KK. Preablation 131-I scans with SPECT/CT in postoperative thyroid cancer patients: what is the impact on staging? J Clin Endocrinol Metab. 2013;98(3):1163–71.

66. Van Nostrand D, Aiken M, Atkins F, Moreau S, Garcia C, Acio E, et al. The utility of radioiodine scans prior to iodine 131 ablation in patients with well-differentiated thyroid cancer. Thyroid. 2009;19(8):849–55.

67. Mitchell G, Pratt BE, Vini L, McCready VR, Harmer CL. False positive 131I whole body scans in thyroid cancer. Br J Radiol. 2000;73(870):627–35.

68. Shapiro B, Rufini V, Jarwan A, Geatti O, Kearfott KJ, Fig LM, et al. Artifacts, anatomical and physiological variants, and unrelated diseases that might cause false-positive whole-body 131-I scans in patients with thyroid cancer. Semin Nucl Med. 2000;30(2):115–32.

69. Dumcke CW, Madsen JL. Usefulness of SPECT/CT in the diagnosis of intrathoracic goiter versus metastases from cancer of the breast. Clin Nucl Med. 2007;32(2):156–9.

70. Jong I, Taubman K, Schlicht S. Bronchiectasis simulating pulmonary metastases on iodine-131 scintigraphy in well-differentiated thyroid carcinoma. Clin Nucl Med. 2005;30(10):688–9.

71. Rachinsky I, Driedger A. Iodine-131 uptake in a menstruating uterus: value of SPECT/CT in distinguishing benign and metastatic iodine-positive lesions. Thyroid. 2007;17(9):901–2.

72. Jammah AA, Driedger A, Rachinsky I. Incidental finding of ovarian teratoma on post-therapy scan for papillary thyroid cancer and impact of SPECT/CT imaging. Arq Bras Endocrinol Metabol. 2011;55(7):490–3.

73. Mebarki M, Menemani A, Medjahedi A, Boualou F, Slama A, Ouguirti S, et al. Radioiodine accumulation in a giant ovarian cystadenofibroma detected incidentally by 131-I whole body scans. Case Rep Radiol. 2012;2012:295617.

74. Sakahara H, Yamashita S, Suzuki K, Imai M, Kosugi T. Visualization of nasolacrimal drainage system after radioiodine therapy in patients with thyroid cancer. Ann Nucl Med. 2007;21(9):525–7.

75. Savas H, Wong KK, Saglik B, Hubers D, Ackermann RJ, Avram AM. SPECT/CT characterization of oral activity on radioiodine scintigraphy. J Clin Endocrinol Metab. 2013;98(11):4410–6.

76. Albano D, Motta F, Baronchelli C, Lucchini S, Bertagna F. 131I whole-body scan incidental uptake due to spermatocele. Clin Nucl Med. 2017;42(11):901–4.

77. Jang HY, Kim BH, Kim WJ, Jeon YK, Kim SS, Kim YK, et al. False-positive radioiodine uptake in a functional ovarian cyst in a patient treated with total thyroidectomy for papillary cancer. Intern Med. 2013;52(20):2321–3.

78. Rizzo A, Zagaria L, Perotti G, Annunziata S, Salvatori M. Accumulation of 131I in esophageal diverticulum diagnosed by SPECT/CT. Clin Nucl Med. 2018;43(11):e410–e1.

79. Oh JR, Ahn BC. False-positive uptake on radioiodine whole-body scintigraphy: physiologic and pathologic variants unrelated to thyroid cancer. Am J Nucl Med Mol Imaging. 2012;2(3):362–85.

80. Glazer DI, Brown RK, Wong KK, Savas H, Gross MD, Avram AM. SPECT/CT evaluation of unusual physiologic radioiodine biodistributions: pearls and pitfalls in image interpretation. Radiographics. 2013;33(2):397–418.
81. Agriantonis DJ, Hall L, Wilson MA. Utility of SPECT/CT as an adjunct to planar whole body I-131 imaging: liver metastasis from papillary thyroid cancer. Clin Nucl Med. 2009;34(4):247–8.
82. Aide N, Lehembre E, Gervais R, Bardet S. Unusual intratracheal metastasis of differentiated thyroid cancer accurately depicted by SPECT/CT acquisition after radioiodine ablation. Thyroid. 2007;17(12):1305–6.
83. Qiu ZL, Luo QY. Erector spinae metastases from differentiated thyroid cancer identified by I-131 SPECT/CT. Clin Nucl Med. 2009;34(3):137–40.
84. von Falck C, Beer G, Gratz KF, Galanski M. Renal metastases from follicular thyroid cancer on SPECT/CT. Clin Nucl Med. 2007;32(9):751–2.
85. Zhao LX, Li L, Li FL, Zhao Z. Rectus abdominis muscle metastasis from papillary thyroid cancer identified by I-131 SPECT/CT. Clin Nucl Med. 2010;35(5):360–1.
86. Barwick T, Murray I, Megadmi H, Drake W, Plowman PN, Akker S, et al. SPECT/CT using Iodine-123 in patients with differentiated thyroid cancer—additional value over whole body planar imaging and SPECT. Eur J Endocrinol. 2010;162(6):1131–9.
87. Wong KK, Sisson JC, Koral KF, Frey KA, Avram AM. Staging of differentiated thyroid carcinoma using diagnostic 131-I SPECT-CT. AJR Am J Roentgenol. 2010;195(3):730–6.
88. Durante C, Haddy N, Baudin E, Leboulleux S, Hartl D, Travagli JP, et al. Long-term outcome of 444 patients with distant metastases from papillary and follicular thyroid carcinoma: benefits and limits of radioiodine therapy. J Clin Endocrinol Metab. 2006;91(8):2892–9.
89. Avram AM, Esfandiari NH, Wong KK. Preablation 131-I scans with SPECT/CT contribute to thyroid cancer risk stratification and 131-I therapy planning. J Clin Endocrinol Metab. 2015;100(5):1895–902.
90. Qiu ZL, Xue YL, Song HJ, Luo QY. Comparison of the diagnostic and prognostic values of 99mTc-MDP-planar bone scintigraphy, 131I-SPECT/CT and 18F-FDG-PET/CT for the detection of bone metastases from differentiated thyroid cancer. Nucl Med Commun. 2012;33(12):1232–42.
91. Oh JR, Byun BH, Hong SP, Chong A, Kim J, Yoo SW, et al. Comparison of (1)(3)(1)I whole-body imaging, (1)(3)(1)I SPECT/CT, and (1)(8)F-FDG PET/CT in the detection of metastatic thyroid cancer. Eur J Nucl Med Mol Imaging. 2011;38(8):1459–68.
92. Bulzacka I, Makarewicz J. Postablative 131I SPECT/CT is much more sensitive than cervical ultrasonography for the detection of thyroid remnants in patients after total thyroidectomy for differentiated thyroid cancer. Clin Nucl Med. 2020;45(12):948–53.
93. Sisson JC, Dewaraja YK, Wizauer EJ, Giordano TJ, Avram AM. Thyroid carcinoma metastasis to skull with infringement of brain: treatment with radioiodine. Thyroid. 2009;19(3):297–303.
94. Song H, He B, Prideaux A, Du Y, Frey E, Kasecamp W, et al. Lung dosimetry for radioiodine treatment planning in the case of diffuse lung metastases. J Nucl Med. 2006;47(12):1985–94.
95. Buck AK, Nekolla SG, Ziegler SI, Drzezga A. SPECT/CT. J Nucl Med. 2008;49(8):1305–19.
96. Gelfand MJ, Lemen LC. PET/CT and SPECT/CT dosimetry in children: the challenge to the pediatric imager. Semin Nucl Med. 2007;37(5):391–8.
97. Kim HY, Gelfand MJ, Sharp SE. SPECT/CT imaging in children with papillary thyroid carcinoma. Pediatr Radiol. 2011;41(8):1008–12.
98. Min JJ, Chung JK, Lee YJ, Jeong JM, Lee DS, Jang JJ, et al. Relationship between expression of the sodium/iodide symporter and 131I uptake in recurrent lesions of differentiated thyroid carcinoma. Eur J Nucl Med. 2001;28(5):639–45.

SPECT/CT in Neuroendrocrine Tumours

6

Torjan Haslerud

6.1 Introduction

Neuroendocrine neoplasms (NENs) comprise a diverse and very heterogeneous group of neoplasms, defined as epithelial neoplasms with predominantly neuroendocrine differentiation. Neuroendocrine cells are present in endocrine glands, as well as diffusely distributed in all body tissues. These cells possess the ability to produce various peptide hormones and bioactive amines [1, 2]. The secretory products are stored in characteristic small intracellular membrane-bound granules (synaptic vesicles) [2]. NENs can produce a great variety of clinical symptoms due to hormone hypersecretion, in addition to the typical carcinoid manifestation with diarrhoea and facial flushing caused by serotonin hypersecretion.

NENs are most frequently located in the gastrointestinal tract and pancreas (GEP-NENs) [3, 4], but can arise in almost every organ. NENs can roughly be categorized into following groups: gastroenteropancreatic tumours, bronchopulmonary tumours, medullary carcinomas of the thyroid, tumours of sympathoadrenal system, tumours caused by the multiple endocrine neoplasia syndrome and pituitary tumours. Primary NENs are frequently present as small tumours and may be difficult to detect with conventional imaging methods, therefore highly sensitive and specific diagnostic imaging methods are essential to locate tumour lesions and metastases. The determination of the accurate extent of disease and potential disease progression is essential to ensure that patients suffering from NEN receive appropriate and correct treatment according to tumour stage and tumour biology.

Due to the growing importance of PRRT and ever-increasing demand for sensitive and specific molecular imaging, especially within oncology, NENs have become an important part of the daily routine within nuclear medicine departments worldwide.

6.2 Epidemiology

Approximately 2.5–5.0 per 100,000 inhabitants are diagnosed with NET in the western world annually [5]. The incidence of NETs has been continuously rising over the last 30 years [5], hence steadily increasing the clinical impact of these neoplasms. Despite the low incidence of NEN in comparison to other cancer entities, NEN has a relatively high prevalence. This is due to the long overall survival patients suffering from well-differentiated NET typically have. Thus, a significant number of patients undergo treatment,

T. Haslerud (✉)
Stavanger University Hospital, Stavanger, Norway

Haukeland University Hospital, Bergen, Norway
e-mail: torjan@haslerud.no

95

staging and surveillance examinations on a yearly basis. About two-thirds of NETs are typical carcinoid tumours and one-third other NETs [3, 4]. Approximately 70% of NENs originate from the gastrointestinal-pancreatic system and the lungs [3, 4]. Additionally, there is a high incidence of very small asymptomatic NETs reported as high as 10% in pancreatic sections [6], which might not be clinically relevant or require any therapeutic intervention.

6.3 Physiology

Neuroendocrine cells possess the ability of amine precursor uptake and have high intracellular concentrations of amino acid decarboxylase (referred to as APUD-cells) [3]. These characteristics enable production of a variety of small peptides and bioactive amines, which are stored in the NEN's characteristic granules [2, 3]. Proteins of these vesicles (Synaptophysin and Chromogranin A) can be used in histological sections to distinguish NENs from other tumours or as serum tumour markers [2]. The cell-lineage and anatomic site of the neuroendocrine cell determine the type of secreted hormone. Table 6.1 shows a selection of different neuroendocrine tumours and corresponding hormones.

Depending on the cell physiology and function, different approaches can be exploited to enable tumour-specific molecular imaging. For tumours of sympathoadrenal lineage (pheochromocytoma, neuroblastoma), the catecholamine pathway is one possible approach to visualize pathologic cell distribution. Metaiodobenzylguanidine (MIBG) labelled with I-123 or I-131 is an adrenaline analogue, which is stored in intracellular vesicles but not further metabolized [7] (more on this subject in Chap. 7 I-MIBG SPECT/CT for tumour imaging).

Another characteristic feature of neuroendocrine tumour cells is the frequent overexpression of somatostatin receptors (sstr) on the cell surface [8, 9]. Of the five known main classes of somatostatin receptors, the subtype sstr2 is predominant in most NENs [8, 9]. Several subtypes may be expressed depending on differentiation, type and anatomic site of primary [8, 9]. Yet there is vast variation in sstr expression even between tumours of the same type.

6.4 Somatostatin

Somatostatin is a small regulatory peptide hormone, which is mainly distributed in the central and peripheral nervous system, endocrine glands, immune system and gastrointestinal tract. Two biologically active forms of somatostatin are known consisting of 14 and 28 amino acids, respectively.

Generally, somatostatin is an inhibitory hormone, which inhibits the release of several secondary hormones. The actions of somatostatin are mainly located at the pituitary where the secretion of growth hormone and TSH is inhibited as well as in the gastrointestinal system, where there release of numerous different gastrointestinal and pancreatic hormones is suppressed. Additionally, somatostatin modulates gastrointestinal motility and immune responses, suppresses the exocrine action of pancreas, shows neuromodulatory functions as well as induces apoptosis.

Table 6.1 Selection of hormone active tumours and corresponding hormone

Tumour	Hormone	Organ
Gastrinoma	Gastrin	Pancreas, duodenum
Insulinoma	Insulin	Pancreas
Glucagonoma	Glucagon	Pancreas
VIPoma	Vasoactive intestinal peptide	Pancreas
Carcinoid	Serotonin, substance P	Small intestine/prox. colon, lung
Medullary thyroid cancer	Calcitonin	Thyroid
Phaeochromocytoma	Norepinephrine	Adrenals
Somatostatinoma	Somatostatin	Pancreas

6.4.1 Somatostatin Receptors

The biologic actions of somatostatin are mediated through one of the six somatostatin receptor subtypes known to date (sstr 1, 2A, 2B, 3, 4 and 5) [3, 10, 11]. These receptors are all G-protein coupled and activate a variety of different intracellular pathways such as inhibition of adenyl cyclase, stimulation of phosphotyrosine phosphatase (PTP) and modulation of mitogen-activated protein kinase (MAPK) [11–13].

After binding of an activating ligand on the receptor, the hormone–receptor complex is internalized in the cell and directed to endosomes. The somatostatin receptor will then be recycled back to the cell membrane or degraded. The degradation of somatostatin receptors can subsequently lead to sstr downregulation on the cell surface [11–13].

Somatostatin receptors are physiologically present in a number of normal human tissues and organs, such as pituitary, brain, gastrointestinal tract, pancreas, kidney, immune cells, blood vessels and peripheral nervous system.

In addition, several other neoplasms (NEN and non-NEN) may express somatostatin receptors [8, 9], and a selection of tumour entities is shown in Table 6.2. Clinically subtype sstr2 is of highest importance as sstr2 is the most frequently overexpressed subtype in NENs [8, 9]. Hence, most somatostatin analogues in clinical use show high/nanomolar affinity to sstr2 [8, 9]. The other sstr subtypes vary in overexpression in NENs as well as in their affinity for synthetic somatostatin derivatives [14].

6.5 Classification

The classification of NENs has been confusing and hitherto no universal consensus has been agreed upon. Several different approaches are in use in order to classify the heterogeneous NENs to ensure optimal prognostic stratification and treatment schemes. Yet no general classification for all NET sites is available. Because NENs predominantly arise in the gastroenteropancreatic or bronchopulmonary system, the following segment will deal mainly with classification of NETs originating from these organ systems.

In general, NENs are classified by histology, grading, proliferation, anatomic site of origin, hormone secretion and/or extent of disease. Because many of the characteristics of the NETs are organ/site specific, location of the primary site can be a relevant factor in the therapy scheme. Therefore, a classification by site of origin can be helpful. The NETs are commonly divided into foregut, midgut and hindgut tumours based upon their embryonic segments and similar biological behaviour. NETs located in the small intestine and proximal colon (midgut) are often associated with typical carcinoid symptoms caused by serotonin hypersecretion whereas NETs in the distal colon and rectum (hindgut) are usually non-functional [2, 15, 16]. Pancreatic and bronchial NETs (foregut) can be associated with hormone hypersecretion, but can be non-functional as well [2, 15, 16].

NETs can be histologically classified as well-differentiated NETs, poorly differentiated NECs and mixed adeno-neuroendocrine carcinomas (MANEC) [17–19]. The well-differentiated NETs are divided into low-grade, intermediate- and high-grade NETs dependent on cell morphology, mitotic rate and/or Ki67 index of "hot

Table 6.2 Neoplasias potentially expressing somatostatin receptors

Gastrinoma
Glucagonoma
Paraganglioma
SCLC
Carcinoid tumours
Merkel cell carcinoma
Neuroblastoma
Pheochromocytoma
Medullary thyroid carcinoma
Pituitary tumours
Breast cancer
Prostate cancer
Lymphoma (NHL and Hodgkin's)
Colon cancer
Ovarian cancer
Melanoma
Sarcoma
Renal cell carcinoma
Astrocytoma

spots" (Table 6.3). The Ki67 index plays an important role in NET classification, due to good correlation between Ki-67 index and survival [20–23]. Additionally, the Ki 67 index has proven to be an independent prognostic factor for survival, regardless of disease extent [24–28]. However, no significant difference in outcome between G1 and G2 carcinoids has been reported. The more aggressive and poorly differentiated NECs are distinguished from NET by using Ki67 index/mitotic rate as well as by presenting with a different pathological appearance. In recent years, a new classification with respect to G3 tumours has emerged (Table 6.4). The division of the earlier NEC G3 into NET G3 and NEC G3 is a natural consequence of increasing knowledge concerning differences in biology, response to platin-based chemotherapy, survival/prognosis and presence of somatostatin receptor expression [29, 30]. The 2019 WHO classification separates NEC into small- and large-cell tumours, regard-

less of Ki-67. This separation does not have impact on the treatment scheme, as NECs are generally treated with a platin-based chemotherapy scheme regardless of cell size (Table 6.5). NECs typically show a more rapid course with shorter survival and generally poor prognosis.

The World Health Organisation guidelines provide a classification for extent of disease using tumour-node-metastasis (TNM) staging. Due to the vast biological diversity of NETs, the extent of the disease alone does not provide an adequate risk stratification or survival data. Many NETs have already metastasized by the time of diagnosis, making a stratification based solely on the TNM system inadequate. For example, NETs of unknown primary are by definition stage IV in

Table 6.3 Grading system for neuroendocrine neoplasms

Grade	Gastrointestinal tract and pancreas (WHO 2010)
Low (G1)	<2 mitoses/10 HPF and Ki-67 index ≤2%
Intermediate (G2)	2–20 mitoses/10 HPF or Ki-67 index 3–20%
High (G3)	>20 mitoses/10 HPF or Ki-67 index >20%

Table 6.4 Nomenclature for high-grade GEP-NEN (NEN G3)

Nomenclature	Morphology	Ki-67-index (%)	Subdivision
NET G3	Well-differentiated	>20	
NEC G3	Poorly differentiated	>20	
	Poorly differentiated	>21–55	Low NEC
	Poorly differentiated	>55	High NEC
NEN G3	Addressing both NET and NEC if uncertain differentiation		

Table 6.5 ENETs stratification proposal for GEP-NETs

Prognosis	Differentiation	Grade	Stage	Potential therapy
Localized tumour				
Very low risk of metastasis	Well-differentiated	G1	T1	Endoscopic resection
Low risk	Well-differentiated	G1	T2	Surgery
Intermediate risk	Well-differentiated	G2	T1	Surgery
High risk	Well-differentiated	G1/G2	T2	Surgery
High risk	Poorly differentiated	G3	T1–T3	Surgery, additional treatment
Nodal metastases				
Slow growth	Well-differentiated	G1	T1–T3, N1	Surgery
Intermediate growth	Well-differentiated	G2	T1–T3, N1	Surgery, additional treatment
Fast growth	Poorly differentiated	G3	T1–T3, N1	Surgery, additional treatment
Nodal and distant metastases				
Slow growth	Well-differentiated	G1	Any T, N1, M1	Surgery, additional treatment
Intermediate growth	Well-differentiated	G2	Any T, N1, M1	Surgery, additional treatment
Fast growth	Poorly differentiated	G3	Any T, N1, M1	Chemotherapy

the TNM system and the histological grade may prove to be the only prognostic parameter.

Functionality may have an impact on prognosis, yet the biological behaviour of most functioning NETs is defined by grade and stage. The clinical symptoms caused by hypersecretion of hormones define the division in functioning or non-functioning NETs. Immunohistological staining is not a defining criterion, yet the presence of typical symptoms are. A functional tumour may be treated differently than a non-functional tumour; therefore, the presence of hormonal production should be included in the tumour nomenclature.

ENETs have come up with a proposal for the stratification of GEP-NETs, which combines TNM stages, grade and growth features (Table 6.5) and suggest potential treatment for the respective groups [31].

6.6 Diagnostical Tracers (Somatostatin Receptor-Based Imaging)

Due to the short half-life of somatostatin in human serum of 2–3 min caused by rapid enzymatic degradation, new somatostatin analogues with longer half-lives were necessary. This led to the development of the cyclooctapeptide octreotide, which is still very much in clinical use today. Non-radioactive "cold" octreotide and lanreotide are used routinely in the treatment of acromegaly as well as for antiproliferative therapy and symptom control of NETs. There are short-acting as well as long-acting products available.

The cyclic peptide additionally served as lead structure for most of the somatostatin analogues developed later such as tyrosine3-octretotide (TOC), tyrosine3-Ocreotate (TATE) and naphtylalanine3-octreotide (NOC). Octreotide and octreotide derivatives show a generally high affinity to sstr2 with varying affinity for the other somatostatin receptor subtypes [32].

The radiolabelled somatostatin analogues generally consist of a biologically active part, usually octreotide, TOC or TATE coupled with a chelator complex (i.e. DTPA, DOTA, EDDA/

HYNIC) and a gamma or positron-emitting radiometal. The internalization of the radioactive ligand–receptor complex with intracellular entrapment of the radiometal is considered to be the mechanism enabling tumour imaging by resulting in high scintigraphic tumour-to-background ratio, especially in delayed images.

The first commercially available tracer enabling visualization of in vivo somatostatin receptor distribution was indium-111–labelled DTPA-Octreotide (OctreoScan), which is arguably still regarded as the gold standard within gamma scintigraphy. Later DOTA- and HYNIC/EDDA-conjugated analogues found their way into the clinical routine. The biggest development with respect to somatostatin receptor imaging has been the emergence of the positron-emitting (i.e. Ga-68, Cu-64) DOTA-labelled derivatives. Due to superior qualities including excellent spatial resolution of PET/CT imaging compared to gammascintigraphy, PET-imaging of sstr have by far outperformed scintigraphic methods in terms of sensitivity and specificity [33]. With the ever-growing density of PET-centres worldwide and introduction of commercial licensed Ga-68-DOTA-labelled derivatives, the latter have inarguably taken over as the gold standard with respect to sstr imaging. However, this modality is still not ubiquitously available, and gamma scintigraphy is still widely in use.

Further developments such as somatostatin analogues with high affinity to multiple/all somatostatin receptors (i.e. pasireotide), somatostatin receptor antagonists (i.e. DOTA-BASS) and novel PET tracers (i.e. Cu-64-SARTATE, fluorine-18 and scandium-44-labelled derivatives) show promising results and may represent the future within sstr imaging [34].

6.6.1 [^{111}In]-DTPA-D-Phe^1-Octreotide

[^{111}In]-DTPA-D-Phe^1-octreotide (or [^{111}In]-pentetreotide) has been commercially available over two decades and is the most frequently used somatostatin analogue within gamma scintigraphy. Due to the relatively long half-life of indium-111 of 2.8 days, sequential multiple-day imaging can be performed. The cyclotron product indium-111 is a gamma-emitting radiometal with two medium-energy photo peaks (173 and 247 keV). Hence, a medium energy collimator is required during imaging, and data from both windows are added.

The recommended intravenously applied activity for adults undergoing a somatostatin receptor study is 185–222 MBq, resulting in an effective dose of around 12 mSv (0.054 mSv/ MBq) [35]. For children, the recommended activity is 5 MBq/kg [35, 36]. The amount of peptide injected is only around 10–20 µg, hence significant pharmacologic effects are not expected. Before administration, a control of the labelling yield according to the manufacturer's instructions is recommended. The radiolabelled product should be applied within 6 h after preparation.

Common indications for somatostatin receptor imaging are staging of patients with NENs, detection and localization of neuroendocrine tumour lesions, follow-up of patients with NENs and evaluation of patients under consideration for peptide receptor radionuclide therapy. In Table 6.6, a selection of tumours (NETs, non-NETs) and non-malignant processes is shown.

[111In]-DTPA-D-Phe1-octreotide is registered for use in scintigraphic localization of primary tumours and to determine the extent of metastatic NET's disease.

Patients undergoing somatostatin receptor imaging should be well hydrated prior to and for at least 1 day after injection, in order to reduce radiation burden. If the patient does not suffer from diarrhoea, a mild laxative should be administered the day before and in the evening on the day of injection. Long-acting somatostatin analogues should be withdrawn 4–6 weeks prior to injection, eventually switching to short-acting preparations until 1 day before the study in order to prevent receptor occupation, potentially leading to false-negative findings. Recent studies, regarding tumour uptake on [68Ga]-DOTATOC/-TATE-PET/CT, have showed that injection of long-acting analogues prior to [68Ga]-DOTATOC/-TATE-PET/CT does not have a neg-

Table 6.6 Sensitivity of somatostatin receptor imaging using [111In]-pentetreotide

Tumour	Sensitivity
Pituitary tumours	High (>75% detection rate)
Gastrinomas	High (>75% detection rate)
Carcinoids	High (>75% detection rate)
Non-functional P-NETs	High (>75% detection rate)
Functional P-NETs except insulinoma	High (>75% detection rate)
Paragangliomas	High (>75% detection rate)
SCLC	High (>75% detection rate)
Merkel cell carcinoma	High (>75% detection rate)
Meningiomas	High (>75% detection rate)
Sarcoidosis and granulomatous diseases	High (>75% detection rate)
Graves' disease and ophthalmopathy	High (>75% detection rate)
Insulinomas	Intermediate (40–75% detection rate)
Medullary thyroid carcinoma	Intermediate (40–75% detection rate)
Differentiated thyroid carcinoma	Intermediate (40–75% detection rate)
Lymphoma (NHL, HL)	Intermediate (40–75% detection rate)
Pheochromocytoma	Intermediate (40–75% detection rate)

ative influence on tumour uptake and thus discontinuation may not prove necessary [37]. Notably these studies have not investigated tumour uptake on scintigraphic sstr imaging. The usual precautions for nuclear medicine studies for pregnant and breastfeeding women apply. [111In]-pentetreotide should not be administered into lines for total parenteral nutrition, because of the possible formation of a complex glycosyl octreotide conjugate.

After injection, [111In]-pentetreotide is rapidly cleared from the plasma; just 35% of the injected radioactivity remains in the bloodstream after 10 min. Twenty-four hours after application, only 1% still remains in the blood. The tracer excretion is almost completely renal; 85% of the administered activity is eliminated with urine within 24 h. Hepatobiliary and faecal excretion account for less than 2% of the total excretion [35, 36, 38]. The biologic half-life of [111In]-pentetreotide is 6 h.

The normal physiologic distribution pattern (Fig. 6.1) of [111In]-DTPA-octreotide features

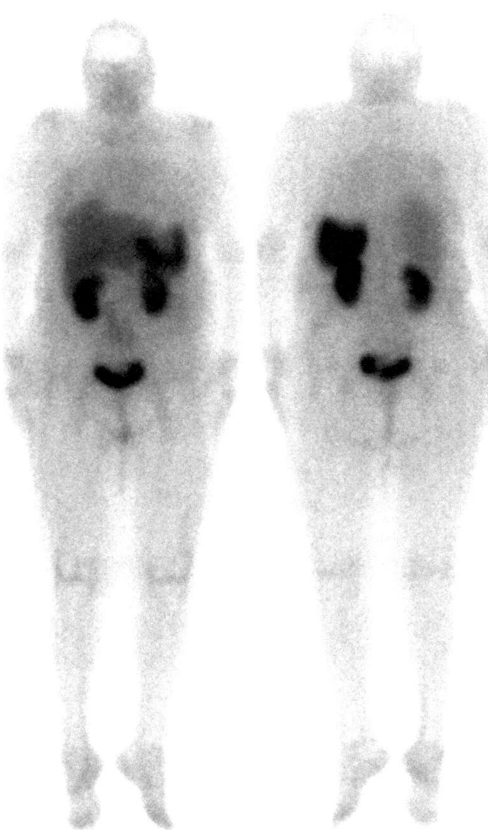

Fig. 6.1 Normal [^{111}In]-pentetreotide whole-body scan with physiologic sstr distribution

Table 6.7 Acquisition protocol for 111In-pentetreotide

Collimator	Medium energy, parallel hole
Energy window	172 and 245 keV with 20% windows summed in the acquisition frames
Planar images (anterior and posterior) 128 × 128 or 256 × 256 matrix	4 h p.i. (7 min), 24 h p.i (10 min), 48 h p.i. (15 min) per view
Whole body (256 × 1024 matrix)	Scanning speed: 4 h p.i.: 10 cm/min, 24 h p.i.: 7 cm/min, 48 h p.i.: 5 cm/min
SPECT or SPECT/CT 128 × 128 acquisition matrix	4 h p.i.: 3° angular sampling, 20 s per projection; 24 h p.i.: 3°, 30 s; 48 h: 6°, 60 s

Table 6.8 Pitfalls and false-positive results causing potential misinterpretation

Radiation pneumonitis	Bacterial pneumonia
Accessory spleen	Cerebrovascular accident
Scar tissue	Granulomatous disease
Gallbladder uptake	Diffuse breast uptake
Nodular goitre	Adrenal uptake
Focal stool collection	Urine contamination
Ventral hernia	Concomitant second tumour
Common cold (nasal uptake)	Respiratory infections

visualization of the thyroid, spleen, liver, kidneys and occasionally the pituitary and adrenals as well as the urinary bladder, gall bladder and bowel. In 15% of female patients diffuse uptake in the breasts can be seen. Additionally, about 15% of patients show benign focal pancreatic head uptake [39]. The tracer uptake in the thyroid, spleen, adrenals and pituitary is somatostatin receptor-mediated, whereas the kidney visualization is caused by re-absorption of the radiotracer in the tubular cells. Normally, bowel uptake is not seen on the early images (4 h after injection), but can occur on delayed images. Therefore, sequential images can be helpful to distinguish between pathological and physiological tracer bowel uptake. A recommended protocol for acquisition parameters is shown in Table 6.7.

The tumour uptake kinetic is relative slow, taking at least 4 h [35, 36, 38]. Therefore, images are acquired 4, 24 and even 48 h after administration. The 4 h images are obtained to evaluate the abdomen before any intestinal activity is visible. Planar whole-body scans provide a good overview of the distribution of the radiopharmaceutical. Due to the lower tumour-to-background ratio compared to delayed imaging, some tumour lesions may not be visible in the early images. Any relevant non-physiological uptake indicates the presence of lesions with overexpression of somatostatin receptors, which is usually suspicious for or concordant with malignant disease. Yet increased focal or diffuse density of somatostatin receptors can be caused by a numerous of benign processes. In Tables 6.8 and 6.9, pitfalls and potential misinterpretation of positive and negative results are shown [35, 36, 38].

Table 6.9 False-negative results causing potential misinterpretation

Presence of unlabelled somatostatin caused by octreotide therapy	Liver metastases may appear iso-intense to normal liver tissue
Presence of unlabelled somatostatin caused by tumour secretion	Variable sstr2 expression of the tumour lesions
Different sstr subtypes of the tumour lesions	Variable tumour differentiation

Table 6.10 Krenning score for visual grading of pathologic uptake

Krenning score	Tumour uptake
0	No uptake
1	Very low
2	= normal liver
3	>normal liver
4	>spleen

Furthermore, the antibiotic/chemotherapeutic agent, bleomycin, may cause local pulmonary accumulation of $[^{111}In]$-pentetreotide.

For imaging of NETs, $[^{111}In]$-DTPA-D-Phe^1-octreotide has occasionally shown higher accuracy than magnetic resonance imaging and CT as well as high-sensitivity ranging from 70% to 90% [14, 40]. The sensitivity is influenced by tumour type, anatomic site of origin and grade of differentiation [7]. Generally, highest sensitivity is achieved in gastroenteropancreatic NETs with reported sensitivities of 80–90% [3, 41]. Insulinomas are the exception with sensitivity of around 70%, which is caused by scarce overexpression of sstr2 [3, 41]. More aggressive tumours located in the gastrointestinalpancreatic system show lower sensitivities [3] and are more suited to undergo an FDG-PET/CT study. The detection of bronchopulmonary NETs is also sufficient with a sensitivity of around 70% [3]. The sensitivity for typical carcinoids of the lung the sensitivity is higher than for atypical carcinoid and small-cell lung cancer. For medullary thyroid cancer, the diagnostic performance of $[^{111}In]$-pentetreotide is poor with a sensitivity of about 50% [3, 42], and only the detection of cervical and mediastinal lymph node metastases is high. The rather low sensitivity in patients with medullary thyroid carcinoma is caused by dedifferentiation and lesional variation in sstr2 expression.

$[^{111}In]$-pentetreotide also possesses a high sensitivity (>90%) for extra-adrenal paragangliomas, especially in the head and neck region. For adrenal pheochromocytomas, $[^{111}In]$-pentetreotide is inferior to MIBG, yet possibly be more sensitive in detecting metastatic disease of phechromocytoma [41, 43]. MIBG is also superior to somatostatin receptor scintigraphy regarding the detection of neuroblastoma [41, 43].

Relevant uptake of $[^{111}In]$-pentetreotide is generally related to tumour manifestations of NET. Yet other tumours such as sarcomas, colon cancer, lymphomas, melanomas, breast cancer, differentiated thyroid cancer and prostate cancer can occasionally show overexpression of sstr2 as well [31]. Additionally, some non-malignant tissues, such as inflammatory or autoimmune processes, sarcoidosis, rheumatoid arthritis and blood vessels or lymphatic tissue can show relevant tracer uptake potentially leading to false-positive findings [31]. Semi-quantitative analysis of the tracer uptake can be performed (tumour-to-background), which seem to correlate with the density of somatostatin receptors on the cell surface. Often a visual scoring system is used to grade the intensity of tumour uptake (Krenning score system, Table 6.10). The extent of the sstr expression might be of prognostic relevance.

In planar images, signals from all depths of the body are registered by the gamma camera. Overprojection from organs and tissues with physiological uptake may completely obscure lesional uptake or by decreasing tumour-to-background ratio making the detection of tumour lesions difficult [31, 44]. Metastases or primaries of NETs can be particularly prone to this kind of observational oversight, as they are frequently small and preferentially located within the abdomen with relatively high background uptake. Therefore, the specificity of planar imaging alone in gastroenteropancreatic NETs is only about 50%. The tumour-to-background ratio is at the highest 24 h after administration; therefore, SPECT imaging should be performed at 24 h, but

SPECT imaging after 48 h can be helpful especially to evaluate potential pathological abdominal activity. SPECT enables visualization of occult lesions caused by organ overprojection. Still the exact location and characterisation of a detected lesion can be difficult due to the lack of morphological and anatomical information.

These drawbacks of SPECT can be overcome by using fused SPECT and CT images, which can ideally be simultaneously acquired using hybrid SPECT/CT cameras. The dual-modality imaging of SPECT/CT enables exact anatomical localization and morphological information combined with the functional data of the nuclear medicine procedure. Additionally, the spatial resolution increases enabling detection of smaller tumour lesions, which may not be visible in planar images or on a sole SPECT image. These advantages in the somatostatin receptor scintigraphy lead to an increased sensitivity and specificity compared to SPECT alone. Sensitivity and specificity ratios have been reported as high as 95% and 92%, respectively [45].

A further advantage of the hybrid imaging compared to SPECT alone is the possibility of reliable attenuation correction of the SPECT images. The effect of CT attenuation correction has been reported to a 2.2% increase in sensitivity as well as significant increase in contrast mostly in lymph nodes followed by bowel, pancreas and liver [46]. Other studies show that single-point SPECT/CT collected after 24 h is as specific and sensitive as traditional strategies (planar imaging and SPECT) using two imaging days [47]. This enhances patient convenience. Additionally, the incorporation of SPECT/CT increases report quality due to improved inter-rater agreement [48].

In Figs. 6.2, 6.3, 6.4, 6.5, and 6.6, a few examples are shown, where the use of SPECT/CT proves helpful and eventually improves diagnostic accuracy.

Various studies have shown that the sensitivity and specificity have most likely been highly overrated. In comparison to [^{68}Ga]-DOTATOC-PET/CT, the sensitivity of [^{111}In]-pentetreotide may be as low as 60% [33]. Figures 6.7 and 6.8 show an example of the superiority of [^{68}Ga]-DOTATOC-PET/CT vs. [^{111}In]-octreoscan SPECT/CT.

Encouraging results have been reported regarding the use of [^{111}In]-pentetreotide in radio-guided surgery [49]. The use of an intraoperative gamma probe enables the detection of lymph node metastases (local and occult) as well as helping in establishing tumour extension. As intestinal-NETs may be multifocal, the use of intraoperative gamma probe can be a supplement to the thorough palpation of the intestines to detect small lesions and ensure complete resection of all tumour manifestations. Hitherto experience in this field is still regarded as limited.

The addition of software tools to SPECT/CT has led to the discovery of useful new image parameters, i.e. tumour heterogeneity, aspheric-

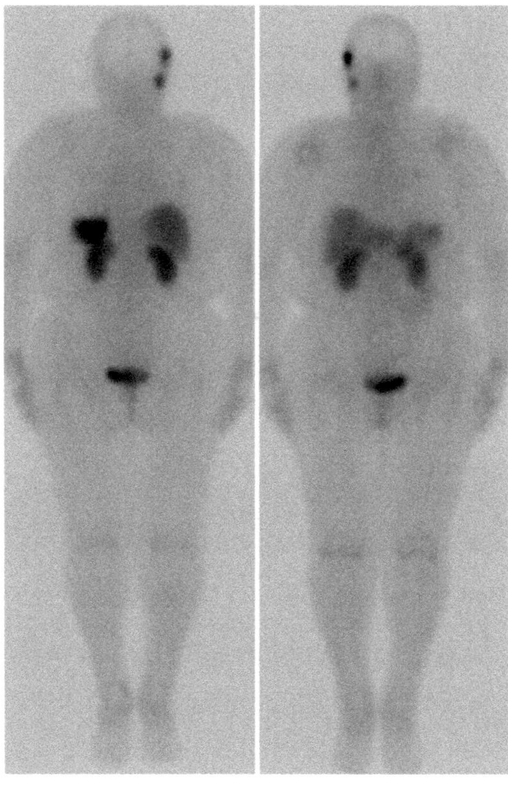

Fig. 6.2 [^{111}In]-pentetreotide of patient with NET (CUP), lymph node metastasis in the right mandibular angle, subcutaneous metastasis in the right temple and faint focal pulmonary uptake in left upper lobe and in the lower left lobe

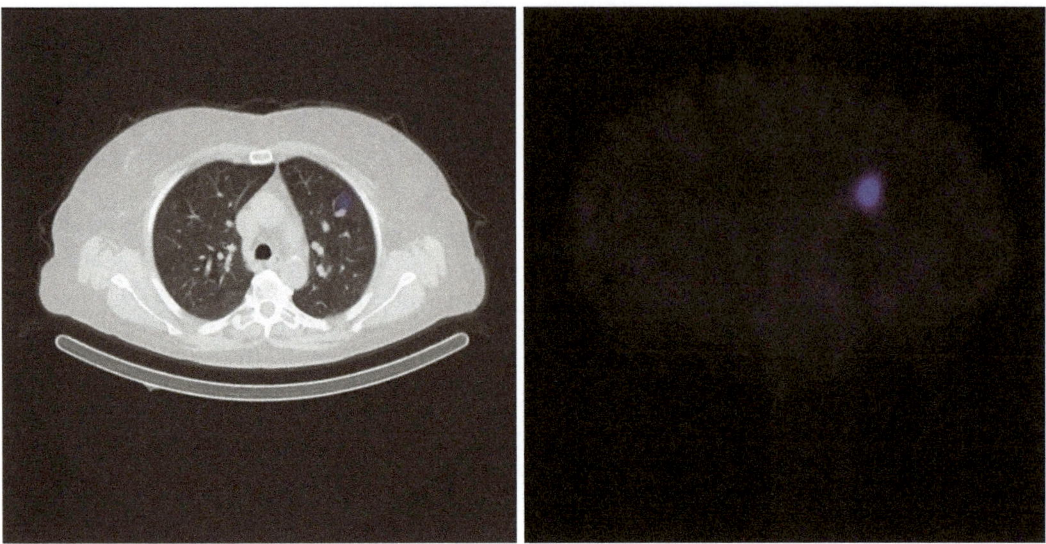

Fig. 6.3 Same patient as is Fig. 6.2 showing a discrete sstr-positive lung metastases in the left upper lobe

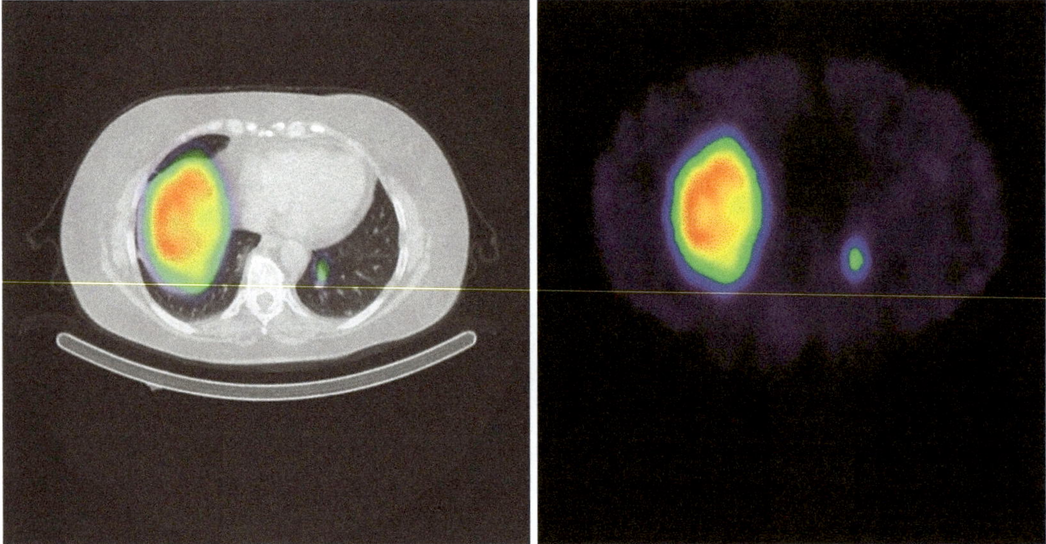

Fig. 6.4 Same patient as is Fig. 6.2 showing a sstr-positive lung metastases in the left inferior lobe

ity and quantitative SPECT/CT as well as a variety of useful semi-quantitative ROI techniques [39, 50].

These new features may among others contribute to predict treatment response prior to PRRT [50].

6.6.2 [^{99m}Tc]-EDDA/HYNIC-Tyr^3-Octreotide ([^{99m}Tc]-TEKTROTYD®)

Tc-99m-labelled radiopharmaceuticals offer many advantages compared to I-123 or In-111-

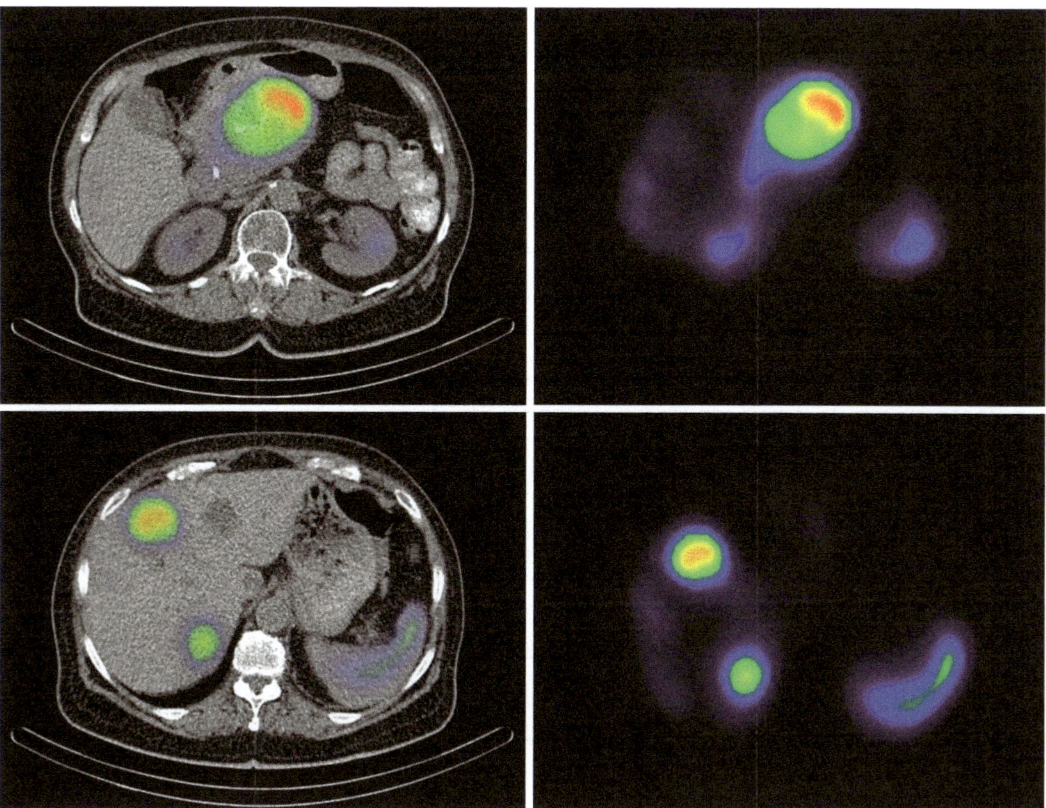

Fig. 6.5 [^{111}In]-pentetreotide SPECT/CT of patient with P-NET and liver metastases prior to PRRT with [^{177}Lu]-DOTA-TATE

labelled compounds. Products labelled with Tc-99m are constantly available and offer improved image quality as well as lower radiation exposure and shorter examination duration. In 2008, [^{99m}Tc]-EDDA/HYNIC-Tyr3-octreotide ([^{99m}Tc]-TEKTROTYD®) was registered for use in diagnostics of pathological lesions with hyperexpression of somatostatin receptors. This is particularly in regard to GEP-NET, pituitary adenomas, tumours of sympathoadrenal lineage and medullary thyroid cancer.

The recommended applied radioactivity is 740–925 MBq in a single intravenous injection, which results in an effective dose of around 4.6 ± 1.1 mSv [51]. The amount of peptide is approximately 20 µg, which again is not expected to cause any relevant side or biological effects.

Indications, precautions and patient preparations are identical to [^{111}In]-pentetreotide.

[^{99m}Tc]-EDDA/HYNIC-TOC is rapidly cleared from the blood after intravenous administration. The activity remaining in the blood is below 5% regardless of time after injection. Binding to blood proteins is lower at earlier time points (2–11% within 5 min after injection) compared to later time points (33–51% after 20 h). Renal elimination is predominant, whereas its hepatobiliary excretion is negligible. Cumulative urine elimination after 4 h is approximately 20% and within the first 24 h in the range of 24–64% of the applied dose [52]. The lesional uptake is usually swift, and after 10 min specific tracer accumulation is visible. The highest tumour-to-background-

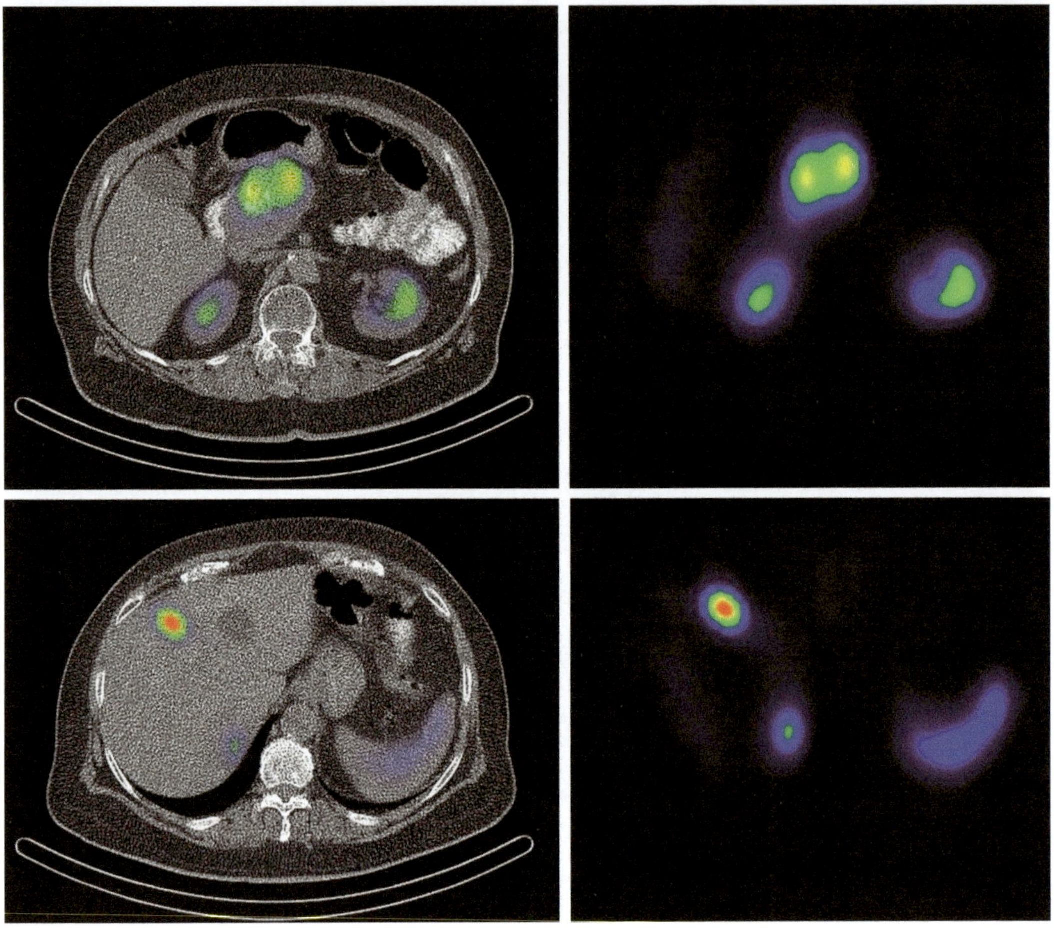

Fig. 6.6 Same patient as in Fig. 6.5 after undergoing 4 cycles of PRRT with [^{177}Lu]-DOTA-TATE, showing a partial remission

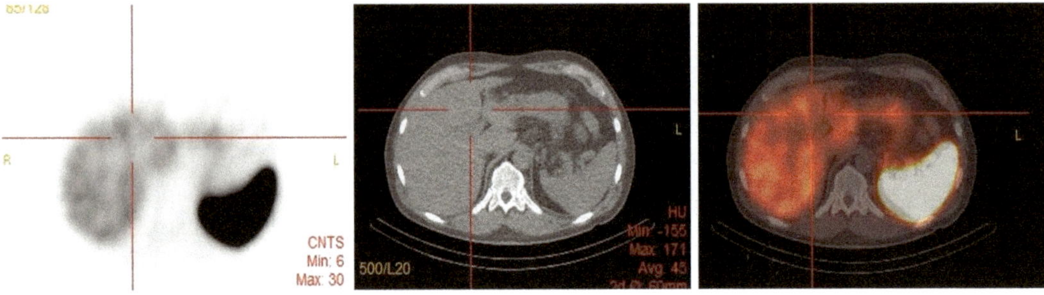

Fig. 6.7 [^{111}In]-Octreoscan-SPECT/CT patient with known liver metastasis in segment IV, but appearing isointense on SPECT/CT (Krenning-score 2)

ratio is seen at 4 h after injection. Lesions are still visible after 24 h, but sensitivity is due to the short half-life of Tc-99m reduced over time. A protocol for acquisition parameters using [^{99m}Tc]-EDDA/HYNIC-TOC is shown in Table 6.11.

The normal scintigraphic distribution pattern (Fig. 6.9) includes moderate to high physiologi-

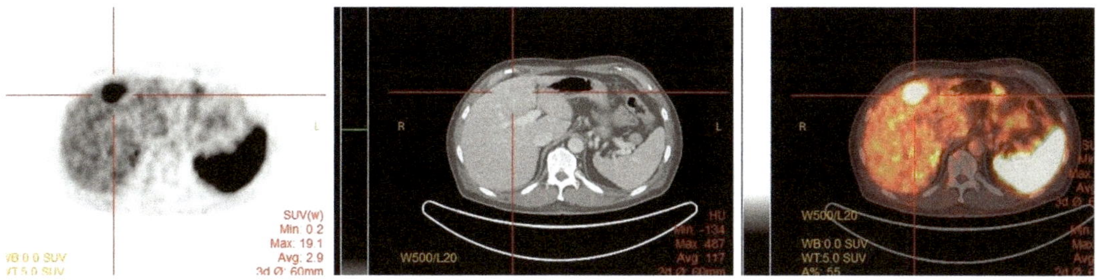

Fig. 6.8 Same patient as in Fig. 6.7 undergoing [Ga^{68}]-DOTATOC-PET/CT showing clearly sstr-positive liver metastasis in segment IV, enabling the patient to undergo PRRT

Table 6.11 Acquisition protocol for 99mTc-EDDA/HYNIC-TOC

Collimator	LEHR, parallel hole
Energy window	140 kEV with 20% window
Planar images (anterior and posterior) 128 × 128 or 256 × 256 matrix	2 h p.i. (5 min), 4 h p.i. (7 min), 24 h p.i. (15 min) per view
Whole body (256 × 1024 matrix)	Scanning speed: 2 h p.i. 15 cm/min, 4 h p.i. 10 cm/min, 24 h p.i. 5 cm/min
SPECT or SPECT/CT 128 × 128 acquisition matrix	360° rotation; 3° angular sampling, 2 h p.i. 20 s per projection, 4 h p.i. 30 s per projection

cal uptake in the kidneys, the liver, and the spleen. Intestinal uptake is weak to moderate. The pituitary or adrenal glands are more frequently seen than with [^{111}In]-pentetreotide. Other organs are visible at different time points as a result of tracer excretion, including the urinary tract, bladder, gallbladder and bowel. As seen with Octreoscan, about 19% of patients show benign pancreatic head uptake [39].

Whole-body scans using low-energy high-resolution (LEHR) collimators are usually performed 1–2 h and 4 h after injection. Delayed imaging (24–48 h) is possible and may prove helpful in interpreting bowel uptake, but the diagnostic sensitivity is reduced at later time points. In addition, SPECT or SPECT/CT (Fig. 6.10) is performed 4 h after injection due to maximal target-to-background ratio. In terms of sensitivity and diagnostic accuracy, SPECT/CT outperforms planar whole-body imaging and SPECT alone [53]. Incorporation

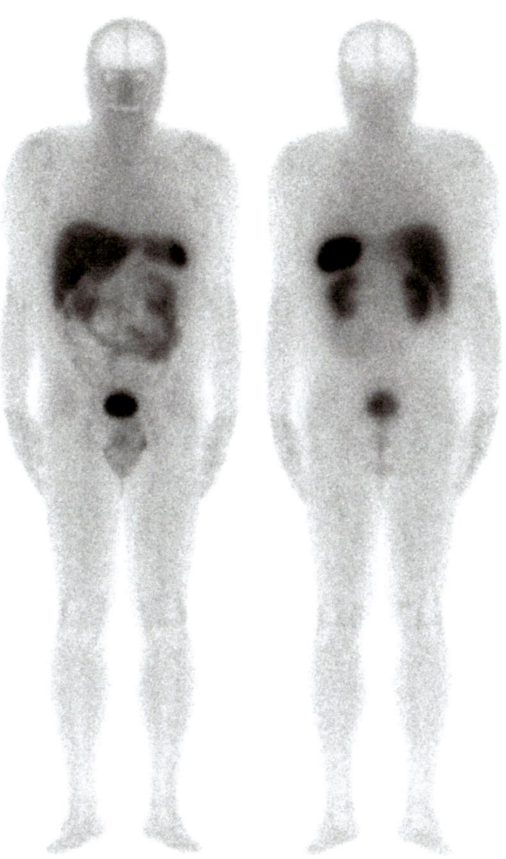

Fig. 6.9 Normal [^{99m}Tc]-EDDA/HYNIC-TOC whole-body scan (4 h p.i.) in anterior and posterior projection with physiologic tracer distribution

of SPECT/CT to the image protocol can enable an omission of early 2-h planar imaging without reducing the diagnostic accuracy [54]. Visual quantification of suspicious lesions is performed using the Krenning score scale (Table 6.10).

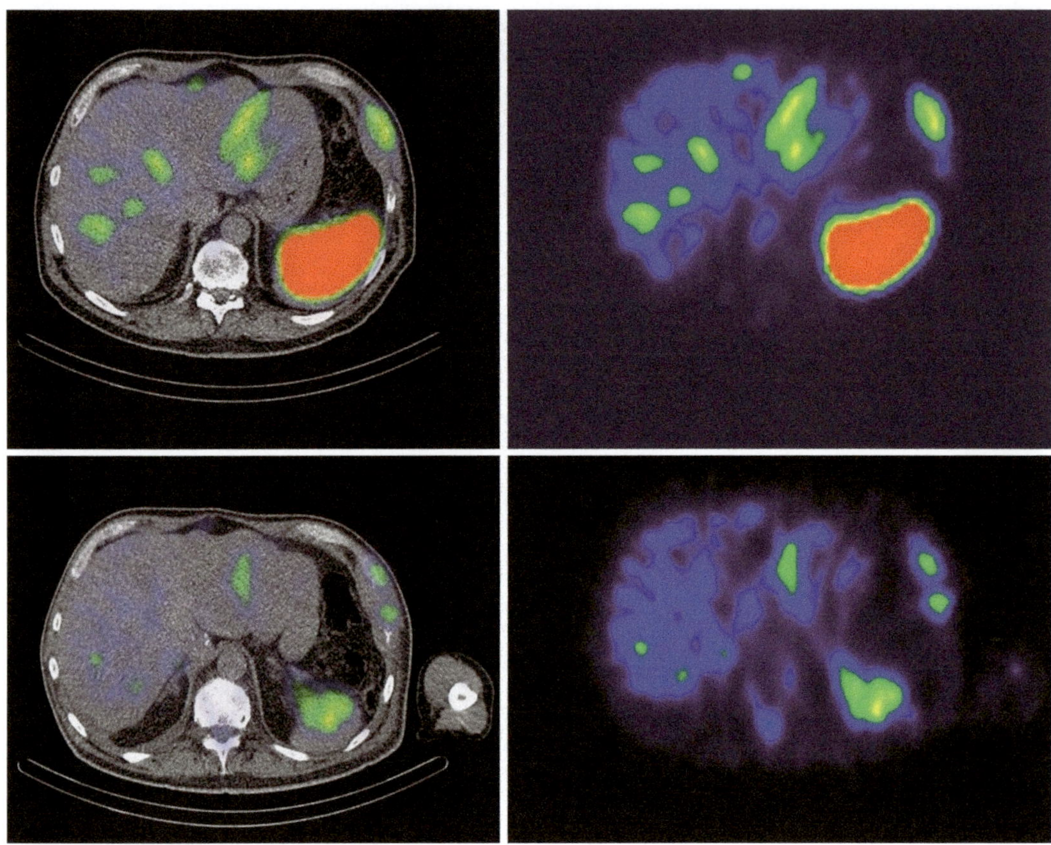

Fig. 6.10 [^{99m}Tc]-EDDA/HYNIC-TOC SPECT/CT 4 h p.i. Patient with hepatic metastases and bone metastases from a carcinoid tumour of the Ileum. The upper images show sstr-positive metastases prior to bilobar selective internal radiotherapy (SIRT). The lower images show a partial remission of the liver metastases 3 months after SIRT

Reports on [^{99m}Tc]-EDDA/HYNIC-TOC are steadily increasing. Early publications reported higher target-to-non-target ratios for [^{99m}Tc]-EDDA/HYNIC-TOC compared to [^{111}In]-pentetreotide [55, 56]. [^{99m}Tc]-EDDA/HYNIC-TOC also showed a higher sensitivity for NET detection in a direct comparison to [^{111}In]-pentetreotide with identification of more lesions, especially smaller liver and lymph node metastases [56]. The sensitivity in abdominal NETs is reported to be around 90%. However, similarly to ^{111}In-pentetreotide, the specificity seems to be rather moderate (40%) [56]. Reports differentiating between the various types of NET are rather scarce.

[^{99m}Tc]-EDDA/HYNIC-TOC possesses a rather moderate sensitivity of 50% for adrenal pheochromocytoma, but a high sensitivity (96%) for extra-adrenal pheochromocytoma [57].

In contrast to [^{111}In]-pentetreotide, a high sensitivity of 80% (specificity 83%) was reported in medullary thyroid cancer [58]. Overall, no significant clinical advantage over the long established [^{111}In]-pentetreotide has been identified.

As with [^{111}In]-pentetreotide, the sensitivity of [^{99m}Tc]-EDDA/HYNIC-TOC is highly overrated when compared to [^{68}Ga]-DOTATOC-PET/CT [59]. Reports are suggesting sensitivities as low as 60%, which is more or less comparable to [^{111}In]-pentetreotide [59]. Yet [^{99m}Tc]-EDDA/

HYNIC-TOC has advantages over [^{111}In]-Octreoscan in terms of lower radiation burden, lower costs, more patient convenient single day imaging as well as constant availability.

6.6.3 [^{99m}Tc]-Depreotide (NeoSPECT®)

The Tc-99m-labelled somatostatin derivative Depreotide (NeoSpect®) was approved to investigate solitary lung nodules suspicious for cancer. The recommended applied dosage is approximately 47 µg depreotide labelled with 555–740 MBq of technetium-99 m. [^{99m}Tc]-depreotide is administered intravenously in a single dose, resulting in an effective radiation dose of 8.88–11.84 mSv for a 70 kg individual. Precautions and patient preparations are identical to the ones for [^{111}In]-pentetreotide.

[^{99m}Tc]-depreotide possesses higher affinity to the somatostatin receptor subtypes sstr3 and sstr5 than [^{111}In]-pentetreotide or [^{99m}Tc]-EDDA/HYNIC-TOC. This characteristic may prove helpful in patients with tumours that are negative on [^{111}In]-pentetreotide scan but that remain highly suspicious for NET. Still [^{99m}Tc]-depreotide shows inferior results compared to [^{111}In]-pentetreotide for abdominal findings [60]. Furthermore, NeoSpect does not seem to add significant value to CECT in the evaluation of pulmonary lesions [61]. For those reasons and due to the infrequent use of NeoSpect for the approved indication, it was consequently withdrawn from the market in 2010 [62]. Due to relatively high uptake in inflammatory processes, [^{99m}Tc]-depreotide has been suggested for scintigraphic imaging of infections and inflammations of the bone [63].

6.6.4 [^{123}I]-MIBG

Some NENs are typically MIBG-avid, especially phaeochromocytomas and neuroblastomas. Further information of the use and relevance of [^{123}I]-MIBG and SPECT/CT can be found in Chap. 7 (I-MIBG SPECT/CT for tumour imaging).

6.6.5 Other Radiolabelled Peptide Receptor Tracers

Due to the diversity of receptors overexpressed by NETs, other imaging approaches have been made, but none are commercially available at the time being. Worth mentioning is the VIP receptor affine compound [^{99m}Tc]-TP3654, which has been studied in the context of gastrointestinal tract tumours [64]. Other studies have dealt with the Bombesin, neuropeptide (NP)-Y or CCK2 (gastrin/cholecystokinin 2) receptors as well as the receptor for glucagon-like peptide-1 (GLP-1R) [3]. Some sstr-negative NETs have been reported to express glucose-dependent insulinotropic polypeptide receptors (GIPR). A synthetic GIP analogue Lys37In-DTPA has shown promising results in visualizing these sstr-negative NENs [65].

6.7 Therapy of Neuroendocrine Neoplasms

The very heterogeneous group of NEN requires an individualized approach to therapy. The therapeutic procedure is determined by a vast range of factors such as primary, differentiation, extent of disease and hormonal activity. In general, potential curative surgical excision should be performed, whenever possible. However, many NENs have already metastasized by the time of diagnosis, making a curable approach impossible. For these NENs, numerous therapeutic alternatives are available. The therapeutic intervention can range from a platin-based chemotherapy scheme for aggressive NECs to biotherapy with unlabelled somatostatin derivatives, Interferon or receptor tyrosine kinase (RTK) inhibitors for the well-differentiated NETs. Another keystone in the therapeutic handling of patients with NET is the peptide receptor radionuclide therapy (PRRT/

PRRNT), which is now performed in numerous hospitals throughout the world. Following the excellent results of PRRT presented in the NETTER-1-trial, PRRT has become an established treatment option for patients suffering from NET [66].

6.7.1 Peptide Receptor-Based Radionuclide Therapy (PRRT/ PRRNT)

PRRT is a molecular-targeted systemic radiation therapy, which exploits the overexpression of receptors of NETs. Though mostly intravenously application of highly affine and specific agonists to the somatostatin receptors, PRRT has been successfully used to treat patients with NETs over the past 20 years [67–75]. The results of the successful phase 3 trial were published in 2017 [66]. The most common compounds used for PRRT are the beta-emitting derivatives [^{177}Lu]-DOTA-TOC/-TATE and [^{90}Y]-DOTA-TOC/-TATE.

Candidates for PRRT are patients with gastroenteropancreatic NET, broncho-pulmonary NET, phaeochromocytoma, paraganglioma, neuroblastoma, medullary thyroid carcinoma, meningioma and radioiodine-negative thyroid carcinoma. Yet not every patient with NET is suited to undergo PRRT, and different selection criterions do apply. PRRT can be performed in patients with histopathologically verified NET and documented sufficient tumoural somatostatin receptor expression (sstr scintigraphy or PET/CT). Sufficient tumour uptake is either defined as a scintigraphic Krenning-score greater than 2 or alternatively using different SUV-parameters on Ga68-DOTATOC/-TATE-PET/CT. In addition, the disease must be inoperable/metastatic and/or cause uncontrollable functional symptoms as well as progress during biotherapy. Another indication can be generally high-tumour load or the potential curative neo-adjuvant approach in initially non-resectable NETs. Furthermore, the Karnofsky performance should exceed 60%, and the tumour differentiation should preferably be grade 1/2 and the Ki-67 index <20%. It is an absolute contraindication to perform PRRT in patients lacking sstr expression, pregnant patients and patients with severe concomitant illness or unmanageable psychiatric disorder. Relative contraindications are breast feeding (if not discontinued), severely reduced kidney function (creatinine >1.7 mg/dl, GFR/TER < 60% of mean age-adjusted normal values) as well as severely compromised bone marrow function.

Before starting the treatment, long-acting "cold" somatostatin preparations should be withdrawn 4–6 weeks prior to PRRT, depending on the clinical symptoms a switch to short-acting formulations can follow. The short-acting analogues have to be discontinued at least 24 h prior to treatment initiation. A blood cell count and a control of kidney function parameters are also obligate. Usually, a 99m-Tc-DTPA and/or 99mTc-MAG3 study is performed to monitor the GFR and/or TER.

Furthermore, due to the proximal reabsorption of the radiolabelled peptide and subsequent retention in the kidney, an infusion in regard to renal protection must be performed. An amino acid solution consisting of arginine and lysine is intravenously administered 30–60 min before and maintained for 4 h after radiopeptide administration to reduce nephrotoxicity. Prior to the application of the amino acid solution, an antiemetic drug (e.g. 5-HT3 antagonist) should be administered and can be repeated if necessary. Corticosteroids can be given as well to prevent nausea or pain caused by radiation inflammation.

The radiopeptide is diluted with saline and intravenously co-infused with the amino acid solution over approximately 30 min. Acute side effects can be nausea, pain caused by tumour lesions or functional symptoms due to excessive hormone release. Electrolyte imbalance (hyperkalaemia, hypernatraemia) caused by the amino acid solution is a possible acute side effect as well. Long-term side effects can be severe nephrotoxicity (<1%), haematoxicity (4–8%) and myelodysplastic syndromes (0.5%). Mild myelosuppression is seen in about 30% of patients [67–75].

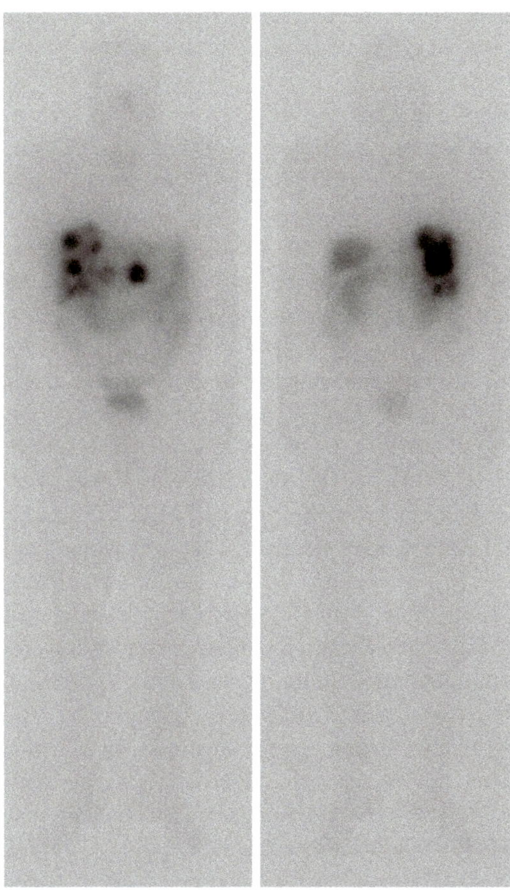

Fig. 6.11 Post-therapy whole-body scan ([¹⁷⁷Lu]-DOTA-TATE) of patient with P-NET and hepatic metastases

During the last years, promising results of intra-arterial application of PRRT in the hepatic artery (Figs. 6.13 and 6.14) have been presented. This approach leads to a higher radiation deposit in liver metastases and reduced radiation exposure for extrahepatic organs [76].

6.7.2 [¹⁷⁷Lu]-DOTA⁰-Tyr³-Octreotate

Lu-177 is a mixed beta and gamma-emitting radioisotope with a half-life of 6–7 days. The beta rays possess a mean range of 0.5 mm in tissue and thus sparing the non-tumorous tissue in near proximity of tumour lesions. Medium-energy gamma rays can be used for post-therapy scans (Figs. 6.11, 6.12, 6.13, and 6.14) and dosimetry. Between 5.55 and 9.25 GBq (150–250 mCi) of Lu-177-labelled DOTA-TOC/-TATE are applied, the standard amount being 7.4 GBq (200 mCi). One patient usually undergoes 3–5 treatment cycles with 6–12 weeks interval between every cycle.

Results following PRRT with [¹⁷⁷Lu]-DOTA-TATE are more than sufficient with reported complete and partial remissions in 30%, minor responses in 15% and stabilization in 35% of treated NET patients. Approximately, 20% of the patients progress while undergoing PRRT. In 310

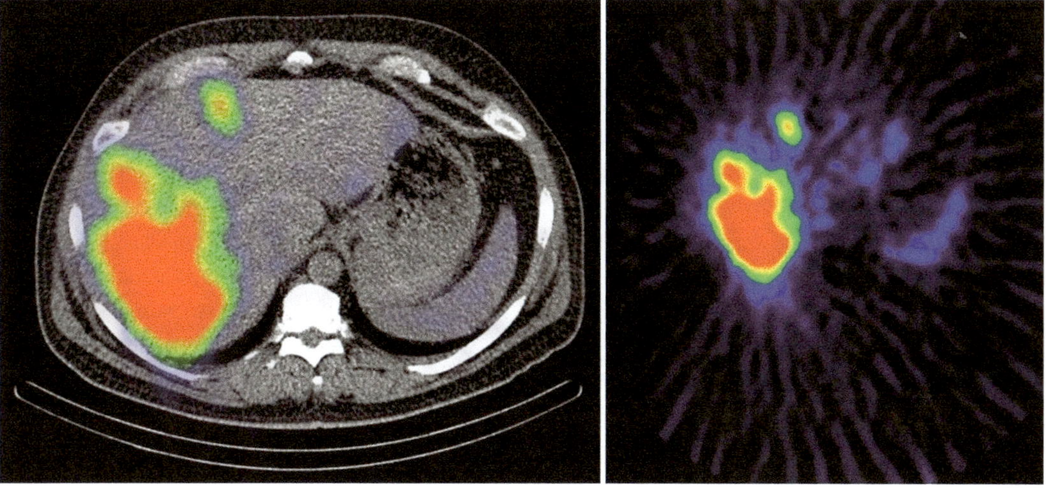

Fig. 6.12 Post-therapy SPECT/CT of the abdomen of same patient as in Fig. 6.11 showing radionuclide uptake in the liver metastases

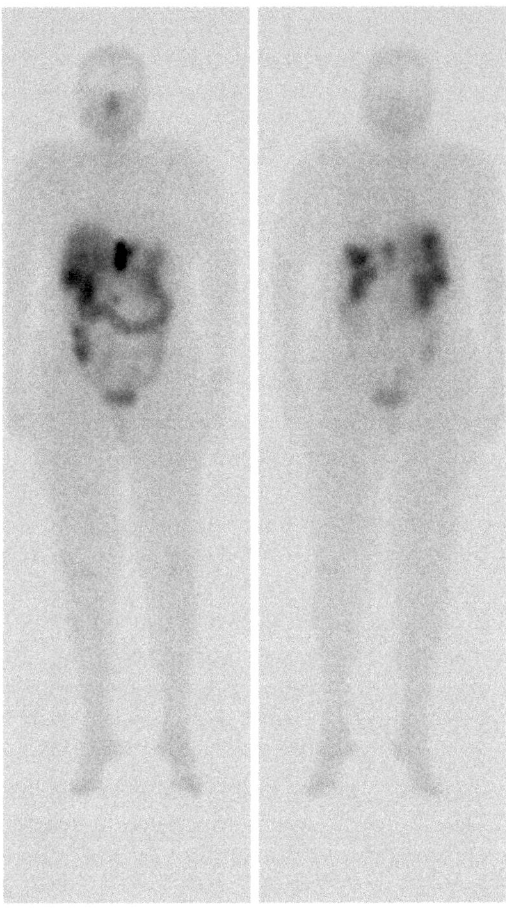

Fig. 6.13 Patient with P-NET and hepatic metastases. Post-therapy whole-body scan after intra-arterial application (hepatic artery) of [^{177}Lu]-DOTA-TATE

patients with gastroenteropancreatic NET, progression-free survival (PFS) was reported to be 33 months with an overall survival of 46 months [67–75]. In the NETTER-1 trial, PFS was initially estimated to 40 months with 18% objective response rate [66].

6.7.3 Dosimetry

Radiation dosimetry of tumour lesions and normal organs provides vital information for optimizing the administration of PRRT. Dosimetry allows maximizing radiation dose delivered to malignant lesions, while minimizing the dose delivered to normal organs, especially kidney and bone marrow. Patient-specific dosimetry should be assessed to provide specific information regarding absorbed dose to certain organs and thus enabling prediction of potential delayed organ toxicity. Following PRRT determination of absorbed dose in organs at risk is recommended and may become mandatory. These parameters can be obtained using SPECT/CT at different time points, dosimetry software and serial blood samples.

Different methods can be applied for radiation dosimetry including data from blood or urine samples or sequent whole-body scans (Figs. 6.11, 6.13, 6.15, and 6.16) and/or SPECT/CT after PRRT. Planar images and/or SPECT/CT at different time points (e.g. 24, 48 and 96 h after treatment) are useful to show pharmacokinetics over a certain time period. The typical biokinetics of radiopeptides with rapid blood clearance and predominant renal excretion determine the information (blood and urine samples, scintigraphic data) required to attain correct dosimetry. In addition, sequential scans enable the possibility of determining absorbed tumour dose, which again may predict treatment response.

SPECT and SPECT/CT (Figs. 6.12, 6.14, and 6.16) images provide insight into organ-specific three-dimensional radioactivity distribution. Especially the hybrid image modality SPECT/CT with the possibility to calculate exact target volume and build reconstruction algorithms with attenuation and scatter correction should enable accurate non-invasive quantitative imaging [77–80]. Reports on quantitative SPECT (QSPECT) of ^{177}Lu sources on a commercially available SPECT/CT system have showed high accuracy in phantom models and after PRRT with [^{177}Lu]-DOTA-TATE [80]. QSPECT can potentially yield more accurate dosimetry data and therefore more accurate therapeutic response assessment [80]. As bremsstrahlung images are difficult to quantify, the dosimetry after PRRT is mainly the domain of [^{177}Lu]-DOTA-TATE.

Hitherto treatment dosimetry rarely influences the therapeutic protocol, due to the lack of solid reliable data with respect to dose thresholds for

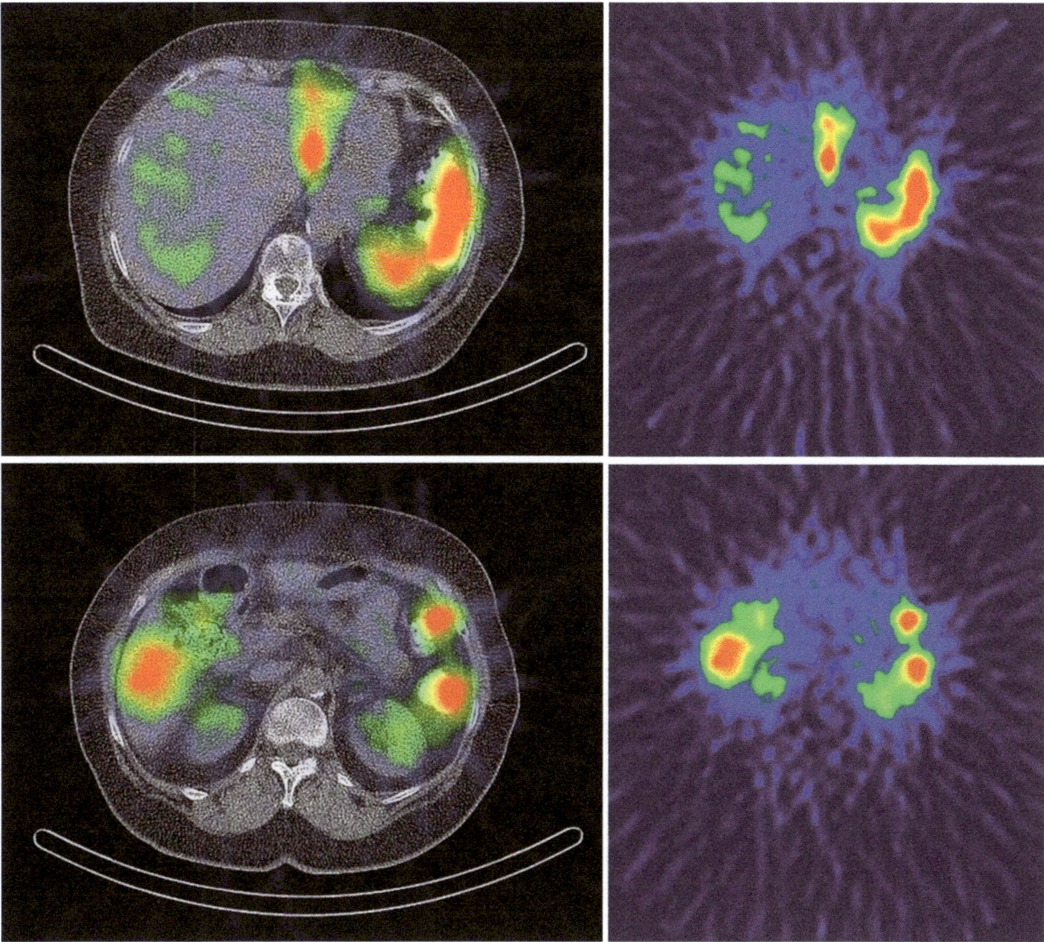

Fig. 6.14 Same patient as in Fig. 6.13. Post-therapy SPECT/CT of the abdomen showing high uptake in the liver metastases

organs-at-risk. Yet the increasing awareness of the importance of dosimetry and availability of software tools may lead to the implementation of a more personal tailored, more effective and safer PRRT in the future.

6.7.4   [⁹⁰Y]-DOTA⁰-Tyr³-Octreotide

PRRT may be performed using beta-emitting [⁹⁰Y]-DOTA-labelled TOC or TATE as well. Y-90 possesses different radiophysical characteristics compared to Lu-177, such as shorter half-life, higher beta energy and lack of gamma emission. The indications and precautions are identical to the one described in the chapter for [¹⁷⁷Lu]-DOTA-TATE. Usually 2–4 cycles with 2.78–4.44 GBq (75–120 mCi) [⁹⁰Y]-DOTA-TOC/-TATE are performed. Following the NETTER-1 trial, the lutetium-labelled compound is more frequently used. Yet promising results have been shown applying a tandem treatment combining [¹⁷⁷Lu]-DOTA-TATE and [⁹⁰Y]-DOTA-TATE [81].

Further information about the relevance of bremsstrahlung imaging and SPECT/CT after PRRT with [⁹⁰Y] compounds can be found in Chap. 13 (?) Bremsstrahlung SPECT/CT.

6.7.5 [⁹⁰Y]-Microspheres and [¹⁶⁶Ho]-Microspheres

NETs often metastasize to the liver, and these metastases are typically hypervascular. Therefore, a local treatment with Y-90- or Ho-166-microspheres by limited (or progressive) disease to the liver can be safely and successfully applied in patients with liver metastases [82–84]. For more information about post-therapy bremsstrahlung imaging and SPECT/CT look in Chap. 12 (?) Therapyplanning with SPECT/CT in Radioembolisation of Liver Tumours and chapter 13 (?) Bremsstrahlung SPECT/CT.

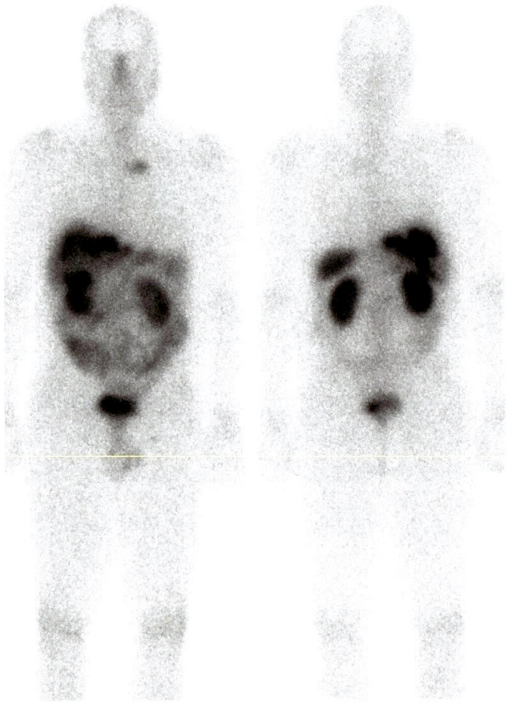

6.7.6 [¹³¹I]-MIBG

Pheochromocytomas and neuroblastomas are able to actively take up MIBG. Further information regarding use and relevance of post-therapeutic I-131-MIBG scintigraphy and SPECT/CT can be found in Chap. 7 (I-MIBG SPECT/CT for tumour imaging).

6.8 Summary

The incidence of neoendocrine neoplasms has steadily been rising and thus enhancing their clinical impact. Somatostatin receptor imaging has proved to be an important tool in the clinical handling of patients with NET. Somatostatin receptor scintigraphy is used for staging, therapy planning, follow-up and treatment monitoring of these patients. Additionally, the presence of somatostatin receptor overexpression is an important prognostic parameter. Furthermore, the introduction of SPECT and SPECT/CT has significantly improved the accuracy of scintigraphic somatostatin receptor imaging. This improvement-enabled 3D imaging and attenuation correction and added much desired morphologic and anatomic information to the functional image modalities. Over the last decade, [68Ga]-DOTATOC/-TATE-PET/CT has taken over as gold standard, by outperforming scintigraphic methods in terms of sensitivity and diagnostic accuracy as well as patient convenience.

Fig. 6.15 Patient with GEP-NET undergoing PRRT with [¹⁷⁷Lu]-DOTATATE with known liver metastases, cervical lymph node metastasis

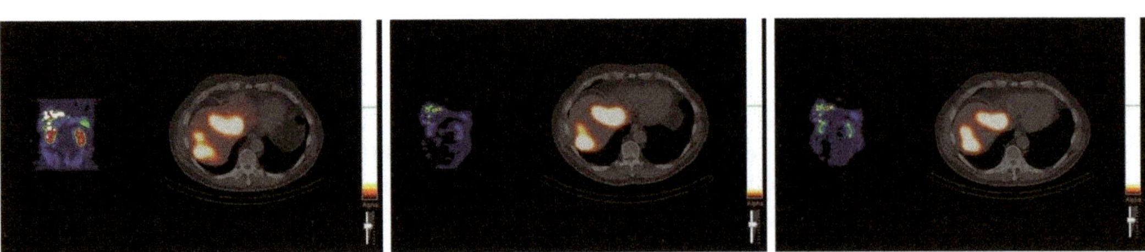

Fig. 6.16 Same patient as in Fig. 6.15 undergoing sequential 3 time point SPECT/CT due determine absorbed dose to kidneys and tumour lesions. SPECT/CT after 24 h, 72 h and 7 days after PRRT administration

PRRT utilizing the beta emitting substances [^{90}Y]-DOTA-TOC/-TATE and [^{177}Lu]-DOTA-TATE/-TOC has become an integral part in the treatment of patients with NET, especially following the superb results in the NETTER-1-trial. This therapeutic alternative has shown good outcomes with prolonged survival and is generally well tolerated. An essential part of the therapeutic handling is patient-specific dosimetry, which helps to optimize PRRT treatment administration. This again could lead to more accurate prediction regarding delayed radiation side effects and therapy outcome. SPECT and SPECT/CT enable 3D imaging of the radionuclide distribution and thus more accurate dosimetry data.

New tools such as quantitative SPECT/CT (QSPECT/CT) and software as well as increasing reports on dosimetry may lead to more frequent use of individualized tailored PRRT, which may be safer and/or more effective. In addition, new image parameters (radiomics) may further enhance the information.

References

1. Gustafsson BI, Kidd M, Modlin IM. Neuroendocrine tumors of the diffuse neuroendocrine system. Curr Opin Oncol. 2008;20:1–12. https://doi.org/10.1097/CCO.0b013e3282f1c595.
2. Modlin IM, Oberg K, Chung DC, Jensen RT, de Herder WW, Thakker RV, et al. Gastroenteropancreatic neuroendocrine tumours. Lancet Oncol. 2008;9:61–72. https://doi.org/10.1016/s1470-2045(07)70410-2.
3. Koopmans KP, Neels ON, Kema IP, Elsinga PH, Links TP, de Vries EG, et al. Molecular imaging in neuroendocrine tumors: molecular uptake mechanisms and clinical results. Crit Rev Oncol Hematol. 2009;71:199–213. https://doi.org/10.1016/j.critrevonc.2009.02.009.
4. Modlin IM, Lye KD, Kidd M. A 5-decade analysis of 13,715 carcinoid tumors. Cancer. 2003;97:934–59. https://doi.org/10.1002/cncr.11105.
5. Lawrence B, Gustafsson BI, Chan A, Svejda B, Kidd M, Modlin IM. The epidemiology of gastroenteropancreatic neuroendocrine tumors. Endocrinol Metab Clin N Am. 2011;40(1):1–18, vii. https://doi.org/10.1016/j.ecl.2010.12.005. Review.
6. Kimura W, Kuroda A, Morioka Y. Clinical pathology of endocrine tumors of the pancreas. Analysis of autopsy cases. Dig Dis Sci. 1991;36(7):933–42.
7. Teunissen JJ, Kwekkeboom DJ, Valkema R, Krenning EP. Nuclear medicine techniques for the imaging and treatment of neuroendocrine tumours. Endocr Relat Cancer. 2011;18(Suppl 1):S27–51. https://doi.org/10.1530/erc-10-0282.
8. Reubi JC, Waser B. Concomitant expression of several peptide receptors in neuroendocrine tumours: molecular basis for in vivo multireceptor tumour targeting. Eur J Nucl Med Mol Imaging. 2003;30:781–93. https://doi.org/10.1007/s00259-003-1184-3.
9. Reubi JC, Waser B, Schaer JC, Laissue JA. Somatostatin receptor sst1-sst5 expression in normal and neoplastic human tissues using receptor autoradiography with subtype-selective ligands. Eur J Nucl Med. 2001;28:836–46.
10. Hoyer D, Bell GI, Berelowitz M, Epelbaum J, Feniuk W, Humphrey PP, et al. Classification and nomenclature of somatostatin receptors. Trends Pharmacol Sci. 1995;16:86–8. S0165614700889889 [pii]
11. Patel YC. Somatostatin and its receptor family. Front Neuroendocrinol. 1999;20:157–98.
12. Volante M, Bozzalla-Cassione F, Papotti M. Somatostatin receptors and their interest in diagnostic pathology. Endocr Pathol. 2004;15:275–91.
13. Patel YC. Molecular pharmacology of somatostatin receptor subtypes. J Endocrinol Investig. 1997;20:348–67.
14. Bombardieri E, Coliva A, Maccauro M, Seregni E, Orunesu E, Chiti A, et al. Imaging of neuroendocrine tumours with gamma-emitting radiopharmaceuticals. Q J Nucl Med Mol Imaging. 2010;54:3–15.
15. Massironi S, Sciola V, Peracchi M, Ciafardini C, Spampatti M, Conte D. Neuroendocrine tumors of the gastro-entero-pancreatic system. World J Gastroenterol. 2008;14(35):5377. https://doi.org/10.3748/wjg.14.5377.
16. Metz DC, Jensen RT. Gastrointestinal neuroendocrine tumors: pancreatic endocrine tumors. Gastroenterology. 2008;135(5):1469–92. https://doi.org/10.1053/j.gastro.2008.05.047.
17. Klimstra DS, Modlin IR, Coppola D, et al. The pathologic classification of neuroendocrine tumors: a review of nomenclature, grading, and staging systems. Pancreas. 2010;39:707.
18. Rindi G, Arnold R, Bosman FT, et al. Nomenclature and classification of neuroendocrine neoplasms of the digestive system. In: Bosman TF, Carneiro F, Hruban RH, Theise ND, editors. WHO classification of tumours of the digestive system. 4th ed. Lyon: International Agency for Research on cancer (IARC); 2010. p. 13.
19. Hruban RH, Pitman MB, Klimstra DS. Tumors of the pancreas. Washington, DC: ARP/AFIP; 2007. p. 422.
20. Panzuto F, Boninsegna L, Fazio N, et al. Metastatic and locally advanced pancreatic endocrine carcinomas: analysis of factors associated with disease progression. J Clin Oncol. 2011;29:2372.
21. La Rosa S, Klersy C, Uccella S, et al. Improved histologic and clinicopathologic criteria for prognostic evaluation of pancreatic endocrine tumors. Hum Pathol. 2009;40:30.

22. von Herbay A, Sieg B, Schürmann G, et al. Proliferative activity of neuroendocrine tumours of the gastroenteropancreatic endocrine system: DNA flow cytometric and immunohistological investigations. Gut. 1991;32:949.

23. La Rosa S, Sessa F, Capella C, et al. Prognostic criteria in nonfunctioning pancreatic endocrine tumours. Virchows Arch. 1996;429:323.

24. Jann H, Roll S, Couvelard A, et al. Neuroendocrine tumors of midgut and hindgut origin: tumor-node-metastasis classification determines clinical outcome. Cancer. 2011;117:3332.

25. La Rosa S, Inzani F, Vanoli A, et al. Histologic characterization and improved prognostic evaluation of 209 gastric neuroendocrine neoplasms. Hum Pathol. 2011;42:1373.

26. Pape UF, Jann H, Müller-Nordhorn J, et al. Prognostic relevance of a novel TNM classification system for upper gastroenteropancreatic neuroendocrine tumors. Cancer. 2008;113:256.

27. Strosberg J, Nasir A, Coppola D, et al. Correlation between grade and prognosis in metastatic gastroenteropancreatic neuroendocrine tumors. Hum Pathol. 2009;40:1262.

28. Yang Z, Tang LH, Klimstra DS. Effect of tumor heterogeneity on the assessment of Ki67 labeling index in well-differentiated neuroendocrine tumors metastatic to the liver: implications for prognostic stratification. Am J Surg Pathol. 2011;35:853.

29. Basturk O, Yang Z, Tang LH, Hruban RH, Adsay V, McCall CM, et al. The high-grade (WHO G3) pancreatic neuroendocrine tumor category is morphologically and biologically heterogenous and includes both well differentiated and poorly differentiated neoplasms. Am J Surg Pathol. 2015;39(5):683–90. https://doi.org/10.1097/PAS.0000000000000408.

30. Sorbye H, Strosberg J, Baudin E, Klimstra DS, Yao JC. Gastroenteropancreatic high-grade neuroendocrine carcinoma. Cancer. 2014;120(18):2814–23. https://doi.org/10.1002/cncr.28721.

31. Delle Fave G, Kwekkeboom DJ, Van Cutsem E, Rindi G, Kos-Kudla B, Knigge U, Sasano H, Tomassetti P, Salazar R, Ruszniewski P. ENETS Consensus Guidelines for the management of patients with gastroduodenal neoplasms. Barcelona Consensus Conference participants. Neuroendocrinology. 2012;95(2):74–87. https://doi.org/10.1159/000335595. Epub 2012 Feb 15.

32. Reubi JC, Schar JC, Waser B, Wenger S, Heppeler A, Schmitt JS, et al. Affinity profiles for human somatostatin receptor subtypes SST1-SST5 of somatostatin radiotracers selected for scintigraphic and radiotherapeutic use. Eur J Nucl Med. 2000;27:273–82.

33. Van Binnebeek S, Vanbilloen B, Baete K, Terwinghe C, Koole M, Mottaghy FM, Clement PM, Mortelmans L, Bogaerts K, Haustermans K, Nackaerts K, Van Cutsem E, Verslype C, Verbruggen A, Deroose CM. Comparison of diagnostic accuracy of (111) In-pentetreotide SPECT and (68)Ga-DOTATOC PET/CT: a lesion-by-lesion analysis in patients with metastatic neuroendocrine tumours. Eur Radiol. 2016;26(3):900–9. https://doi.org/10.1007/s00330-015-3882-1. Epub 2015 Jul 12.

34. Pauwels E, Cleeren F, Bormans G, Deroose CM. Somatostatin receptor PET ligands - the next generation for clinical practice. Am J Nucl Med Mol Imaging. 2018;8(5):311–31.

35. Kwekkeboom DJ, Krenning EP, Scheidhauer K, Lewington V, Lebtahi R, Grossman A, Vitek P, Sundin A, Plöckinger U. ENETS Consensus Guidelines for the Standards of Care in Neuroendocrine Tumors: somatostatin receptor imaging with (111) In-pentetreotide. Mallorca Consensus Conference participants; European Neuroendocrine Tumor Society. Neuroendocrinology. 2009;90(2):184–9. https://doi.org/10.1159/000225946. Epub 2009 Aug 28.

36. Balon HR, Brown TL, Goldsmith SJ, Silberstein EB, Krenning EP, Lang O, et al. The SNM practice guideline for somatostatin receptor scintigraphy 2.0. J Nucl Med Technol. 2011;39:317–24. https://doi.org/10.2967/jnmt.111.098277.

37. Aalbersberg EA, de Wit-van der Veen BJ, Versleijen MWJ, Saveur LJ, Valk GD, Tesselaar MET, Stokkel MPM. Influence of lanreotide on uptake of ^{68}Ga-DOTATATE in patients with neuroendocrine tumours: a prospective intra-patient evaluation. Eur J Nucl Med Mol Imaging. 2019;46(3):696–703. https://doi.org/10.1007/s00259-018-4117-x. Epub 2018 Aug 10.

38. Bombardieri E, Ambrosini V, Aktolun C, Baum RP, Bishof-Delaloye A, Del Vecchio S, et al. 111In-pentetreotide scintigraphy: procedure guidelines for tumour imaging. Eur J Nucl Med Mol Imaging. 2010;37:1441–8. https://doi.org/10.1007/s00259-010-1473-6.

39. Derakhshan JJ, Farwell MD. Prevalence and quantitative analysis of In-111 pentetreotide (Octreoscan) uptake in the pancreatic head on SPECT/CT imaging: establishing an ROI-based pathological uptake threshold. Nucl Med Commun. 2019;40(7):727–33. https://doi.org/10.1097/MNM.0000000000001022.

40. Pepe G, Moncayo R, Bombardieri E, Chiti A. Somatostatin receptor SPECT. Eur J Nucl Med Mol Imaging. 2012;39(Suppl 1):S41–51. https://doi.org/10.1007/s00259-011-2019-2.

41. Rufini V, Calcagni ML, Baum RP. Imaging of neuroendocrine tumors. Semin Nucl Med. 2006;36:228–47. https://doi.org/10.1053/j.semnuclmed.2006.03.007.

42. Mariani G, Bruselli L, Kuwert T, Kim EE, Flotats A, Israel O, et al. A review on the clinical uses of SPECT/CT. Eur J Nucl Med Mol Imaging. 2010;37:1959–85. https://doi.org/10.1007/s00259-010-1390-8.

43. van der Harst E, de Herder WW, Bruining HA, Bonjer HJ, de Krijger RR, Lamberts SW, et al. [(123)I]metaiodobenzylguanidine and [(111)In]octreotide uptake in benign and malignant pheochromocytomas. J Clin Endocrinol Metab. 2001;86:685–93.

44. Zanzonico P. Principles of nuclear medicine imaging: planar, SPECT, PET, multi-modality, and autoradiography systems. Radiat Res. 2012;177:349–64.
45. Perri M, Erba P, Volterrani D, Lazzeri E, Boni G, Grosso M, et al. Octreo-SPECT/CT imaging for accurate detection and localization of suspected neuroendocrine tumors. Q J Nucl Med Mol Imaging. 2008;52:323–33.
46. Steffen IG, Mehl S, Heuck F, Elgeti F, Furth C, Amthauer H, Ruf J. Attenuation correction of somatostatin receptor SPECT by integrated low-dose CT: is there an impact on sensitivity? Clin Nucl Med. 2009;34(12):869–73. https://doi.org/10.1097/RLU.0b013e3181becfcb.
47. Wong KK, Wynn EA, Myles J, Ackermann RJ, Frey KA, Avram AM. Comparison of single time-point [111-In] pentetreotide SPECT/CT with dual time-point imaging of neuroendocrine tumors. Clin Nucl Med. 2011;36(1):25–31. https://doi.org/10.1097/RLU.0b013e3181feedc0.
48. Apostolova I, Riethdorf S, Buchert R, Derlin T, Brenner W, Mester J, Klutmann S. SPECT/CT stabilizes the interpretation of somatostatin receptor scintigraphy findings: a retrospective analysis of inter-rater agreement. Ann Nucl Med. 2010;24(6):477–83. https://doi.org/10.1007/s12149-010-0383-9. Epub 2010 May 7.
49. Bombardieri E, Coliva A, Maccauro M, Seregni E, Orunesu E, Chiti A, Lucignani G. Imaging of neuroendocrine tumours with gamma-emitting radiopharmaceuticals. Q J Nucl Med Mol Imaging. 2010;54(1):3–15.
50. Christoph W, Apostolova I, Steffen IG, Hofheinz F, Furth C, Kupitz D, Ruf J, Venerito M, Klose S, Amthauer H. Predictive value of asphericity in pretherapeutic [111In]DTPA-octreotide SPECT/CT for response to peptide receptor radionuclide therapy with [177Lu]DOTATATE. Mol Imaging Biol. 2017;19(3):437–45. https://doi.org/10.1007/s11307-016-1018-x.
51. Grimes J, Celler A, Birkenfeld B, Shcherbinin S, Listewnik MH, Piwowarska-Bilska H, Mikolajczak R, Zorga P. Patient-specific radiation dosimetry of 99mTc-HYNIC-Tyr3-octreotide in neuroendocrine tumors. J Nucl Med. 2011;52(9):1474–81. https://doi.org/10.2967/jnumed.111.088203. Epub 2011 Jul 27.
52. Institute of Atomic Energy (Poland). 99mTc-Tektrotyd summary of product characteristics. 2007.
53. Trogrlic M, Težak S. Incremental value of (99m)Tc-HYNIC-TOC SPECT/CT over whole-body planar scintigraphy and SPECT in patients with neuroendocrine tumours. Nuklearmedizin. 2017;56(3):97–107. https://doi.org/10.3413/Nukmed-0851-16-10. Epub 2017 Feb 6.
54. Al-Chalabi H, Cook A, Ellis C, Patel CN, Scarsbrook AF. Feasibility of a streamlined imaging protocol in technetium-99m-Tektrotyd somatostatin receptor SPECT/CT. Clin Radiol. 2018;73(6):527–34. https://doi.org/10.1016/j.crad.2017.12.019. Epub 2018 Feb 2.
55. Decristoforo C, Mather SJ, Cholewinski W, Donnemiller E, Riccabona G, Moncayo R. 99mTc-EDDA/HYNIC-TOC: a new 99mTc-labelled radiopharmaceutical for imaging somatostatin receptor-positive tumours; first clinical results and intra-patient comparison with 111In-labelled octreotide derivatives. Eur J Nucl Med. 2000;27:1318–25.
56. Gabriel M, Decristoforo C, Donnemiller E, Ulmer H, Watfah Rychlinski C, Mather SJ, et al. An intra-patient comparison of 99mTc-EDDA/HYNIC-TOC with 111In-DTPA-octreotide for diagnosis of somatostatin receptor-expressing tumors. J Nucl Med. 2003;44:708–16.
57. Chen L, Li F, Zhuang H, Jing H, Du Y, Zeng Z. 99mTc-HYNIC-TOC scintigraphy is superior to 131I-MIBG imaging in the evaluation of extraadrenal pheochromocytoma. J Nucl Med. 2009;50:397–400. https://doi.org/10.2967/jnumed.108.058693.
58. Czepczynski R, Parisella MG, Kosowicz J, Mikolajczak R, Ziemnicka K, Gryczynska M, et al. Somatostatin receptor scintigraphy using 99mTc-EDDA/HYNIC-TOC in patients with medullary thyroid carcinoma. Eur J Nucl Med Mol Imaging. 2007;34:1635–45. https://doi.org/10.1007/s00259-007-0479-1.
59. de Camargo Etchebehere ECS, de Oliveira Santos A, Gumz B, Vicente A, Hoff PG, Corradi G, Ichiki WA, de Almeida Filho JG, Cantoni S, Camargo EE, Costa FP. 68Ga-DOTATATE PET/CT, 99mTc-HYNIC-octreotide SPECT/CT, and whole-body MR imaging in detection of neuroendocrine tumors: a prospective trial. J Nucl Med. 2014;55(10):1598–604. https://doi.org/10.2967/jnumed.114.144543. Epub 2014 Aug 28.
60. Lebtahi R, Le Cloirec J, Houzard C, Daou D, Sobhani I, Sassolas G, et al. Detection of neuroendocrine tumors: 99mTc-P829 scintigraphy compared with 111In-pentetreotide scintigraphy. J Nucl Med. 2002;43:889–95.
61. Harders SW, Madsen HH, Hjorthaug K, Rehling M, Rasmussen TR, Pedersen U, Pilegaard HK, Meldgaard P, Baandrup UT, Rasmussen F. Limited value of 99mTc depreotide single photon emission CT compared with CT for the evaluation of pulmonary lesions. Br J Radiol. 2012;85(1015):e307–13. https://doi.org/10.1259/bjr/10438644.
62. Brandon D, Alazraki A, Halkar RK, Alazraki NP. The role of single-photon emission computed tomography and SPECT/computed tomography in oncologic imaging. Semin Oncol. 2011;38:87–108. https://doi.org/10.1053/j.seminoncol.2010.11.003.
63. Papathanisou ND, Rondogianni PE, Pianou NK, Karampina PA, Vlontzou EA, Datseris IE. 99m-Tc-depreotide in the evaluation of bone infection and inflammation. Nucl Med Commun. 2008;29:239–46.
64. Pallela VR, Thakur ML, Chakder S, Rattan S. 99mTc-labeled vasoactive intestinal peptide receptor agonist: functional studies. J Nucl Med. 1999;40:352–60.
65. Willekens SMA, Joosten L, Boerman OC, Brom M, Gotthardt M. Characterization of 111In-labeled glucose-dependent insulinotropic polypeptide

as a radiotracer for neuroendocrine tumors. Sci Rep. 2018;8(1):2948. https://doi.org/10.1038/s41598-018-21259-3.

66. Strosberg J, El-Haddad G, Wolin E, Hendifar A, Yao J, Chasen B, Mittra E, Kunz PL, Kulke MH, Jacene H, Bushnell D, O'Dorisio TM, Baum RP, Kulkarni HR, Caplin M, Lebtahi R, Hobday T, Delpassand E, Van Cutsem E, Benson A, Srirajaskanthan R, Pavel M, Mora J, Berlin J, Grande E, Reed N, Seregni E, Öberg K, Lopera Sierra M, Santoro P, Thevenet T, Erion JL, Ruszniewski P, Kwekkeboom D, Krenning E. Phase 3 trial of (177)Lu-Dotatate for midgut neuroendocrine tumors. N Engl J Med. 2017;1(2):125–35. https://doi.org/10.1056/NEJMoa1607427.

67. Kwekkeboom DJ, Bakker WH, Kooij PP, et al. [177 Lu-DOTA 0 Tyr 3]octreotate: comparison with [111 In-DTPA 0] octreotide in patients. Eur J Nucl Med. 2001;28:1319–25.

68. Esser JP, Krenning EP, Teunissen JJ, Kooij PP, van Gameren AL, Bakker WH, Kwekkeboom DJ. Comparison of [(177) Lu-DOTA (0), Tyr (3)] octreotate and [(177) Lu-DOTA (0), Tyr (3)] octreotide: which peptide is preferable for PRRT? Eur J Nucl Med Mol Imaging. 2006;33:1346–1351.16.

69. Kwekkeboom DJ, De Herder WW, Kam BL, et al. Treatment with the radiolabeled somatostatin analog [177 Lu-DOTA 0, Tyr 3]octreotate: toxicity, efficacy, and survival. J Clin Oncol. 2008;26:2124–30.

70. Otte A, Herrmann R, Heppeler A, et al. Yttrium-90 DOTATOC: first clinical results. Eur J Nucl Med. 1999;26:1439–47.

71. Waldherr C, Pless M, Maecke HR, Haldemann A, Mueller-Brand J. The clinical value of [90 Y-DOTA]-D-Phe 1-Tyr 3-octreotide (90 YDOTATOC) in the treatment of neuroendocrine tumours: a clinical phase II study. Ann Oncol. 2001;12:941–5.

72. Waldherr C, Pless M, Maecke HR, et al. Tumor response and clinical benefit in neuroendocrine tumors after 7.4 GBq (90)Y-DOTATOC. J Nucl Med. 2002;43:610–6.

73. Hörsch D, Ezziddin S, Haug A, Gratz KF, Dunkelmann S, Krause BJ, Schümichen C, Bengel FM, Knapp WH, Bartenstein P, Biersack HJ, Plöckinger U, Schwartz-Fuchs S, Baum RP. Peptide receptor radionuclide therapy for neuroendocrine tumors in Germany: first results of a multi-institutional cancer registry. Recent Results Cancer Res. 2013;194:457–65. https://doi.org/10.1007/978-3-642-27994-2_25.

74. Ezziddin S, Sabet A, Heinemann F, Yong-Hing CJ, Ahmadzadehfar H, Guhlke S, Höller T, Willinek W, Boy C, Biersack HJ. Response and long-term control of bone metastases after peptide receptor radionuclide therapy with (177)Lu-octreotate. J Nucl Med. 2011;52(8):1197–203. https://doi.org/10.2967/jnumed.111.090373. Epub 2011 Jul 15.

75. Forrer F, Waldherr C, Maecke HR, Mueller-Brand J. Targeted radionuclide therapy with 90Y-DOTATOC in patients with neuroendocrine tumors. Anticancer Res. 2006;26(1B):703–7.

76. van Vliet EI, Teunissen JJ, Kam BL, de Jong M, Krenning EP, Kwekkeboom DJ. Treatment of gastroenteropancreatic neuroendocrine tumors with peptide receptor radionuclide therapy. Neuroendocrinology. 2013;97(1):74–85. https://doi.org/10.1159/000335018. Epub 2012 Jan 10.

77. Shcherbinin S, Piwowarska-Bilska H, Celler A, Birkenfeld B. Quantitative SPECT/CT reconstruction for ^{177}Lu and ^{177}Lu/^{90}Y targeted radionuclide therapies. Phys Med Biol. 2012;57(18):5733–47. https://doi.org/10.1088/0031-9155/57/18/5733. Epub 2012 Sep 5.

78. Shcherbinin S, Celler A, Belhocine T, Vanderwerf R, Driedger A. Accuracy of quantitative reconstructions in SPECT/CT imaging. Phys Med Biol. 2008;53(17):4595–604. https://doi.org/10.1088/0031-9155/53/17/009. Epub 2008 Aug 4.

79. Garkavij M, Nickel M, Sjögreen-Gleisner K, Ljungberg M, Ohlsson T, Wingårdh K, Strand SE, Tennvall J. 177Lu-[DOTA0,Tyr3] octreotate therapy in patients with disseminated neuroendocrine tumors: analysis of dosimetry with impact on future therapeutic strategy. Cancer. 2010;116(4 Suppl):1084–92. https://doi.org/10.1002/cncr.24796.

80. Beauregard JM, Hofman MS, Pereira JM, Eu P, Hicks RJ. Quantitative (177)Lu SPECT (QSPECT) imaging using a commercially available SPECT/CT system. Cancer Imaging. 2011;11:56–66. https://doi.org/10.1102/1470-7330.2011.0012.

81. Kunikowska J, Zemczak A, Kołodziej M, Gut P, Łoń I, Pawlak D, Mikołajczak R, Kamiński G, Ruchała M, Kos-Kudła B, Królicki L. Tandem peptide receptor radionuclide therapy using ^{90}Y/^{177}Lu-DOTATATE for neuroendocrine tumors efficacy and side-effects - polish multicenter experience. Eur J Nucl Med Mol Imaging. 2020;47(4):922–33. https://doi.org/10.1007/s00259-020-04690-5.

82. Ezziddin S, Meyer C, Kahancova S, Haslerud T, Willinek W, Wilhelm K, Biersack HJ, Ahmadzadehfar H. 90Y Radioembolization after radiation exposure from peptide receptor radionuclide therapy. J Nucl Med. 2012;53(11):1663–9. https://doi.org/10.2967/jnumed.112.107482. Epub 2012 Sep 17.

83. Ahmadzadehfar H, Biersack HJ, Ezziddin S. Radioembolization of liver tumors with yttrium-90 microspheres. Semin Nucl Med. 2010;40(2):105–21. https://doi.org/10.1053/j.semnuclmed.2009.11.001. Review.

84. Rajekar H, Bogammana K, Stubbs RS. Selective internal radiation therapy for gastrointestinal neuroendocrine tumour liver metastases: a new and effective modality for treatment. Int J Hepatol. 2011;2011:404916. https://doi.org/10.4061/2011/404916. Epub 2011 Nov 15.

$^{123/131}$I-MIBG SPECT/CT for Tumour Imaging

Hojjat Ahmadzadehfar and Marianne Muckle

7.1 Introduction

Metaiodobenzylguanidine (mIBG) is an aralkyl-guanidine norepinephrine analogue, which was clinically introduced in 1981 and developed to visualize tumours of the adrenal medulla [1]. It enters the neuroendocrine cells of postganglionic sympathetic neurons by an active uptake mechanism via the epinephrine transporter and is stored in the neurosecretory granule without being metabolized. This leads to a difference in the concentration compared to cells of other tissues [2, 3], whereas the storage intensity of mIBG-avid tissue is dependent on tissue uptake, and the storage capacity is proportional to the quantity of catecholamine-containing vesicles in the tumour and tracer turnover [4–6].

7.2 Physical Properties of ^{123}I and ^{131}I

^{123}I is a pure gamma-emitting radionuclide used only for diagnostic imaging. The physical half-life of ^{123}I is 13.13 h, and its principal gamma

photon is emitted at 159 keV (83% abundance). It also emits multiple low-abundance, high-energy photons. ^{131}I emits a principal gamma photon of 364 keV (81% abundance) with a physical half-life of 8.04 days and also beta particles with a maximum energy of 0.61 MeV (mean 0.192 MeV) [2, 5].

mIBG can be labelled with ^{131}I or ^{123}I and allows scintigraphic delineation of neuroectodermal tumours [2, 5]. Although ^{131}I-mIBG can be applied for diagnostics, it is mostly used for therapeutic purposes. Its utilization for diagnostics is possible whether ^{123}I-mIBG is commercially unavailable (as was the case in several countries such as the USA until 2008) or in the case of estimation of tumour uptake for mIBG therapy planning [7].

Nonetheless, for diagnostic issues, ^{123}I-mIBG has some advantages over ^{131}I-mIBG, namely, its better physical characteristics, which result in better image quality. Its gamma energy (159 keV) is more appropriate for imaging than the 360 keV gamma photons of ^{131}I. Its higher photon efficiency in combination with shorter half-life (13.13 h vs. 8.04 days) induces a more suitable radiation dosimetry and lower radiation burden and therefore allows injection of higher tracer activities, resulting in higher count rates. In addition, the duration between injection and imaging is shorter (4–24 h) than with ^{131}I-mIBG scintigraphy (48–72 h), because, with ^{131}I-mIBG, delayed images may be required for optimal

H. Ahmadzadehfar (✉)
Department of Nuclear Medicine, Klinikum
Westfalen, Dortmund, Germany
e-mail: hojjat.ahmadzadehfar@ruhr-uni-bochum.de,
hojjat.ahmadzadehfar@klinikum-westfalen.de

M. Muckle
Radiology am Rhein, Bad Honnef, Germany

H. Ahmadzadehfar et al. (eds.), *Clinical Applications of SPECT-CT*,
https://doi.org/10.1007/978-3-030-65850-2_7

target-to-background ratios [6, 8]. Finally, ^{123}I-mIBG is the radiopharmaceutical of choice concerning diagnostic imaging, even if its use may be limited due to higher costs and inferior availability [3, 5].

7.3 Indications for mIBG Scan

There are several non-oncological indications for ^{123}I-mIBG scintigraphy, such as disorders of the sympathetic innervation of the myocardium (cardiomyopathy), differentiation between idiopathic Parkinson's disease and multisystem atrophy or hyperplasia of the adrenal medulla, which are not addressed in this chapter [3]; however, there is a wide spectrum of different oncological indications, especially for imaging of neuroendocrine neoplasms (e.g. neuroendocrine tumours (NET)/ neuroendocrine carcinomas (NEC), phaeochromocytomas/paragangliomas, neuroblastoma and medullary thyroid carcinoma) [2].

7.4 Patient Preparation

Pre-treatment with a saturated solution of sodium perchlorate is required to protect the thyroid from ablation and absorption of free iodine, especially as the infantile thyroid is very sensitive to radiation. Thyroid blockade (130 mg/day of potassium iodide; equivalent to 100 mg of iodine) should be started 1 day before tracer injection and continued for 1–2 days for ^{123}I-mIBG or 2–3 days for ^{131}I-mIBG. In the case of intolerance of sodium perchlorate, potassium perchlorate (SSKI) should be applied (administered 4 h before tracer injection and continued for 2 days; 400–600 mg/day) [3]. After appropriate thyroid blocking, a slow intravenous injection (over about 1 min) reduces side effects such as hypertensive crisis and tachycardia, which can occur as rare side effects rather concerning with catecholamine-producing tumours such as phaeochromocytomas. Adverse allergic reactions are not expected.

7.5 Interfering Drugs

There are some drugs known to interfere with mIBG uptake, such as tricyclic antidepressants (amitriptyline, imipramine), sympathomimetics (phenylephrine, phenylpropanolamine, ephedrine, xylometazoline and cocaine) and also antihypertensive medications such as labetalol, reserpine or calcium channel blockers. If possible, these medications should be discontinued for sufficient time prior to scintigraphy [5, 9–12].

The use of non-prescription drugs should also be considered, especially in children, and the use of the nasal drops or sprays containing xylometazoline or bronchodilators such as fenoterol, salbutamol, sultanol and terbutaline.

However, there are no precise data as to whether there is an influence of the abovementioned drugs on mIBG uptake. Therefore, it is unknown how often false-negative mIBG scans occur because of these medications [3].

7.6 Contraindications

Pregnancy is with very few exceptions classified as absolute contraindication. After an mIBG scintigraphy with ^{123}I, breastfeeding should be discontinued for 48 h, and the milk should be pumped out and discarded. After investigation with ^{131}I, ablactation is recommended. There is not any known contraindication in children [3].

7.7 Dose Calculation

The recommended activities in adults are 200–400 MBq for ^{123}I-mIBG and 40–80 MBq for ^{131}I-mIBG. The activity administered to children should be calculated on the basis of a reference dose for an adult, scaled to body weight according to the schedule proposed by the EANM Paediatric Task Group [13].

7.8 Image Acquisition

The particular strength of mIBG scan lays in providing a whole-body evaluation with one single administration of the radiotracer. ^{123}I-mIBG scans are usually obtained 20–24 h after tracer injection. Selected delayed images (never later than day 2) may be useful in the case of equivocal findings on day 1. Early static images at 4–6 h after injection can be performed optionally to assess the dynamics of the tracer accumulation. Scanning with ^{131}I-mIBG is performed 1 and 2 days after injection and can be repeated at day 3 or later [3].

Planar and tomographic (SPECT/CT) images are performed with a multiple-head gamma camera with a large field of view. A high-energy parallel hole collimator is used for ^{131}I-mIBG and a low-energy high-resolution collimator (LEHR) for ^{123}I-mIBG. Whole-body imaging with additional spot images should be performed. With ^{123}I-mIBG, a total body scan with a speed of 5 cm/min or both anterior and posterior static spot views of the head and neck, chest, abdomen, pelvis and upper and lower extremities with about 500 k counts or 10–15 min acquisition per image using a 256 × 256 matrix or 128 × 128 matrix with zoom, and a 20% window centred at the 159 keV photo peak is usually performed. More useful information regarding acquisition, reconstruction parameters and camera settings for whole body and planar spot imaging have been described in detail elsewhere [2].

7.9 Acquisition of SPECT/CT

mIBG SPECT/CT should cover the region of interest (e.g. pelvis, abdomen or thorax), especially the anatomical regions showing pathological tracer uptake on planar images or reported suspected lesions by other modalities such as MRI.

Generally, SPECT images are obtained for a 360° orbit in 120 projections (128 × 128 matrix,

6° angle steps, 30–45 s per step or in 3° steps in continuous or step and shoot mode, 25–35 s per step). In the case of noncompliant patients or children, it is possible to reduce acquisition time (6° steps or a 64 × 64 matrix with shorter time per frame) [14, 15]. If only one mIBG SPECT/CT scan can be performed, acquisition at 24 h is preferred because of a higher target-to-background ratio.

SPECT/CT imaging is performed with co-registered CT images (100–130 keV, mAs modulation recommended) with high resolution in order to have a better characterization of the anatomical surroundings. This enables attenuation correction and facilitates precise localization of any focus of increased tracer uptake, which is particularly useful over the abdomen and head and neck region. Despite additional radiation burden of the (low-dose) CT, regardless, SPECT/CT should be performed in children in case of equivocal findings that, by SPECT alone, cannot be ascertained. Sedation of children is often necessary and is taken into account.

7.10 Reconstruction of SPECT/CT

Iterative reconstruction or other validated reconstruction protocols that allow accurate visualization of lesions and a CT-based attenuation correction should be performed. Scatter correction methods using spectral analysis can be used to improve the accuracy of quantification. Iterative reconstruction with a low-pass post-filter often provides better images than filtered back-projection. Any reporting should clearly state the methodology adopted for image processing and quantification [2].

7.11 Radiation Exposure

The radiation exposure depends on amount of the applied activity, which should be limited according to weight and age (for paediatric patients, see guidelines for radioiodinated mIBG scintigraphy in children) [16].

The effective doses are 0.013 mSv/MBq for ^{123}I-mIBG and 0.14 mSv/MBq for ^{131}I-mIBG in adults and 0.037 mSv/MBq for ^{123}I-mIBG and 0.43 mSv/MBq for ^{131}I-mIBG in children (5 years old) [17, 18]; for example, a 5-year-old child's radiation exposure is about 5.6 mSv (18 kg for 124 MBq ^{123}I-mIBG) [3, 19]. Additional SPECT with low-dose CT implicates increased radiation dose (volume CT dose index: 3–5 mGy, depending on acquisition parameters).

7.12 Physiological mIBG Uptake and Distribution

mIBG is normally taken up mainly by the liver; lower levels of uptake have been described in the spleen, lungs, salivary glands, skeletal muscles and heart, based on the extensive sympathetic innervation of these tissues and/or catecholamine excretion [5].

One of the other variants in biodistribution of ^{123}I-mIBG is its accumulation in brown fat tissue in children which is more common in cold weather than in warm weather [20, 21]. This may be seen mainly in the neck and supraclavicular regions [21].

Therefore, evaluation and interpretation of mIBG scans should be considered thoroughly, especially if unknown suspicious findings are next to those regions or organs with physiological uptake, avoiding false-positive or false-negative results, e.g. in the liver with its diffuse, inhomogeneous tracer uptake, the discrimination between physiological enhancement and focal suspicious tracer accumulation is sometimes challenging, particularly in the case of small liver lesions.

Concerning the adrenal glands, symmetrical mIBG uptake less than or equivalent to liver uptake is described to be physiological. Normal, non-enlarged adrenal glands are sometimes difficult to localize on planar mIBG scans. The majority of mIBG is excreted unaltered by the kidneys (50% of the injected dose is recovered in the urine within 24 h), while faecal elimination is weak. In patients with phaeochromocytoma and paraganglioma, uptake in the heart and liver is significantly lowered by about 40% [22].

7.13 The Importance of mIBG SPECT and SPECT/CT

Many studies indicate a high sensitivity and specificity of mIBG scintigraphy detecting tumours of the sympathetic nerve system. For neuroblastoma, sensitivity is about 80% for determining neuroblastoma lesions, while specificity is nearly 100% in the guidelines [3].

These data are mostly based on performing planar and whole-body images in many previous studies, as modern hybrid systems such as SPECT or SPECT/CT were not yet available [23, 24].

Based on these data, it could be concluded that whole-body imaging and planar imaging are sufficient enough, and additional diagnostic tools such as SPECT or SPECT/CT are not required to achieve good diagnostic results with respect to mIBG scintigraphy.

However, the use and benefit of SPECT for achieving better diagnostic accuracy has already been described in several studies and highlighted in the guidelines when it comes to smaller tumour lesions or suspicious findings next to organs, which physiologically accumulate mIBG, such as the urinary bladder or liver.

But despite this diagnostic benefit, SPECT is not sufficient in all cases and cannot achieve adequate diagnostic accuracy since differentiation between physiological structures and the findings is not always possible because of absent anatomical correlations.

Such difficulties occur regularly and require the best care and attention by the nuclear medicine physicians, as the interpretation of the findings in the mIBG scan often has far-reaching consequences and the results of an mIBG scan might influence the running therapy.

One way to overcome these limitations is the additional advantage of SPECT with potential of fusion with other radiological imaging methods (MRI/CT scan) [3, 14, 15, 25]. However, this option may suffer from the problem that SPECT and MRI/CT images sometimes cannot be fused exactly, as the slices do not match to each other.

A way out of this dilemma is newly available hybrid SPECT/CT cameras, which enable direct correlation of anatomic and functional information [26–30]. Physiological activities can be delineated properly, which otherwise would have required additional imaging. With the help of low-dose CT of SPECT/CT, more accurate spatial resolution than using SPECT alone can be achieved. This results in a better localization and clearer delineation of small tumour lesions [31].

Besides detailed anatomic evaluation of suspicious findings such as mIBG avide or non-avide lesions, there is the above-mentioned possibility of fusion or co-registration SPECT/low-dose CT with diagnostic CT or MRI, whereas low-dose CT serves as a bridging tool for anatomical orientation. As a consequence, SPECT/CT findings may guide the diagnostic CT or MRI concerning equivocal findings. To summarize, SPECT/CT bridges the gap between mIBG scintigraphy and diagnostic CT or MRI scans, with guidance of diagnostic CT/MRI and characterization of its findings [30].

7.14 MIBG SPECT/CT in Neuroblastoma

Neuroblastoma is the third most common malignant solid tumour in childhood and the most common extra cranial malignant tumour (8–10%). This tumour entity arises in the adrenal gland (65%) or the sympathetic nervous system, as its cells are derived from the embryonic neural crest and remain as autonomous nervous tissue-neuroblasts in an immature state [32–34].

About 40% of children are diagnosed in the first year; the incidence decreases with age. Ninety percent of patients are younger than 6 years. The median age at diagnosis is 2 years. In a many of cases, there are already metastases of neuroblastoma at the time of diagnosis. It metastasizes to the liver, adrenal glands, lymph nodes, bone marrow and bone, whereas the pri-

mary can be localized at the cervical, thoracic and abdominal trunk, as well as the paraganglia [34, 35].

Approximately 40% of patients are at stage 4 (INSS classification) at the time of diagnosis with detection of distant metastases. Since the spread of the disease correlates with the prognosis and thus affects the extent of therapy, an accurate detection of all tumour foci is essential to determine the spread of the disease [3, 33, 34, 36].

In addition to the conventional radiological diagnostic modalities, such as ultrasound and CT, MRI plays an important role and may provide important information regarding to the basic staging, the tumour locations and choosing appropriate site for bioptic assurance.

Staging is completed with performing a ^{123}I-mIBG scan, which has the advantage of whole-body evaluation with one single administration of the radiotracer. This can provide important information about tumour localization and thus has an influence on the treatment planning with regard to chemotherapy strategy or possible operation plans [5]. The specificity of mIBG for detecting tumours of the sympathetic nervous system is nearly 100%. The sensitivity for the detection of an individual neuroblastoma lesion is stated to be 80% [3, 32, 37–44]. By using SPECT/CT, the sensitivity can be increased to 98% [45]. A recent published study reported that by using SPECT/CT in the follow-up of patients with high-risk neuroblastoma, the interpretation of planar imaging can be improved significantly and in 39% of cases SPECT/CT provided additional information [46].

7.14.1 Interpretation of the Findings: What Is Physiological?

To distinguish true-positive from false-positive findings, the knowledge of physiological distribution of mIBG in different organs or localizations is of importance (see above). Approximately 10% of patients show (usually symmetric) mIBG uptake in brown adipose tissue of the neck and shoulder area [3]. Tracer uptake in the myocardium can be relatively high, especially in children under 1 year. At other ages, comparable mIBG-storage can also be found in the liver, which may complicate the detection and distinction of suspicious liver lesions, especially if whole-body imaging and planar imaging are performed without any additional SPECT/CT.

In addition, free iodine causes thyroid uptake and storage in the gastrointestinal tract. The bony skeleton has no mIBG storage. In the extremities, only slight activity is found in the muscles and the bones, whereas the knees and joints can be seen as cold areas [3, 20, 21].

7.14.2 Image Interpretation

7.14.2.1 False-Negative Findings
Lesions may be overlooked due to anatomical or physiological reasons: small lesions that are close to the primary tumour, next to large metastases or in regions with high physiological uptake (myocardium, thyroid, salivary glands, liver, kidney, bladder and colon) maybe overlooked [3, 43, 47]. These limitations can be solved by using SPECT/CT (Figs. 7.1 and 7.2).

7.14.2.2 False-Positive Findings
There are different benign accumulations which could cause false-positive results including accumulation in the lung correlating with pneumonia or because of atelectasis, mIBG uptake in the focal nodular hyperplasia, intense uptake in the liver because of prior radiation, because of accessory spleen [48] and also because of contamination, most often urine contamination or any other contamination (salivary secretion). Using SPECT/CT can avoid misinterpretation of these findings.

7.14.3 SPECT/CT: Reducing False-Negative and -Positive Results

As mentioned, SPECT/CT allows better anatomical localization of mIBG-avide findings, which is essential in most cases. In particular, fusion of SPECT with other imaging modalities (MRI/diagnostic CT) improves diagnostic accuracy, while low-dose CT of mIBG-SPECT/CT serves as anatomical orientation [30] (Fig. 7.3).

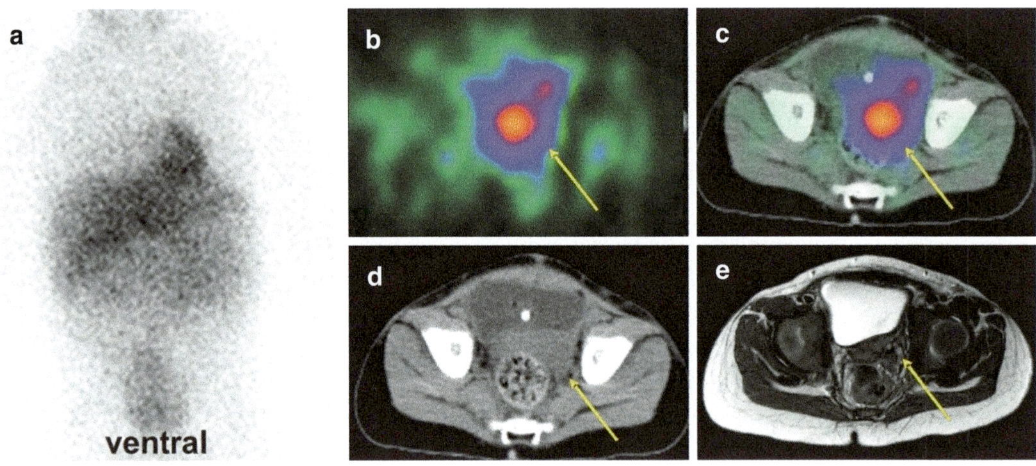

Fig. 7.1 A 2-year-old patient with retrovesical neuroblastoma (**e**: MRI, yellow arrow) underwent ¹²³I-mIBG scan, for evaluation of treatment possibility with ¹³¹I-mIBG. (**a**) Planar scan was inconclusive because of bladder activity. (**b–d**) Exact localization, differentiation of the bladder and evaluation of mIBG uptake were made possible only by SPECT/CT (yellow arrows). A Foley catheter was used for emptying the bladder

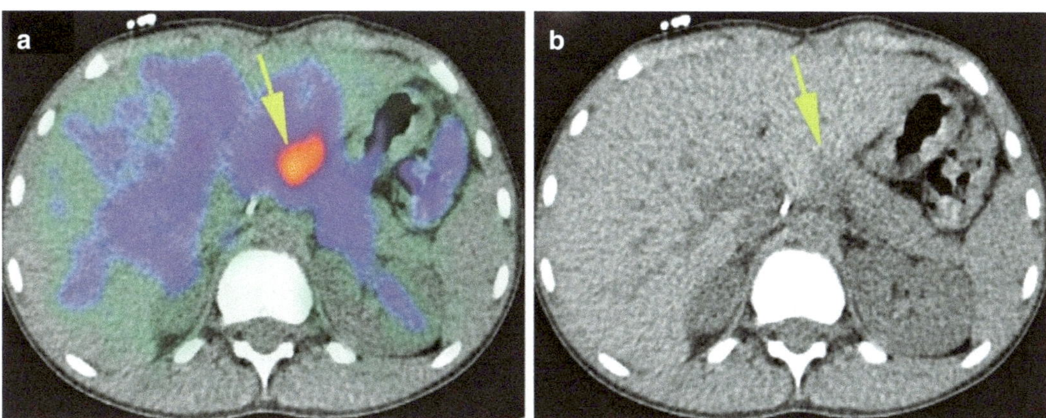

Fig. 7.2 A 9-year-old patient with stage IV neuroblastoma received ^{123}I-mIBG scan for restaging after chemotherapy. SPECT/CT revealed a suspected uptake beside the liver (yellow arrow), which had been overlooked by MRI. The patient underwent an operation. Histopathology showed a lymph node metastasis. (**a**) SPECT/CT transversal view, (**b**) CT transversal view

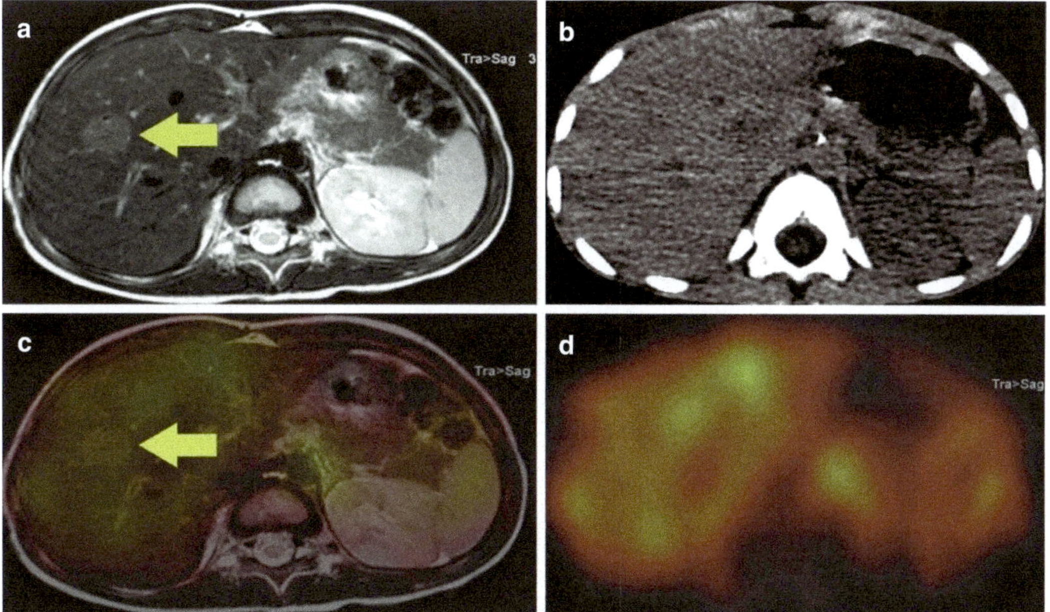

Fig. 7.3 A 3-year-old patient with suspected, new occurred liver lesion in MRI (**a**, yellow arrow), which was detected in his restaging examination after chemotherapy. The lesion showed no pathological ^{123}I-mIBG uptake (**c**, yellow arrow and **d**), reported as benign, which was confirmed by biopsy as FNH. A fusion with MRI (**c**) was possible with the help of the low-dose CT (**b**) of the SPECT/CT

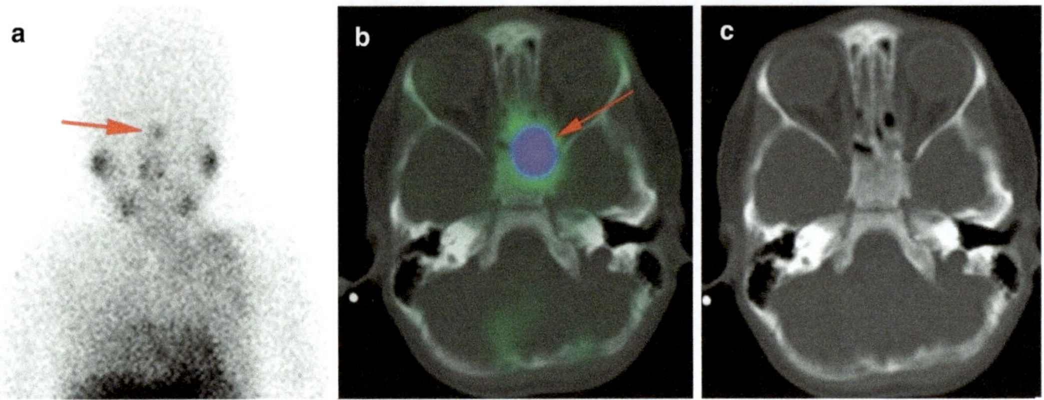

Fig. 7.4 A 4-year-old patient with tracer accumulation in the region of nasal mucosa (**a**, red arrow). SPECT/CT (**b**, **c**) revealed sphenoid bone involvement confirmed with MRI. This result resulted in further chemotherapy

Detection of small foci, which would have been mostly overlooked with planar imaging alone, is possible by using SPECT/CT (Fig. 7.4).

7.15 MIBG SPECT/CT in Pheochromocytoma and Paraganglioma

The pheochromocytoma is a catecholamine-secreting tumour of the chromaffin cells, and it is localized in the adrenal medulla to 85% and occurs with an incidence of 1/100,000 people p.a.

Its characteristic symptoms are episodic headaches, palpitations, diaphoresis and paroxysmal or sustained hypertension [7]. The pheochromocytoma occurs in isolation or as part of a syndrome, e.g. MEN 2 syndrome, von-Hippel-Lindau syndrome or neurofibromatosis type 1 (M. Recklinghausen). With widespread use of cross-sectional imaging, an increasing number of pheochromocytomas are diagnosed incidentally, without the presence of symptoms or complaints by the patient. Incidental tumours, as well as tumours detected while screening patients with hereditary syndromes, tend to be smaller than symptomatic ones.

The first diagnostic method is plasma or urine measurements of catecholamines and their metabolites [7, 49]. If there is positive biochemical testing, further imaging is required, such as ultrasound, CT of the abdomen or MRI.

mIBG scintigraphy for detecting pheochromocytomas or paragangliomas has been widely used for more than 25 years and have a reported high sensitivity and specificity of about 83–100% and 85–100%, respectively [50]. In the last 5 years, however, image quality and spatial resolution of other imaging methods, such as MRI with a high sensitivity for detection of tumours in the adrenal gland (which are usually hyper-intense on T2-weighted images and hypointense on T1-weighted images), increased significantly [7, 51]; in addition, other functional imaging modalities such as ^{18}F-DOPA PET/CT have been increasingly applied. Regarding this, some studies have been published compared sensitivity and specificity of those other imaging methods to mIBG SPECT. They all share a significantly lower sensitivity for mIBG scintigraphy, from which it might be concluded that the mIBG scan has lost its monopoly position as the gold standard functional imaging method for pheochromocytoma/paraganglioma. Critics find fault in its low-spatial resolution, the long examination time of 24 h, the necessity of thyroid blockade, the interference with several medications and the significant tracer-uptake in the normal adrenal medulla [52].

The disadvantage of the low spatial resolution may be largely compensated by the use of mIBG SPECT/CT; however, the other "disadvantages" remain. Additionally, limitations in

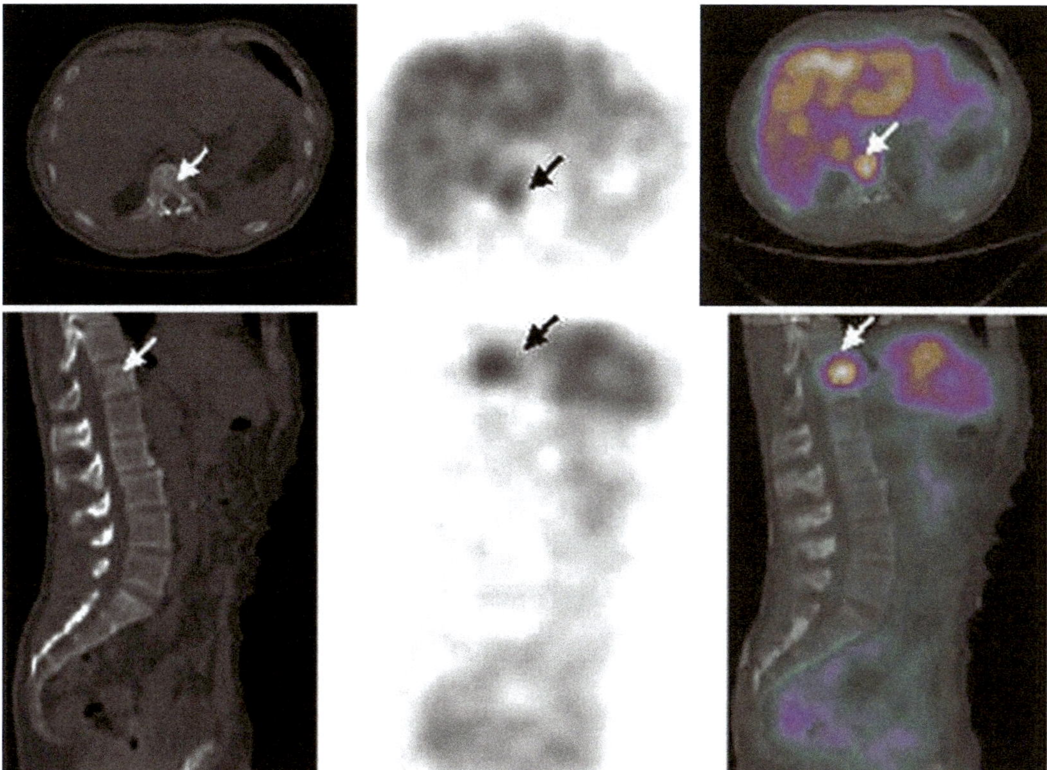

Fig. 7.5 CT, mIBG SPECT and fused mIBG SPECT/CT images of phaeochromocytoma metastasis to the body of T12 vertebra (white arrow). (With kind permission from Springer Science + Business Media: Meyer-Rochow et al. [29]. Fig. 1B)

terms of decreased sensitivity and specificity exist in several diseases, such as MEN2-related phaeochromocytoma, extra-adrenal, multiple or hereditary paragangliomas or metastatic disease, which may lead to a significant underestimation of the extent of disease in the mIBG-scan with potentially inappropriate management. The particular strengths of mIBG SPECT/CT are detection of local recurrence, small extra-adrenal pheochromocytomas, multifocal tumours or the presence of metastatic disease [29]. In patients with clinical or biochemical suspicion of pheochromocytoma, SPECT/CT, compared to SPECT and planar imaging, has a significantly higher accuracy (Fig. 7.5) [53]. ^{123}I-mIBG scintigraphy, precisely with assistance of SPECT/CT, can serve for evaluation and dose calculation for ^{131}I-mIBG therapy, from which patients may benefit [7, 54, 55].

7.15.1 Interpretation of the Findings

In some cases, there are quite unequivocal true-positive findings with a convincing focal mIBG-uptake, matched to an obvious size of adrenal masses in additional imaging such as CT. These unequivocal findings can even be detected only by using whole-body and planar imaging. In such cases, SPECT/CT may be useful to rule out any extra-adrenal manifestations; otherwise, does not have any additional benefit.

Concerning less conclusive accumulations or small masses in the adrenal, low-dose CT of SPECT/CT serves as an anatomical landmark. In SPECT/CT, the left adrenal is often detected much more easily than the right adrenal due to the anatomical location of the liver and large vessels, such as vena cava, with their physiological uptake. Especially for the detection of the right adrenal, the use of SPECT/CT is very valuable;

even when it only provides an inconspicuous finding, this can thus be diagnosed.

Additionally, there are several other difficulties and challenges besides localization, namely the distinction between a significantly increased uptake, therefore interpreted as pathological, and a mildly enhanced uptake, slightly above or similar to that of the liver. This is because there are no cut-off values from which an uptake can be considered significantly positive for a pathological finding. A dissociation of benign findings, such as adrenal adenoma with a moderate uptake, is not always easy.

The risk of misinterpreting any positive uptake as pathologic may lead to an increased rate of false-positive findings. On the other hand, smaller or extra-adrenal findings bear a great challenge, precisely because they can be easily overlooked, particularly if planar imaging is performed or if the findings are located next to physiological accumulations or organs.

It should be noted at least that larger adrenal masses, already considered to be suspicious in other imaging tools such as MRI because of their density, might show no or very low mIBG uptake. In such cases, an adrenal carcinoma cannot be ruled out. An operation with histological confirmation is so far the only opportunity to definitively assure diagnosis.

Some hints to reduce false-positive or -negative results:

- Correct patient selection criteria are required, which means positive biochemical testing and/or evaluation of suspicious masses of the adrenal in other imaging modalities.
- In utilization of SPECT/CT, the particular strengths of mIBG SPECT/CT are detection of local recurrence, small extra-adrenal pheochromocytomas and multifocal tumours (Fig. 7.6).

7.16 mIBG SPECT/CT in Medullary Thyroid Carcinoma

Medullary thyroid carcinoma (MTC) is a quite rare thyroid tumour which occurs in 5–10% of all thyroid carcinomas and arises from thyroid para-follicular C cells, which are embedded in the thyroid, but do not belong to the thyrocytes. It releases calcitonin, CEA and several other substances, such as chromogranin, serotonin, somatostatin and gastrin-releasing peptide.

A sensitive and specific marker for the occurrence of MTC is calcitonin, which is produced by the C-cells. An elevated calcitonin level (hypercalcitoninaemia) reflects a disorder, a reactive stimulation of the C-cells or impaired/disturbed degradation for calcitonin. There is a wide range of differential diagnoses for increased calcitonin levels, such as alcohol consumption, intake of various drugs (calcium, proton pump inhibitor, medication with calcitonin), hypercalcaemia and andrenal insufficiency. Also, a severe bacterial infection, a serious illness or a para-neoplastic syndrome can also cause a hypercalcitoninaemia. If reasons such as these are excluded, only C-cell hyperplasia (CCH, C-cell hyperplasia) and MTC remain as the two most frequent diagnoses. It should be noted that C-cell hyperplasia is associated specifically with males, in combination with autoimmune thyroiditis, or hyperparathyroidism-associated hyper-gastrinaemia.

The reference values for basal calcitonin are higher in men than in women. Hypercalcitoninaemia should be confirmed in a second measurement. The interpretation of an elevated calcitonin level between 10 and 100 pg/ml is ambiguous; only a basal calcitonin level >100 pg/ml is almost always accompanies an MTC. If available, for further diagnosis, a pentagastrin test should be carried out. If pentagastrin stimulation is not available, stimulation can also be performed with calcium, noting that after calcium stimulation, false-positive findings appear to be more common in female patients and patients with thyroiditis and thyroid neoplasia, other than MTC [56]. $^{131/123}$I-mIBG uptake in MTC appears via the same molecular mechanisms, just as in other neuroendocrine tumours such as pheochromocytoma [7].

7.16.1 Imaging Procedures

Cross-sectional imaging studies employing neck, chest and three-phase abdominal CT scans or

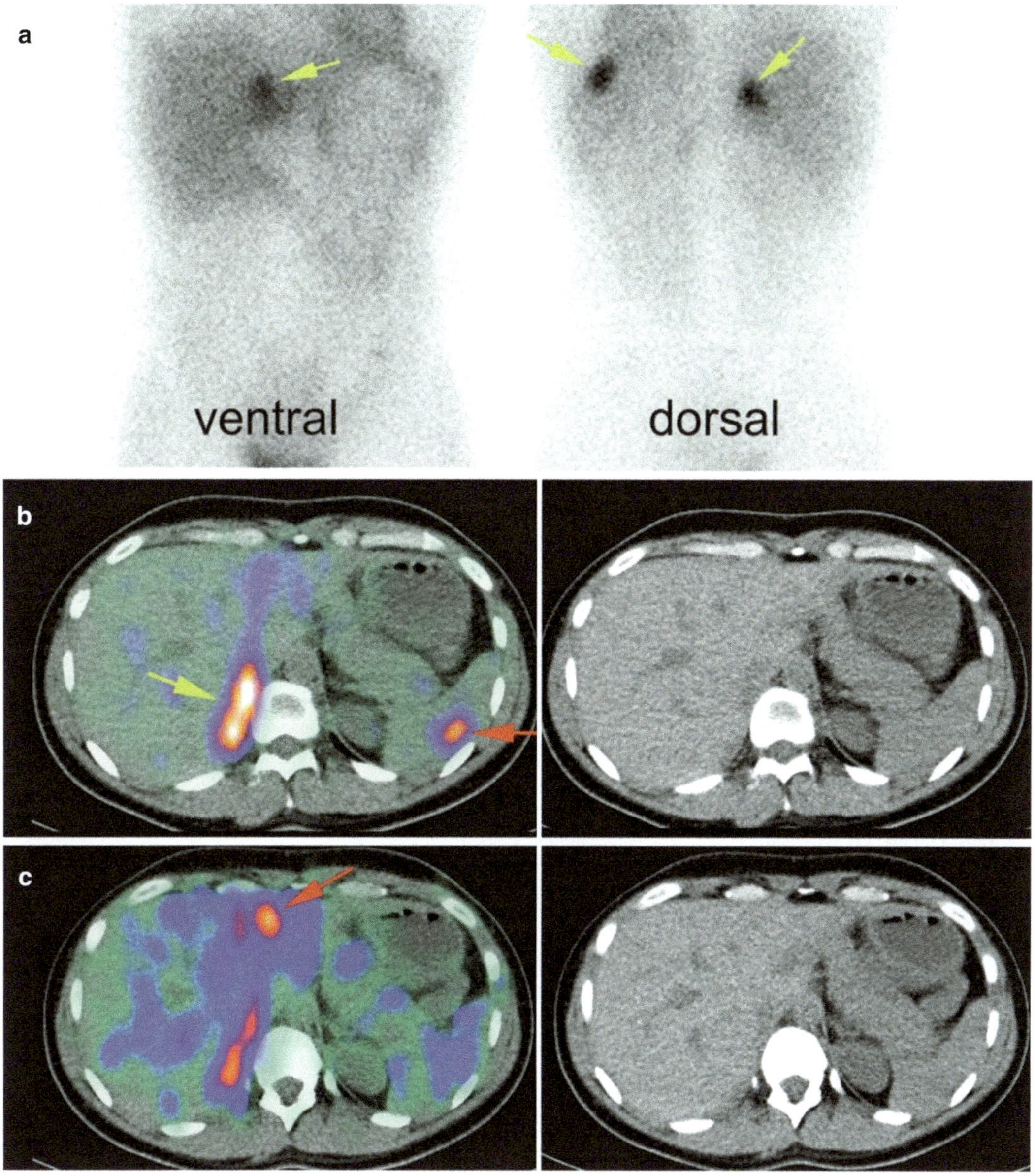

Fig. 7.6 Planar images of a patient with suspected recurrence of phaeochromocytoma showed three suspected abdominal uptake (**a**, yellow arrows). SPECT/CT revealed the exact anatomical localization of these uptakes (**b**, **c**) local recurrence (yellow arrow), a spleen metastasis and a liver metastasis (red arrows)

contrast-enhanced MRIs are recommended to rule-out distant metastases, especially when suspicious lymph nodes are identified or when calcitonin levels are >400 pg/ml [57, 58].

There are also several radiotracers to mention, such as ^{99}Tc-DMSA, ^{123}I-mIBG, ^{111}In-labelled somatostatin analogue and the PET pharmaceuticals ^{18}F-FDG, ^{68}Ga-DOTATOC and ^{18}F-DOPA [59].

The use of ^{123}I-mIBG in MTC is not the gold standard procedure because of its low sensitivity, which is said to be approximately 35% especially for familial/MEN-associated MTC. For sporadic MTC, data are superior. The specificity of mIBG is quite high and is approximately 95% [59–63].

In summary, the role of $^{131/123}$I-mIBG in the diagnostic evaluation of MTC is limited, but it still serves as an evaluation method for tentative therapy with ^{131}I-mIBG [7].

Moreover, a combined diagnosis of $^{131/123}$I-mIBG scan and somatostatine receptor scintigraphy (SRS) increases the sensitivity up to 100% and seems to be the best practice to choose the most effective radiopharmaceutical with regard to therapy options [59].

The use of $^{131/123}$I-mIBG SPECT/CT can serve as a follow up to individual metastases and their responses to therapy, as SPECT/CT, more than planar imaging, simplifies localization and evaluation of the tumour burden.

References

1. Nakajo M, Shapiro B, Copp J, Kalff V, Gross MD, Sisson JC, et al. The normal and abnormal distribution of the adrenomedullary imaging agent m-[I-131]iodobenzylguanidine (I-131 MIBG) in man: evaluation by scintigraphy. J Nucl Med. 1983;24:672–82.
2. Bombardieri E, Giammarile F, Aktolun C, Baum RP, Bischof Delaloye A, Maffioli L, et al. 131I/123I-metaiodobenzylguanidine (mIBG) scintigraphy: procedure guidelines for tumour imaging. Eur J Nucl Med Mol Imaging. 2010;37:2436–46.
3. Taieb D, Timmers HJ, Hindie E, Guillet BA, Neumann HP, Walz MK, et al. EANM 2012 guidelines for radionuclide imaging of phaeochromocytoma and paraganglioma. Eur J Nucl Med Mol Imaging. 2012;39:1977–95.
4. Berglund AS, Hulthen UL, Manhem P, Thorsson O, Wollmer P, Tornquist C. Metaiodobenzylguanidine (MIBG) scintigraphy and computed tomography (CT) in clinical practice. Primary and secondary evaluation for localization of phaeochromocytomas. J Intern Med. 2001;249:247–51.
5. Niederle B, Heinz-Peer G, Kaczirek K, Kurtaran A. The value of adrenal imaging in Adrenal surgery. In: Linos D, van Heerden J, editors. Adrenal glands, diagnostic aspects and surgical therapy. New York: Springer; 2005. p. 41.
6. Shapiro B, Fig L, Gross MD, Shulkin BL, Sisson JC. Neuroendocrine tumors. In: Aktolun C, Tauxe W, editors. Nuclear oncology. New York: Springer; 1999. p. 3–31.
7. Ilias I, Divgi C, Pacak K. Current role of metaiodobenzylguanidine in the diagnosis of pheochromocytoma and medullary thyroid cancer. Semin Nucl Med. 2011;41:364–8.
8. Shapiro B, Gross MD. Radiochemistry, biochemistry, and kinetics of 131I-metaiodobenzylguanidine (MIBG) and 123I-MIBG: clinical implications of the use of 123I-MIBG. Med Pediatr Oncol. 1987;15:170–7.
9. Khafagi FA, Shapiro B, Fig LM, Mallette S, Sisson JC. Labetalol reduces iodine-131 MIBG uptake by pheochromocytoma and normal tissues. J Nucl Med. 1989;30:481–9.
10. Kloos RT, Gross MD, Francis IR, Korobkin M, Shapiro B. Incidentally discovered adrenal masses. Endocr Rev. 1995;16:460–84.
11. Solanki KK, Bomanji J, Moyes J, Mather SJ, Trainer PJ, Britton KE. A pharmacological guide to medicines which interfere with the biodistribution of radiolabelled meta-iodobenzylguanidine (MIBG). Nucl Med Commun. 1992;13:513–21.
12. Tobes MC, Fig LM, Carey J, Geatti O, Sisson JC, Shapiro B. Alterations of iodine-131 MIBG biodistribution in an anephric patient: comparison to normal and impaired renal function. J Nucl Med. 1989;30:1476–82.
13. Lassmann M, Chiesa C, Flux G, Bardies M. EANM Dosimetry Committee guidance document: good practice of clinical dosimetry reporting. Eur J Nucl Med Mol Imaging. 2011;38:192–200.
14. Rufini V, Fisher GA, Shulkin BL, Sisson JC, Shapiro B. Iodine-123-MIBG imaging of neuroblastoma: utility of SPECT and delayed imaging. J Nucl Med. 1996;37:1464–8.
15. Rufini V, Giordano A, Di Giuda D, Petrone A, Deb G, De Sio L, et al. [123I]MIBG scintigraphy in neuroblastoma: a comparison between planar and SPECT imaging. Q J Nucl Med. 1995;39:25–8.
16. Olivier P, Colarinha P, Fettich J, Fischer S, Frokier J, Giammarile F, et al. Guidelines for radioiodinated MIBG scintigraphy in children. Eur J Nucl Med Mol Imaging. 2003;30:B45–50.
17. Radiation dose to patients from radiopharmaceuticals (addendum 2 to ICRP publication 53). Ann ICRP. 1998;28:1–126.
18. Radiation dose to patients from radiopharmaceuticals. A report of a Task Group of Committee 2 of the International Commission on Radiological Protection. Ann ICRP. 1987;18:1–377.
19. Stabin MG, Gelfand MJ. Dosimetry of pediatric nuclear medicine procedures. Q J Nucl Med. 1998;42:93–112.
20. Okuyama C, Ushijima Y, Kubota T, Yoshida T, Nakai T, Kobayashi K, et al. 123I-Metaiodobenzylguanidine uptake in the nape of the neck of children: likely visualization of brown adipose tissue. J Nucl Med. 2003;44:1421–5.
21. Gelfand MJ. 123I-MIBG uptake in the neck and shoulders of a neuroblastoma patient: damage to sympathetic innervation blocks uptake in brown adipose tissue. Pediatr Radiol. 2004;34:577–9.
22. Sinclair AJ, Bomanji J, Harris P, Ross G, Besser GM, Britton KE. Pre- and post-treatment distribution pattern of 123I-MIBG in patients with phaeochromocytomas and paragangliomas. Nucl Med Commun. 1989;10:567–76.
23. Feine U, Muller-Schauenburg W, Treuner J, Klingebiel T. Metaiodobenzylguanidine (MIBG) labeled with 123I/131I in neuroblastoma diagnosis and follow-up

treatment with a review of the diagnostic results of the International Workshop of Pediatric Oncology held in Rome, September 1986. Med Pediatr Oncol. 1987;15:181–7.

24. Hoefnagel CA, Voute PA, de Kraker J, Marcuse HR. Radionuclide diagnosis and therapy of neural crest tumors using iodine-131 metaiodobenzylguanidine. J Nucl Med. 1987;28:308–14.

25. Gelfand MJ, Elgazzar AH, Kriss VM, Masters PR, Golsch GJ. Iodine-123-MIBG SPECT versus planar imaging in children with neural crest tumors. J Nucl Med. 1994;35:1753–7.

26. Muckle M, Simon B, Sabet A, Habibi E, Biersack H, Ezziddin S, et al. The added value of 123I-MIBG SPECT/CT in the diagnosis of pheochromocytoma compared to planar imaging. J Nucl Med Meeting Abstracts. 2013;54:1911.

27. Derlin T, Busch JD, Wisotzki C, Schoennagel BP, Bannas P, Papp L, et al. Intraindividual comparison of 123I-mIBG SPECT/MRI, 123I-mIBG SPECT/CT, and MRI for the detection of adrenal pheochromocytoma in patients with elevated urine or plasma catecholamines. Clin Nucl Med. 2013;38:e1–6.

28. Fukuoka M, Taki J, Mochizuki T, Kinuya S. Comparison of diagnostic value of I-123 MIBG and high-dose I-131 MIBG scintigraphy including incremental value of SPECT/CT over planar image in patients with malignant pheochromocytoma/paraganglioma and neuroblastoma. Clin Nucl Med. 2011;36:1–7.

29. Meyer-Rochow GY, Schembri GP, Benn DE, Sywak MS, Delbridge LW, Robinson BG, et al. The utility of metaiodobenzylguanidine single photon emission computed tomography/computed tomography (MIBG SPECT/CT) for the diagnosis of pheochromocytoma. Ann Surg Oncol. 2010;17:392–400.

30. Rozovsky K, Koplewitz BZ, Krausz Y, Revel-Vilk S, Weintraub M, Chisin R, et al. Added value of SPECT/CT for correlation of MIBG scintigraphy and diagnostic CT in neuroblastoma and pheochromocytoma. AJR Am J Roentgenol. 2008;190:1085–90.

31. Edmund Kim E, Mar MV, Inoue T, Chung J. Sectional anatomy: PET/CT and SPECT/CT. New York: Springer; 2007.

32. Kushner BH. Neuroblastoma: a disease requiring a multitude of imaging studies. J Nucl Med. 2004;45:1172–88.

33. Wilson LM, Draper GJ. Neuroblastoma, its natural history and prognosis: a study of 487 cases. Br Med J. 1974;3:301–7.

34. Shimada H, Ambros IM, Dehner LP, Hata J, Joshi VV, Roald B. Terminology and morphologic criteria of neuroblastic tumors: recommendations by the International Neuroblastoma Pathology Committee. Cancer. 1999;86:349–63.

35. Brisse HJ, McCarville MB, Granata C, Krug KB, Wootton-Gorges SL, Kanegawa K, et al. Guidelines for imaging and staging of neuroblastic tumors: consensus report from the International Neuroblastoma Risk Group Project. Radiology. 2011;261:243–57.

36. Young JL Jr, Ries LG, Silverberg E, Horm JW, Miller RW. Cancer incidence, survival, and mortality for children younger than age 15 years. Cancer. 1986;58:598–602.

37. Franzius C, Hermann K, Weckesser M, Kopka K, Juergens KU, Vormoor J, et al. Whole-body PET/CT with 11C-meta-hydroxyephedrine in tumors of the sympathetic nervous system: feasibility study and comparison with 123I-MIBG SPECT/CT. J Nucl Med. 2006;47:1635–42.

38. Gelfand MJ. Meta-iodobenzylguanidine in children. Semin Nucl Med. 1993;23:231–42.

39. Jacobs A, Delree M, Desprechins B, Otten J, Ferster A, Jonckheer MH, et al. Consolidating the role of *I-MIBG-scintigraphy in childhood neuroblastoma: five years of clinical experience. Pediatr Radiol. 1990;20:157–9.

40. Kushner BH, Cheung NK. Exploiting the MIBG-avidity of neuroblastoma for staging and treatment. Pediatr Blood Cancer. 2006;47:863–4.

41. Kushner BH, Yeh SD, Kramer K, Larson SM, Cheung NK. Impact of metaiodobenzylguanidine scintigraphy on assessing response of high-risk neuroblastoma to dose-intensive induction chemotherapy. J Clin Oncol. 2003;21:1082–6.

42. Lumbroso JD, Guermazi F, Hartmann O, Coornaert S, Rabarison Y, Leclere JG, et al. Meta-iodobenzylguanidine (mIBG) scans in neuroblastoma: sensitivity and specificity, a review of 115 scans. Prog Clin Biol Res. 1988;271:689–705.

43. Parisi MT, Greene MK, Dykes TM, Moraldo TV, Sandler ED, Hattner RS. Efficacy of metaiodobenzylguanidine as a scintigraphic agent for the detection of neuroblastoma. Investig Radiol. 1992;27:768–73.

44. Perel Y, Conway J, Kletzel M, Goldman J, Weiss S, Feyler A, et al. Clinical impact and prognostic value of metaiodobenzylguanidine imaging in children with metastatic neuroblastoma. J Pediatr Hematol Oncol. 1999;21:13–8.

45. Muckle M, Sabet A, Simon B, Ezziddin S, Dilloo D, Biersack HJ, et al. The significance of iodine 123 MIBG SPECT/CT for the diagnosis and treatment planning in neuroblastoma. J Nucl Med Meeting Abstracts. 2012;53:2209.

46. Liu B, Servaes S, Zhuang H. SPECT/CT MIBG imaging is crucial in the follow-up of the patients with high-risk neuroblastoma. Clin Nucl Med. 2018;43:232–8.

47. Bonnin F, Lumbroso J, Tenenbaum F, Hartmann O, Parmentier C. Refining interpretation of MIBG scans in children. J Nucl Med. 1994;35:803–10.

48. Sharp SE, Trout AT, Weiss BD, Gelfand MJ. MIBG in neuroblastoma diagnostic imaging and therapy. Radiographics. 2016;36:258–78.

49. Elsayes KM, Menias CO, Siegel CL, Narra VR, Kanaan Y, Hussain HK. Magnetic resonance characterization of pheochromocytomas in the abdomen and pelvis: imaging findings in 18 surgically proven cases. J Comput Assist Tomogr. 2010;34:548–53.

50. Fottner C, Helisch A, Anlauf M, Rossmann H, Musholt TJ, Kreft A, et al. 6-18F-fluoro-

L-dihydroxyphenylalanine positron emission tomography is superior to 123I-metaiodobenzylguanidine scintigraphy in the detection of extraadrenal and hereditary pheochromocytomas and paragangliomas: correlation with vesicular monoamine transporter expression. J Clin Endocrinol Metab. 2010;95:2800–10.

51. Jacobson AF, Deng H, Lombard J, Lessig HJ, Black RR. 123I-meta-iodobenzylguanidine scintigraphy for the detection of neuroblastoma and pheochromocytoma: results of a meta-analysis. J Clin Endocrinol Metab. 2010;95:2596–606.

52. Lev I, Kelekar G, Waxman A, Yu R. Clinical use and utility of metaiodobenzylguanidine scintigraphy in pheochromocytoma diagnosis. Endocr Pract. 2010;16:398–407.

53. Sharma P, Dhull VS, Jeph S, Reddy RM, Singh H, Naswa N, et al. Can hybrid SPECT-CT overcome the limitations associated with poor imaging properties of 131I-MIBG?: comparison with planar scintigraphy and SPECT in pheochromocytoma. Clin Nucl Med. 2013;38(9):e346–53.

54. Giammarile F, Chiti A, Lassmann M, Brans B, Flux G. EANM procedure guidelines for 131I-meta-iodobenzylguanidine (131I-mIBG) therapy. Eur J Nucl Med Mol Imaging. 2008;35:1039–47.

55. Scholz T, Eisenhofer G, Pacak K, Dralle H, Lehnert H. Clinical review: current treatment of malignant pheochromocytoma. J Clin Endocrinol Metab. 2007;92:1217–25.

56. Lorenz K, Elwerr M, Machens A, Abuazab M, Holzhausen HJ, Dralle H. Hypercalcitoninemia in thyroid conditions other than medullary thyroid carcinoma: a comparative analysis of calcium and pentagastrin stimulation of serum calcitonin. Langenbecks Arch Surg. 2013;398:403–9.

57. Tuttle RM, Ball DW, Byrd D, Daniels GH, Dilawari RA, Doherty GM, et al. Medullary carcinoma. J Natl Compr Cancer Netw. 2010;8:512–30.

58. Strosberg JR. Update on the management of unusual neuroendocrine tumors: pheochromocytoma and paraganglioma, medullary thyroid cancer and adrenocortical carcinoma. Semin Oncol. 2013;40:120–33.

59. Castellani MR, Seregni E, Maccauro M, Chiesa C, Aliberti G, Orunesu E, et al. MIBG for diagnosis and therapy of medullary thyroid carcinoma: is there still a role? Q J Nucl Med Mol Imaging. 2008;52:430–40.

60. Rufini V, Salvatori M, Garganese MC, Di Giuda D, Lodovica Maussier M, Troncone L. Role of nuclear medicine in the diagnosis and therapy of medullary thyroid carcinoma. Rays. 2000;25:273–82.

61. Papotti M, Kumar U, Volante M, Pecchioni C, Patel YC. Immunohistochemical detection of somatostatin receptor types 1–5 in medullary carcinoma of the thyroid. Clin Endocrinol. 2001;54:641–9.

62. Wafelman AR, Hoefnagel CA, Maes RA, Beijnen JH. Radioiodinated metaiodobenzylguanidine: a review of its biodistribution and pharmacokinetics, drug interactions, cytotoxicity and dosimetry. Eur J Nucl Med. 1994;21:545–59.

63. Baulieu JL, Guilloteau D, Delisle MJ, Perdrisot R, Gardet P, Delepine N, et al. Radioiodinated meta-iodobenzylguanidine uptake in medullary thyroid cancer. A French cooperative study. Cancer. 1987;60:2189–94.

Bone SPECT/CT in Oncology

Kanhaiyalal Agrawal and Gopinath Gnanasegaran

8.1 Introduction

Bone scintigraphy is a routine nuclear medicine procedure mainly used to detect bone metastases in a cancer patient. Bone scintigraphy has traditionally been the mainstay of whole-body screening for bone metastases. A planar bone scan is sensitive in detecting osteoblastic bone metastasis but has limited specificity due to non-specific uptake in benign bone conditions. Almost half of the solitary focus on planar bone scintigraphy in patients with a malignancy history may be benign abnormalities. Hence, radiological correlation is necessary in some of the cases showing radiotracer uptake in bones. Hybrid SPECT/CT can provide:

- Functional and morphological data in one examination.
- Increasing the specificity of bone scintigraphy.
- Avoiding indeterminate findings and additional investigation.

8.2 Radiopharmaceutical for Bone Scintigraphy/SPECT-CT

SPECT tracers used in bone scintigraphy are Technetium-99m (99mTc) based. The tracers are 99mTc methylene diphosphonate (99mTc MDP), 99mTc hydroxymethylene diphosphonate (99mTc HDP or HMDP), 99mTc hydroxyethylidene diphosphonate (99mTc HEDP) and 99mTc pyrophosphate.

The bone imaging agents are either phosphates or diphosphonates. The P-O-P bond in phosphate is easily broken down by phosphatase enzyme and is less stable in vivo than a stable P-C-P bond in diphosphonate. Therefore, diphosphonate is a commonly used radiopharmaceutical in bone imaging [1]. The diphosphonate agents are usually available in kit form. Labelling occurs by adding pertechnetate to the cold kit and mixing. Generally, the oxidation state of 99mTc in bone kits is 3+. The uptake in bone is due to ion exchange phenomena. 99mTc diphosphonate binding occurs by chemisorption in the hydroxyapatite mineral component of the bone matrix. Both tracers are primarily excreted through kidneys.

K. Agrawal
Department of Nuclear Medicine, All India Institute of Medical Sciences (AIIMS), Bhubaneswar, India

G. Gnanasegaran (✉)
Royal Free NHS Foundation Trust, London, UK
e-mail: gopinath.gnanasegaran@nhs.net

© The Author(s), under exclusive license to Springer Nature Switzerland AG 2022
H. Ahmadzadehfar et al. (eds.), *Clinical Applications of SPECT-CT*,
https://doi.org/10.1007/978-3-030-65850-2_8

8.3 Radiopharmaceutical Activity

An adult's recommended activity is intravenous injection of 740–1110 MBq (20–30 mCi) of 99mTc-labelled agents. For obese patients, the administered tracer activity is increased to 11–13 MBq/kg (300–350 µCi/kg). In kids, the recommended dose is 9–11 MBq/kg (250–300 µCi/kg), with a minimum of 20–40 MBq (0.5–1.0 mCi) [2].

8.4 Bone SPECT/CT Patient Preparation

The patient preparation for bone SPECT/CT is similar to bone scintigraphy. In general, before making an appointment for bone scintigraphy and SPECT/CT, pregnancy and active breastfeeding should be ruled out in female patients. No specific patient preparation is required for bone scintigraphy. Unless contraindicated, the patient should be well hydrated before and during the study. The Nuclear medicine team should document relevant medical history related to the investigation before radiotracer administration. In particular, the referral cause, current symptoms, history of trauma or fractures, prior bone scintigraphy results, any history of allergy, renal impairment, etc., should be recorded. Past medical history of surgery, chemotherapy or radiotherapy to the patient must be documented. Any recent nuclear medicine studies which may impair bone scintigraphy image quality must be reported [3].

In between administration of tracer and study acquisition, the patient should void frequently and immediately before the scan. All metallic objects must be removed during imaging unless contraindicated. The non-removable metallic objects like pacemakers must be documented before study.

8.5 Image Acquisition Protocol

Always bone SPECT/CT is preceded by planar bone scintigraphy image acquisition. In planar whole-body imaging, anterior and posterior view images are acquired. The whole-body scan is acquired to obtain more than 1.5 million total counts. The table rate should be adjusted depending on the equipment manufacturer's specification. The energy window should be centred at 140 keV. Window width is kept at 15–20%. Matrix size is 256 × 1024 or higher. If needed, spot view may be acquired depending upon the clinical indications and should be 500K–1000K per image (less for skull and extremities). Additional three-phase acquisition, lateral, oblique or special (frog-leg views of the hips) views may be acquired if necessary.

SPECT acquisition has the following parameters: Contoured orbit, 64 × 64 or greater matrix, 3–6° intervals, 10–40 s/stop. SPECT image reconstruction is done with 3D iterative OSEM (ordered-subsets expectation-maximization) with ideally 3–5 iterations and 8–10 subsets. CT acquisition parameters are 120 kV, 30–100 mA/slice (or intensity-modulated), and slice thickness depends on the body part imaged (1.5–2 mm) [4]. Usually, a contrast medium is not necessary for SPECT-CT of bones. Literature evidence suggests that even low-dose CT protocols with low-tube current-time products in the range of 2.5–30 mAs give good diagnostic accuracy [5].

SPECT-CT is usually done with a CT field of view restricted to the equivocal or indeterminate tracer uptake seen on the planar study called SPECT-guided low-dose CT or targeted SPECT-CT. This procedure gives less extra average radiation dose to the patient (generally additional 2–3 mSv depending on CT protocol used). However, some researchers have shown better accuracy of whole-body SPECT-CT, which is discussed later in this chapter.

8.6 Role of SPECT-CT in Bone Metastases

Early and accurate detection of bone metastases is crucial for better management of cancer patients and preventing complications. The most common bone metastasis sites are the vertebral column and pelvic bones due to the high proportion of red marrow in these bones [4]. Approximately 60–80% of patients with breast and prostate cancer develop bone metas-

Table 8.1 Different responses from bone metastasis in various malignancies

Predominantly osteoblastic	Predominantly osteolytic	Mixed osteoblastic and lytic
Prostate cancer	Thyroid cancer	Breast cancer
Hodgkin lymphoma	Renal cell carcinoma	Stomach cancer
Carcinoid	Non-small cell lung cancer	Colon cancer
Small cell lung cancer	Multiple myeloma	Urinary bladder cancer
Medulloblastoma	Melanoma	Squamous cancers
	Langerhans-cell histiocytosis	

tases [6]. About 90% of patients with multiple myeloma develop osteolytic bone metastases [7]. According to the plain radiographic appearances, bone metastases are generally classified as lytic, sclerotic, or mixed. Wherever bone resorption predominates with little new bone formation, the metastases will have a lytic appearance. Table 8.1 mentions different types of responses to bone metastases in various malignancies. Literature evidence of biochemical markers of bone turnover indicates that all three types of radiological metastases are associated with biochemical evidence of increased bone turnover [8]. Complex endocrine interactions with tumour biology have led to a greater understanding of bone metastases and allowed several novel interventions for metastases and treatment-related osteoporosis [8]. Lytic lesions are particularly interesting as successful therapy leads to progressive sclerosis of the lesions [9], which in scintigraphy studies manifests as the 'flare' phenomenon [10].

8.7 Radiological Imaging

The plain film is a relatively insensitive method for evaluating bony metastatic disease in the absence of symptoms. It is crucial as a screening tool in multiple myeloma. The principal advantage of the plain film is that its findings may help to identify the primary tumour, exclude benign conditions and predict the risk of pathological fracture, mostly if more than 50% of the cortex has been destroyed by the tumour [11].

While CT scanning is more sensitive than conventional radiography, it is not an appropriate investigation for screening the entire skeleton. The CT scan's great strength lies in confirming suspicious lesions that are apparent on either plain film or bone scintigraphy with clarification of the anatomic site and extent of cortical destruction.

MRI is highly sensitive for detecting skeletal metastases at a nascent level when the tumour deposits have infiltrated bone marrow. The normal fat cells in the bone marrow are displaced by tumour cells. The T1-weighted study will demonstrate low-signal intensity at infiltration sites and high-signal intensity on fat-suppressed images. Metastases also have a bright T2 signal around them [11]. Diffusion-weighted whole-body MRI has shown similar sensitivity to skeletal scintigraphy in detecting metastases from prostate, breast cancer or non-small cell cancer of the lung [12, 13].

8.8 Bone Scintigraphy

Bone scintigraphy detects bone metastases when there is a reactive increase in bone formation. The advantage of bone scintigraphy is screening the entire skeleton with extremely high sensitivity for detecting metastases, particularly in prostate and breast cancer. Literature evidence demonstrated that bone scan sensitivity in detecting metastases is 85–96% [14–16]. However, the diagnostic accuracy of planar and SPECT bone scintigraphy is limited due to the non-specific nature of radiopharmaceutical in bone disease and relatively poor spatial resolution. The specificity of bone scintigraphy in detecting bone metastases is low because many benign bone diseases show abnormal radiotracer accumulation leading to false-positive diagnosis (Table 8.2) [17]. However, SPECT/CT leads to characterization of tracer uptake leading to improved bone scintigraphy specificity.

Further, the lesion may be missed if it is tiny in size on planar bone scan [18]. Planar bone

Table 8.2 Metastatic patterns on planar bone scintigraphy

Metastasis	Benign uptake mimicking metastasis
• Randomly scattered multifocal uptake • Diffuse heterogeneous uptake in skeleton • A cold defect with peripheral rim uptake (lytic lesion) • Photopenic defect • Asymmetric uptake in growth plates of long bones in children in neuroblastoma	• Multifocal uptake in contiguous ribs could be post-traumatic • Multifocal uptake may be seen in polyostotic bone dysplasia • Multifocal uptake in the facet joints/endplate region of spine could be degenerative changes • Diffuse uptake in the long bones due to hypertrophic pulmonary osteoarthropathy

Table 8.3 Advantages and disadvantages of bone SPECT-CT

Advantages	Disadvantages
1. Provides both anatomical and functional data in one study, therefore increasing the sensitivity and specificity of the planar study	1. Increase in radiation burden to patient
2. Avoiding additional investigation due to equivocal findings in planar study, which could be time consuming and uncomfortable for the patient and also leads to delay in diagnosis	2. Increase in scan time leading to patient discomfort and decrease in output of the department
3. Attenuation correction by CT data	3. Expensive equipment
4. Incremental value due to incidental findings	4. Non-uniform protocols

scintigraphy has low sensitivity in detecting purely lytic lesions seen in renal cancer, lymphoma and breast cancer. CT component of the SPECT/CT helps detect small and lytic lesions, increasing the sensitivity of the investigation.

8.9 Bone SPECT-CT

SPECT-CT helps increase the planar bone scintigraphy's sensitivity by detecting tracer non-avid lytic lesions or small lesions missed on planar study. The specificity of planar and SPECT study is augmented by accurate localization and characterization of the tracer uptake by SPECT-CT. Moreover, in the staging of disease, the leading utility of SPECT-CT lies in differentiating degenerative disease in the spine common in the elderly patient from metastatic disease. For this purpose, localization of tracer uptake with low-dose CT protocol is sufficient for accurate differentiation of nature of uptake. The advantages and disadvantages of SPECT-CT in bone metastases are mentioned in Table 8.3.

8.10 Artifacts on SPECT/CT

There are different types of image artifacts on SPECT/CT, as mentioned in Table 8.4 [19].

8.11 Literature Evidence on the Role of Bone SPECT/CT in Metastases

There is published literature evaluating SPECT/CT's role in detecting bone metastases in indeterminate or equivocal lesions on planar bone scans. A meta-analysis studying the role of SPECT/CT in classifying indeterminate bone lesions on planar bone scintigraphy, the pooled sensitivity and specificity of SPECT/CT was reported as 93% [95% confidence interval (CI) 0.91–0.95] and 96% [95% CI 0.94–0.97], respectively [20]. The summary of the articles is mentioned in Tables 8.5 and 8.6. SPECT/CT characterizes most of the equivocal findings on planar bone scan with acceptable accuracy in all the studies. SPECT/CT's sensitivity and specificity were found better than planar and SPECT

Table 8.4 Artifacts in SPECT-CT

Artifacts	Effect on image quality
Artifacts on CT component	
• Motion during CT acquisition	Blurring of the contours, disturbances in whole image
• Beam hardening artifacts (Fig. 8.1)	Streaks between bone structures
• Partial volume effects due to structures which are only partially included in the slice	Dark and light streak artifacts
Artifacts on SPECT-CT	
• Misregistration due to poor calibration of isocentres, patient movement (Fig. 8.2a–c)	Wrong localization of tracer uptake leading to misinterpretation, wrong attenuation correction leading to false visualization of uptake
• Truncation artifacts if field of view is too small or patient is too large or patient arm is extended outside selected field of view (Fig. 8.1)	Leads to streak artifacts and hyperdense areas on CT
• High attenuation foreign bodies, e.g. metal artifacts, CT contrast agent, barium (Fig. 8.3)	Leads to low photon counts and high noise, streak artifacts and inaccurate attenuation coefficient measurement
• CT noise due to large patient or low-dose CT protocol (Fig. 8.4)	Low photon counts, error in defining of the CT numbers, loss of smaller details

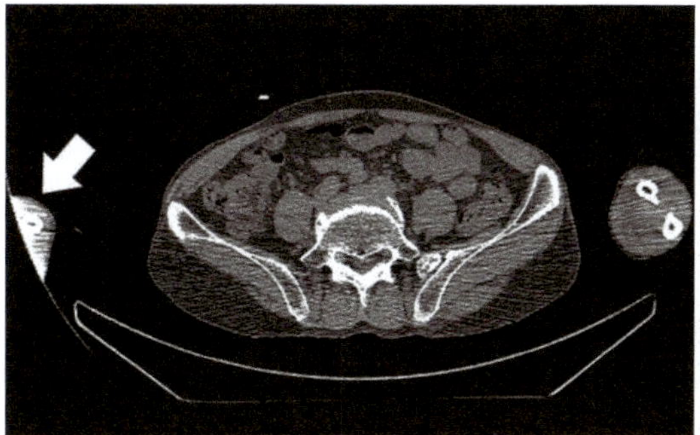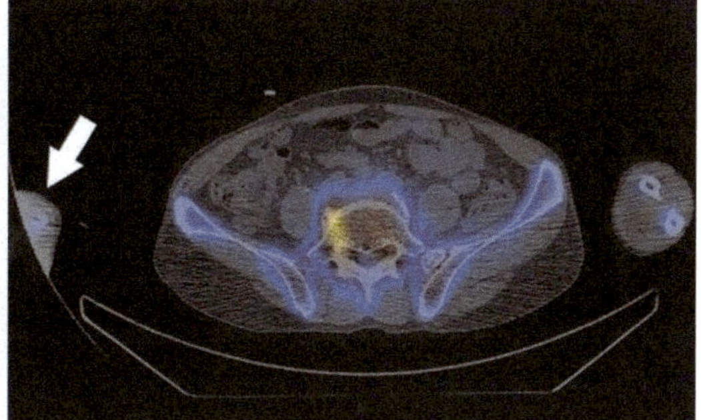

Fig. 8.1 Truncation artifact on CT leading to hyperdense area in the region of right forearm bones (arrow) and streak artifacts due to truncation as well as beam hardening

bone scintigraphy to detect metastases in almost all research.

A new perspective for bone SPECT/CT is whole-body SPECT/CT rather than targeted SPECT/CT. Some studies have shown higher sensitivity, but similar specificity to one-field-of-view targeted SPECT/CT [33]. However, there is a marginal incremental diagnostic value for whole-body SPECT/CT compared to one-field-of-view SPECT/CT [34]. With the availability of faster acquisition protocols for SPECT/CT, whole-body bone SPECT/CT could be widely used [35].

Different scenarios where bone SPECT/CT is contributary in bone metastases evaluation.

(a) Differentiation of degenerative bone diseases/fracture from metastases:

SPECT/CT localizes and characterizes the abnormal tracer uptake leading to differentiation of degenerative changes, facetal arthropathies, enthesopathies, fractures and osteoporotic collapse from metastases (Figs. 8.5, 8.6, 8.7, 8.8, 8.9, 8.10, 8.11, 8.12, and 8.13), and this is the most common use of bone SPECT/CT in oncology.

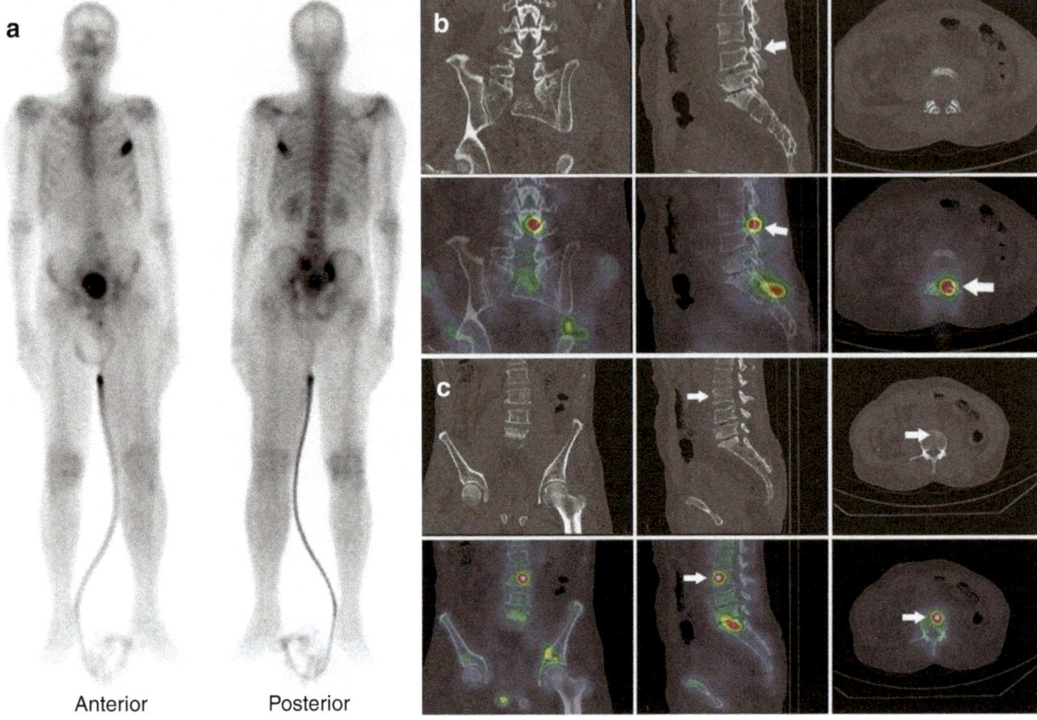

Fig. 8.2 (a–c) Misregistration: Known carcinoma prostate, whole-body bone scan (a) shows multifocal uptake in the left rib, lower lumbar spine and pelvic bones. SPECT/CT of the lumbar spine and pelvis (b) localizes the uptake in the lumbar region to the left L3–L4 facet joint (arrow); however, fused coronal image shows gross misregistration between CT and SPECT images. On inquiry, the technologist informed that patient moved during image acquisition. However, as some anatomical landmarks were available, manual registration of images localizes the uptake to the L3 vertebral body (arrow) and sacrum showing minimal sclerosis (c) suggestive of metastasis

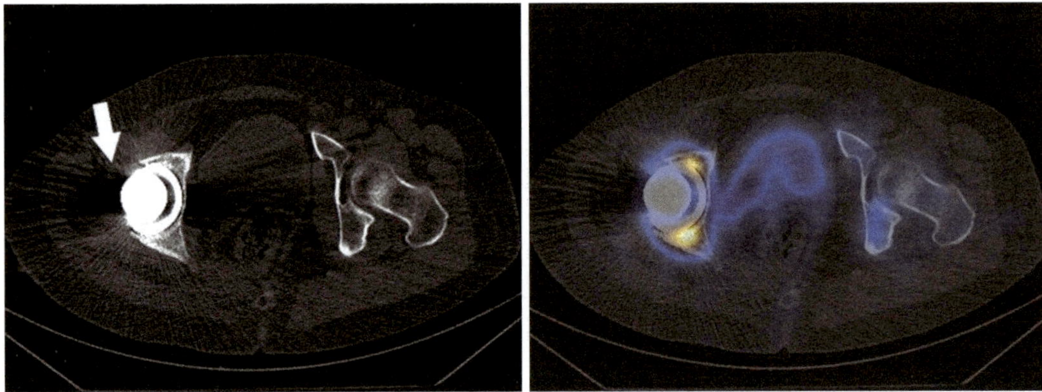

Fig. 8.3 Metal artifact due to hip prosthesis shows darkening adjacent to the metal and streak artifact leading to poor image quality

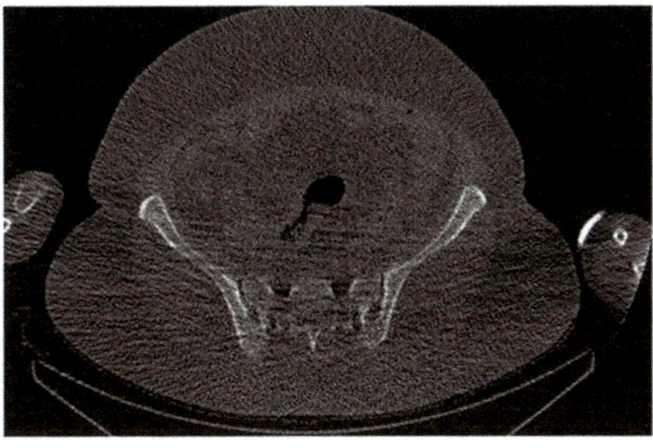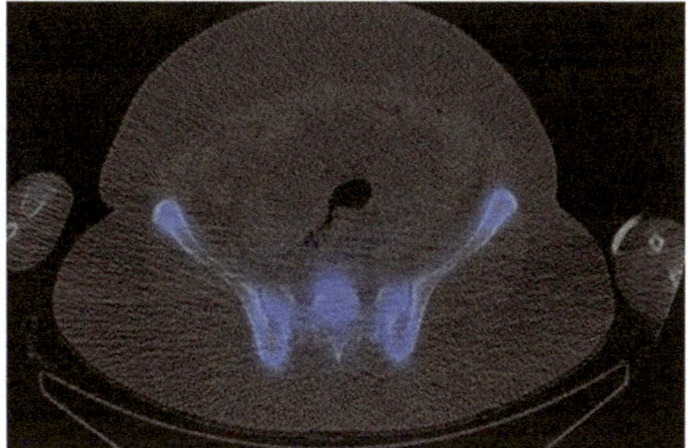

Fig. 8.4 Low-dose CT protocol with 10 mAs and 120 kV in an obese patient leading to high noise and poor image quality

(b) Differentiation of benign bone diseases from metastases:

Several benign bone diseases mimic metastases on planar bone scintigraphy, e.g. Paget's disease (Fig. 8.14), fibrous dysplasia, exostosis, haemangioma (Fig. 8.15), hypertrophic osteoarthropathy. Although some of these entities produce typical appearance on planar bone scintigraphy, other correlative anatomical imaging is required. SPECT/CT acts as one-stop-shop imaging for differentiation of these benign bone entities from metastases.

(c) Extra-skeletal uptake:

There could be extra-skeletal uptake of radiotracer in a bone scan which may mimic bone uptake. Transplant and ectopic pelvic kidney may resemble abnormal uptake in the pelvic bones (Fig. 8.16). Non-osseous tracer uptake is seen in splenic infarct, liver metastasis (Fig. 8.17), lung metastasis (Fig. 8.18), ascites (Fig. 8.19), urinary bladder stones, physiological bowel uptake (Fig. 8.20), etc. Sometimes, the primary tumour shows tracer uptake and should be differentiated from metastases, e.g. neuroblastoma primary, lung cancer, soft-tissue Ewing sarcoma (Fig. 8.21).

(d) Differentiation of local bone infiltration of primary from metastases:

The uptake in the bone could be due to primary local infiltration or secondaries in the bone. This dilemma often occurs if the uptake is seen in a bone close to the primary site. SPECT/CT is usually helpful in this scenario (Fig. 8.22). Differentiation of local infiltration from metastatic bone involvement leads to change in management.

(e) Lytic metastases and metabolically inactive disease:

A planar bone scan has lower sensitivity in the detection of lytic bone metastasis. CT component of the SPECT/CT detects the small lytic lesions, hence increasing the bone scan's sensitivity (Figs. 8.23 and 8.24). Further, SPECT, due to increasing spatial resolution, may detect mildly increased tracer uptake due to bone reaction secondary to lytic metastases not seen on planar scintigraphy. Some authors suggest that the areas that cause pain and a high likelihood of metastases should be included in SPECT/CT, even if planar bone scintigraphy is negative [36]. Sometimes, the sclerotic lesions may not show tracer uptake or show very low-grade uptake on planar study if the patient is on treatment, where SPECT/CT increases the diagnostic sensitivity (Figs. 8.25 and 8.26).

(f) Prognostication value:

The abnormally increased tracer uptake on bone scintigraphy could be due to pure sclerotic or mixed lytic sclerotic metastases [36]. However, both have different prognos-

Table 8.5 Studies evaluating role of SPECT/CT in indeterminate bone lesions on planar bone scan—lesion-based evaluation

Author (year)	Number of patients included in study	Study design	Radiotracer used	Parts of body SPECT-CT	CT used in SPECT-CT	CT radiation dose mAs and kV	Sensitivity (%)	Specificity (%)	Comment
Gayed et al. (2011) [21]	19	Retrospective	MDP	Targeted	6 slice	90, 130	100	92	Evaluation of solitary skull lesions
Sharma et al. (2012) [22]	50	Retrospective	MDP	Targeted	6 slice	100, 130	96 and 98[a]	89	Only lung cancer patients
Sharma et al. (2012) [23]	102	Retrospective	MDP	Targeted	6 slice	100, 130	83	98	Only breast cancer patients, improvement mostly in lytic lesion
Sharma et al. (2014) [24]	32	Retrospective	MDP	Targeted	6 slice	100, 130	95	100	SPECT-CT in isolated skull uptake on bone scan (1–2 lesions) in underlying malignancy patient
Rager et al. (2018) [25]	19	Retrospective	HDP	Whole body	6 slice	40 with intensity modulation, 110	86	96	Breast cancer patient
Zhang et al. (2020) [26]	120	Retrospective	MDP	Targeted	16 slice	Not reported	100	42 and 58[a]	

[a]By two reviewers

Table 8.6 Studies evaluating role of SPECT/CT in indeterminate bone lesions on planar bone scan—patient-based evaluation

Author (year)	Number of patients included in study	Study design	Radiotracer used	Parts of body SPECT-CT	CT used in SPECT-CT	CT radiation dose in mAs (kV)	Sensitivity (%)	Specificity (%)	Comments
Palmedo et al. (2014) [27]	308	Prospective	MDP	Whole body	4 and 2 slice	2.5–20, 120	97	94	Only breast and prostate cancer patients
Fonager et al. (2017) [28]	37	Prospective	MDP/HDP	Whole body	2 and 16 slice	30–100, 130	89	100	In high-risk prostate cancer patient
Teyateeti et al. (2017) [29]	80	Prospective	MDP	Whole body	4 and 16 slice	20, 120	97	100	
Fleury et al. (2018) [30]	328	Retrospective	HMDP	Trunk SPECT-CT	2 and 16 slice	Modulation mA, 130–140	100	97	Breast and prostate cancer patients
Mavriopoulou et al. (2018) [31]	257	Prospective	HDP	Whole body	1 and 4 slice	2.5, 140	97	87.5	Breast cancer patient
Rager et al. (2018) [25]	19	Retrospective	HDP	Whole body	6 slice	40 with intensity modulation, 110	92	100	Breast cancer patient
Leiris et al. (2020) [32]	115	Retrospective	MDP	Whole body	2 slice	Not reported, 130	87	99	Prostate cancer patients

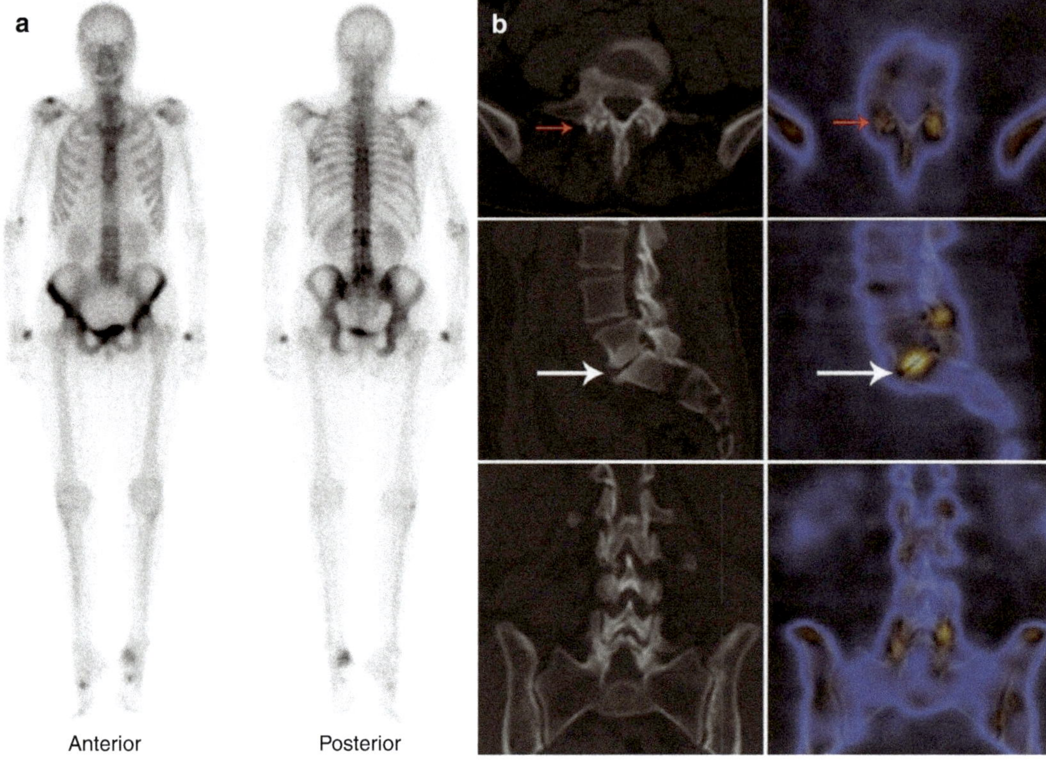

Fig. 8.5 (**a**, **b**) Lung carcinoma with diffuse heterogeneous uptake of tracer in the thoraco-lumbar vertebrae on whole-body bone scan (**a**) could be metastatic involvement. However, SPECT/CT (**b**) localizes the tracer uptake to degenerative changes in the facet joints (red arrow) and endplate changes (white arrow), therefore ruling out metastatic involvement

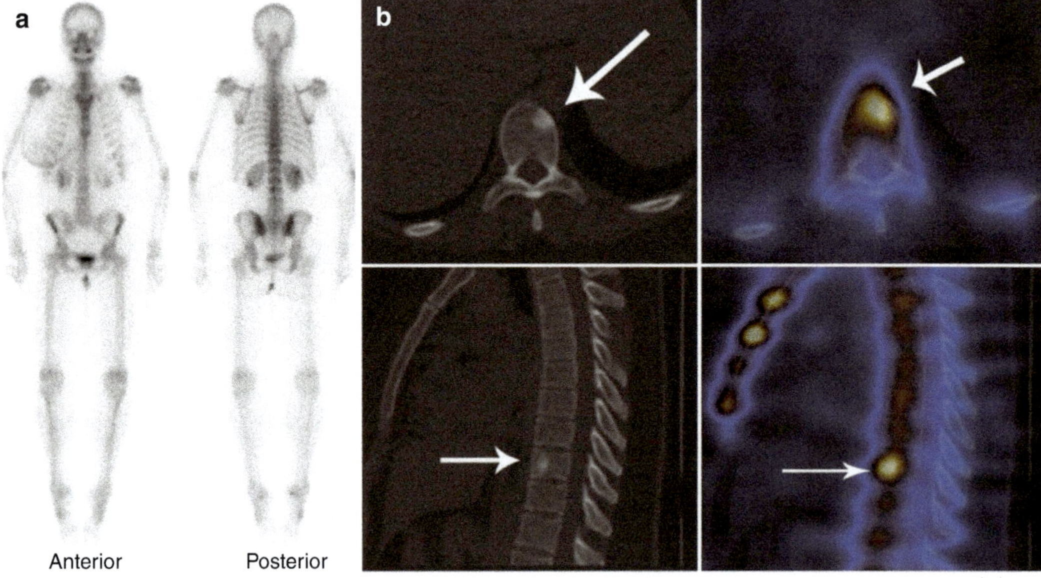

Fig. 8.6 (**a**, **b**) Breast cancer post-neoadjuvant chemotherapy. Whole-body bone scan (**a**) shows mild focal uptake of tracer in the D10 vertebra. Only planar imaging findings could be misinterpreted as degenerative changes. However, SPECT-CT of spine (**b**) localizes the uptake in the D10 vertebra to a sclerotic lesion, consistent with metastatic disease. Teaching point: SPECT-CT increases sensitivity of bone scan in determination of metastasis

tic values. Literature evidence suggests that lytic bone lesions have a relatively worse prognosis. SPECT/CT confirms the metastatic involvement of bone and classifies the lesions as pure sclerotic or mixed sclerotic-lytic, which is not always possible on planar scintigraphy due to lack of anatomical data. Further, SPECT/CT's CT component helps in detecting additional complications like impending fracture, spinal cord involvement and vertebral collapse.

(g) Increases diagnostic confidence:

Sometimes, tracer uptake is seen on the planar bone scintigraphy is confused with surface contamination of tracer (Fig. 8.27). Although cleaning the area with water and reimaging is standard protocol in suspected surface contamination, the uptake persists, leading to a diagnostic dilemma. SPECT/CT often clarifies the difficulty with certainty. Conversely, surface contamination in atypical location could be misinterpreted as sinister

pathology, and SPECT/CT helps in the accurate image interpretation (Fig. 8.28). Further, in many other conditions, the SPECT/CT increases the diagnostic confidence of the reader (Figs. 8.29, 8.30, and 8.31).

(h) Incidental findings:

There could be incidental findings on a SPECT/CT performed to clarify equivocal uptake on planar bone scintigraphy. These findings might be unknown and incidentally detected, impacting patient management, e.g. detection of an ectopic kidney, soft-tissue metastases (Figs. 8.17 and 8.18), lung nodules (Fig. 8.32) and aortic aneurysm.

8.11.1 Primary Bone Malignancy

The role of bone scintigraphy is limited to the evaluation of primary bone malignancy. The bone sarcomas such as osteosarcoma, Ewing's sarcoma, chondrosarcoma show non-specific tracer

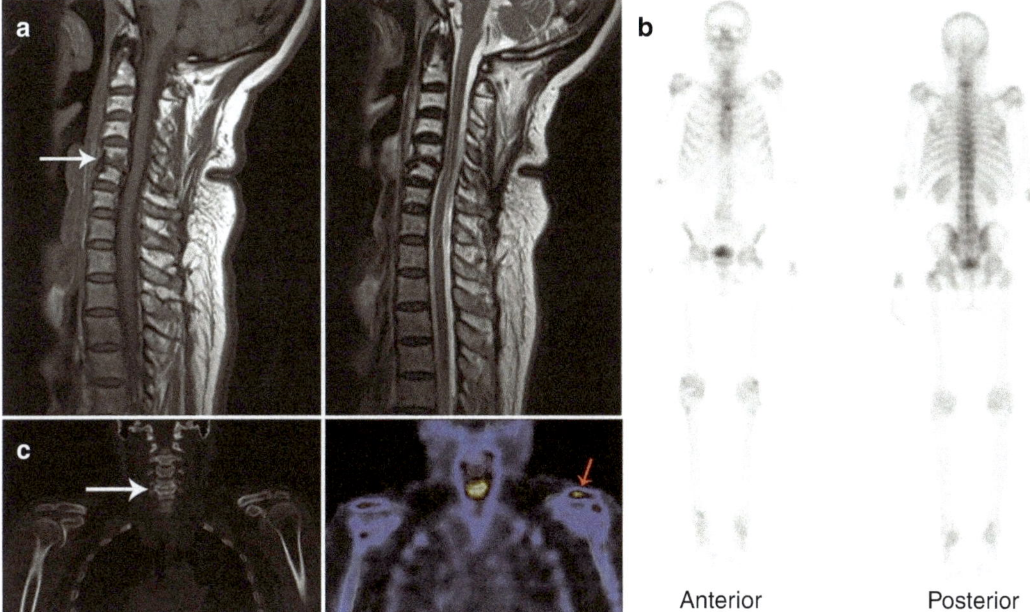

Fig. 8.7 (**a–c**) A patient with supraglottic carcinoma, post-radiotherapy, presented with numbness in upper and lower limbs. MRI cervical spine (**a**) shows radiotherapy changes in the C2–C6 vertebral bodies. A low-signal lesion is seen in the C5 vertebral body (arrow), likely degenerative changes. To confirm the finding and rule out metastasis, bone scan was performed. Linear tracer uptake is seen in the mid cervical spine (posterior image in **b**), which on SPECT-CT localizes to endplate degenerative changes at C5–C6 vertebrae (white arrow in **c**), thus ruling out metastatic involvement. The uptake in left acromioclavicular joint (red arrow **c**) is degenerative in nature

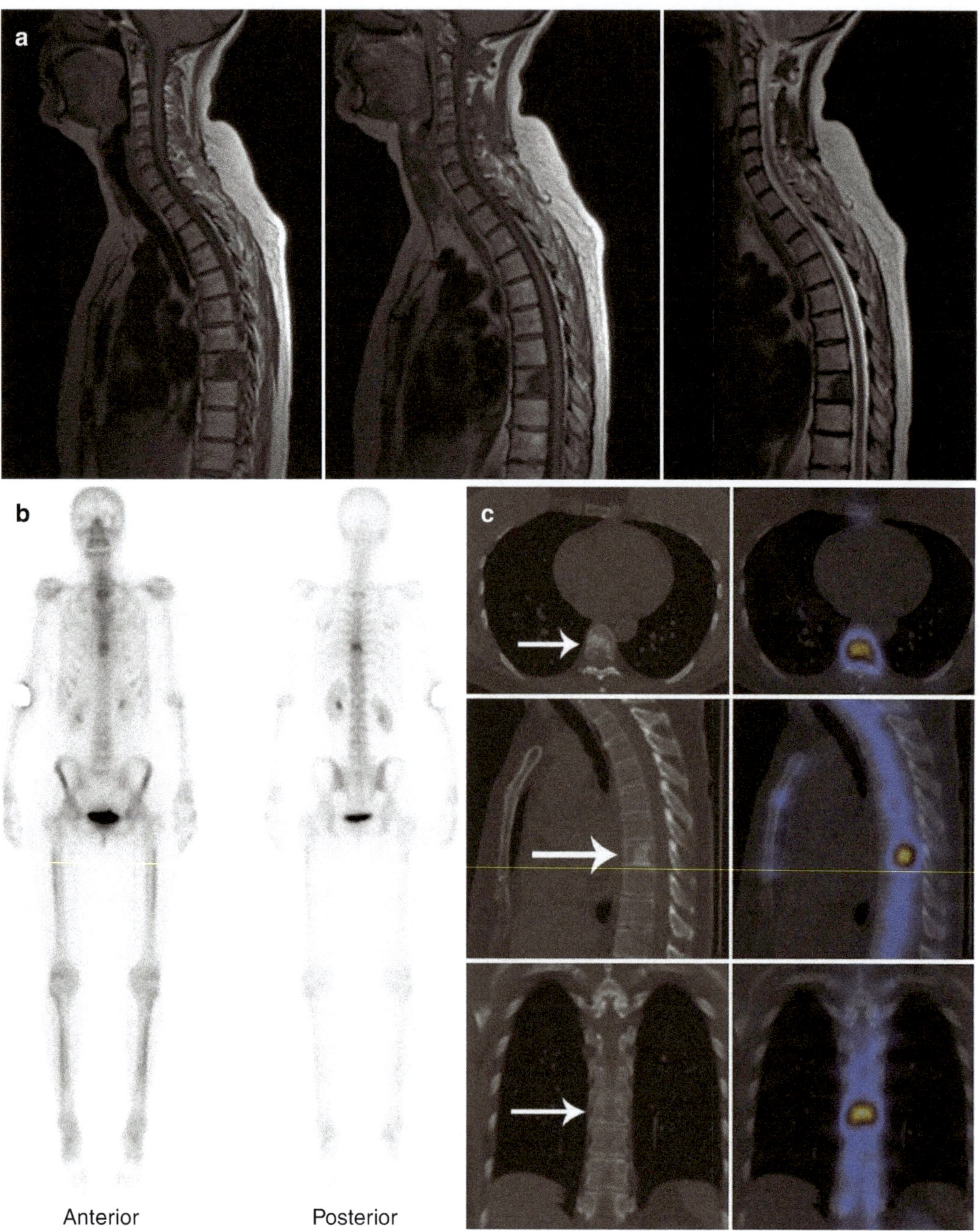

Fig. 8.8 (**a–c**) A 51-year-old lady with known breast carcinoma, status post-mastectomy, presented with pain in the thoracic and lumbar vertebrae, worse at night. (**a**) MR images of spine (T1, T2 and STIR sagittal sequences) show low-signal intensity lesion in the D8 vertebral body, which raises possibility of a metastasis. (**b**) Whole-body bone scan shows focal increased tracer uptake in the D8 vertebra. (**c**) SPECT-CT of thoracic spine localizes the abnormal tracer uptake seen in whole-body study to a sclerotic lesion in the D8 vertebral body (arrows), compatible with solitary bone metastasis

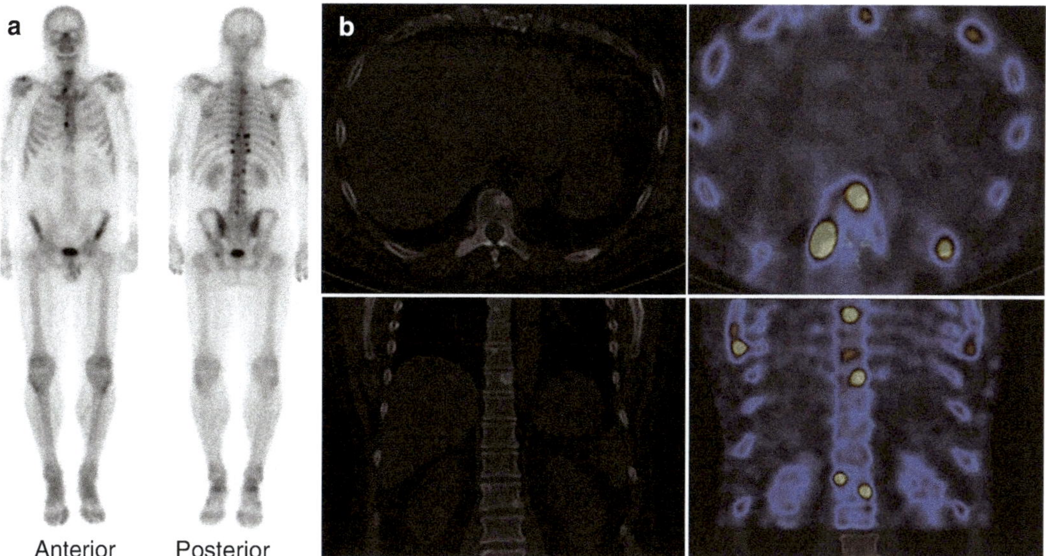

Fig. 8.9 (**a**, **b**) Prostate carcinoma with PSA level 108 ng/mL. The whole-body bone scan (**a**) shows increased tracer uptake along multiple costovertebral junctions, which could be due to degenerative changes. Similarly, low-grade uptake in the ribs could be traumatic fracture as seen in previous case. There is focal tracer uptake in the sternum and left hip joint, which are indeterminate. SPECT-CT of thorax (**b**) shows multiple sclerotic lesions in the thoraco-lumbar vertebrae involving the body and transverse process. There is also sclerotic lesion in the rib showing increased uptake of tracer. The findings are consistent with multifocal skeletal metastases

uptake on bone scintigraphy. SPECT-CT is helpful in the diagnosis of primary, mostly due to the CT component characterizing the lesion type.

However, the planar bone scan tends to overestimate the tumour extent in these tumours (Fig. 8.33). Often, SPECT-CT helps in the estimation of the accurate extent of the disease (Fig. 8.33). Whole-body bone scintigraphy has a role in detecting skip lesions in osteosarcoma and detecting osseous metastases in polyostotic tumour.

A bone scan has limited sensitivity in multiple myeloma and histiocytosis. Multiple myeloma shows lytic lesions with a lack of reactive osteoblastic reaction, so it may not be visible on a planar bone scan. Similarly, in leukaemia and lymphoma, the bone scan has limited utility. There may be increased focal uptake in the marrow in patients with marrow infiltration; however, diffuse increased osteoblastic activity may be seen in patients with blast crises.

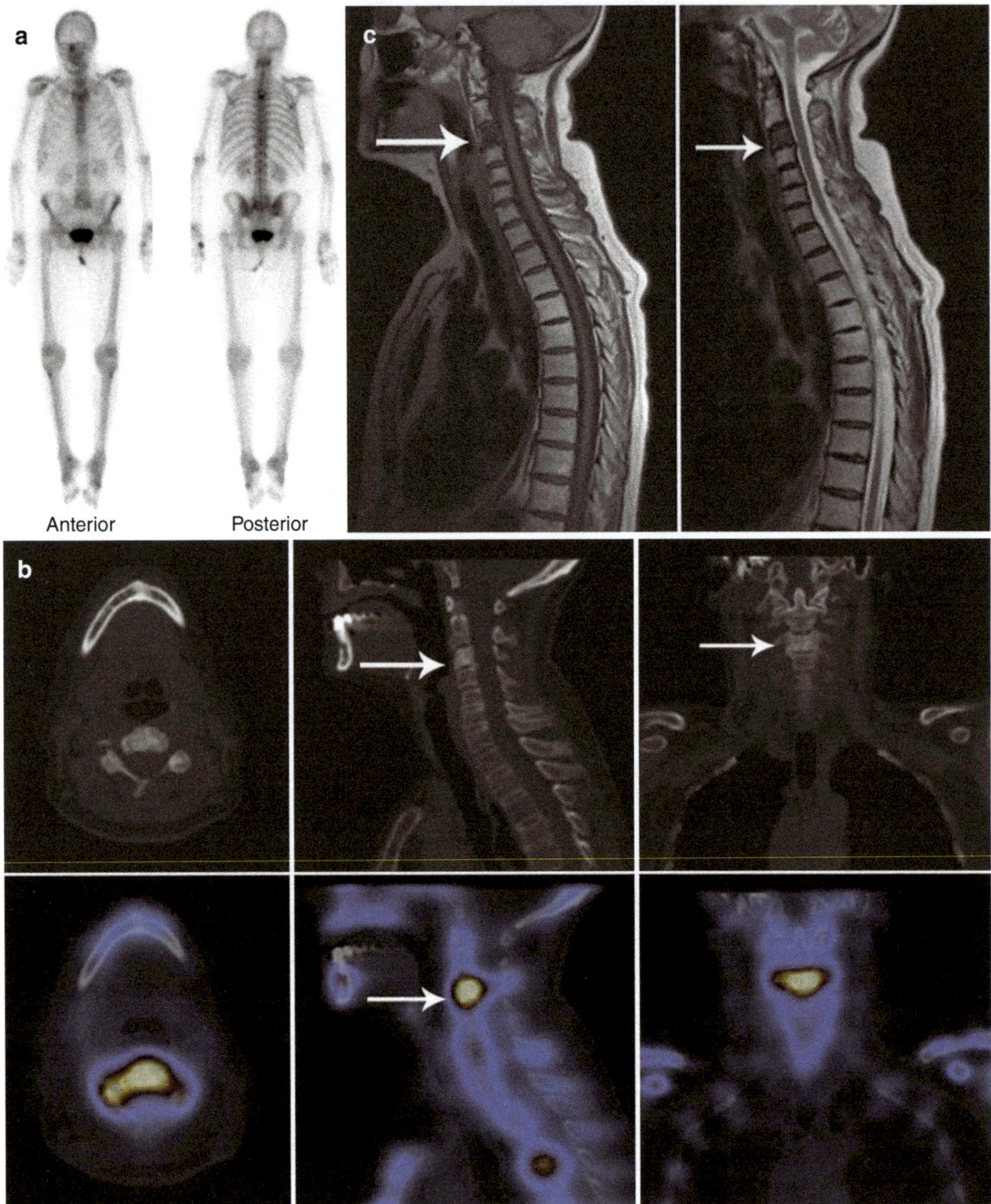

Fig. 8.10 (**a–c**) Lung cancer treated with radical radiotherapy and radiofrequency ablation. PET-CT scan showed uptake in C3 vertebra? which was indeterminate. Whole-body bone scan (**a**) shows mild heterogeneous tracer uptake in the upper cervical region, D4 vertebra, left lumbosacral region and right sacroiliac joint. SPECT-CT of cervical spine (**b**) localizes uptake in the cervical region to a sclerotic C3 vertebra and extends from the vertebral body into both lateral masses (arrows). The uptake in D4 vertebra localizes to partial collapse, which is new comparison to PET-CT study, morphologically favouring osteoporotic collapse. Overall, the findings are suggestive of malignant infiltration of C3 vertebra. This finding was supported by MRI cervical spine done after few days, which shows diffuse low T1-weighted and T2-weighted signal change within C3 vertebra (arrow in **c**)

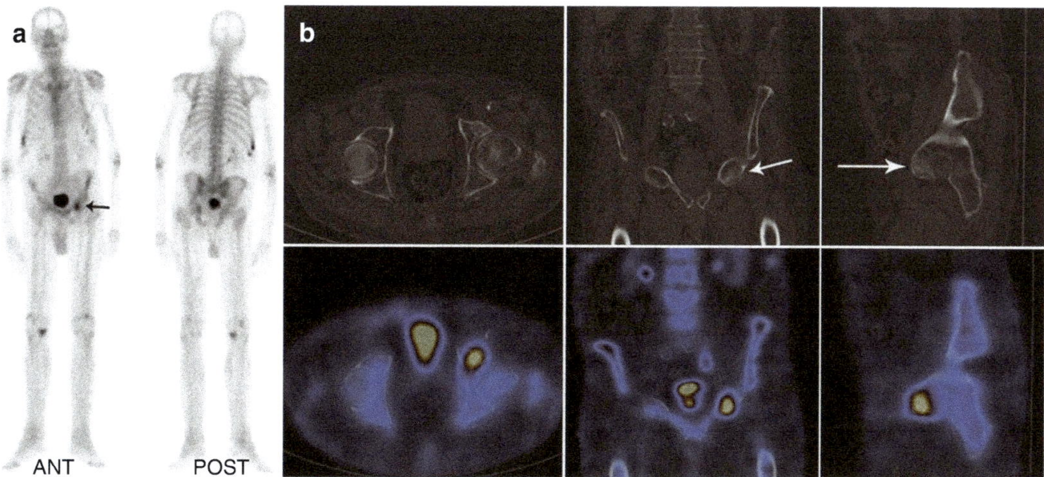

Fig. 8.11 (**a**, **b**) Patient with prostate cancer. Whole-body bone scan (**a**) shows multiple foci of increased tracer uptake in the left 6th–8th ribs and right 9th–11th ribs which are likely due to fractures. There is intense uptake of tracer in the left hip joint region (arrow). This could be due to metastatic disease. However, SPECT-CT of pelvis (**b**) localizes the uptake of tracer to the anterior column of the left acetabulum where there is a breach of cortex (arrow) and is consistent with a fracture. The findings on SPECT-CT suggested likely insufficiency fracture in the left acetabulum as there are similar fractures in the ribs; however, MRI was suggested for further evaluation

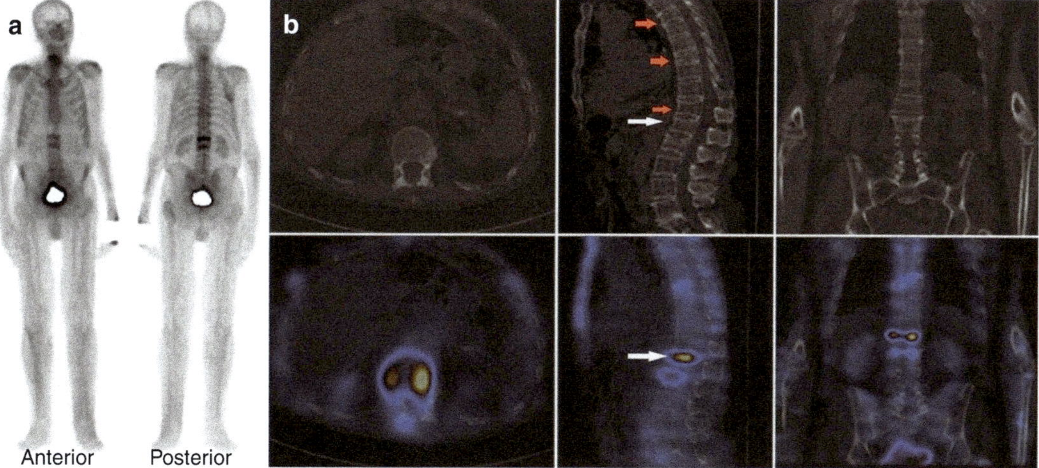

Fig. 8.12 (**a**, **b**) A 64-year-old gentleman with history of prostate cancer presented with sudden onset back pain. The patient had previous history of traumatic vertebral fracture, and exact level could not be known from the history. Bone scan was performed to identify cause of pain. Whole-body bone scan (**a**) demonstrates intense linear tracer uptake in the L1 vertebral region with more moderate linear uptake in the L2 vertebral region. Moderate tracer uptake is associated with the right aspect of the mid cervical vertebra. SPECT-CT of the thoracolumbar spine (**b**) shows marked osteoporotic changes within the thoracolumbar spine. The epicentre of the increased uptake in L1 vertebra corresponds to superior endplate of L1 where there is minor degree of endplate compression consistent with a fracture (white arrows). Mild metabolic activity in L2 is associated with more significant superior endplate compression at L2 vertebra. There are established wedge compression fractures at T6, T9 and T12 vertebrae which are metabolically inactive (red arrows). The findings are suggestive of an acute osteoporotic superior endplate compression fracture of L1 (which is likely cause of acute pain), with a previous, chronologically older compression fracture at L2

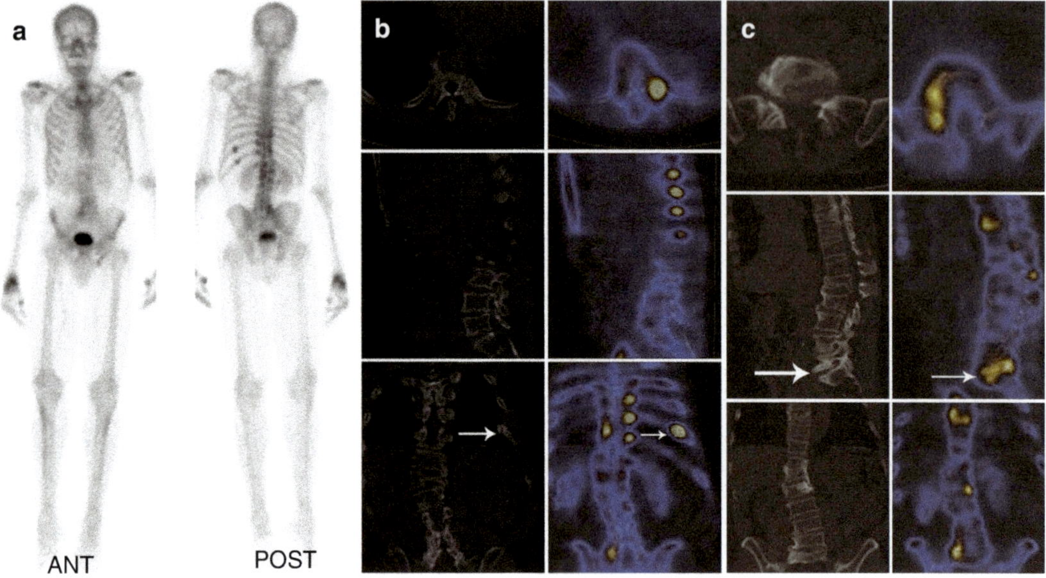

Fig. 8.13 (a–c) Prostate carcinoma with Gleason score 4 + 5 and PSA level 24 ng/mL and new onset back pain. Whole body bone scan (**a**) to look for metastatic disease shows focal tracer uptake in the left 10th and 11th ribs posteriorly, increased tracer uptake in D9–L2 vertebrae and at the right lumbosacral junction. The overall findings are suspicious for metastatic disease. There is further increased tracer uptake in the right wrist, which is likely benign in nature. However, SPECT-CT of thoracolumbar spine (**b**) localizes the tracer uptake in the left 10th and 11th ribs to site of fracture (arrow). Further, SPECT-CT of thoracolumbar spine (**b**, **c**) localizes uptake in the D9–L2 vertebrae and at right lumbosacral junction to degenerative changes (arrow in **c**). Note is also made of several collapsed vertebrae with normal tracer uptake suggestive of old traumatic/osteoporotic collapse. Overall, SPECT-CT helped in ruling out metastatic disease and identified cause of pain to be likely degenerative changes or rib fracture

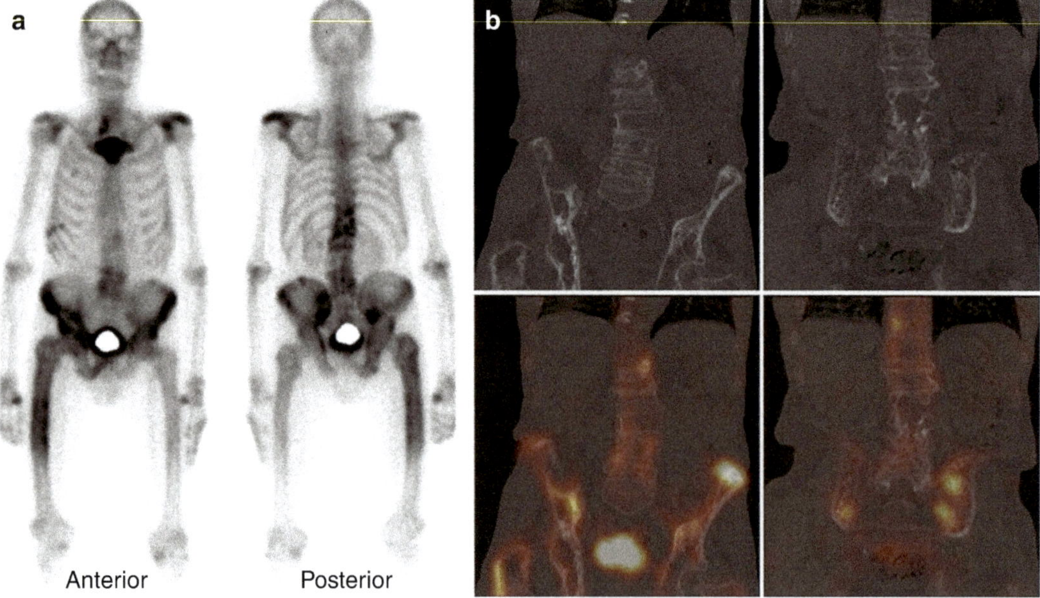

Fig. 8.14 (**a**, **b**) Bone scan was acquired from the vertex to the knees in a patient with prostate cancer. The planar bone scan shows (**a**) intense tracer uptake in the manubrium and left shoulder. Patchy tracer localization is seen in the lower thoracic and lumbar vertebrae, pelvis and bilateral femora (right side more than left). Foci of uptake in the right-side lower ribs are likely due to fractures. SPECT-CT of lower thoracic and lumbar spine and pelvis (**b**) shows marked coarsening of the trabecular pattern and cortical thickening particularly in the pelvic bones. Thus, the bone scan appearances along with SPECT-CT findings are most in keeping with extensive Paget's disease

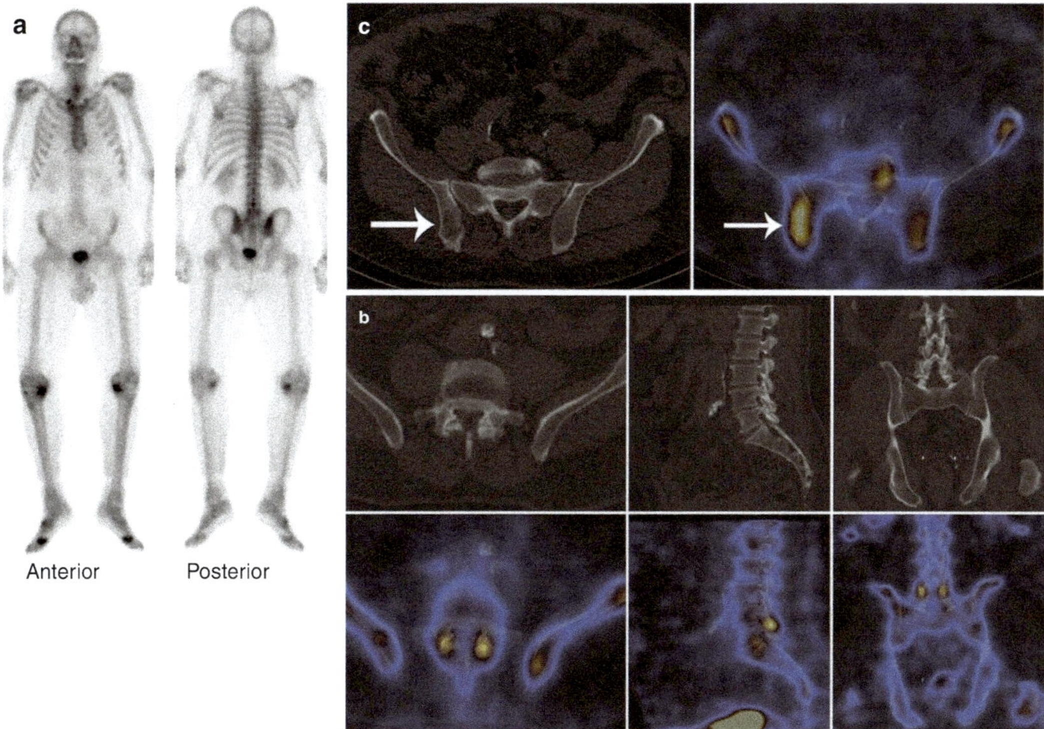

Fig. 8.15 (**a–c**) Patient with prostate cancer presented with 6-month history of worsening buttock pain. Whole-body bone scan (**a**) shows mild heterogeneous tracer uptake in the lower lumbar spine and right sacroiliac joint. The uptake of tracer in the knees and feet is likely due to degenerative changes. SPECT-CT of lumbar spine and pelvis (**b**) demonstrates increased tracer uptake in bilateral L4–L5 facet joints showing degenerative change on CT, which could be pain generator. Increased uptake of tracer is seen at the L5–S1 endplate changes (**b**). Further, the uptake in the right sacroiliac joint localizes to area of decreased bone attenuation in the right iliac bone (arrow in **c**). The SPECT-CT appearances of right iliac bone lesion are atypical for metastasis. MRI of pelvis showed well-defined T2 hyperintense lesion in the right ilium adjacent to the sacroiliac joint suggestive of a haemangioma (not shown)

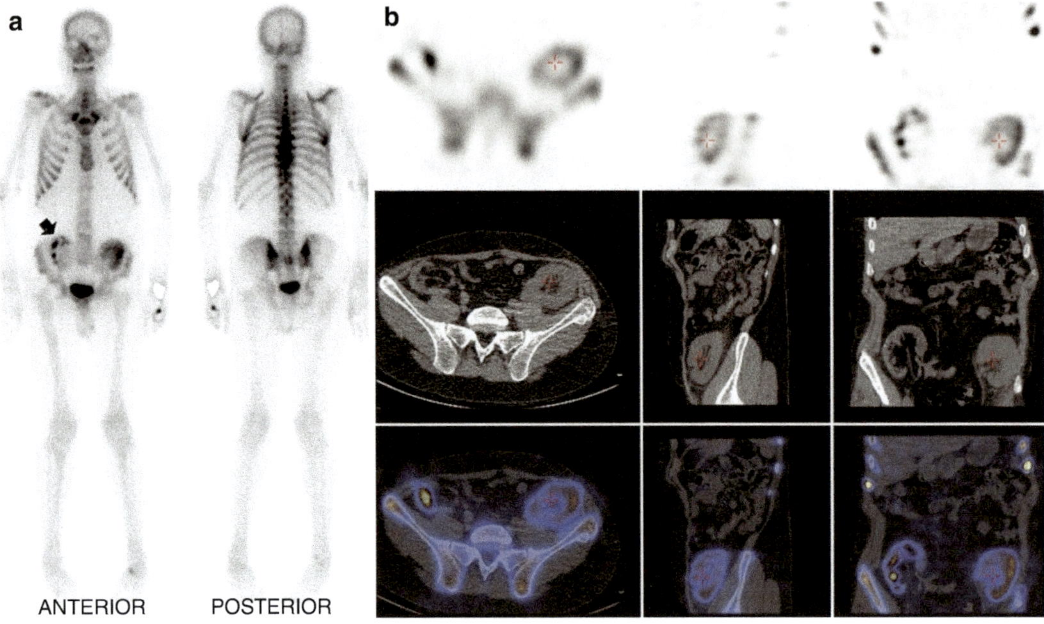

Fig. 8.16 (**a**, **b**) Patient with prostate cancer and low back pain underwent a bone scan. Whole-body bone scan (**a**) shows no abnormal tracer uptake in the lumbar spine. Abnormal tracer accumulation in the bilateral iliac fossa region in anterior image (arrow in **a**) localizes to bilateral renal transplant on SPECT-CT (**b**), suggestive of physiological tracer excretion. Heterogeneous tracer uptake in thoracic vertebrae is suggestive of degenerative changes

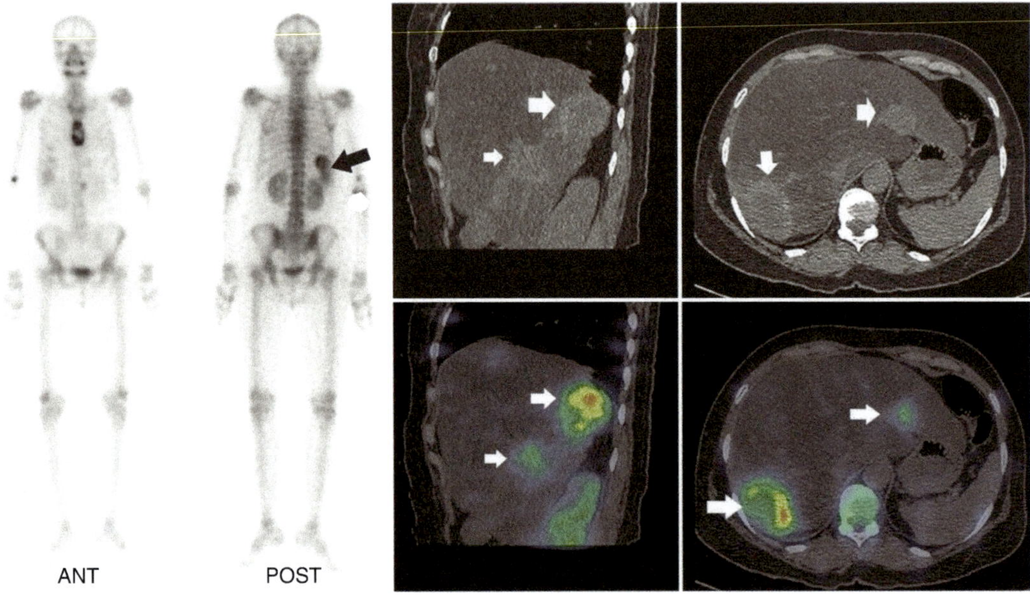

Fig. 8.17 Known carcinoma breast, whole-body bone scan shows increased uptake in the right lower thoracic region prominent on posterior view image (black arrow) as well as increased osteoblastic activity in sternum (lytic metastasis). SPECT-CT localizes the uptake in thoracic region to the hyperdense lesions in the liver (white arrows) suggestive of metastatic deposits

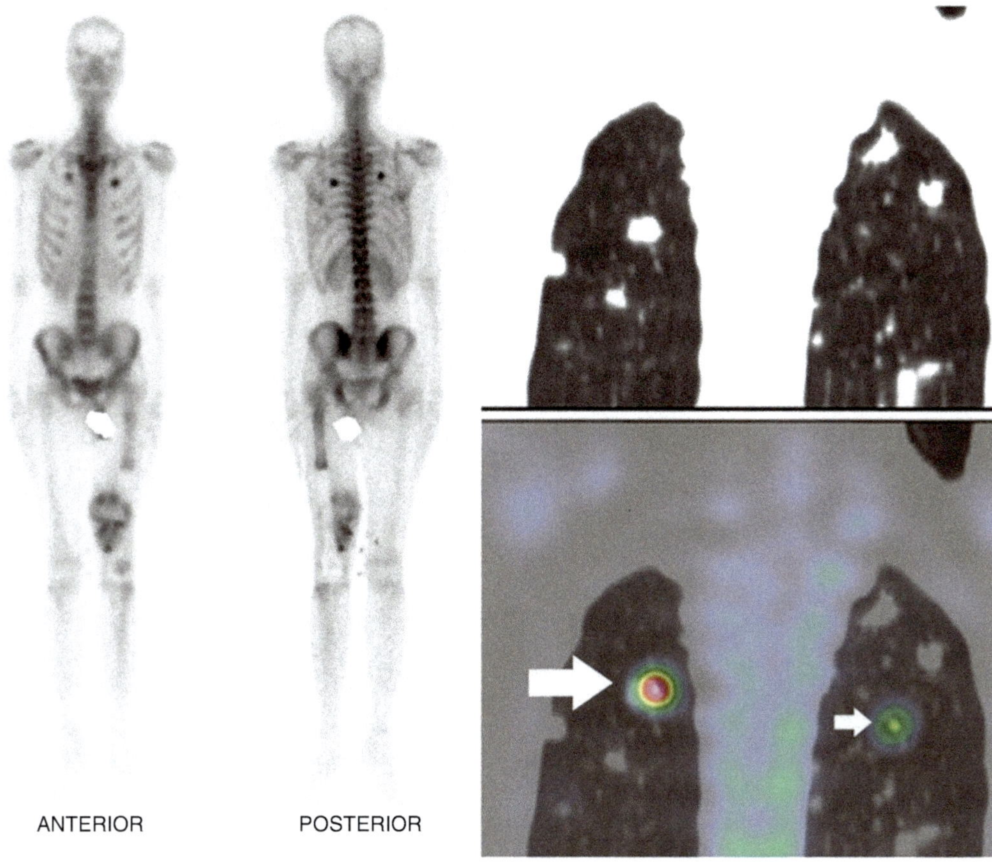

Fig. 8.18 Twenty-three-year-old male with known osteosarcoma of the left lower femur, post-surgery recurrence, bone scan shows increased heterogenous uptake at the primary site with two prominent foci of uptake in the chest could be rib metastases. However, SPECT-CT localizes the uptake to calcified lung nodules (arrows) suggestive of metastasis along with other tracer non-avid lung nodules [Teaching point: lung metastasis from osteosarcoma may show calcification leading to tracer uptake on a bone scan]

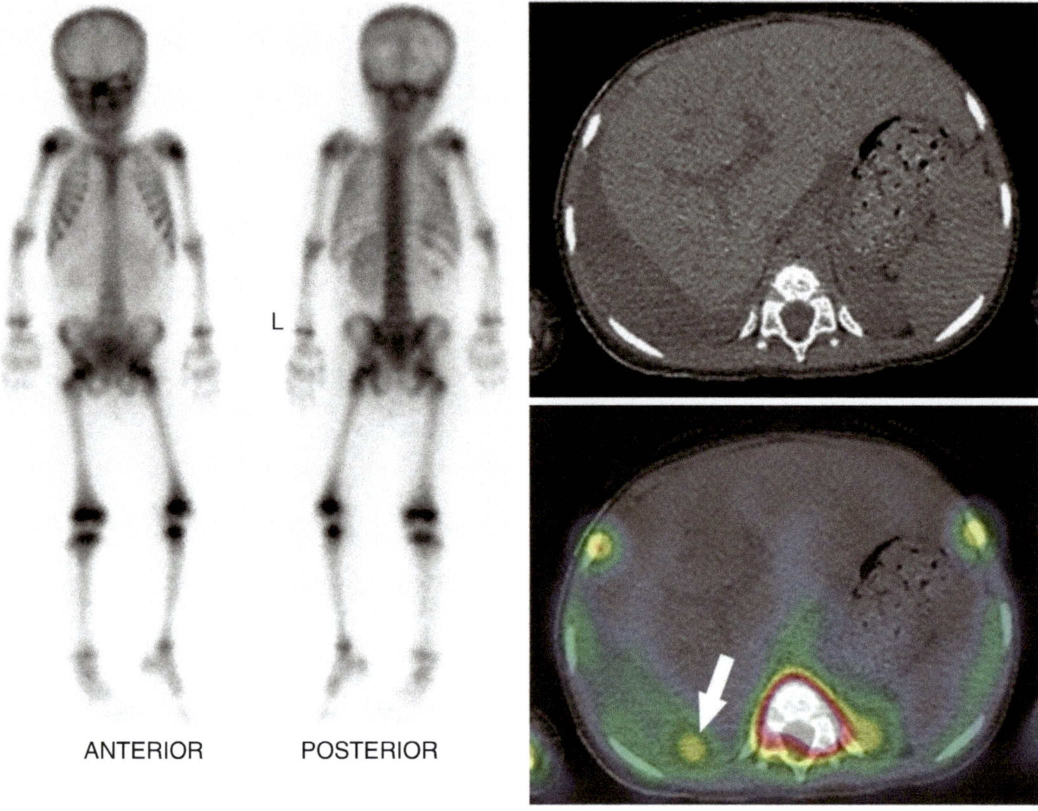

Fig. 8.19 Four-year-old boy with known Wilms tumour shows heterogeneous tracer uptake in the right lower ribs on planar bone scan, which on SPECT-CT localizes to uptake in ascitic fluid adjacent to the ribs (arrows) ruling out bone metastasis

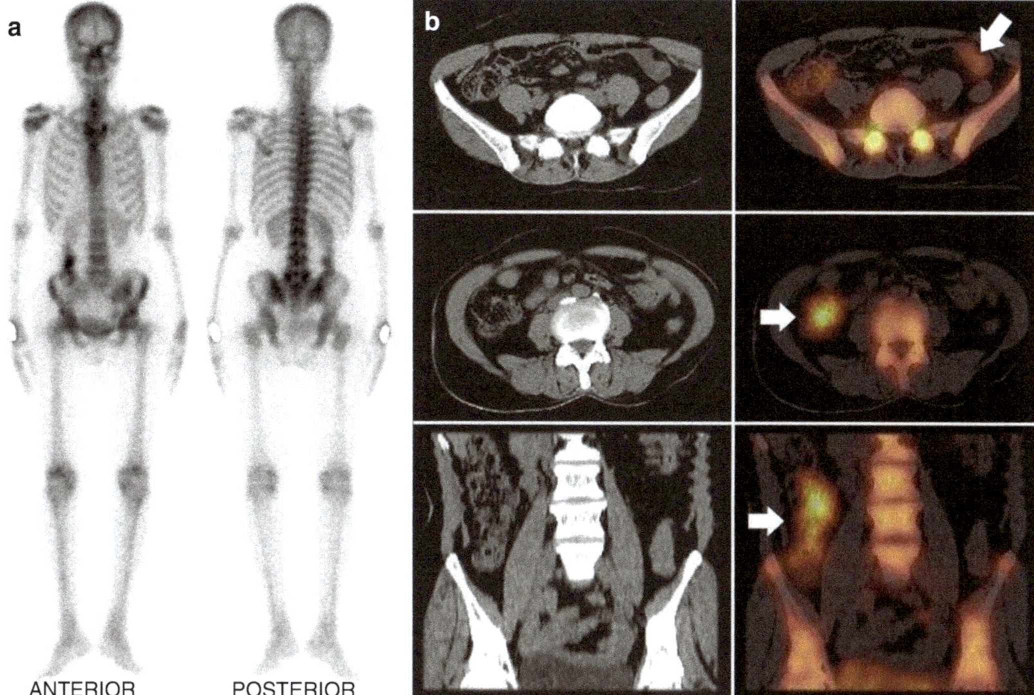

Fig. 8.20 (**a**, **b**) A patient with prostate cancer shows abnormal tracer uptake in bilateral iliac fossa on whole-body bone scan (**a**). The uptake on planar bone scan could be misinterpreted as metastasis in the left iliac bone. However, SPECT-CT of abdomen and pelvis (**b**) localizes tracer uptake in iliac fossa region to intestinal loops (arrows) suggestive of altered biodistribution of tracer. SPECT-CT helps in avoiding false-positive interpretation in cancer patient

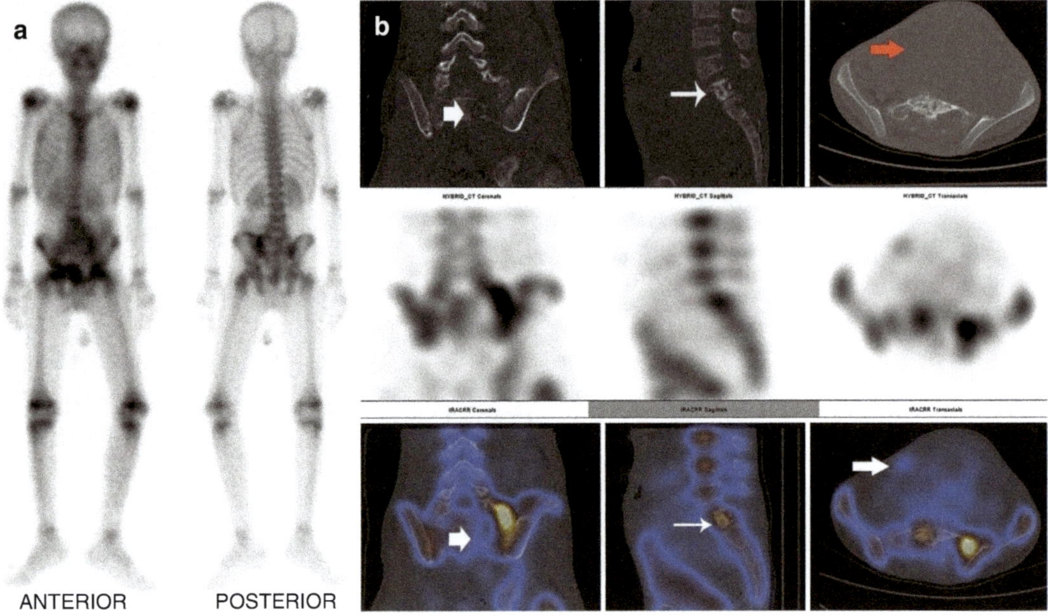

Fig. 8.21 (**a**, **b**) Known Ewing's sarcoma pelvic mass, planar bone scan (**a**) shows heterogeneous tracer uptake in the pelvis region which could be due to uptake in primary or secondary bone disease. SPECT-CT of pelvis (**b**) demonstrates uptake in the primary soft-tissue mass with uptake in the L5 and sacrum with local bone infiltration by primary mass showing lytic sclerotic lesion

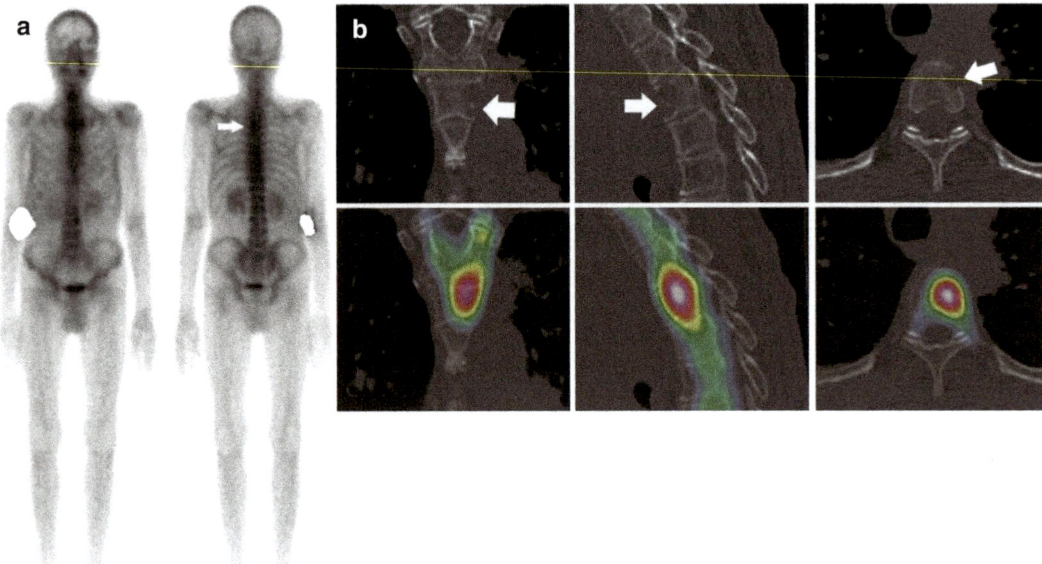

Fig. 8.22 (**a**, **b**) Known lung carcinoma in a 68-year-old male, whole-body bone scan (**a**) shows doubtful focus of uptake in the region of left sternoclavicular joint. On SPECT-CT (**b**), the uptake localizes to lytic changes in the thoracic vertebra due to local infiltration of the left lung mass (arrows)

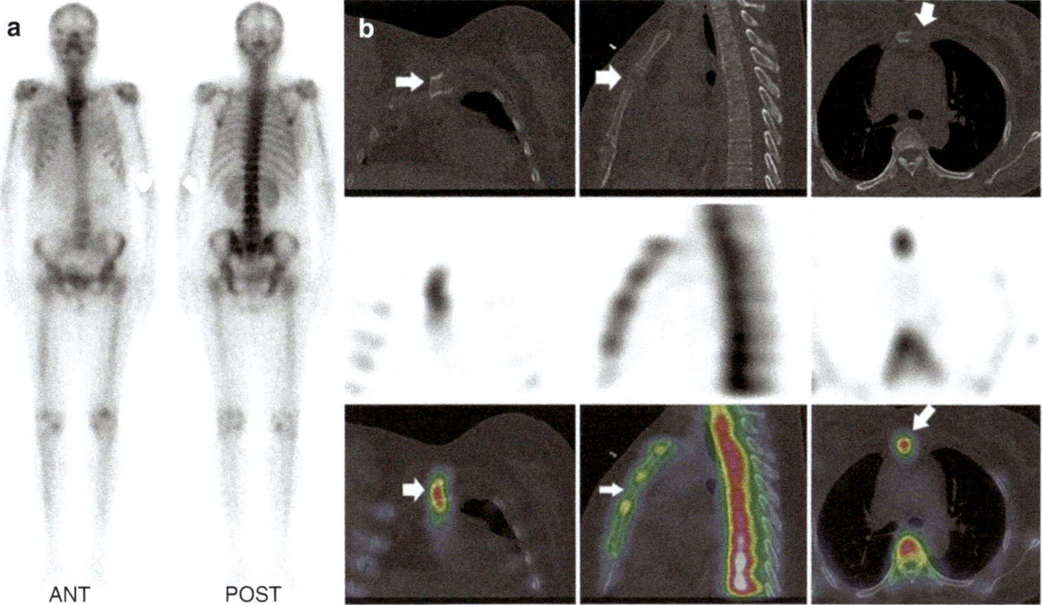

Fig. 8.23 (**a**, **b**) Forty-six-year-old female with known breast carcinoma shows mild heterogeneous uptake at the manubriosternal joint region on whole-body scan (**a**). SPECT-CT of sternum demonstrates focal lytic lesion with soft-tissue component just below manubriosternal joint suggestive of metastasis

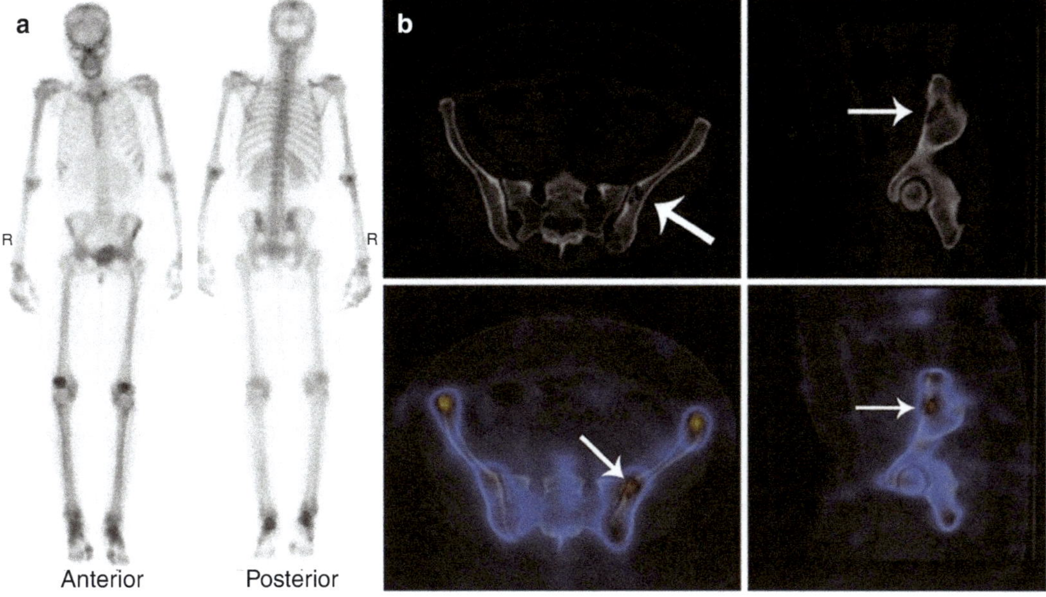

Fig. 8.24 (**a**, **b**) Whole-body bone scan (**a**) of a patient referred for metastatic evaluation shows increased tracer uptake in the knees, ankles and feet suggestive of degenerative changes. On planar imaging, no abnormal tracer uptake is seen anywhere in the skeleton to suggest metastasis. However, SPECT-CT of the pelvis (**b**) demonstrates mild tracer uptake in the left iliac bone showing two lytic lesions (arrows) suggestive of metastatic disease

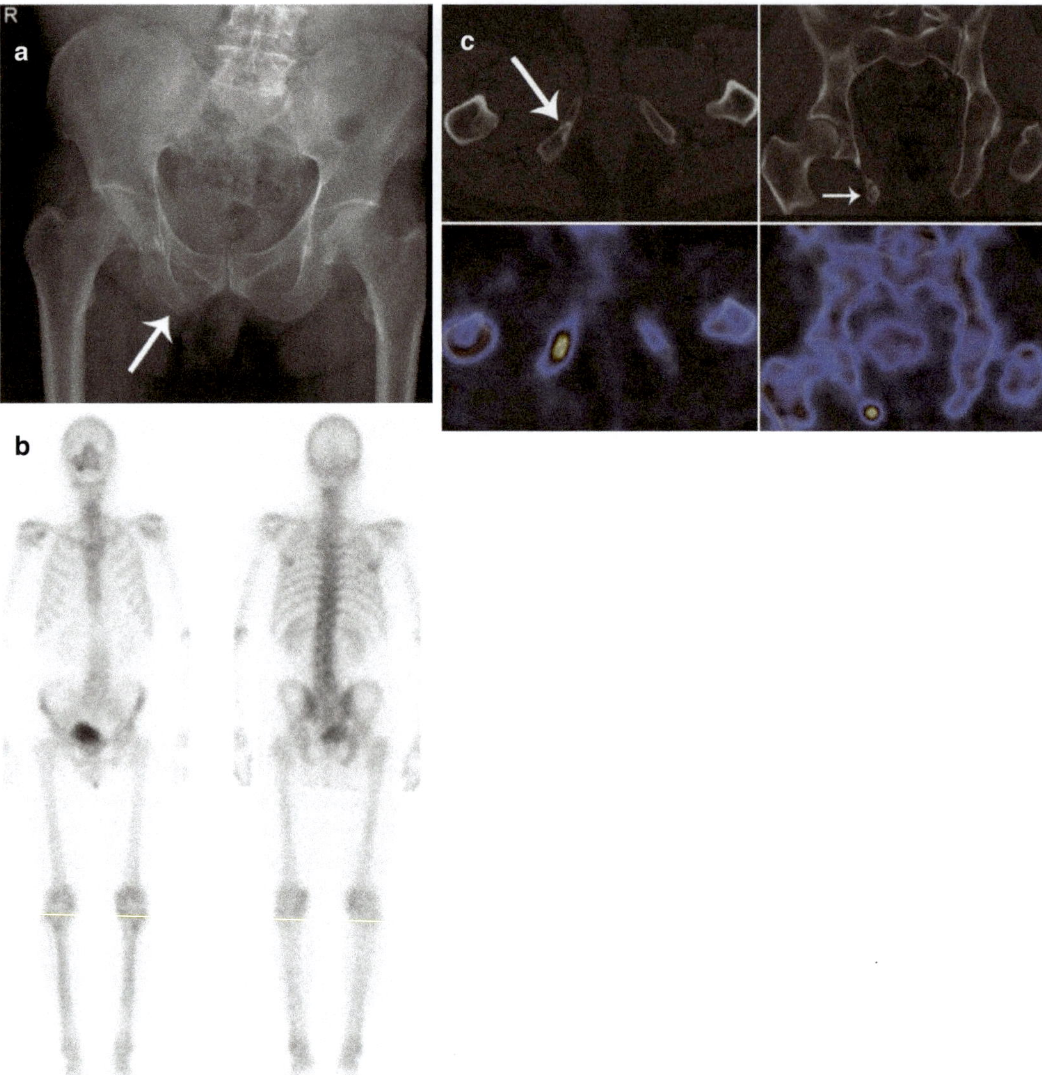

Fig. 8.25 (**a–c**) Patient with prostate cancer. X-ray pelvis shows a sclerotic lesion in the right ischium (arrow in **a**). Bone scan was done to rule out metastasis. Whole-body bone scan (**b**) shows no abnormal tracer uptake in the pelvic bones. However, SPECT-CT of pelvis (**c**) shows mild tracer uptake in a sclerotic lesion in the right ischium (arrows), suspicious for metastasis. In this particular example, SPECT-CT has increased sensitivity compared to planar bone scan in detection of bone lesions

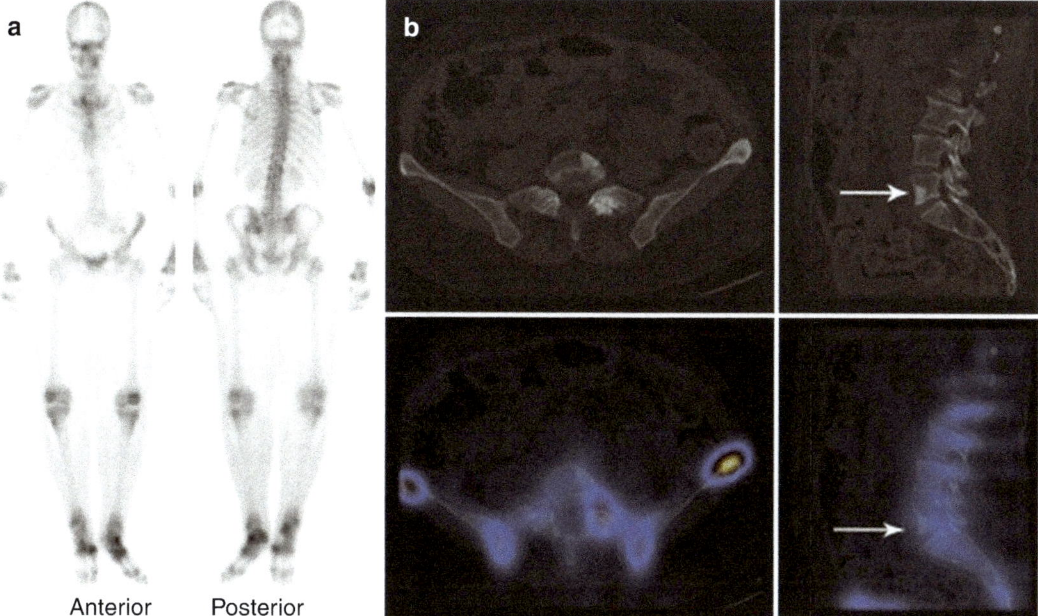

Fig. 8.26 (**a**, **b**) A patient with breast cancer underwent a bone scan with SPECT-CT for staging. The whole-body study (**a**) shows increased tracer uptake in the cervical spine, elbows, wrists, knees, ankles and feet, likely due to degenerative changes. Increased tracer uptake is seen in the sternum and left iliac bone. SPECT-CT of lumbar spine and pelvis (**b**) shows increased tracer uptake in the left iliac bone corresponding to sclerotic lesion suggestive of metastasis. Moreover, there is a sclerotic lesion in the L5 vertebral body with no tracer uptake (arrow in **b**). The findings are suggestive of bone metastases in the sternum, L5 vertebrae and left iliac bone. SPECT-CT helps in identifying metabolically inactive metastasis in this patient

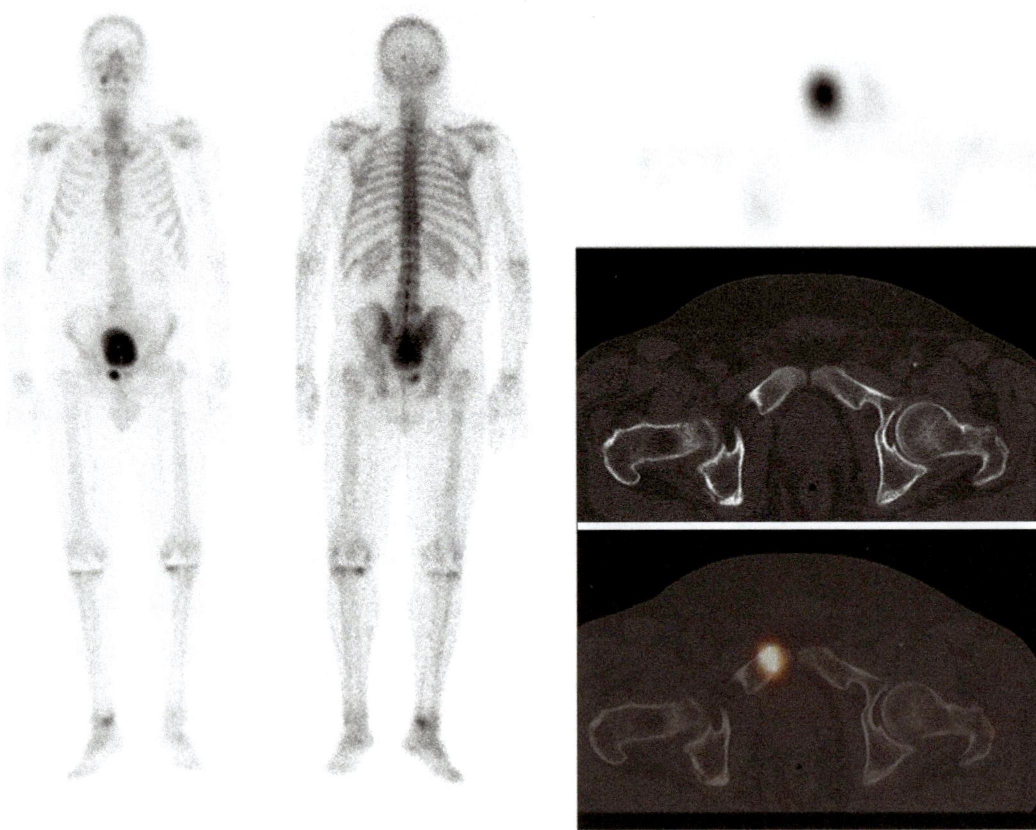

Fig. 8.27 Whole-body bone scan of a prostate cancer patient with serum PSA level 88 ng/mL shows intense focal tracer uptake at the right pubic ramus which is suspicious for metastasis, but could be due to urine contamination. Two subtle foci of tracer uptake are seen in the skull posteriorly, which is non-specific and likely benign. Note is made of bilateral knee replacement. SPECT-CT of the pelvis localizes focal uptake at the right pubic symphysis to subtle sclerosis on CT component of the study, suggestive of early bone metastasis

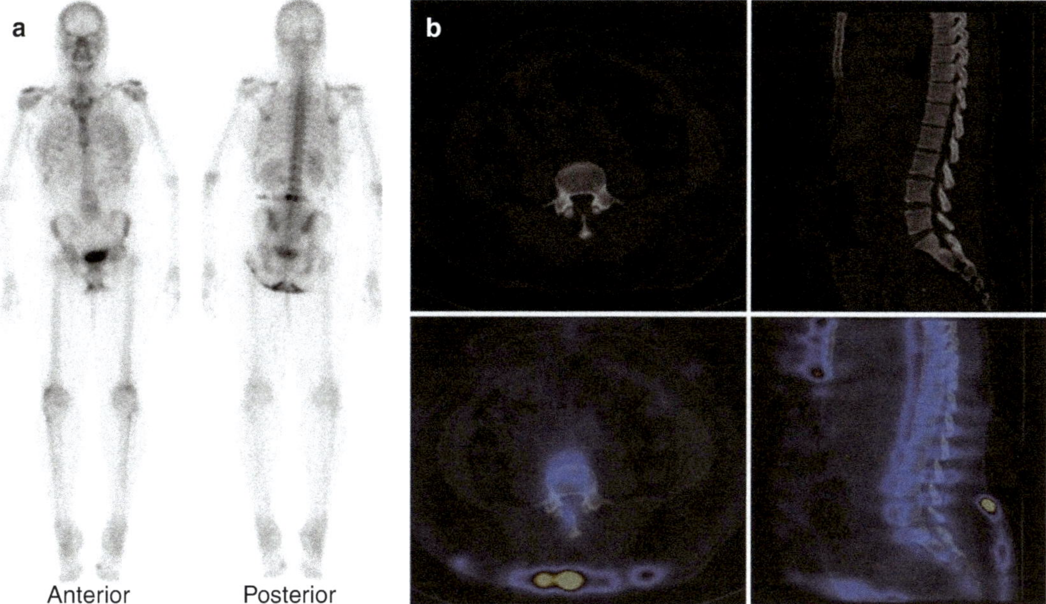

Fig. 8.28 (a, b) Breast cancer with back pain. Whole-body bone scan (a) shows increased tracer uptake in the region of lower lumbar vertebrae. SPECT-CT of lumbar spine (b) localizes the uptake to skin contamination. No morphological abnormality is seen in the lumbar vertebrae

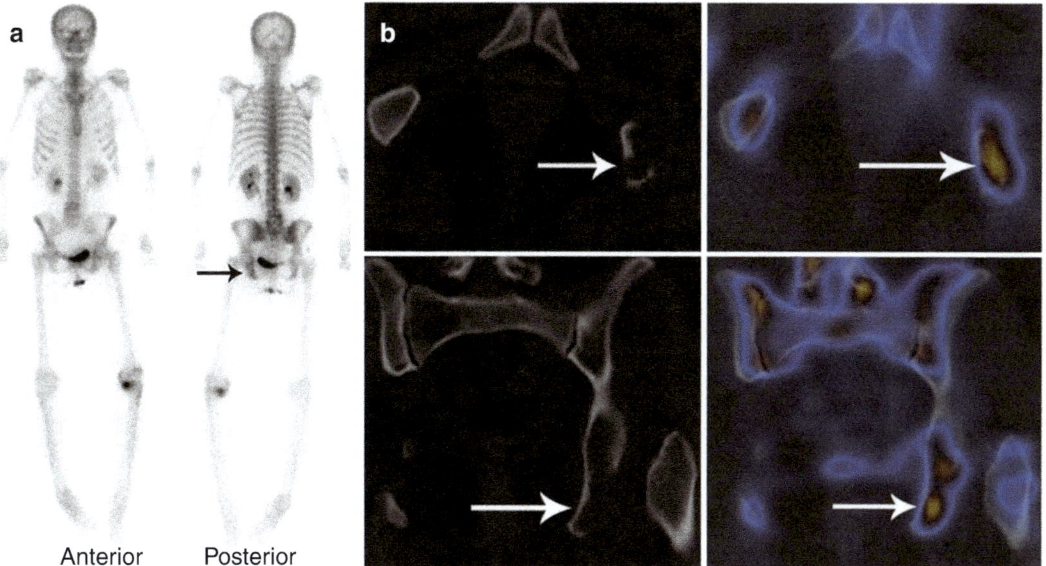

Fig. 8.29 (a, b) Patient with lung carcinoma. On whole-body bone scan (a), there is low-grade patchy uptake of tracer in the left ischium (arrow). This is equivocal for a skeletal metastasis. SPECT-CT of pelvis (b) localizes tracer uptake in the left ischium to a lytic lesion with soft-tissue component suggestive of metastasis. Further increased tracer uptake in the left knee (a) localizes to a lytic lesion in the medial aspect of the left tibial plateau with soft-tissue component (not shown). In this particular case, SPECT-CT was useful in increasing the confidence of the scan reader

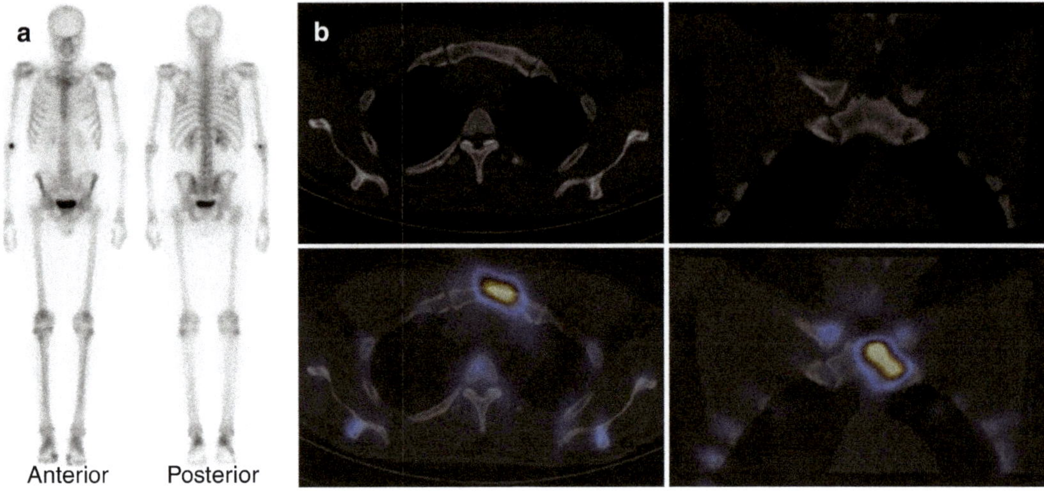

Fig. 8.30 (**a**, **b**) Prostate cancer on hormonal treatment. Increased tracer uptake is seen in the manubrio sternum on whole-body bone scan (**a**), which is not typical for metastasis. However, SPECT-CT (**b**) localizes the tracer uptake to sclerosis on CT component of the study. Although, the appearances are non-specific on planar study, it is strongly suspicious for metastasis on SPECT-CT study

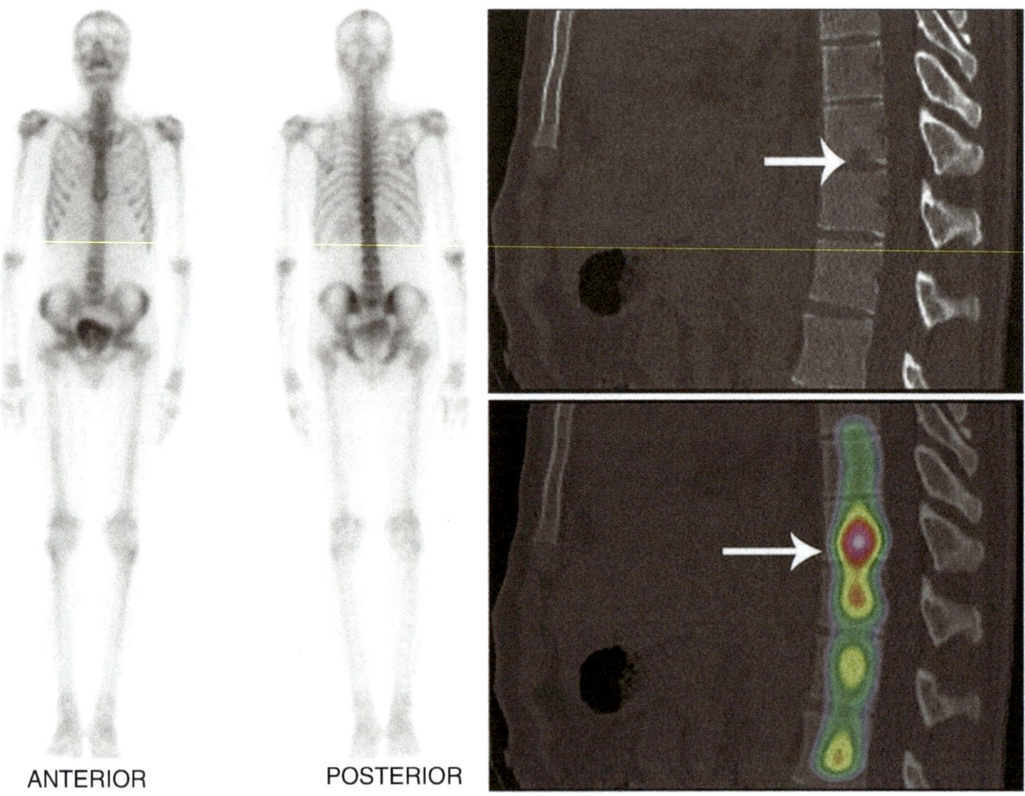

Fig. 8.31 Known lung carcinoma, whole-body bone scan shows solitary minimal increased osteoblastic activity in D10 vertebral region on whole-body study posterior view which could be metastasis but needs further anatomical correlation. The uptake localizes to a small lytic lesion in D10 vertebral body on SPECT-CT confirming metastasis (arrows)

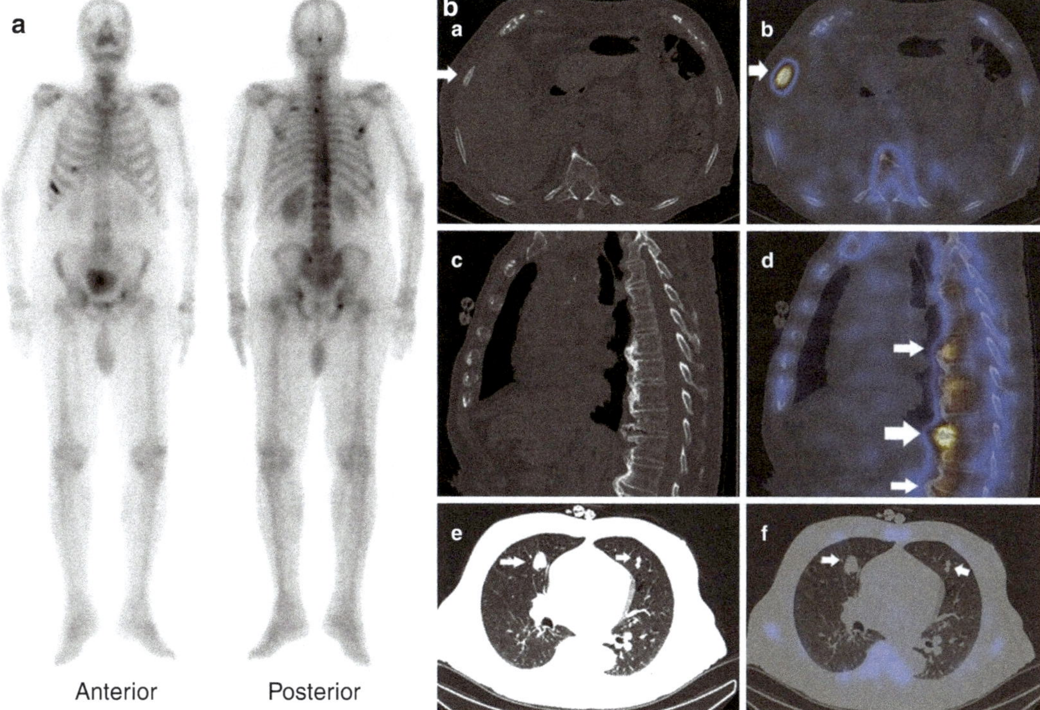

Fig. 8.32 (**a, b**) Sixty-year-old male patient with known prostate carcinoma shows multifocal uptake in the pelvis and thorax, and heterogeneous tracer uptake in the vertebrae (**a**). On SPECT-CT of thorax (**b**), the uptake in rib localizes to sclerotic lesion (a, b) suggestive of metasta-ses, and uptake in vertebrae localizes to degenerative osteophytic changes (c, d). Moreover, there is incidental lung nodules on low-dose CT component of SPECT-CT (e, f), which could be metastatic and needs further evaluation

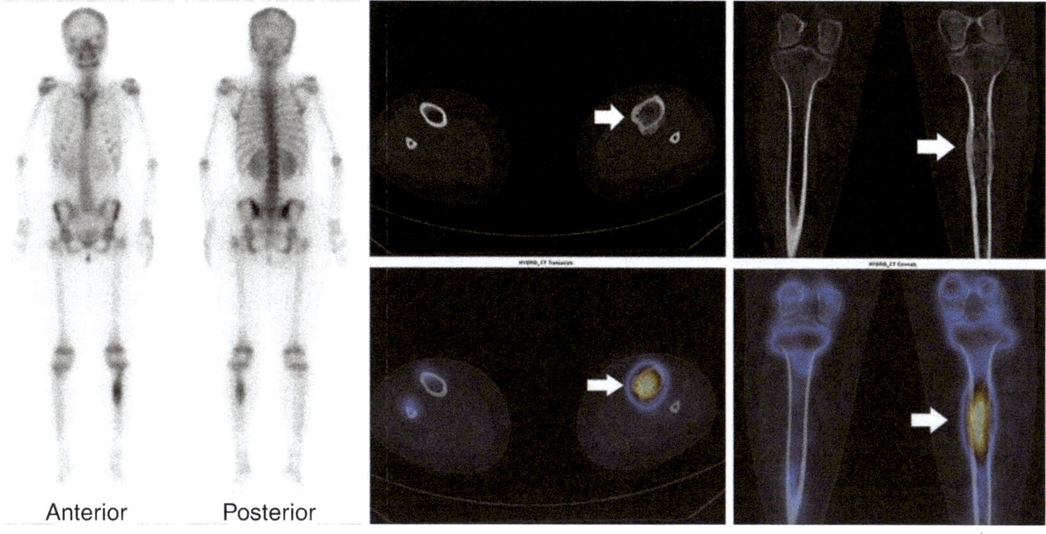

Fig. 8.33 A known case of left tibial Ewing's sarcoma, whole-body bone scan shows increased osteoblastic activity in the proximal left tibia possibly extension up to the proximal epiphysis. However, SPECT-CT localizes the uptake to intramedullary sclerosis with thick periosteal reaction (arrows) in the proximal diaphysis sparing the epiphysis and metaphysis, which is helpful in knee preserving surgery

References

1. Saha GB, editor. Fundamentals of nuclear pharmacy. 5th ed. New York: Springer; 2004.
2. Donohoe KJ, Brown ML, Collier BD, et al. Society of Nuclear Medicine procedure guideline for bone scintigraphy. Society of Nuclear Medicine website. Accepted 20 Jun 2003.
3. Van den Wyngaert T, Strobel K, Kampen WU, Kuwert T, van der Bruggen W, Mohan HK, Gnanasegaran G, Delgado-Bolton R, Weber WA, Beheshti M, Langsteger W, Giammarile F, Mottaghy FM, Paycha F, EANM Bone & Joint Committee and the Oncology Committee. The EANM practice guidelines for bone scintigraphy. Eur J Nucl Med Mol Imaging. 2016;43(9):1723–38.
4. Gnanasegaran G, Barwick T, Adamson K, Mohan H, Sharp D, Fogelman I. Multislice SPECT/CT in benign and malignant bone disease: when the ordinary turns into the extraordinary. Semin Nucl Med. 2009;39(6):431–42.
5. Kuwert T. Skeletal SPECT/CT: a review. Clin Transl Imaging. 2014;2:505–17.
6. Poon M, Zeng L, Zhang L, Lam H, Emmenegger U, Wong E, et al. Incidence of skeletal-related events over time from solid tumour bone metastases reported in randomised trials using bone-modifying agents. Clin Oncol (R Coll Radiol). 2013;25(7):435–44.
7. Melton LJ III, Kyle RA, Achenbach SJ, Oberg AL, Rajkumar SV. Fracture risk with multiple myeloma: a population-based study. J Bone Miner Res. 2005;20(3):487–93.
8. Hofbauer LC, Rachner TD, Coleman RE, Jakob F. Endocrine aspects of bone metastases. Lancet Diabetes Endocrinol. 2014;2(6):500–12.
9. Fogelman I, Cook G, Israel O, Van der Wall H. Positron emission tomography and bone metastases. Semin Nucl Med. 2005;35(2):135–42.
10. Coleman RE, Mashiter G, Whitaker KB, Moss DW, Rubens RD, Fogelman I. Bone scan flare predicts successful systemic therapy for bone metastases. J Nucl Med. 1988;29(8):1354–9.
11. Rosenthal DI. Radiologic diagnosis of bone metastases. Cancer. 1997;80(8 Suppl):1595–607.
12. Gutzeit A, Doert A, Froehlich JM, Eckhardt BP, Meili A, Scherr P, et al. Comparison of diffusion-weighted whole body MRI and skeletal scintigraphy for the detection of bone metastases in patients with prostate or breast carcinoma. Skelet Radiol. 2010;39(4):333–43.
13. Takenaka D, Ohno Y, Matsumoto K, Aoyama N, Onishi Y, Koyama H, et al. Detection of bone metastases in non-small cell lung cancer patients: comparison of whole-body diffusion-weighted imaging (DWI), whole-body MR imaging without and with DWI, whole-body FDG-PET/CT, and bone scintigraphy. J Magn Reson Imaging. 2009;30(2):298–308.
14. Davila D, Antoniou A, Chaudhry MA. Evaluation of osseous metastasis in bone scintigraphy. Semin Nucl Med. 2015;45:3–15.
15. Azad GK, Taylor B, Rubello D, Colletti PM, Goh V, Cook GJ. Molecular and functional imaging of bone metastases in breast and prostate cancers: an overview. Clin Nucl Med. 2016;41:e44–50.
16. Cook GJ, Azad GK, Goh V. Imaging bone metastases in breast cancer: staging and response assessment. J Nucl Med. 2016;57(Suppl 1):27s–33s.
17. Agrawal K, Marafi F, Gnanasegaran G, Van der Wall H, Fogelman I. Pitfalls and limitations of radionuclide planar and hybrid bone imaging. Semin Nucl Med. 2015;45(5):347–72.
18. Israel O, Pellet O, Biassoni L, De Palma D, Estrada-Lobato E, Gnanasegaran G, Kuwert T, la Fougère C, Mariani G, Massalha S, Paez D, Giammarile F. Two decades of SPECT/CT - the coming of age of a technology: an updated review of literature evidence. Eur J Nucl Med Mol Imaging. 2019;46(10):1990–2012.
19. Gnanasegaran G, Cook G, Adamson K, Fogelman I. Patterns, variants, artifacts, and pitfalls in conventional radionuclide bone imaging and SPECT/CT. Semin Nucl Med. 2009;39(6):380–95.
20. Mohd Rohani MF, Zanial AZ, Suppiah S, Phay Phay K, Mohamed Aslum Khan F, Mohamad Najib FH, Mohd Noor N, Arumugam M, Amir Hassan SZ, Vinjamuri S. Bone single-photon emission computed tomography/computed tomography in cancer care in the past decade: a systematic review and meta-analysis as well as recommendations for further work. Nucl Med Commun. 2021;42(1):9–20.
21. Gayed IW, Kim EE, Awad J, Joseph U, Wan D, John S. The value of fused SPECT/CT in the evaluation of solitary skull lesion. Clin Nucl Med. 2011;36:538–41.
22. Sharma P, Kumar R, Singh H, Bal C, Julka PK, Thulkar S, Malhotra A. Indeterminate lesions on planar bone scintigraphy in lung cancer patients: SPECT, CT or SPECT-CT? Skelet Radiol. 2012;41:843–50.
23. Sharma P, Singh H, Kumar R, Bal C, Thulkar S, Seenu V, Malhotra A. Bone scintigraphy in breast cancer: added value of hybrid SPECT-CT and its impact on patient management. Nucl Med Commun. 2012;33:139–47.
24. Sharma P, Jain TK, Reddy RM, Faizi NA, Bal C, Malhotra A, Kumar R. Comparison of single photon emission computed tomography-computed tomography, computed tomography, single photon emission computed tomography and planar scintigraphy for characterization of isolated skull lesions seen on bone scintigraphy in cancer patients. Indian J Nucl Med. 2014;29:22–9.
25. Rager O, Lee-Felker SA, Tabouret-Viaud C, Felker ER, Poncet A, Amzalag G, et al. Accuracy of whole-body HDP SPECT/CT, FDG PET/CT, and their combination for detecting bone metastases in breast cancer: an intrapersonal comparison. Am J Nucl Med Mol Imaging. 2018;8:159–68.
26. Zhang Y, Li B, Wu B, Yu H, Song J, Xiu Y, Shi H. Diagnostic performance of whole-body bone scintigraphy in combination with SPECT/CT for detection of bone metastases. Ann Nucl Med. 2020;34:549–58.

27. Palmedo H, Marx C, Ebert A, Kreft B, Ko Y, Türler A, et al. Whole-body SPECT/CT for bone scintigraphy: diagnostic value and effect on patient management in oncological patients. Eur J Nucl Med Mol Imaging. 2014;41:59–67.

28. Fonager RF, Zacho HD, Langkilde NC, Fledelius J, Ejlersen JA, Haarmark C, et al. Diagnostic test accuracy study of 18F-sodium fluoride PET/CT, 99mTc-labelled diphosphonate SPECT/CT, and planar bone scintigraphy for diagnosis of bone metastases in newly diagnosed, high-risk prostate cancer. Am J Nucl Med Mol Imaging. 2017;7:218–27.

29. Teyateeti A, Tocharoenchai C, Muangsomboon K, Komoltri C, Pusuwan P. A comparison of accuracy of planar and evolution SPECT/CT bone imaging in differentiating benign from metastatic bone lesions. J Med Assoc Thail. 2017;100:100–10.

30. Fleury V, Ferrer L, Colombié M, Rusu D, Le Thiec M, Kraeber-Bodéré F, et al. Advantages of systematic trunk SPECT/CT to planar bone scan (PBS) in more than 300 patients with breast or prostate cancer. Oncotarget. 2018;9:31744–52.

31. Mavriopoulou E, Zampakis P, Smpiliri E, Spyridonidis T, Rapti E, Haberkorn U, et al. Whole body bone SPET/CT can successfully replace the conventional bone scan in breast cancer patients. A prospective study of 257 patients. Hell J Nucl Med. 2018;21:125–33.

32. de Leiris N, Leenhardt J, Boussat B, Montemagno C, Seiller A, Phan Sy O, et al. Does whole-body bone SPECT/CT provide additional diagnostic information over [18F]-FCH PET/CT for the detection of bone metastases in the setting of prostate cancer biochemical recurrence? Cancer Imaging. 2020;20:58.

33. Rager O, Nkoulou R, Exquis N, Garibotto V, Tabouret-Viaud C, Zaidi H, et al. Whole-body SPECT/CT versus planar bone scan with targeted SPECT/CT for metastatic workup. BioMed Res Intern. 2017;2017:7039406.

34. Guezennec C, Keromnes N, Robin P, Abgral R, Bourhis D, Querellou S, et al. Incremental diagnostic utility of systematic double-bed SPECT/CT for bone scintigraphy in initial staging of cancer patients. Cancer Imaging. 2017;17:16.

35. Abikhzer G, Gourevich K, Kagna O, Israel O, Frenkel A, Keidar Z. Whole-body bone SPECT in breast cancer patients: the future bone scan protocol? Nucl Med Commun. 2016;37:247–53.

36. Tuncel M, Lay Ergun E, Caglar Tuncali M. Clinical impact of SPECT-CT on bone scintigraphy in oncology: pattern approach. J BUON. 2016;21(5):1296–306.

Bone SPECT/CT in Orthopaedics

9

Kanhaiyalal Agrawal, Girish Kumar Parida,
Hans Van der Wall, and Gopinath Gnanasegaran

9.1 Introduction

Bone scintigraphy, commonly known as a bone scan, has proven its utility in the metastatic workup and benign bone diseases. However, planar scintigraphy is only a two-dimensional representation of the image. For better localization, a three-dimensional SPECT modality was used previously. Though SPECT became a milestone in this search, it could not completely solve the purpose due to the persistent lack of specificity of bone SPECT. The lack of specificity on conventional planar bone scan and SPECT led to developement of hybrid imaging modality like SPECT/CT. The functional information can be obtained from the SPECT, and the precise anatomic localization and characterization can be assessed on the CT component of the study. SPECT/CT bone scan has significantly increased sensitivity and specificity when compared to planar bone scintigraphy. In the previous chapter, we have discussed the role of bone scan with SPECT/CT in oncology. Here, we will discuss the orthopaedic applications of bone SPECT/CT.

9.1.1 Indications

Metastatic workup has been the most common use of skeletal scintigraphy. However, there are many benign bone conditions including infective/inflammatory diseases, where the bone scan has shown its significance. Following are the benign conditions where the bone scan is being used [1, 2]:
- Enchondroma
- Shin splints
- Avascular necrosis
- Arthropathies
- Paget's disease
- Fibrous dysplasia
- Hypertrophic osteoarthropathy
- Trauma
- Prosthesis complications
- Complex regional pain syndrome (reflex sympathetic dystrophy)
- Bone infarction
- Heterotopic ossification
- Condylar hyperplasia
- Bone graft viability

K. Agrawal · G. K. Parida
Nuclear Medicine, All India Institute of Medical
Sciences, Bhubaneswar, India

H. Van der Wall
CNI Molecular Imaging, Notre Dame University in
Sydney, Chippendale, NSW, Australia

G. Gnanasegaran (✉)
Nuclear Medicine, Royal Free London NHS Hospital
Trust, London, UK

University College London, London, UK
e-mail: gopinath.gnanasegaran@nhs.net

© The Author(s), under exclusive license to Springer Nature Switzerland AG 2022
H. Ahmadzadehfar et al. (eds.), *Clinical Applications of SPECT-CT*,
https://doi.org/10.1007/978-3-030-65850-2_9

- Vertebral collapse
- Spondylodiscitis
- Intraosseous disc herniation

9.1.2 Radiopharmaceuticals

Benign bone pathologies can be broadly classified into two groups, non-infective and infective pathologies. For non-infective pathologies, 99mTc methylene diphosphonate (99mTc MDP), 99mTc hydroxymethylene diphosphonate (99mTc HDP or HMDP) and 99mTc hydroxyethylidene diphosphonate (99mTc HEDP) are used. However, in infective conditions, bone SPECT tracers like 67Ga-Citrate, 99mTc or 111In-labelled WBC and radiolabelled anti-granulocyte antibody are used and shown in Table 9.1 [3].

9.1.3 Radiopharmaceutical Activity

An adult's recommended activity is intravenous injection of 740–1110 MBq (20–30 mCi) of 99mTc-labelled bone seeking agents. For obese patients, the administered tracer activity is increased to 11–13 MBq/kg (300–350 µCi/kg). In kids, the recommended dose is 9–11 MBq/kg (250–300 µCi/kg), with a minimum of 20–40 MBq (0.5–1.0 mCi) [1–3].

9.2 Bone SPECT/CT: Patient Preparation

The patient preparation for bone SPECT/CT is similar to bone scintigraphy. In general, before making an appointment for bone scintigraphy and SPECT/CT, pregnancy and active breastfeeding should be excluded. No specific patient preparation is required for bone scintigraphy. Unless contraindicated, the patient should be well hydrated before and during the study. The nuclear medicine team should document relevant medical history related to the investigation before radiotracer administration. In particular, the referral cause, current symptoms, history of trauma or fractures, prior bone scintigraphy results, any history of allergy, renal impairment, etc., should be recorded. History of previous surgery must be documented. Any recent nuclear medicine studies which may impair bone scintigraphy image quality must be reported [1, 2]. In between radiotracer administration and imaging, the patient should be advised to void frequently and immediately before the scan. All metallic objects must be removed during imaging unless contraindicated. The non-removable metallic objects like pacemakers must be documented before the study to avoid misinterpretation of scan findings.

Table 9.1 SPECT tracers used in bone inflammation/infection

Radiopharmaceutical	Targeting mechanism	Pathophysiological process	Administered dose (MBq)
^{99m}Tc-HMPAO/^{111}In-oxine WBCs	Cell migration for chemotaxis	Enhanced vascular permeability, chemotaxis, cell recruitment, immune response	200/18.5
^{67}Ga-citrate	Transferrin and lactoferrin receptor-binding, siderophores bacteria	Enhanced vascular permeability	185
^{99m}Tc-polyclonal human Iimmunoglobulins	Extravasation from bloodstream	Local hyperemia, enhanced vascular permeability	555
^{99m}Tc-anti SSEA-1 IgM, falonesomab (Leu-Tech, NeutroSpec)	Antigen binding	Targeting, immune response	370–740

9.3 Image Acquisition Protocol

In benign bone diseases, three-phase bone scan is often required. In SPECT/CT, the SPECT image reconstruction is done with 3D iterative OSEM (ordered-subsets expectation-maximization) with ideally 3–5 iterations and 8–10 subsets. The CT parameters typically include a 512×512 matrix, a tube voltage of 120 kV, an intensity–time product of 2.5–300 mAs (depending on the anatomy or site being imaged) and a high-resolution application filter to the final image. A single SPECT/CT field of view is usually 40 cm, and several separate or contiguous fields of view can be used when the desired area of investigation is large. Fused three-dimensional SPECT/CT images are usually displayed as two-dimensional orthogonal (axial, coronal and sagittal) and maximum-intensity projections [1]. Different institutes follow different protocols in the acquisition of SPECT-CT. Table 9.2 shows one of such accepted protocols for different regions [2, 3].

9.4 Bone SPECT/CT in Different Benign Bone Conditions

9.4.1 Enchondroma

Enchondroma is benign intramedullary cartilage neoplasm. It could be solitary or involves multiple bones. It represents approximately 20% of all cartilage tumours of bone and is generally discovered in the third or fourth decade of life [4]. Enchondromas are second to osteochondromas in frequency amongst benign cartilage tumours (30%) [4]. These benign tumours are thought to arise from embryonic rests derived from the epiphyseal growth plate, which are displaced into the metaphysis [5]. A majority of these benign tumours are located centrally in short tubular bones, the proximal femur and the humerus, proximal phalanx being the most common area of involvement. Most of the enchondromas are discovered incidentally during metastatic workup on bone scan. Hence, knowledge of CT and bone

Table 9.2 Summary of acquisition parameters (Adapted from [3])

	Spine	Hand and wrists	Hips and pelvis	Knees	Ankles and feet
SPECT acquisition	LEHR collimators Matrix 128×128 128 angles 20 s/angle Step mode Non-circular rotation	LEHR collimators Matrix 128×128 128 angles 20 s/angle Step mode Non-circular rotation	LEHR collimators Matrix 128×128 128 angles 20 s/angle Step mode Non-circular rotation	LEHR collimators Matrix 128×128 128 angles 20 s/angle Step mode Non-circular rotation	LEHR collimators Matrix 128×128 128 angles 20 s/angle Step mode Non-circular rotation
Localization CT or for attenuation correction	2.5–40 mA 80–130 keV 1–5 mm slice thickness	2.5–40 mA 80–130 keV 1–5 mm slice thickness	2.5–40 mA 80–130 keV 1–5 mm slice thickness	2.5–40 mA 80–130 keV 1–5 mm slice thickness	2.5–40 mA 80–130 keV 1–5 mm slice thickness
Diagnostic CT	100 mA/slice 120 kV 1.5 mm slice thickness	150 mA/slice 140 kV 0.8 mm slice thickness	100 mA/slice 120 kV 1.5 mm slice thickness	100 mA/slice 120 kV 1.5 mm slice thickness	100 mA/slice 120 kV 1.5 mm slice thickness

N.B. Routine early blood pool and delayed static images of region are recommended for the afore-mentioned indications, and CT settings are variable depending on local requirements/protocols/cameras etc. The use of dose reduction features is recommended if available

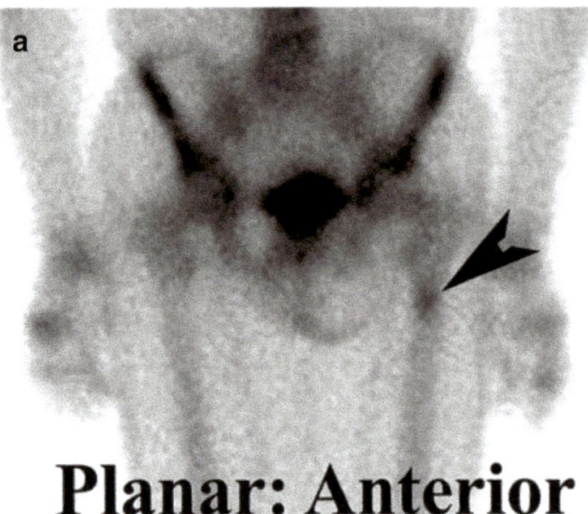

Fig. 9.1 Enchondromatosis: Incidentally discovered region of increased uptake in the left femoral meta-diaphysis (arrowhead in **a**), while the patient was being screened for lower back pain. Figures (**b**, **c**) representing CT and fused SPECT/CT images, respectively, showing multiple calcified nodules within the medullary cavity with diffuse uptake, in the typical pattern of enchondromatosis

scan appearance is essential to avoid misinterpretation. Often, they are asymptomatic. However, enchondromas of hand and feet may present with pain. Further, two syndromes are associated with multiple enchondromas: Ollier's disease and Maffucci syndrome (Fig. 9.1).

CT Appearance Variable punctate or linear calcification of the enchondroma may be apparent without significant thickening or cortical breach. However, there may be mild endosteal scalloping of the cortex. There is a narrow zone of transition and sharply defined margins. In general, no periosteal reaction and no soft-tissue mass.

SPECT Generally, the enchondromas show low- to moderate-grade tracer uptake in the bone scintigraphy. With SPECT-CT, further anatomic characterization with the CT component is possible. Enchondroma with no tracer uptake in the bone scan has not been reported in the literature to our knowledge. Therefore, if a calcific lesion in the metaphysis demonstrates no significant tracer uptake, then a calcified lipoma or bone infarct should be suspected. While the bone scan appearances are non-specific, the study is essential in assessing the entire skeleton for multiple enchondromatosis (Ollier's disease). Distinguishing benign from malignant transformation by the degree of uptake in an enchondroma is not possible.

9.4.2 Shin Splint

The term shin splints is described as medial tibial stress syndrome (MTSS) [6, 7]. It is a form of stress injury that usually occurs in the medial tibia and is characterized by pain, tenderness, swelling and warmth of the skin overlying the attachments of the involved muscles to the tibia. Aetiology remains the traction injury involving the soleus and flexor hallucis longus and possibly the flexor digitorum longus with a claw-toe deformity [8]. While the history and physical examination may yield the diagnosis, the critical issue is to exclude a stress fracture. One-leg hop test is the clinical test to distinguish shin splint from a stress fracture, but a three-phase bone scan helps determine these two conditions objectively. A linear, longitudinal uptake along the affected tibial cortex's periosteal surface is seen on the bone scan [9, 10]. Further, the first two phases of the bone scan show normal appearances in shin splint (Fig. 9.2).

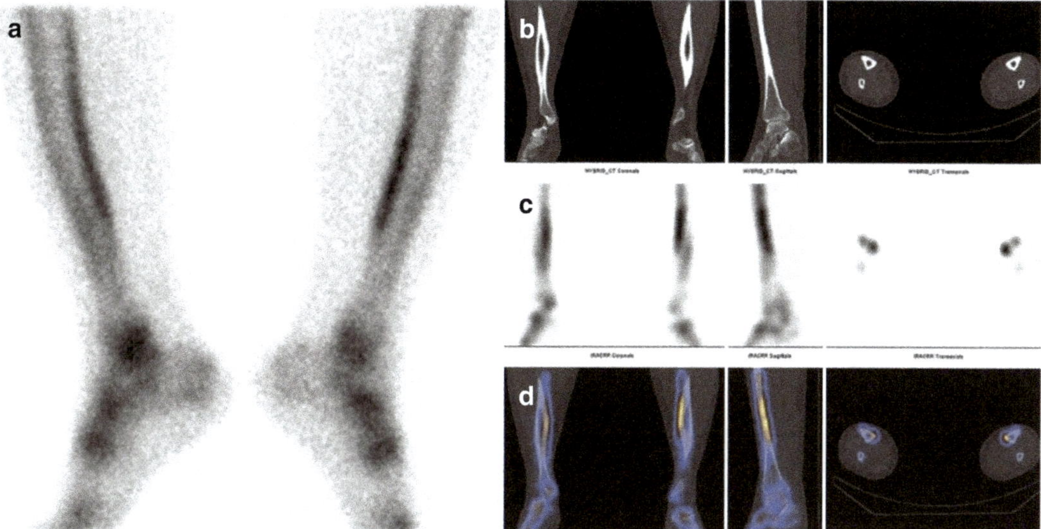

Fig. 9.2 Shin splint: 17-year-old male athlete presented with pain in bilateral lower limbs since few months. Bone scan shows linear increased tracer uptake in posteromedial cortex of bilateral tibia suggestive of shin splint on planar (**a**) with corresponding CT, SPECT and SPECT/CT images, respectively, showing mild periosteal reaction related to site of uptake (**b–d**)

9.4.2.1 SPECT-CT Findings

CT CT is not sensitive in MTSS. The earliest manifestation of the MTSS is mild posteromedial tibial cortical osteopenia. There is no definite fracture line as seen in stress fracture.

SPECT The planar image shows intense long-segment uptake along the posterior/posteromedial cortex of both distal tibiae. The SPECT images show the long-segment sub-periosteal pattern of uptake in the posterior or posteromedial cortices of both distal tibiae, without a focal abnormality to suggest a stress fracture [9, 10].

9.4.3 Avascular Necrosis

Avascular necrosis (AVN) is defined as massive bone and marrow necrosis due to disruption of the blood supply. AVN might be the result of a local or a systemic process [11]. The local causes include infection, trauma or localized field radiation ther-apy. The systemic causes of AVN are multifactorial and include barotrauma, corticosteroid use, genetic and haematological (sickle-cell anaemia). The pathophysiology of AVN relates to an interruption of the blood supply to bone, leading to ischemia. AVN has a propensity for yellow marrow sites with a large proportion of adipocytes such as the femoral head [12]. Necrosis leads to loss of the normal biomechanical property of bone, and a secondary fracture often occurs together with subchondral dissection and collapse of the necrotic segment, which is when the condition becomes symptomatic [13]. The most common site for AVN is the femoral head. AVN might also be seen in the scaphoid, capitate, humeral head, vertebral body, talus and knee.

The Association Research Circulation Osseous system is widely accepted for staging of AVN [14]. It extends from stage 0 (where there is no imaging evidence of avascular necrosis) to stage IV (where there is a collapse of the necrotic region with joint space narrowing and destruction of the joint) [14] (Fig. 9.3).

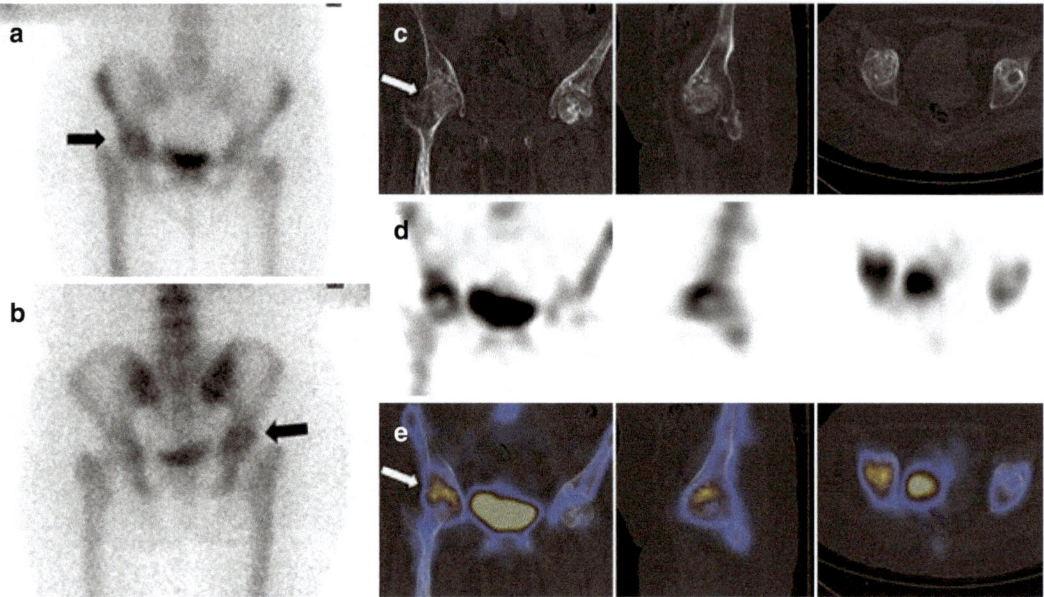

Fig. 9.3 Avascular necrosis: 26-year-old male underwent bone scan for right hip pain. Flow and pool images show no significant abnormality. Delayed bone scan shows focal increased tracer uptake in right femoral head (**a**, **b**, black arrow). SPECT-CT images show increased tracer uptake at the right femoral head associated with corre-sponding sclerosis and absorption of the head of femur on CT (**c**–**e**, respectively representing CT, SPECT and SPECT/CT images, white arrows), suggesting avascular necrosis. In SPECT images (**d**), central photopenia is well appreciated compared to planar images.

9.4.3.1 SPECT-CT Findings

CT: The earliest CT sign of avascular necrosis is osteopenia. In the intermediate stage, there may be trabecular condensation and sclerosis of the region. In the later stages, subchondral micro fractures and reactive bone formation will lead to the crescent sign (subchondral lucency) followed by fracture and the necrotic region's collapse. CT is less sensitive in the early stage of the disease.

SPECT: Bone scan is a highly sensitive investigation in AVN. Although MRI is the gold standard, a bone scan is a choice in a patient with sickle cell disease where multiple sites of involvement need to be ruled out. Bone scan in early disease usually shows a cold area representing the disruption of the blood supply. Later in the disease process, a photopenic region surrounded by high uptake (due to surrounding hyperaemia and osteoblastic bone reaction—Doughnut sign) is seen. There is subsequent revascularization at the interface between necrotic and normal bone, leading to a progressive increase in uptake of tracer with bony remodelling leading to a progressive increase in uptake within the necrotic territory. SPECT imaging has higher sensitivity than planar bone scan as photopenia could be masked in two-dimensional planar imaging due to low-grade tracer uptake in the overlapping structures. SPECT-CT not only provides accurate localization but also provides an anatomic characterization of the lesions.

9.4.4 Sacroiliitis

Arthropathies are a varied group of inflammatory rheumatic diseases, ranging from reactive arthritis to ankylosing spondylitis, enteropathic arthritis, facet joint arthropathies and other undifferentiated arthropathies [15].

Arthropathies are associated with synovitis, spondylitis, dactylitis and enthesitis at ligament, tendon or capsular insertions into bone. The commonly encountered arthropathies in the bone scan are facet joint arthropathies and sacroiliitis, which can be falsely considered metastases. Sacroiliitis is generally regarded as a form of

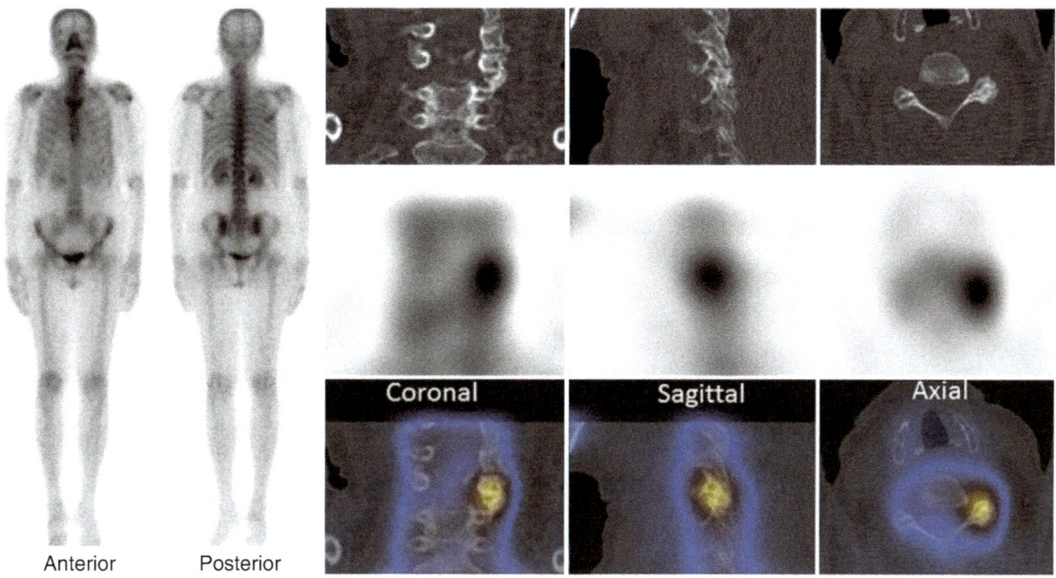

Fig. 9.4 Facet joint arthropathy: 58-year-old female with carcinoma lung for metastatic workup. Bone scan showed focal tracer uptake in the cervical vertebra which on SPECT-CT localized to a facet joint arthropathy

synovitis but erosive changes to the joint may occur in the upper third, adjacent to the interosseous ligament, which contains no synovium [16, 17] (Fig. 9.30).

9.4.4.1 SPECT-CT Findings

CT: Radiologically, it has five grades in the New York criteria [18]. Grade 0 is a normal sacroiliac joint (SIJ). Grade 1 is a suspicious joint without a definite abnormality. Grade 2 is minimal sacroiliitis, which indicates sclerosis and minor erosions but no loss of joint space. Grade 3 is moderate sacroiliitis with definite sclerosis on both sides of the joint, erosions and widening of the interosseous space. Grade 4 is consistent with complete joint obliteration or ankylosis with or without residual sclerosis.

SPECT: The SPECT part shows increased uptake around the joints with arthropathy. MRI is probably the earliest marker of sacroiliitis as it detects disease at the cartilaginous level, before the bony changes occur. The current generation of SPECT/CT devices can challenge the role of MRI, as preliminary experience has shown [19].

9.4.5   Paget's Disease

Paget's disease of the bone is a common metabolic skeletal disorder of older persons [20]. This condition is often asymptomatic, identified incidentally on radiological studies for other purposes. Any bone may be affected, although polyostotic involvement of the axial skeleton is most commonly observed (monostotic disease accounts for only 10–35% of cases) [21, 22]. The pelvis is most commonly involved, followed by the lumbar spine, thoracic spine and skull [23]. Localized bone pain is the most common feature in symptomatic patients, whilst deformity (typically bowing of long bones), osteoarthritic changes (secondary to Pagetoid bony remodelling within a joint) and neurologic complications (secondary to compression of adjacent neural structures by expansile bone remodelling) might also occur. Histologically, the disease is characterized by several non-inflammatory phases of bone remodelling, initiated by an initial osteolytic phase of excess osteoclast activity [24]. This is later accompanied by osteoblast and fibroblast activation leading to an intermediate phase of simultaneous bone resorption and formation. Osteoblastic bone formation later predominates

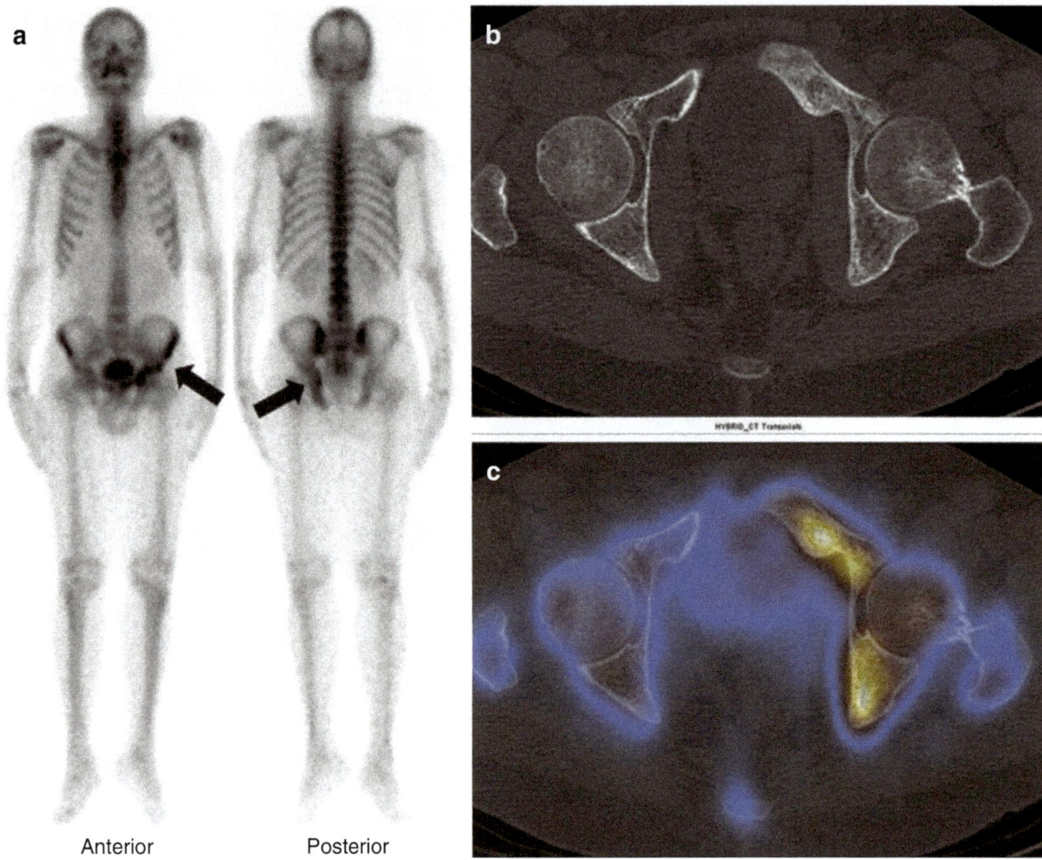

Fig. 9.5 Paget's disease: 56-year-old male was incidentally detected to have Paget's disease. Bone scan shows diffuse increased tracer uptake in left hemipelvis (arrows in **a**) which on SPECT-CT showed diffuse sclerosis with cortical thickening (**b**, **c**, respectively, shows CT and fused SPECT/CT images)

with the net deposition of structurally weak woven and lamellar bone in a disordered manner leading to bone expansion and thickening of trabeculae. The final burn-out phase is characterized by a reduction in osteoblast activity and bone turnover [24] (Figs. 9.5 and 9.29).

9.4.5.1 SPECT-CT Findings

CT: Characteristics of the initial osteolytic phase are regions of well-defined osteolysis, often with a leading edge advancing from the subarticular/metaphyseal bone towards the diaphysis ('blade of grass' sign) [25]. The intermediate phase of osteolysis/osteosclerosis demonstrated bony expansion, cortical thickening and coarsening of the trabecular pattern (referred to as 'picture-frame vertebra' within the spine—bone-in-bone

appearance of thick peripheral trabeculae and lucent inner aspect of the vertebral body) [22]. In the late burn-out phase, affected bones are markedly sclerotic ('ivory vertebrae'). CT is usually beneficial in defining the anatomy of symptomatic cases with neurological involvement (e.g. skull base, neural foramina). Lytic lesions demonstrate avid enhancement. The typical pelvic involvement features are cortical thickening and sclerosis of the iliopectineal and ischiopubic lines, acetabular protrusion and enlargement of the pubic rami and ischium.

SPECT: Bone scan shows superior sensitivity to plain radiography and demonstrates the extent of polyostotic involvement [26]. Characteristically, there is marked uptake, particularly in symptomatic lesions, although late phase burnt-out lesions

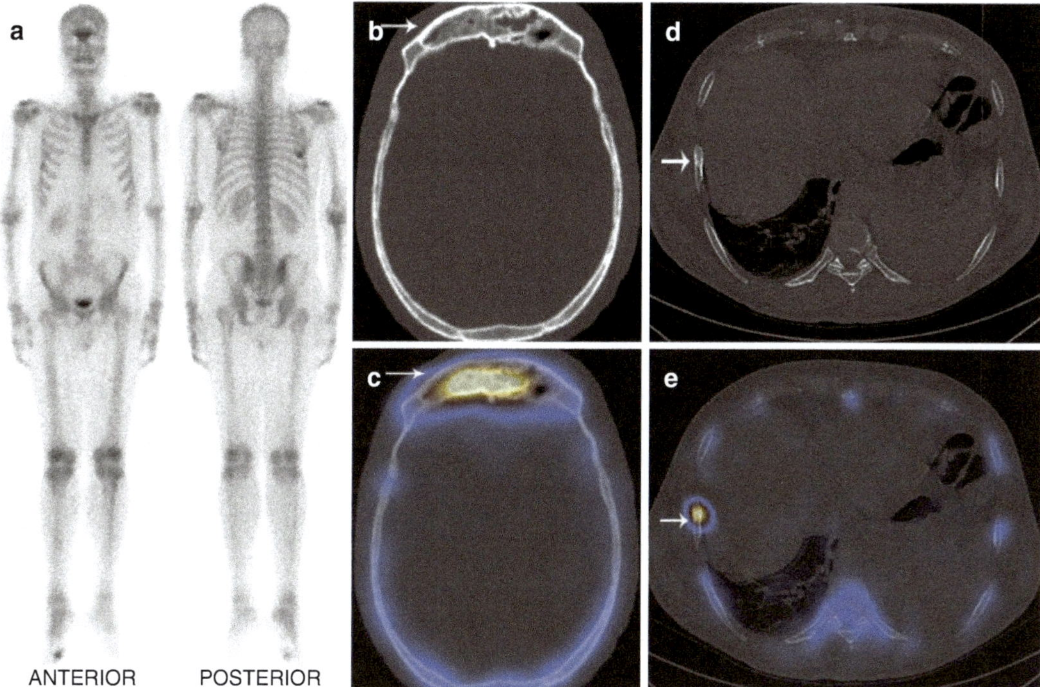

Fig. 9.6 Fibrous dysplasia: Whole-body bone scan shows linear tracer uptake in the frontal bone and prominent focal uptake in the right seventh rib. SPECT-CT localizes the uptake in the frontal bone and right rib to ground-glass opacities with expansion of bones suggestive of polyostotic fibrous dysplasia

may not show increased uptake [26]. Early lytic lesions may demonstrate peripheral uptake only. Combined SPECT-CT has significantly higher sensitivity and specificity than either of the individual modalities.

9.4.6 Fibrous Dysplasia

Fibrous dysplasia was first described in 1938 by Lichtenstein [27]. The true incidence and prevalence are difficult to estimate, but the condition is not rare and is thought to represent approximately 5–7% of all benign bone tumours [28]. Fibrous dysplasia may present in either one bone (monostotic) or multiple bones (polyostotic). The basic pathophysiology is thought to be a failure in the remodelling of primitive bone to mature lamellar bone and the failure of the bone to realign in response to mechanical stress

[29]. The failure of maturation results in isolated trabeculae enmeshed in dysplastic fibrous tissue, which slows turn over and is metabolically active. Most lesions are monostotic and incidentally discovered on imaging. Fibrous dysplasia is associated with several syndromes, such as McCune-Albright and Mazabraud diseases (Fig. 9.6).

9.4.6.1 SPECT-CT Findings
CT: Normal bone is generally replaced by a radiolucent ground-glass pattern, homogeneous with no visible trabeculation. The extent of the lesion is readily apparent, and the cortical boundaries are more clearly delineated. The thickness of the native bony cortex, endosteal scalloping and periosteal new-bone reaction is best demonstrated with CT.

SPECT: Whole-body bone scintigraphy helps demonstrate the extent of the disease. There is generally intense uptake of tracer in adolescence and throughout life due to the continuing bony turnover. Combined SPECT-CT better characterizes the lesions.

9.4.7 Hypertrophic Pulmonary Osteoarthropathy

Hypertrophic pulmonary osteoarthropathy (HPOA) is a clinical condition characterized by clubbing of the digits, long bone periostitis and polyarthropathy. HPOA manifests clinically as diffuse bone and joint pain. It is classified as a primary and secondary disease, and the vast majority of cases (>90%) are secondary. Over 90% of cases of HPOA have been described in association with intrathoracic pathology, of which 80% are lung cancers [30]. There are numerous reports of the HPOA resolving after-treatment of lung cancer [31] (Fig. 9.7).

9.4.7.1 SPECT-CT Findings

CT: CT is more sensitive than plain X-ray at demonstrating early changes of sub-periosteal bone formation or changes at the terminal digits.

SPECT: Scintigraphy is probably the most sensitive method for detecting periostitis in the long bones, digital clubbing and arthropathy in HPOA. Several case reports [32] demonstrate disease identified by bone scintigraphy that is not apparent on the MRI or plain film. The typical SPECT-CT appearance is increased uptake in a peri cortical distribution in the diametaphysis or the distal phalanges (clubbing) with or without evidence of synovitis.

9.4.8 Trauma

The majority of skeletal fractures are clinically and radiologically evident. However, a few circumstances under which plain film radiography and even CT may not identify an occult fracture. These occur in high-speed trauma, where a whole-body study is essential to evaluate the presence of occult fractures apart from the apparent presenting fractures/soft-tissue injuries and is of particular importance in small children and unconscious patients. Fractures without significant displacement may also lead to confusion, particularly so of the wrist and hip. Occasionally, the degree of trauma may not cause an apparent cortical infraction, but instead will lead to significant damage in the form of microtrabecular fractures (bone bruising). This 'bone bruise' can be visible on scintigraphy as increased sub-cortical uptake and on the MRI as bone marrow oedema. The plain film and CT are invariably normal in these circumstances. If the force exceeds the cortical bone's elastic limits, a breach in the cortex or fracture will occur (Figs. 9.8, 9.21, 9.23, 9.24, 9.25, and 9.26).

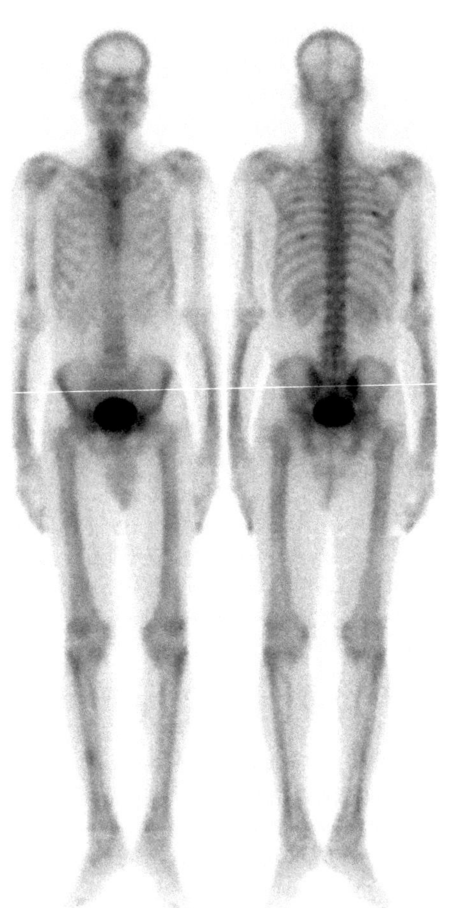

Fig. 9.7 Hypertrophic pulmonary osteoarthropathy: 59-year-old female with carcinoma lung for metastatic workup. Bone scan showed diffuse heterogeneously increased tracer uptake in the upper and lower limb bones—suggestive of hypertrophic pulmonary osteoarthropathy (HPAO)

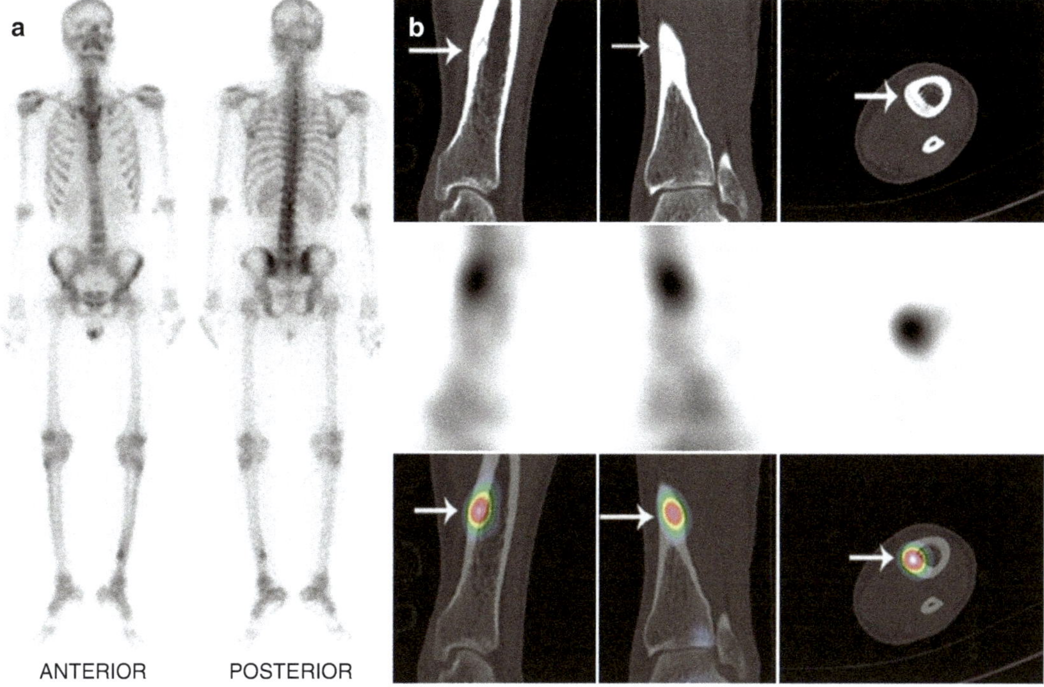

Fig. 9.8 Stress fracture: 24-year-old athlete presented with pain in left distal tibia. Planar bone scan (**a**) showed focal increased tracer uptake in the shaft of left distal tibia, which on SPECT-CT (**b**) localized to a linear break in the posterior cortex—suggestive of stress fracture

9.4.8.1 SPECT-CT Findings

CT: Multi-detector CT adds a significant level of sensitivity for the detection of occult fractures by showing subtle fracture lines, significant articular injury, bone loss and surgically important staging information [33]. It helps to exclude occult malignancy and infection. Volumetric reconstruction helps in planning surgery in complex acetabular, foot, ankle and shoulder fractures.

SPECT: Scintigraphy has traditionally been the modality of choice for detecting occult fractures of the wrist, hip and pelvis, although it currently has been supplanted by MRI in most instances. The advent of hybrid SPECT and CT devices has allowed SPECT/CT to establish itself as an essential modality in assessing occult fractures. The high sensitivity of bone scintigraphy fused with CT's high-spatial resolution has allowed for significant improvements in overall specificity [34].

9.4.9 Identification of Pain Generator (Prosthesis Related)

Contemporary joint arthroplasty procedures began less than 75 years ago when the modern-day hip replacement's predecessor was introduced. Similarly, the predecessor of the modern-knee prosthesis developed about 40 years ago. With time, these prostheses have undergone a significant amount of improvement [35]. These prostheses are anchored to bone by various methods, including polymethylmethacrylate and osseous ingrowth into the device's surface. Some devices are coated with hydroxyapatite which induces new bone formation and attaches to newly produced periprosthetic osseous tissue [35].

Currently, the most common cause of prosthetic failure is aseptic loosening and occurs in more than a quarter of these devices. Aseptic loosening results from an inflammatory reaction induced by the prosthetic components [36, 37], and the inflammatory

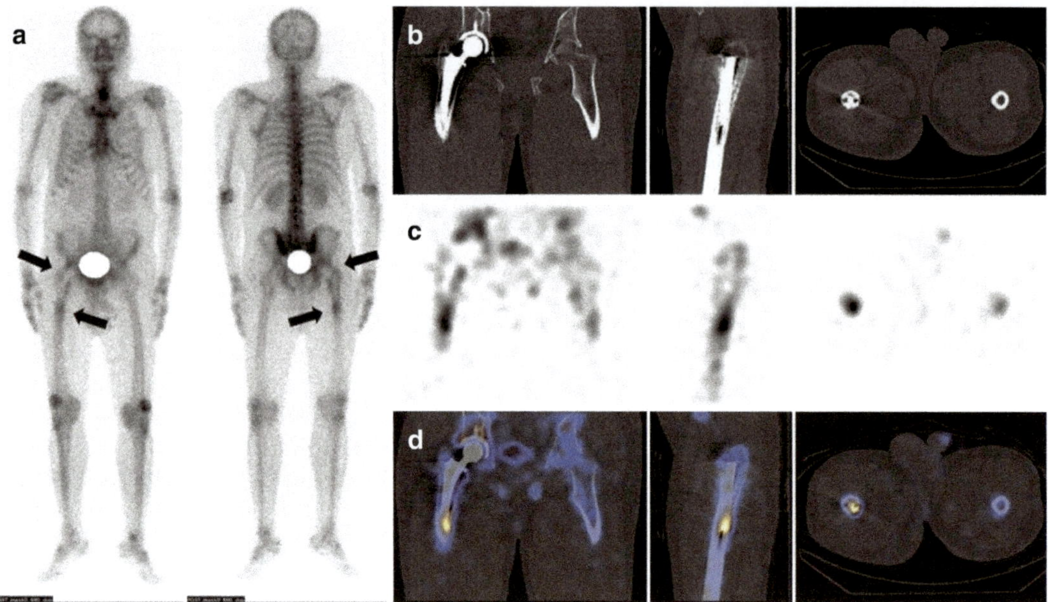

Fig. 9.9 Aseptic loosening: 53-year-old male had undergone total hip replacement 2 years ago, presented with pain in the hip since few days. Bone scan shows mild focal tracer uptake adjacent to the prosthesis only on delayed images (arrows in **a**). Figures (**b–d**) represent corresponding CT, SPECT and SPECT-CT images showing focal tracer uptake at the femoral tip and acetabular component of the hip prosthesis—suggestive of aseptic loosening

reaction is characterized by an influx of various types of leukocytes [38–40]. Most cases of aseptic loosening are treated with surgery. Prosthesis infection is less common and occurs in up to 2% of primary implants, and up to 5% revision. The management approach often depends on the accurate diagnosis of aseptic loosening and infection. This differentiation is not always obvious. Signs and symptoms, except for pain, frequently are lacking. Laboratory tests may be suggestive but are not diagnostic of infection. The definitive preoperative test's joint aspiration with culture is specific, but sensitivity is variable [41, 42] (Figs. 9.9 and 9.35). Further, bone scan with SPECT-CT is helpful in identification of pain generators in spine (Figs. 9.4 and 9.15), wrists (Figs. 9.16, 9.17, 9.19, and 9.20), hip (Figs. 9.21, 9.22, 9.23, 9.24, 9.25, 9.26, 9.27, and 9.28), knee (Figs. 9.31, 9.32, 9.33, and 9.34) and foot pain (Figs. 9.37, 9.38, and 9.39).

9.4.9.1 SPECT-CT Findings

Lucency around the prosthesis or migration of the prosthesis is the classical sign of loosening [43]. It is normal to identify a thin, linear lucent zone at the prosthesis cement interface, especially at the stem's proximal lateral aspect [44]. A normal bone scan essentially excludes a prosthetic complication.

On bone scintigraphy, focal abnormalities (not diffuse) in two or more zones or intense uptake in one zone about the prosthesis indicate loosening. However, in uncemented prostheses, an increased tracer activity can still be seen in some at the distal tip at 2 years [45].

In infection, classically, the three-phase bone scan shows diffusely increased periprosthetic activity on delayed images associated with infection (as opposed to loosening in which there is a focal abnormality identified about the prosthesis) [45, 46]. Unfortunately, the bone scan findings are nonspecific, and there is considerable overlap between infection and loosening [45]. SPECT-CT can help in such a situation, and additional CT findings help in making an accurate diagnosis (Fig. 9.35).

SPECT-CT with a combination of either white blood cell-tagged Tc99m or Tc99m-sulesamab with bone marrow imaging can reduce the false-positive scans and further increases the diagnostic accuracy up to 90% [45–47]. Any spatially incongruent area of In-111 WBC tracer activity which does not match marrow activity should be considered as infection (regardless of the intensity of the tracer uptake) [45]. Sequential bone-gallium imaging can also be used to evaluate prosthesis infection, but the overall accuracy (70–80%) is significantly less than that of combined

Table 9.3 Summary of clinical applications in identification of pain generator and evolving evidence [47–70]

	Spine	Hand and wrists	Hips and pelvis	Knees	Ankles and feet
Clinical application	-Localization of metabolically active facet joints -Localization of alternate pain generators -Assessment of complications related to post-operative spine	-Localizing abnormal metabolic active sites -Detecting post-traumatic bone remodelling -Detecting occult fractures which are often missed or equivocal other modalities	-Evaluation of painful joint prosthesis -Evaluating aseptic and septic loosening of hip prosthesis -Identifying potential pain generators -Identifying potential alternate pain generators -Evaluation of bone viability	-Evaluation of painful joint prosthesis -Evaluating aseptic and septic loosening of knee prostheses -Identifying potential pain generators	-Localization and characterization of abnormal increased tracer uptake in the foot and ankle joints -Localizing alternate metabolically active pain generators -Assessment of post-operative complications
When to use SPECT-CT	-If planar imaging is non-diagnostic -To help identify patients with low back pain who would benefit from facet joint infiltration -In the post-surgery setting (with or without implants)	-If planar imaging is non-diagnostic and accurate localization and characterization are challenging	-If planar imaging is non-diagnostic, usually late-phase SPECT/CT -Particularly useful for evaluation of hip prosthesis	-If planar imaging is non-diagnostic, usually late-phase SPECT/CT. Particularly useful for the evaluation of knee prosthesis	-If planar imaging is non-diagnostic and accurate localization and characterization is challenging
Summary of current evidence	-Identifies other potential causes of recurrent low back pain -Precise localization of focal increased metabolic activity -Guides therapy -Compliment's clinical diagnosis -Procedure of choice for patients with low back pain after lumbar fusion surgery -Highly sensitive and specific tool for the exclusion of screw loosening	-Lesion detection is relatively greater when compared to standard X-rays or planar bone scans -Good inter-observer agreement -Significant impact on patient management -Beneficial to integrate into the diagnostic imaging algorithm	-Increased diagnostic accuracy in the evaluation of aseptic or septic loosening in hip prosthesis -Significantly better than planar scanning in assessing acetabular cup loosening but not for the femoral stem	-Increased diagnostic accuracy in the evaluation of aseptic and septic loosening of knee prosthesis -Significantly better than planar scanning in assessment femoral component with superior results in assessment of tibial component -Ideal imaging modality for evaluation of patellofemoral disorders after knee replacements	-Complementary to conventional imaging modalities -Comparable diagnostic performance with MRI -Useful in localizing and characterizing impingement syndrome and soft-tissue pathology

In-111 WBC and Tc-99m marrow scintigraphy [45, 46]. The summary of clinical application and evolving clinical evidence is discussed in Table 9.3 [47–70].

9.4.10 Complex Regional Pain Syndrome

Complex regional pain syndrome (CRPS) is a disorder showing continuous pain, characterized by sensory, vasomotor, sudomotor or motor symptoms and signs [71, 72]. It can be due to surgery, trauma or minor injury [72, 73], and nerve damage is the standard for classifying CRPS type I and II [71–74]. The diagnostic criteria of CRPS were developed by the International Association for the Study of Pain (IASP) through The Budapest Clinical Diagnostic Criteria for Complex Regional Pain Syndrome in 1994 [75]. However, the criteria of IASP tended to over-diagnose CRPS, and it has difficulty discriminating between CRPS and other neuropathic pain [76]. The revised criteria presented a sensitivity of 85% and a specificity of 69% and reduced false-positive diagnosis [77]. Although diagnostic procedures such as three-phase bone scintigraphy, magnetic resonance imaging (MRI), X-ray and skin temperature differences were not included in the revised criteria of CRPS, they could provide additional information to diagnose CRPS [78, 79]. The usefulness of bone scintigraphy for extremity pain has not been well studied. However, as the study of single-photon emission computed tomography/computed tomography (SPECT/CT) has increasing, studies regarding SPECT/CT in patients with extremity pain have been performed (Fig. 9.18).

9.4.10.1 SPECT-CT Findings

Although triple-phase bone scan findings vary depending on the disease's duration, the typical pattern of bone scan in CRPS is increased uptake in blood flow, blood pool and delayed phases. In SPECT-CT, the tracer uptake is localized in the periarticular region. Schürmann et al. [80] compared the diagnostic performance of bone scan with thermography and MRI. The sensitivity of bone scan and MRI was 19% and 43% at 8 weeks, 14% and 13% at 16 weeks after the trauma, showing both modalities' poor sensitivity. However, the specificity of bone scan and MRI was 96% and 78% at 8 weeks, 100% and 98% at 16 weeks after the trauma, potentially ruling out CRPS. According to a meta-analysis by Cappello et al. [78], the bone scan had a significantly higher sensitivity and negative predictive value than MRI (Fig. 9.18).

9.4.11 Bone Infarct

Bone infarcts are often thought to be in the same disease spectrum as osteonecrosis occurs within the metaphysis or diaphysis of the long bone. The cause of bone infarct can be trauma, sickle cell disease, thalassemia, connective tissue disorders, Gaucher's disease and steroid use. The pathophysiology is an interruption of blood supply by intrinsic or extrinsic factors. Usually, they are asymptomatic and are found incidentally (Fig. 9.10).

9.4.11.1 SPECT-CT Findings

Usually, the lesions are present in the medulla, with a CT finding of sheet-like central lucency surrounded by sclerosis with a serpiginous border. A bone scan can show increased uptake in late stage; however, it is not specific for infarct.

9.4.12 Heterotopic Ossification

Heterotopic ossification (HO) is a condition of abnormal osteogenesis in non-skeletal tissue. Although it is not a malignant condition, the sequelae associated with HO can range from asymptomatic to severe ankylosis of the joint with loss of range of motion [81].

Other conditions, such as infection, including osteomyelitis, thrombophlebitis, cellulitis, deep vein thrombosis and benign and malignant tumours, can mimic heterotopic bone formation clinically, and imaging studies should differentiate these [81–83]. In imaging studies, precise localization of abnormalities is crucial for proper detection of HO. The diagnosis of heterotopic ossification is based on radiographic findings; however, X-rays can be normal for up to 4 weeks or longer even after the condition's onset. Bone scintigraphy is considered the method of choice for the earliest detection of heterotopic ossification and for assessing its maturity [84, 85].

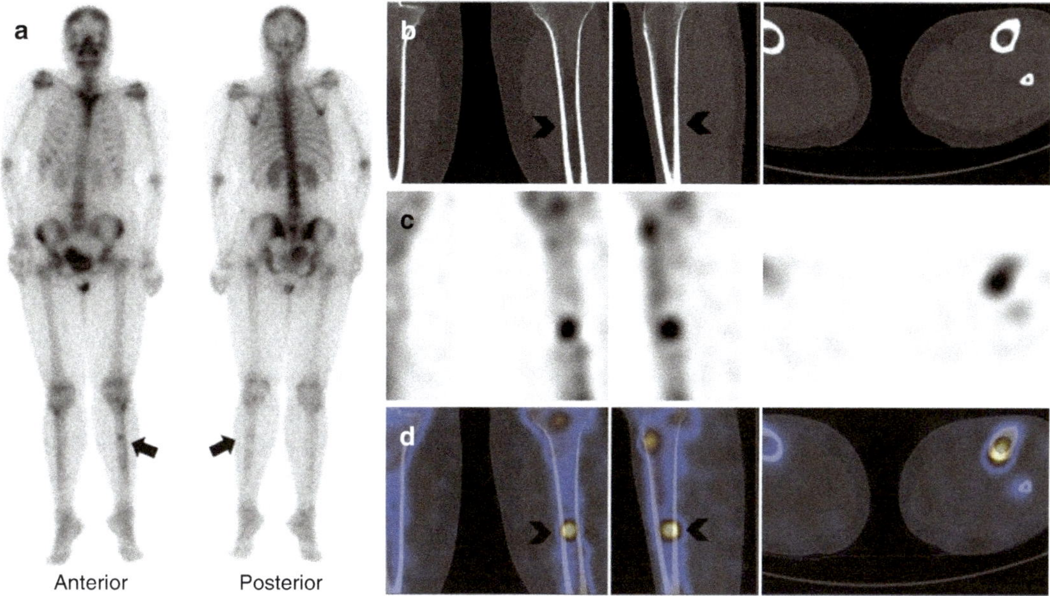

Fig. 9.10 Bone infarct: 17-year-old female presented with sudden onset of pain in shaft of left tibia since few days. X-ray was non-suggestive. Bone scan showed focal increased tracer uptake in the shaft (arrows in **a**). SPECT-CT localized it to a subtle irregular marrow sclerosis (arrow heads in **b–d**), suggestive of bone infarct

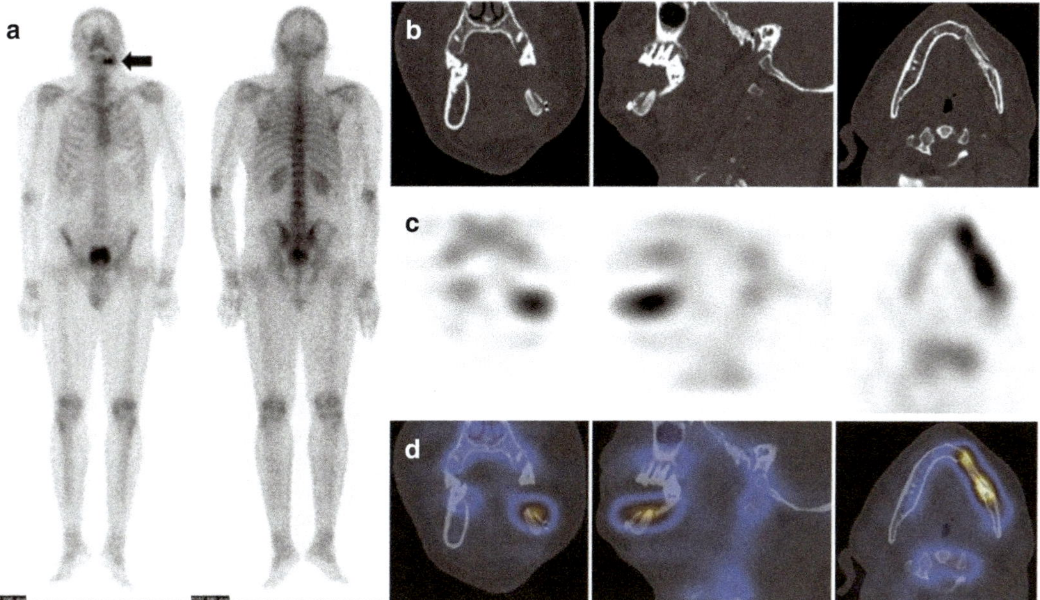

Fig. 9.11 Viable bone: 38-year-old male post left hemi-mandibulectomy for a tumour and repaired with an autologous bone graft, came for viability evaluation. Bone scan showed tracer uptake in the bone graft (arrow in **a**) with SPECT-CT localizing the uptake to graft showing normal bone attenuation (**b–d**), suggestive of viable bone

9.4.12.1 SPECT-CT Findings

Accurate localization of the uptake on bone scintigraphy is the key to differentiating the condition from other pathologies. Bone scan shows increased tracer uptake in the ossification site. However, the localization may be less accurate on planar bone scintigraphy. The addition of

SPECT imaging of the area of concern can help to localize the uptake. Registering the acquired data from SPECT with low-dose CT images obtained from the new hybrid systems SPECT-CT can also provide better activity localization.

9.4.13 Condylar Hyperplasia

Condylar hyperplasia is a rare disease that manifests as non-neoplastic overgrowth of the mandibular condyle. This disorder usually unilateral and often results in facial asymmetry, deformity and malocclusion and is sometimes associated with obvious pain and dysfunction. Condylar hyperplasia is common and frequently occurs in groups during the growth phase, especially in adolescence [86]. Females also appear to be more sensitive to condylar hyperplasia than males [87, 88]. Appropriate therapeutic decisions are mainly based on subjective clinical evaluation and are supported by bone scans [89, 90]. Although condylar hyperplasia is a self-limiting condition, it is characterized by progressive and independent growth that always results in the bone volume of one condyle being greater than that of the other. According to the growth state, condylar hyperplasia is divided into an active phase and stationary phase. The activity level of the condyle is considered to be highly correlated with mandibular asymmetry [91, 92]. When making a therapeutic plan, it is essential to determine whether there is an excessive condylar activity, for example with skeletal scintigraphy [92], which has recently been used in the diagnosis of condylar hyperplasia. Routine imaging examinations, such as X-ray and CT, can detect anatomical changes and not condylar growth activity.

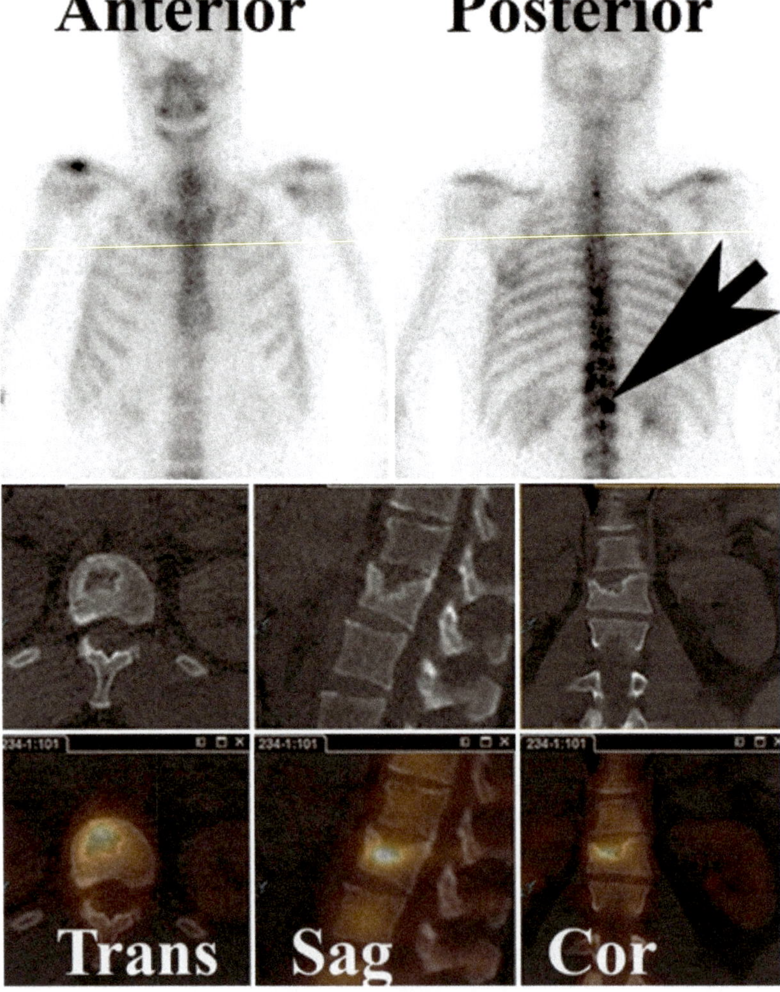

Fig. 9.12 Central disc herniation: 26-year-old male presented with the sudden onset of pain in the lower thoracic region after doing a water ski jump and landing awkwardly before pitching forwards. The patient underwent bone scan. Delayed study showed increased uptake at the L1 vertebra (arrow). SPECT/CT images, however, demonstrated a lucent central superior endplate defect of L1 with sclerotic margins best appreciated in the sagittal projection. There was intense uptake at the site of central disc herniation

9.4.13.1 SPECT-CT Findings

Single-photon emission computed tomography (SPECT) has been commonly used to evaluate metabolism in several tissue types [93–95]. Importantly, SPECT-CT could provide both functional and morphological information associated with condylar hyperplasia [96]. Using a bone-seeking radiopharmaceutical agent, areas of increased osteoblastic activity can be highlighted so that condylar activity can be examined. Because clinical and radiographic presentations in patients with condylar hyperplasia are highly diverse, condylar growth activity assessment has a vital role in managing these patients [97].

9.4.14 Graft Viability Evaluation

Autogenous bone grafts are the gold standard for osseous defect regeneration in the craniofacial region due to osteogenicity, osteoinductivity, osteoconductivity and eventual replacement by natural bone [98]. The free bone grafts are associated with bone resorption, rejection and sinus formation. Therefore, early assessment of the graft is vital for future prediction of graft. It is also critical to assess the viability of bone after bone graft surgeries. The viability can be assessed by angiography, duplex sonography and radiography. One of the methods of graft monitoring is bone scintigraphy using technetium-99m-labelled methylene diphosphonate status [99] (Fig. 9.11).

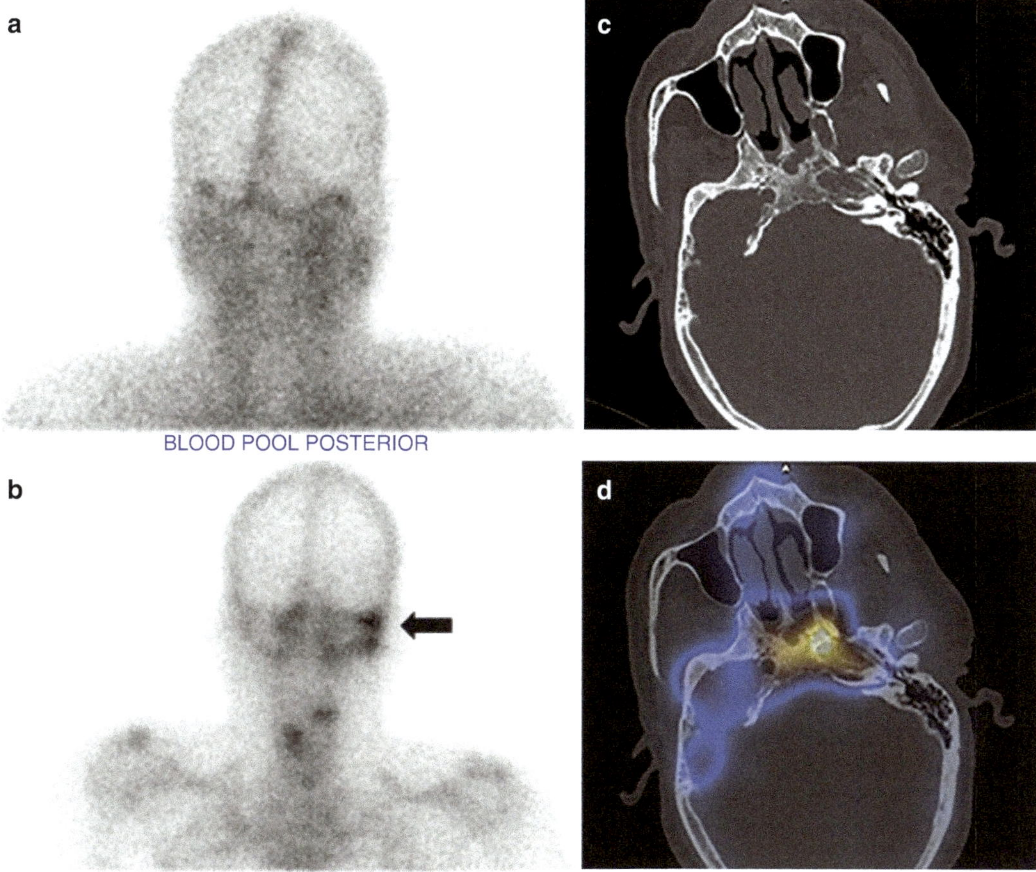

Fig. 9.13 Residual skull base osteomyelitis: 59-year-old male with right-sided malignant otitis externa was having pain and pus discharge. Blood pool image shows no subtle increased tracer uptake in right side of face (arrow in **a**). Delayed bone scan showed increased tracer uptake in the right temporal region and base of skull (arrow in **b**). SPECT-CT localized the uptake to sclerosis with erosions in right petrous temporal bone, sphenoid bone, clivus and left petrous temporal bone (**c**, **d**) suggestive of residual skull base osteomyelitis

9.4.14.1 SPECT-CT Findings

Bone scan using 99mTc MDP is an important tool in the assessment of the bone flap viability. It is a simple, non-invasive method but still not routinely performed in hospitals. 99mTc MDP uptake in bone flap reflects the flap's blood flow and metabolic activity, which is indirect evidence of bone survival. Bone SPECT-CT imaging increases the diagnostic accuracy for detecting bone flap viability. The increased accuracy is due to better signal-to-noise ratio by removing superimposed activity, especially in the immediate post-operative period and when overlying skin necrosed, leading to surrounding soft-tissue hyperaemia [100, 101].

9.4.15 Vertebral Compression Fracture

Vertebral compression fractures are commonly observed in the context of elderly patients in the absence of trauma. While osteoporosis is the most common cause of vertebral compression fracture, the spine represents the most common bony metastases (39% of all bone metastases). So, this can frequently result in pathological fracture [102]. Differentiation between such benign and malignant fractures can pose a significant diagnostic dilemma, given that both fracture types can be observed in the elderly population.

Besides that, benign compression fractures can co-exist in up to one-third of patients with bone metastases [103] (Fig. 9.14).

9.4.15.1 SPECT-CT Findings

CT: CT demonstrates an associated paraspinal or epidural mass due to a metastatic lesion's soft-tissue extension. A convex posterior border of the vertebral body is also suggestive of a malignant fracture. In contrast, posterior bone fragments' retropulsion into the spinal canal is more typical of benign osteoporotic fracture [104].

SPECT: SPECT usually shows increased tracer uptake irrespective of the cause of the collapse. And so, hybrid SPECT-CT imaging has improved the diagnostic accuracy of the bone scintigraphy.

9.4.16 Spondylodiscitis

Spondylodiscitis is the infection of the intervertebral disc, which can spread to the nearby bone. The incidence of post-operative spondylodiscitis has been reported to vary between 0.1 and 3% of patients. The diagnosis should be suspected in severe back pain with or without fever, and elevated serum CRP levels. Treatment usually consists of long-term antibiotics and should be initiated as early as possible to reduce the risk of severe deformities, such as kyphosis [105, 106].

Fig. 9.14 (**a, b**) Vertebral fracture: A patient with previous history of Non-Hodgkin lymphoma and being treated with steroid long back presented with lower thoracic back pain since 10 months. X-ray and MR images (**a**) of lower thoracic and lumbar spine show multi-level loss of height of vertebral bodies in the lower thoracic and lumbar spine. On MR images (**a**), the cortical outline of the vertebral bodies is intact and there is no associated soft tissue or intraspinal abnormalities, favouring a benign aetiology. However, exact cause of recent pain generator could not be ascertained. A whole-body scan was performed, which showed intense focal uptake in the T7 vertebra, faint uptake of tracer in T9-T11 vertebral region (not shown). SPECT-CT of the thoracic spine (**b**) localizes intense tracer uptake in T7 vertebra to collapsed vertebral body, suggestive of metabolically active vertebral fracture and likely cause of pain. Minimal tracer uptake is seen in the collapsed T6, T9, T10 and T11 vertebrae suggestive of resolved fractures (arrows in **b**). No tracer uptake is seen in the collapsed T12, L1 and L2 vertebrae suggestive of old fractures

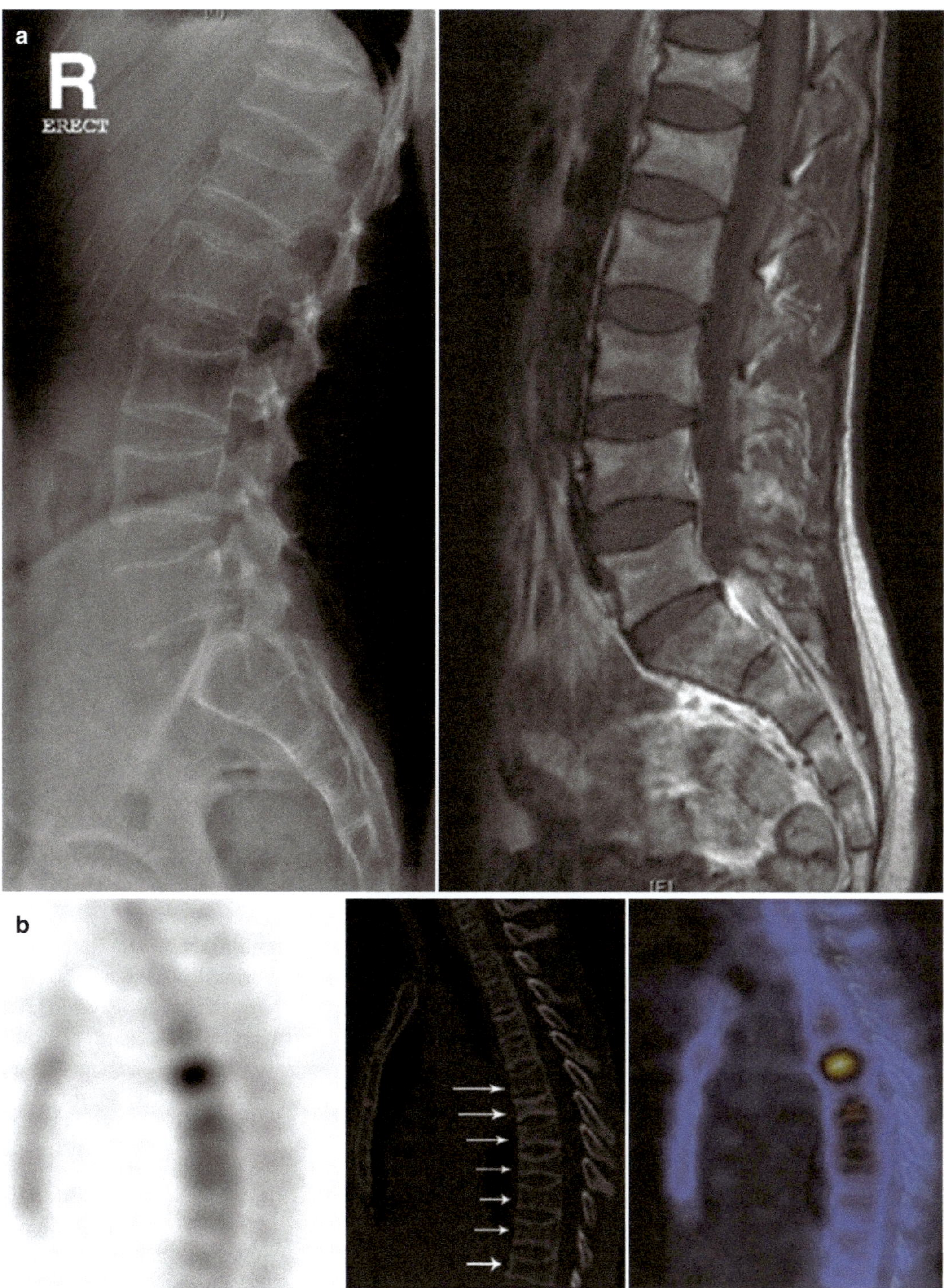

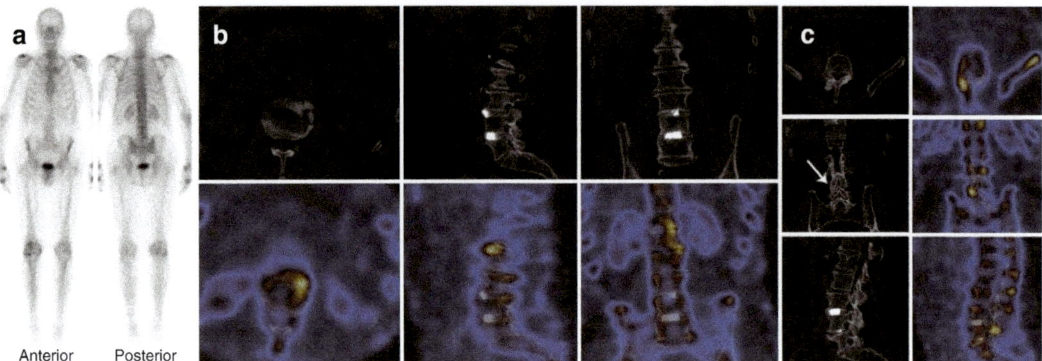

Fig. 9.15 (**a, b**) Facet joint arthropathy: Patient with previous L3-L4 and L4-L5 anterior cage fusion presented with increasing back pain. X-ray showed possible appearance of pseudoarthrosis. Bone scan (**a**) performed to identify cause of pain shows focal uptake of tracer at the left aspect of D12 vertebra with lower grade patchy uptake in remainder of lumbar spine. SPECT-CT of the lumbar spine (**b**) shows no abnormal tracer uptake in the region of fixation. The uptake mostly localizes to D12-L1 and L1-L2 osteophytosis. Further increased tracer uptake is seen in the degenerative changes at the right L4-L5 facet joint (arrow in **c**). SPECT-CT ruled out origin of pain from the disc prosthesis. Hence, cause of pain could be facetal arthropathy or osteophytosis

9.4.16.1 SPECT-CT Findings

CT: It provides better assessment of local bone damage and can be used to guide tissue biopsy. It is reported to have approximately 90% accuracy in post-surgical patients.

SPECT: It is usually considered to be an adjunct technique that can be used in case of equivocal MRI findings. Labelled white blood cell imaging has no role in spondylodiscitis. Combined gallium and bone SPECT/CT imaging can be used in the post-operative setting, with the differential intensity of both tracers' uptake, allowing some differentiation between infection or secondary changes [107, 108].

9.4.17 Intraosseous Disc Herniation

Acute intraosseous disc herniation is a rare cause of the sudden onset of back pain, usually after forced flexion/compression injury or minor trauma in osteoporotic patients. The most common site of disease extends from T10 to L1 [109]. It is thought to be the aetiology of the later development of Schmorl's nodes, which has been reported in approximately 19% of the population [110, 111]. Pathophysiology is herniation of the nucleus pulposus through the central vertebral endplate into the trabecular bone, either above and/or below the disc [112]. This process elicits significant marrow oedema around the site of herniation. These herniations may become organized to form Schmorl's nodes and, if vascularised, lead to chronic lower back pain. The condition should not be confused with the limbus vertebra, where the herniation occurs through the superior and anterior aspect of the ring apophysis [113] (Fig. 9.12).

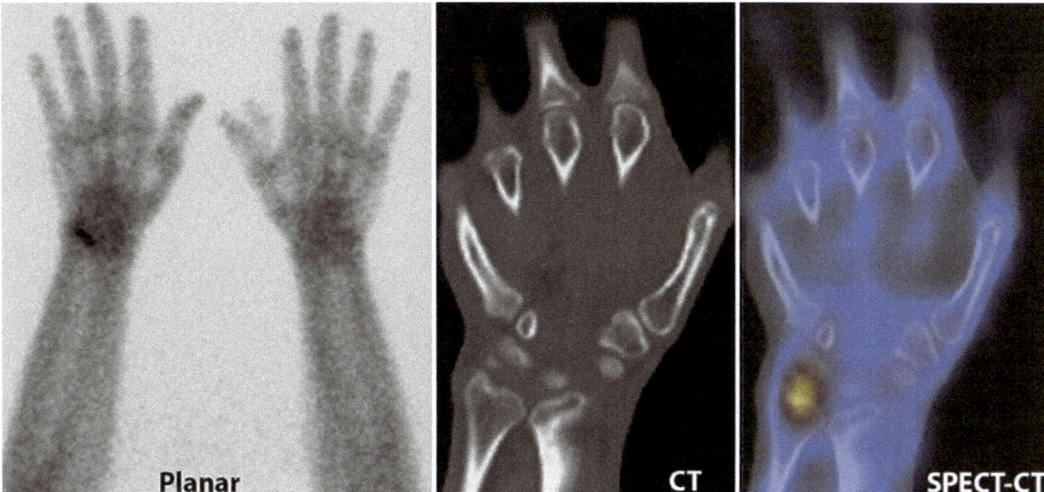

Fig. 9.16 Ulna-triquetral abutment syndrome: A man sustained a fractured ulna styloid 6 years prior to imaging and complains of continued ulna-sided wrist pain. Focal uptake within the ulna side of the wrist joint on planar imaging is accurately localized by SPECT-CT to active pathology on both sides of the ulna-triquetral articulation and diagnosed as ulna-triquetral abutment secondary to non-union of a previously fractured ulna styloid. This is one of many treatable causes of ulna-sided wrist pain, the majority of which can be differentiated accurately by SPECT-CT. Whilst MRI is the superior modality in evaluating the triangular fibrocartilagenous complex, SPECT-CT will provide complementary and often more specific information regarding cortical bone pathology

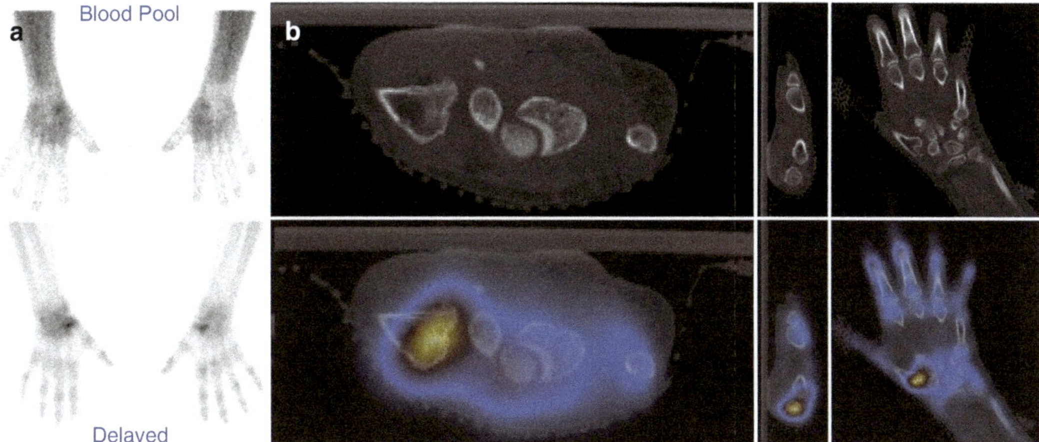

Fig. 9.17 (**a, b**) Post carpal excisional instability and degeneration: Pain in left wrist post Trapeziectomy. Two-phase bone scan (**a**) shows increased tracer uptake in bilateral first CMC joint region on both blood pool and delayed phases. SPECT-CT of the left wrist (**b**) localizes the tracer uptake to the base of the first metacarpal showing cystic changes suggestive of degenerative changes. Note is made of Trapeziectomy and multiple small bone fragments. The scan findings are likely due to post carpal excisional instability and degeneration

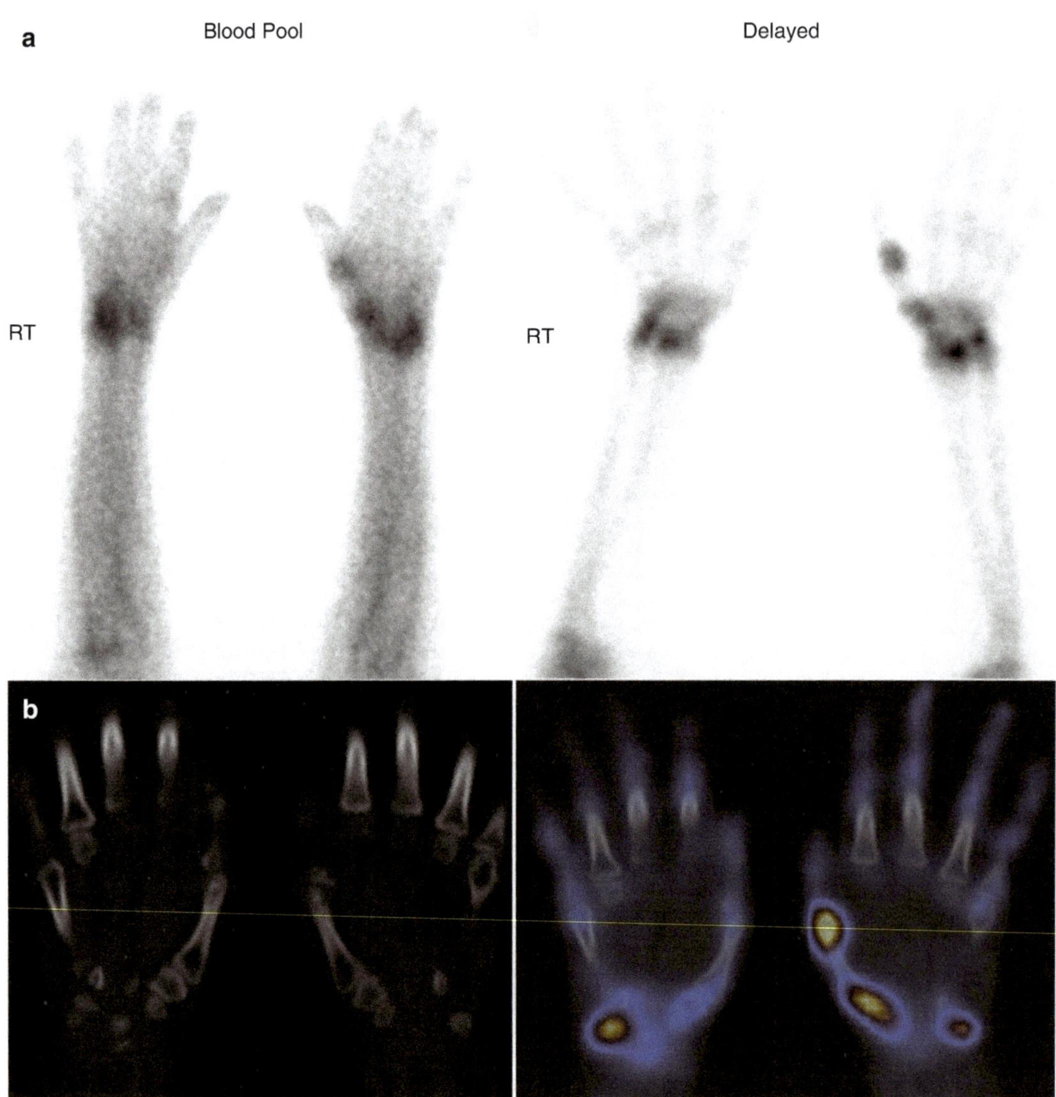

Fig. 9.18 (**a, b**) Complex regional pain syndrome: Injury to bilateral wrist, since then pain in the left wrist, patient has large cubitus valgus of the left elbow. Two-phase bone scan (**a**) shows increased tracer uptake in bilateral wrists and also at the left first CMC and MCP articulations on both phases. SPECT-CT of the wrists and hands (**b**) localizes the tracer to bilateral radio-carpal region, left triquetral, left first MCP joints with no obvious CT abnormalities. The findings are suggestive of complex regional pain syndrome

Fig. 9.19 (**a, b**) Biomechanical stress: This patient presented with ongoing pain following previous internal fixation of a fractured second metacarpal. A small, intense focus of tracer uptake in the mid-shaft of the second metacarpal region on planar bone scan (**a**) is accurately localized by SPECT-CT (**b**) to the position of the proximal screw, with a concordant rim of osteopenia demonstrable on CT (arrow). Only minor uptake is seen at the remainder of the fracture site (which was relatively long as it was a spiral/oblique fracture), and good callus formation was confirmed on CT. Minor uptake was also seen at the radio-scaphoid articulation with minor degenerative changes seen on CT. The features are compatible with ongoing biomechanical stress related to the proximal screw with satisfactory healing of the fracture by CT criteria. The removal of the culprit screw led to improved symptoms. In this case, SPECT-CT directly impacted upon management and led to improved symptoms and also identified low-grade secondary pathology at the wrist joint

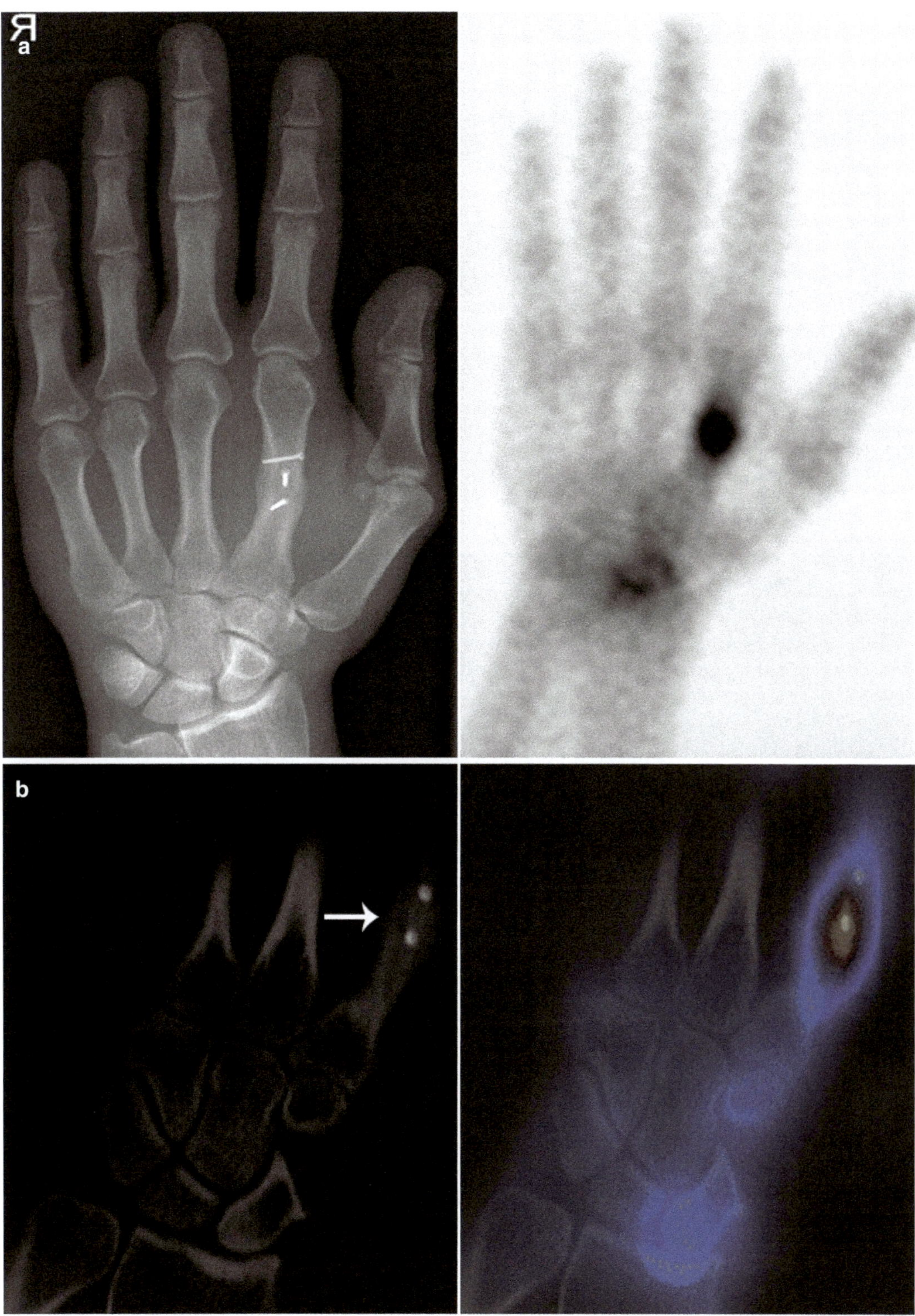

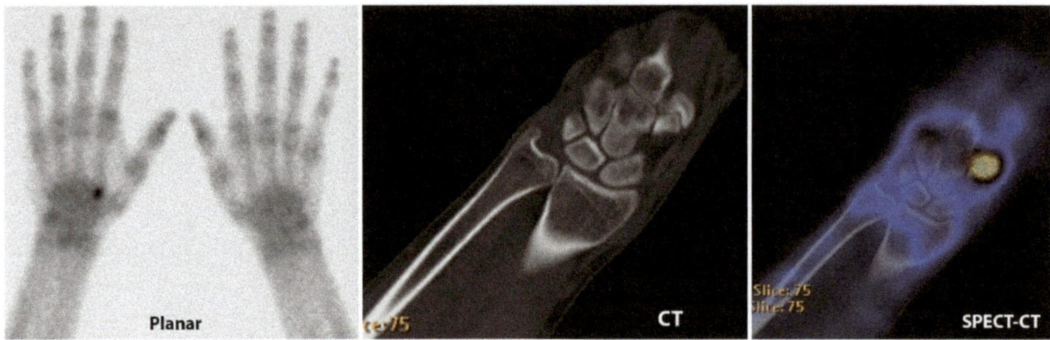

Fig. 9.20 Accessory ossicle with degenerative change. This patient presents with non-traumatic pain at the right hand especially involving the base of the index finger. X-rays were suggestive of minor degenerative change. An isolated focus of moderate tracer uptake with low-grade hyperaemia was seen on planar bone scan, which was localized by SPECT-CT to the second carpo-metacarpal joint. CT not only demonstrates degenerative changes at this joint but also an accessory ossicle (os styloideum) with an associated pseudo-arthrosis, the likely cause of symptoms. Accessory ossicles in the hand and wrist are common but are usually asymptomatic and when an os styloideum is symptomatic, it is termed Carpal Boss Syndrome. When they cause pain or altered function, they can be treated conservatively (medication and immobilization) or with surgical resection

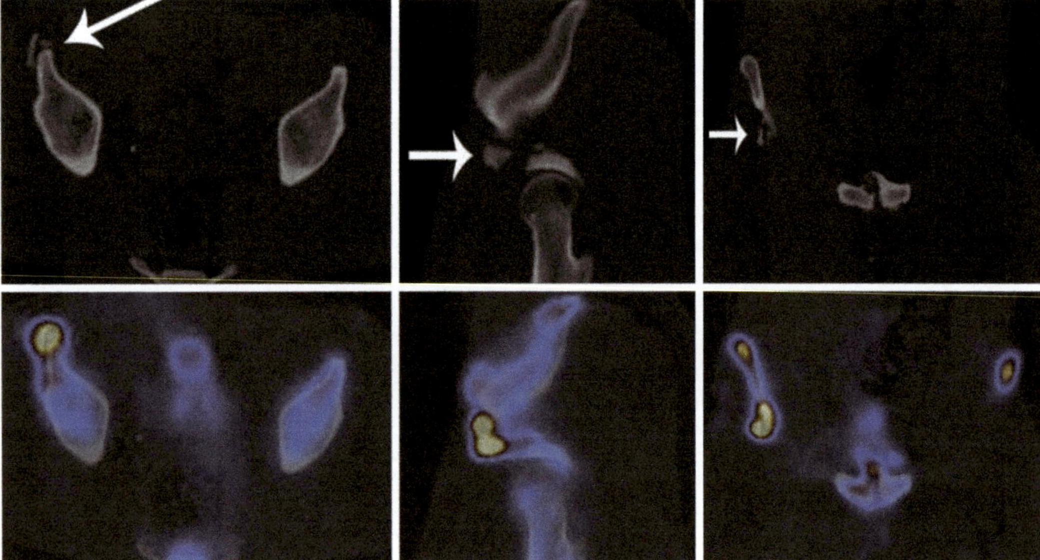

Fig. 9.21 A patient after traction injury presented with hip pain. Two-phase bone scan showed focal uptake of tracer at the right hemi pelvis on delayed image with increased uptake at the same site on the blood pool image (not shown here). However, due to non-specific character of uptake, SPECT-CT of pelvis was performed. SPECT-CT of pelvis shows the uptake is localized to bony spurs which are fragmented and arising from the anterior inferior iliac spine of the right iliac crest (arrows). The findings are suggestive of an **avulsion injury at the muscle insertion of the anterior inferior iliac spine**. Further uptake is seen at the symphysis pubis where there are osteophytes arising superiorly, likely due to osteitis pubis

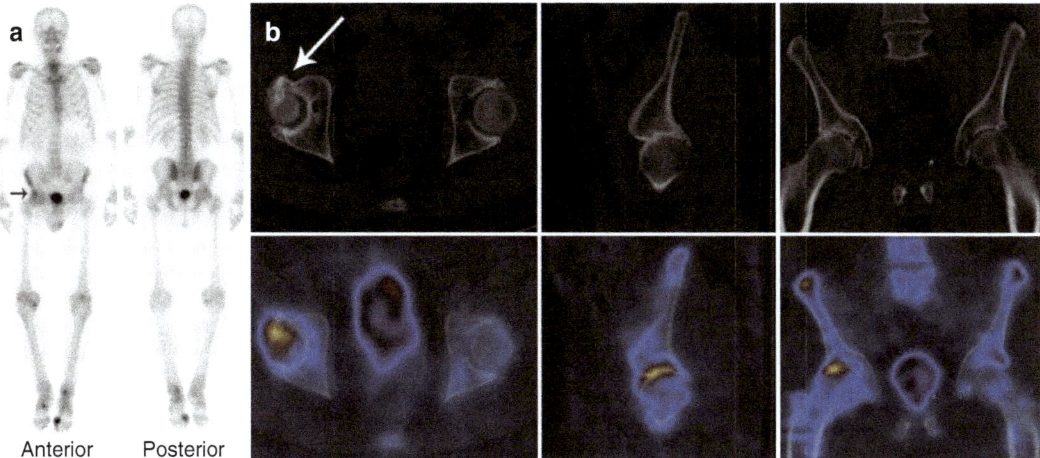

Fig. 9.22 (**a**, **b**) Patient with prostate cancer and rising PSA level presented with painful hip joint. Whole-body bone scan (**a**) shows focal tracer uptake in the right hip joint (arrow). Multiple foci of tracer uptake in the knees, left ankle and both feet are likely due to degenerative changes/arthropathy. SPECT-CT of the pelvis (**b**) localizes tracer uptake in the right hip to the joint between superior aspect of the acetabulum and the right femoral head (arrow), where there is joint reduction, acetabular sclerosis and subarticular cystic changes. There are bilateral osseous bumps noted at the femoral head/neck junction suggestive of **CAM type of femoroacetabular impingement**

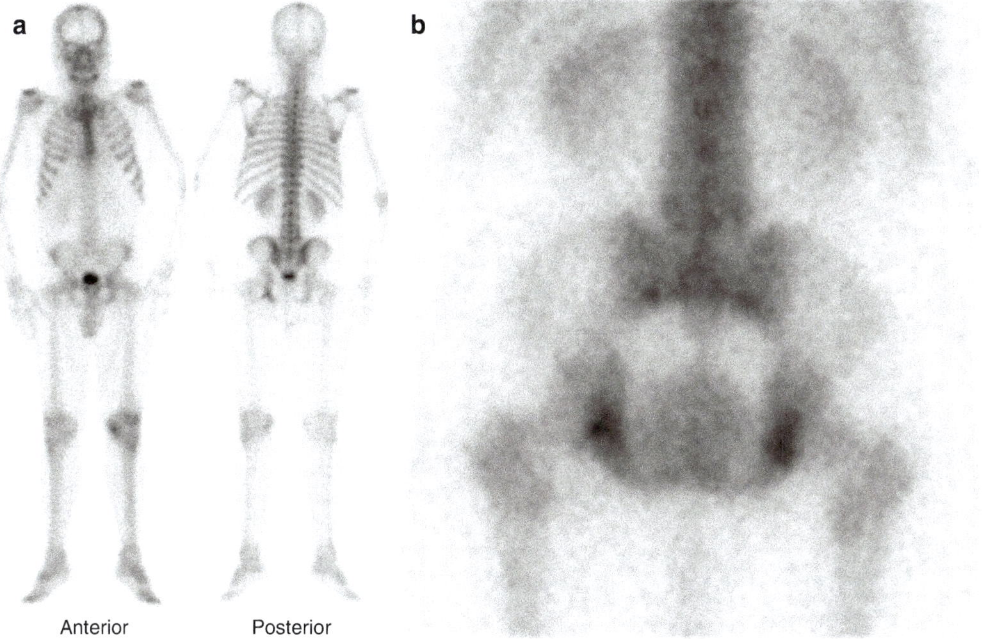

Fig. 9.23 (**a–c**) Prostate cancer patient with recent trauma and hip pain shows low-grade tracer uptake in the bilateral ischium on planar bone scan (**a**, **b**) which is likely due to enthesopathy. But SPECT-CT of pelvis (**c**) shows a discrete focus of abnormal uptake in the **coccyx showing a fracture** (arrow) which is not perceptible in planar imaging

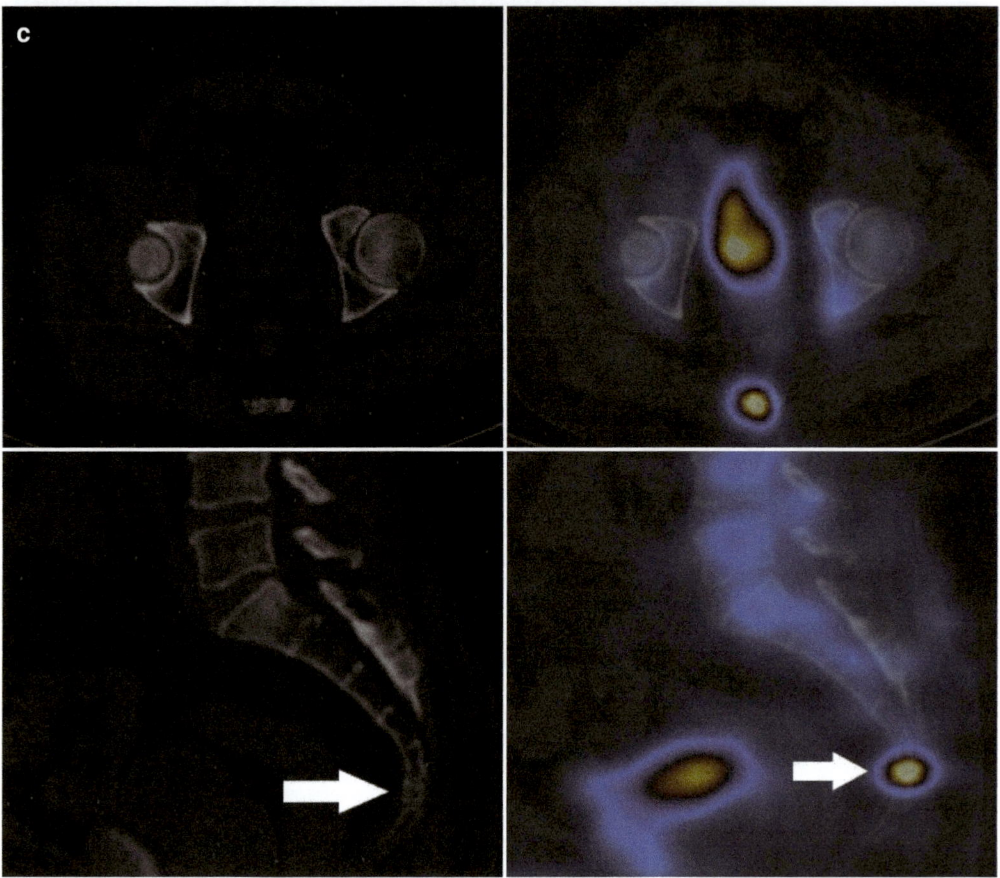

Fig. 9.23 (continued)

9.4.17.1 SPECT-CT Findings

CT: An evident defect is apparent in the vertebral endplate with a lucency in the trabecular bone immediately adjacent to the defect.

SPECT: The blood pool image is primarily normal, with the delayed image showing increased uptake around the affected endplate. The SPECT/CT images usually demonstrate a lucent defect in the

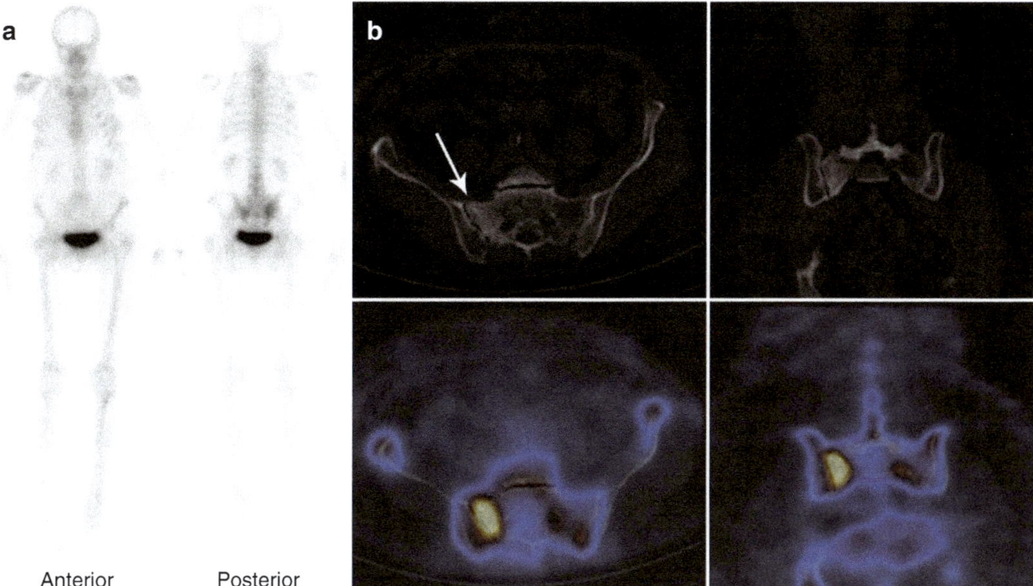

Fig. 9.24 (**a, b**) A patient with breast cancer presented with pain in the right sacroiliac region which is failing to settle. She had a history of fall about 4 months ago. The left hip prosthesis is stable on clinical examination. A bone scan was done to rule out metastatic disease. On planar images (**a**), there is intense tracer uptake seen within both sacroiliac joints (right > left). No abnormal tracer uptake is seen in the left hip prosthesis. SPECT-CT of the hip (**b**) localizes the tracer uptake in the right sacroiliac joint to the sacrum showing sclerosis (arrow) and vertical linear lucency suggestive of **sacral fracture**. Similar appearance with lesser severity was noted on the left side in SPECT-CT (not shown)

affected endplate with intense uptake around the adjacent lucency that extends into the vertebral body [114, 115]. It is essential to distinguish compression fracture from the vertebral endplate (Fig. 9.12).

9.4.18 Osteomyelitis

Acute and chronic osteomyelitis is a heterogeneous group of infectious disease entities. The

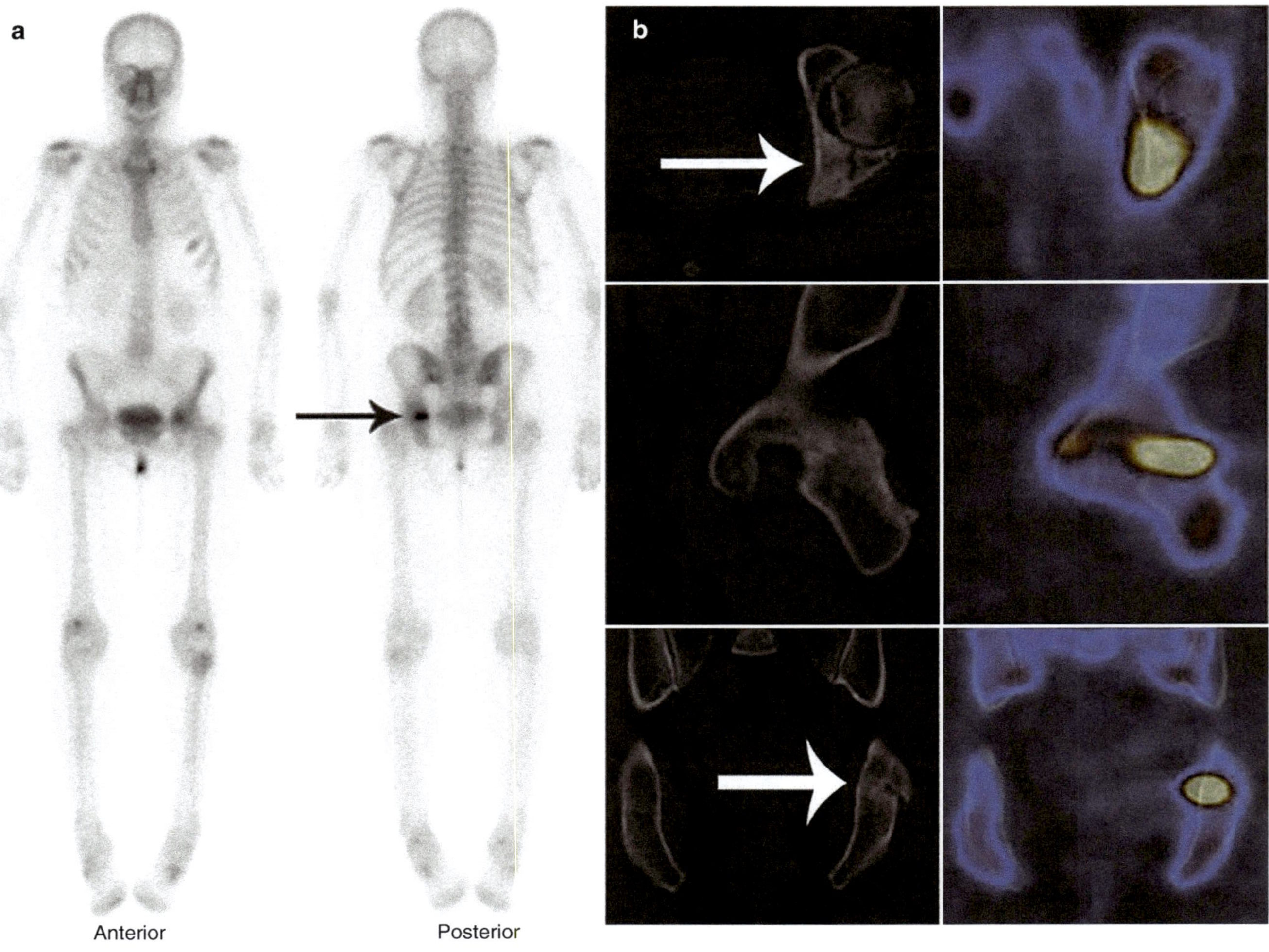

Fig. 9.25 (**a**, **b**) Patient with left hip pain. Whole-body bone scan (**a**) shows tracer uptake in the left hip joint (arrow) which could be degenerative in nature. But, SPECT-CT of hip (**b**) localizes the uptake to a **fracture in the posterior column of the left acetabulum** (arrows) and identifies the site of pain generator

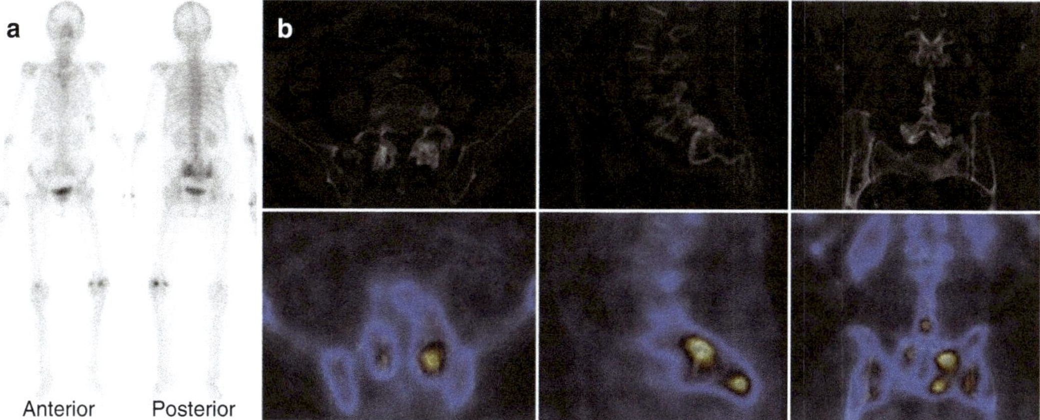

Fig. 9.26 (**a**, **b**) A patient with severe osteoporosis on DEXA scan presented with new onset right hip pain. Bone scan was done to find out new site of fractures. Patchy increased tracer uptake is seen in the sacroiliac joints with tracer uptake in the left side of sacrum and left L5-S1 facet joint (**a**). Low-grade increased tracer uptake in the left side lower ribs could be due to old fractures. SPECT-CT of the lumbar spine and pelvis (**b**) localizes tracer activity in the lumbar spine to left L5-S1 facet joint showing degenerative changes. The uptake in the sacrum localizes to sclerotic change in the left side of the sacrum in keeping with resolving **fracture**. Mild uptake in bilateral sacroiliac joint is likely due to degenerative changes

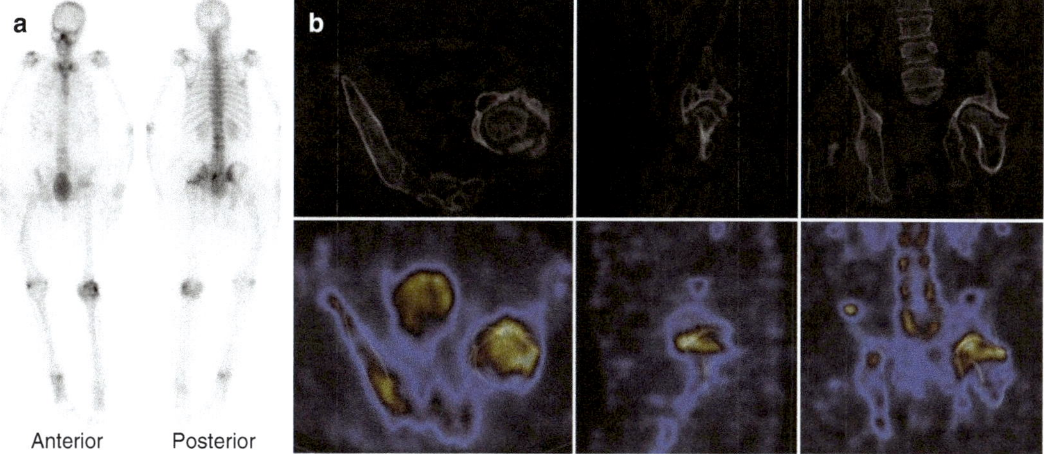

Fig. 9.27 (**a**, **b**) Patient with history of road traffic accident (7 years ago) and extensive hip injuries now presented with hip pain. Bone scan was done to rule out infection or non-union. Whole-body bone scan (**a**) shows increased tracer uptake in the left acetabulum and left femoral head. However, no significant tracer accumulation is seen at these sites on blood pool images (not shown). SPECT-CT of hip (**b**) shows significantly increased tracer uptake in the left acetabulum showing striking degenerative changes and further uptake in the left femoral head. Protrusio of left hip is seen. The two-phase bone scan findings rule-out acute infection. However, the findings on SPECT-CT could be due to **chronic septic arthritis or could be due to post-traumatic synovitis**. In-111-labelled white cell scan showed no scan evidence of acute infection in the left hip (not shown)

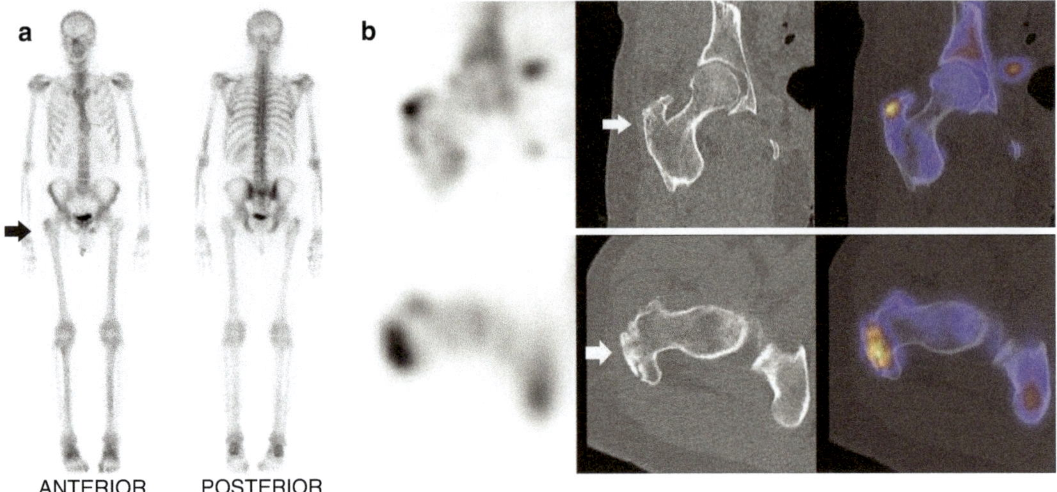

Fig. 9.28 (**a**, **b**) A patient with right lateral hip pain underwent bone scan (**a**) which shows increased tracer uptake in the right greater trochanter region (arrow). On SPECT-CT (**b**), the uptake corresponds to cortical irregularity and mild sclerosis at the right greater trochanter (arrows), suggestive of right **greater trochanter bursitis**

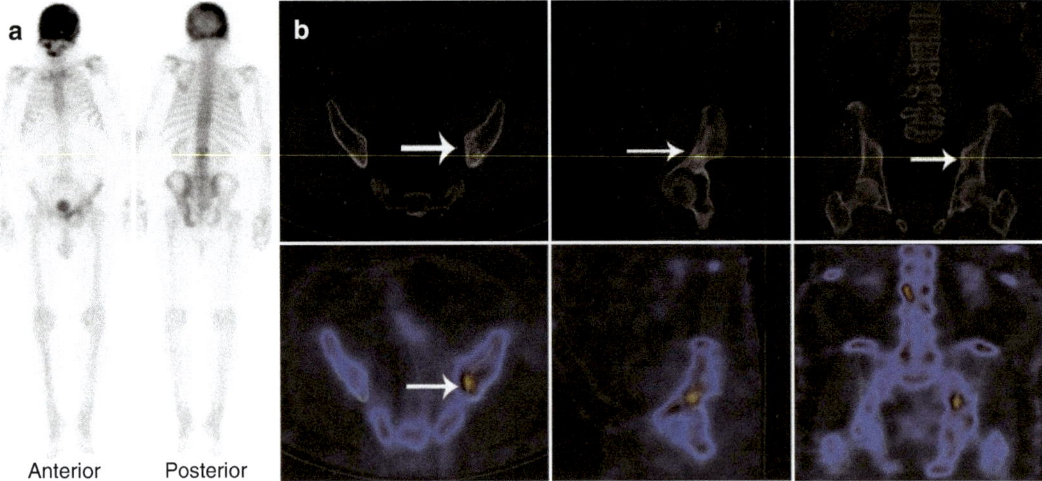

Fig. 9.29 (**a**, **b**) Prostate cancer patient with left lower thoracic pain and tenderness. Whole-body bone scan (**a**) shows diffusely increased tracer uptake in the skull bone with subtle increased tracer uptake in the upper lumbar spine and left hemipelvis. The uptake in the skull bone could be due to Paget's disease. However, uptake in the lumbar spine and left hemipelvis could be due to metastasis. SPECT-CT of the pelvis localizes the uptake in the left iliac bone showing coarsened trabeculae with sclerosis on CT (arrows in **b**). Within the lumbar spine, there is increased tracer uptake involving the right side of L2 vertebral body showing coarsened trabeculae. The overall scan appearance is in keeping with **Paget's disease** and rules out metastatic involvement

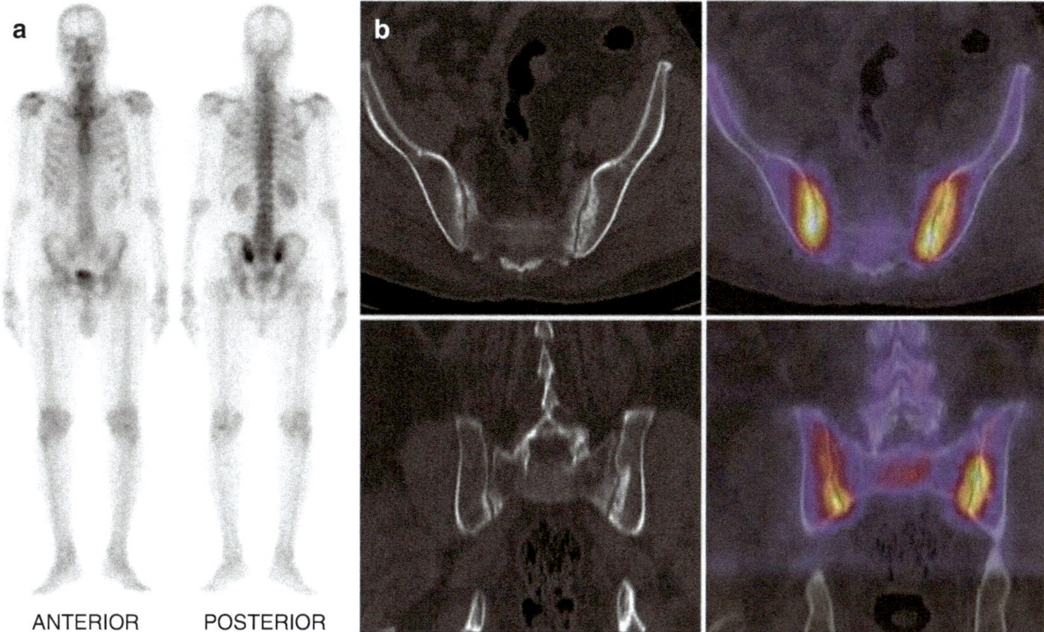

Fig. 9.30 (**a**, **b**) A patient with urinary bladder cancer and hip pain underwent bone scan to rule out metastases. Whole-body bone scan (**a**) shows increased tracer uptake at the inferior part of bilateral sacroiliac joints. SPECT-CT of pelvis (**b**) localizes increased tracer uptake to sclerosis and irregular margin of sacrum and iliac bones adjacent to bilateral sacroiliac joints, suggestive of **bilateral sacroiliitis**

patient's history, subjective symptoms and biochemical and physical findings are often inconclusive, particularly in the early stages. Osteomyelitis may not become visible on a plain X-ray until 10–21 days after onset. Because at least 30–50% loss of bone density is required before radiographs can detect the disease [116]. Detailed anatomical imaging with computed tomography (CT) or magnetic resonance imaging (MRI) is often unable to detect osteomyelitis at an early stage of the disease. Early detection is crucial in this disease for adequate treatment [117]. Functional imaging might have some advantages over anatomical imaging in detecting osteomyelitis before anatomical changes (Figs. 9.13 and 9.36).

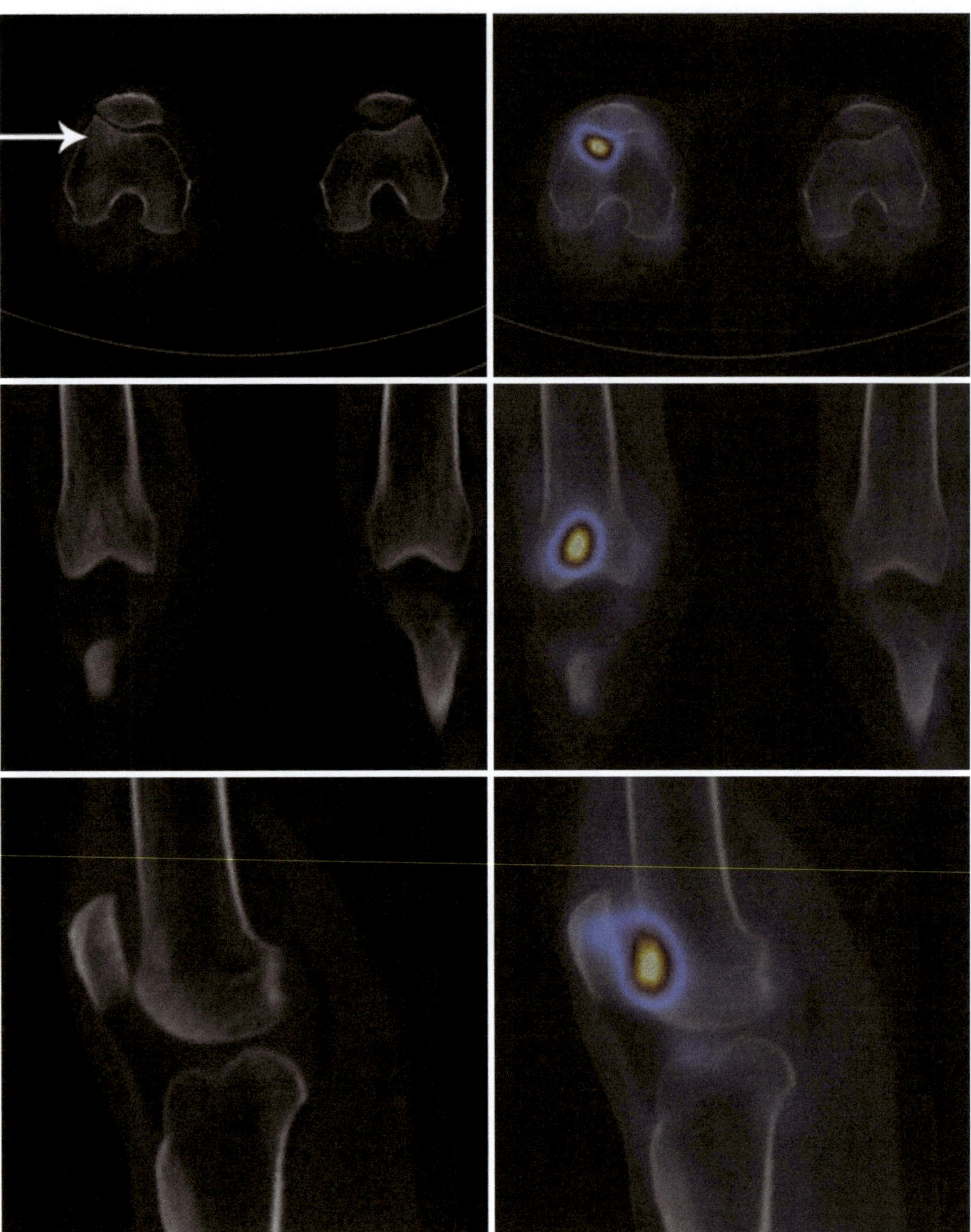

Fig. 9.31 Case of metastatic renal cancer with new onset right knee pain. Bone scan was performed to rule out metastatic disease. Focal tracer uptake was seen in the right knee on whole-body study (not shown), which on SPECT-CT localizes to a subchondral sclerotic area with lucent centre in the right lateral femoral condyle (arrow). The findings are suggestive of a **chondral defect** in the right lateral femoral condyle. There is no evidence of metastatic disease

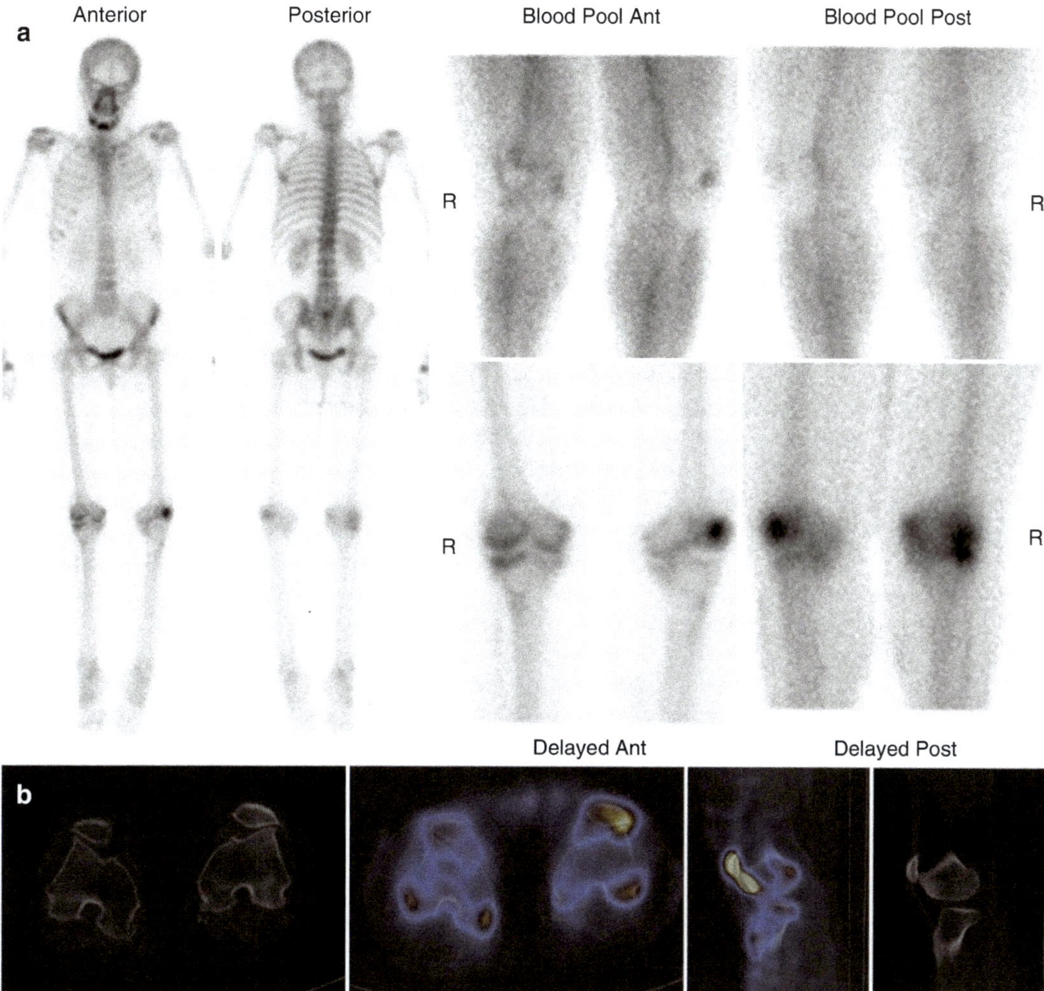

Fig. 9.32 (**a**, **b**) Patient with history of breast cancer presented with new onset left side knee pain post chemotherapy. Bone scan was performed to rule-out metastatic disease or AVN. Two-phase bone scan (**a**) shows intense focal tracer uptake in the lateral condylar region of the left femur with mild increase in the vascularity. Further increased uptake of tracer is seen in the lateral compartment of the right knee. SPECT-CT (**b**) localizes the tracer uptake in the left femoral condyle region to the **patellar maltracking** with degenerative changes. There is also right side patellar maltracking with normal tracer uptake. Thus, SPECT-CT definitely ruled out metastasis and diagnosed patellar maltracking with associated degenerative changes as the cause of pain

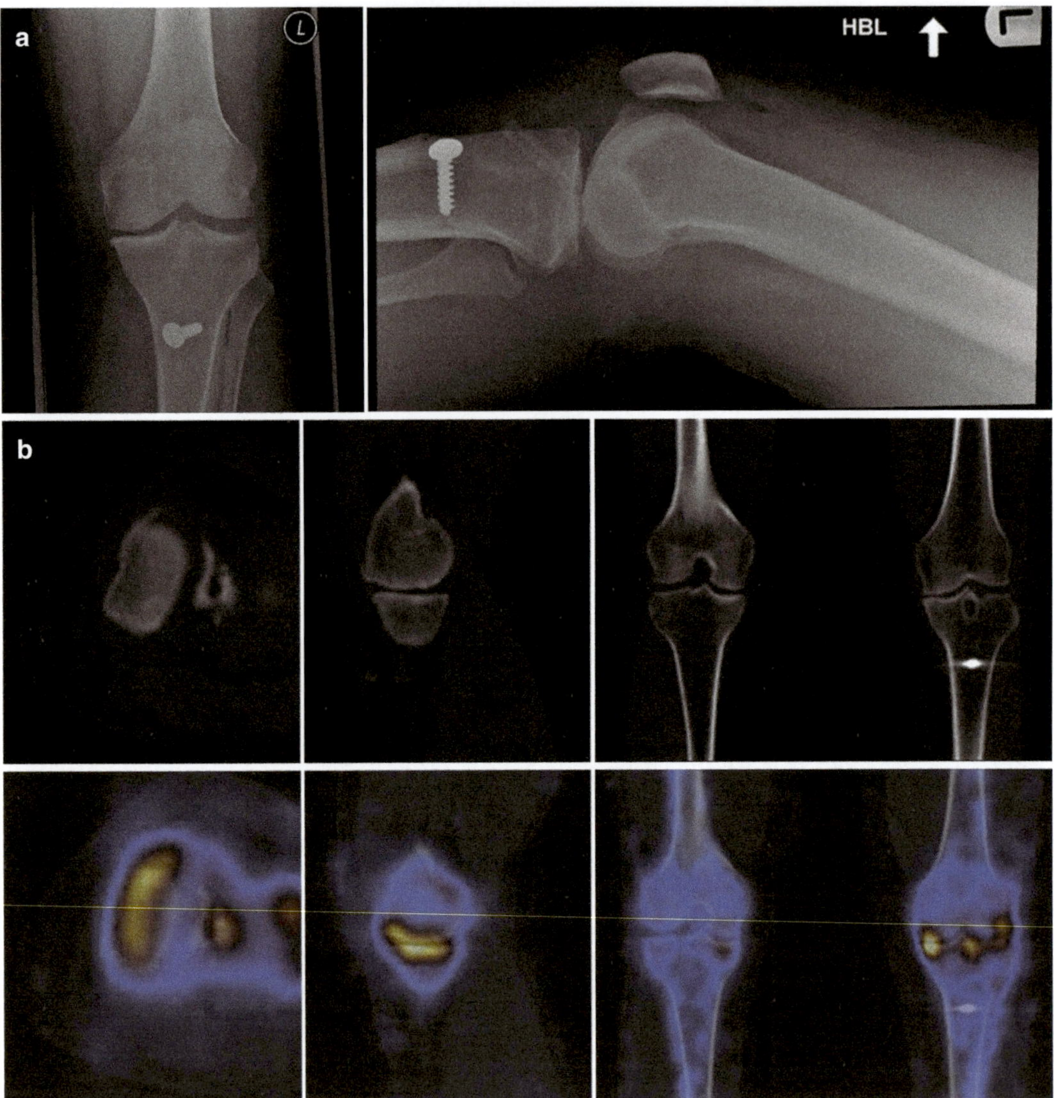

Fig. 9.33 (**a**, **b**) Previous **ACL reconstruction** on the left side. The patient complained of new onset pain in the left knee. X-ray of the left knee shows narrowing of medial joint space (**a**). Two-phase bone scan showed increased tracer uptake in the left knee, more on the medial side on both phases of study (not shown). SPECT-CT (**b**) shows channels for previous ACL reconstruction in the left knee. Increased uptake in the medial compartment localizes to the loss of joint space with subarticular irregularities particularly along the medial plateau. The findings are suggestive of metabolically active **degenerative changes**

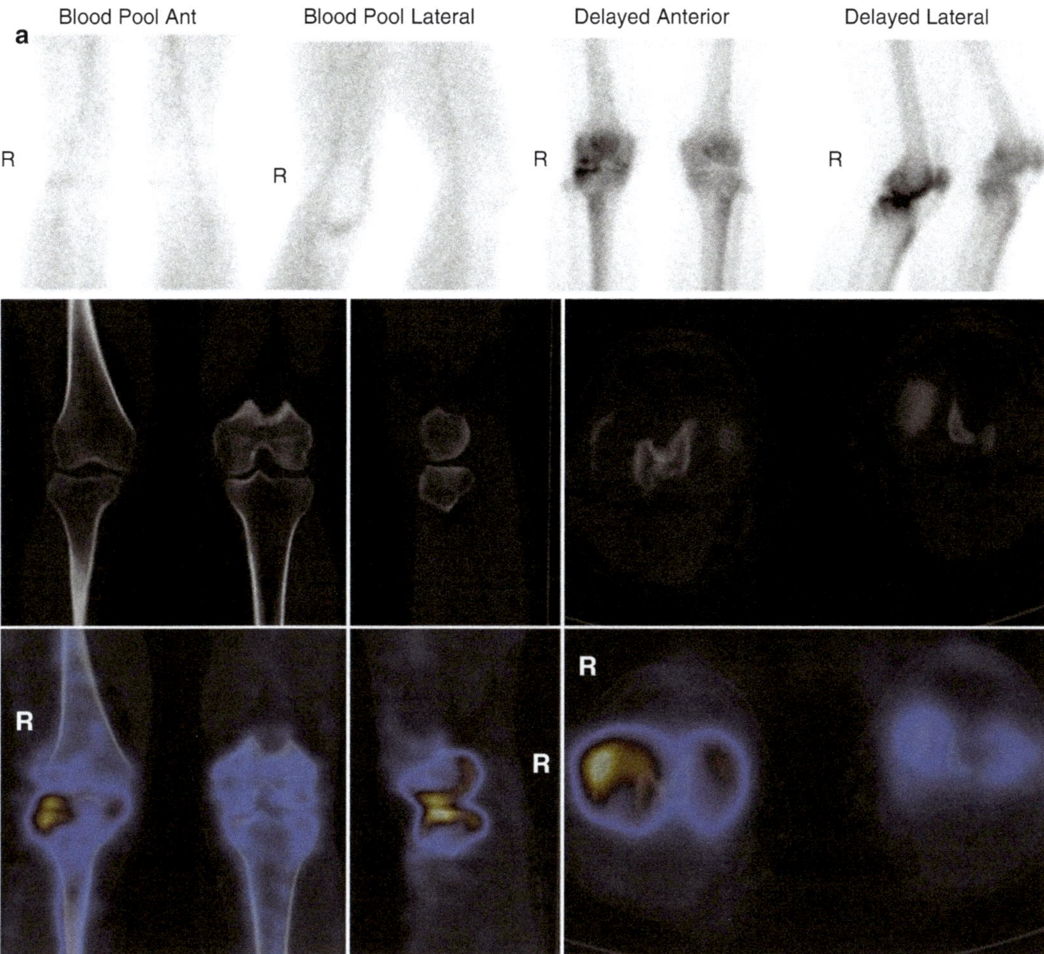

Fig. 9.34 (**a**, **b**) Right knee lateral meniscectomy. Patient is considered for meniscal transplant, and bone scan was performed to see metabolic activity elsewhere. Two-phase bone scan (**a**) shows increased tracer uptake in the lateral compartment and patella of the right knee without increase in vascularity. On SPECT-CT (**b**), the uptake in the lateral compartment localizes to the post-operative changes in the right knee in a crescentic pattern. The uptake in the patella localizes to the degenerative changes (not shown)

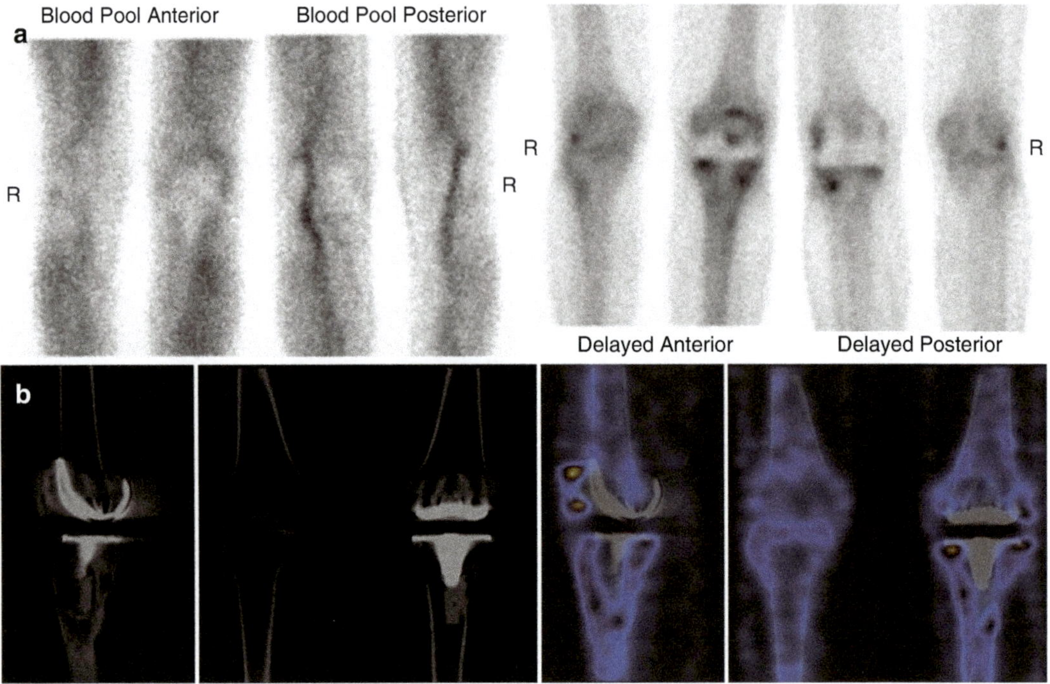

Fig. 9.35 (a, b) **Painful left knee prosthesis**, post 1 year after replacement. Two-phase bone scan (**a**) shows mild tracer uptake in the medial and lateral aspects of the left proximal tibia and in the left lateral femoral condyle region without corresponding increase in vascularity. SPECT-CT of the knees (**b**) demonstrates tracer uptake in the **left patellofemoral joint showing degenerative changes**. The tracer uptake at the left tibial plateau shows no evidence of loosening on CT and could be due to post-surgical changes

9.4.18.1 SPECT-CT Findings

The role of SPECT in bone and joint infections has been investigated using a series of radiopharmaceuticals. These radiopharmaceuticals include 67Ga-citrate, 99mTc-MDP, 111In-WBC and 99mTc-WBC, 99mTc-labelled anti granulocyte antibodies, and 99mTc-sulfur colloid. SPECT imaging of 99mTc-MDP alone [118, 119] showed a reasonable level of sensitivity (78–84%), but specificity remained low (33–50%) [118, 119]. In hybrid SPECT/CT, however, the specificity increased appreciably higher, i.e. 86%, due to better anatomical localization by adding CT [119]. Therefore, activity on the 111In-WBC image without related activity on the 99mTc-sulfur colloid image was considered positive for infection. Any other pattern was considered a negative study for infection. This combined 111In-WBC and bone marrow imaging with 99mTc-sulfur colloid showed a 100% sensitivity and 98% specificity in 50 patients with suspected infected total hip arthroplasty [120]. With 99mTc-anti-NCA-95 IgG, Horger et al. [121] showed in 27 patients that sensitivity for detection of relapsing posttraumatic osteomyelitis was excellent and identical for SPECT and hybrid SPECT/CT (100%). In contrast, specificity improved from 78% with SPECT to 89% when using hybrid SPECT/CT (Figs. 9.13 and 9.36).

Fig. 9.36 (**a–c**) Painful swelling in the left proximal leg, past history of chronic distal leg lump. Two-phase bone scan (**a**) shows increased vascularity and intense delayed phase uptake in the left proximal tibia starting from the tibial plateau up to the junction of upper and mid third of the tibia. SPECT-CT (**b**) of the leg localizes the intense uptake to the coarse cortical thickening of the left proximal tibia. There is endosteal scalloping. However, marked cortical thickening in the middle third of tibia is not showing tracer uptake. The findings are suggestive of acute on **chronic osteomyelitis of the left proximal tibia**. MRI of the left tibia (**c**) shows a lobulated lesion in the proximal tibia, which is low signal on T1 and high signal on proton density images. There is a sinus seen breaching the cortical surface, which extends into the surrounding soft tissues. There is extensive bone marrow oedema noted surrounding this lesion. The appearances are consistent with a Brodie's abscess with a sinus

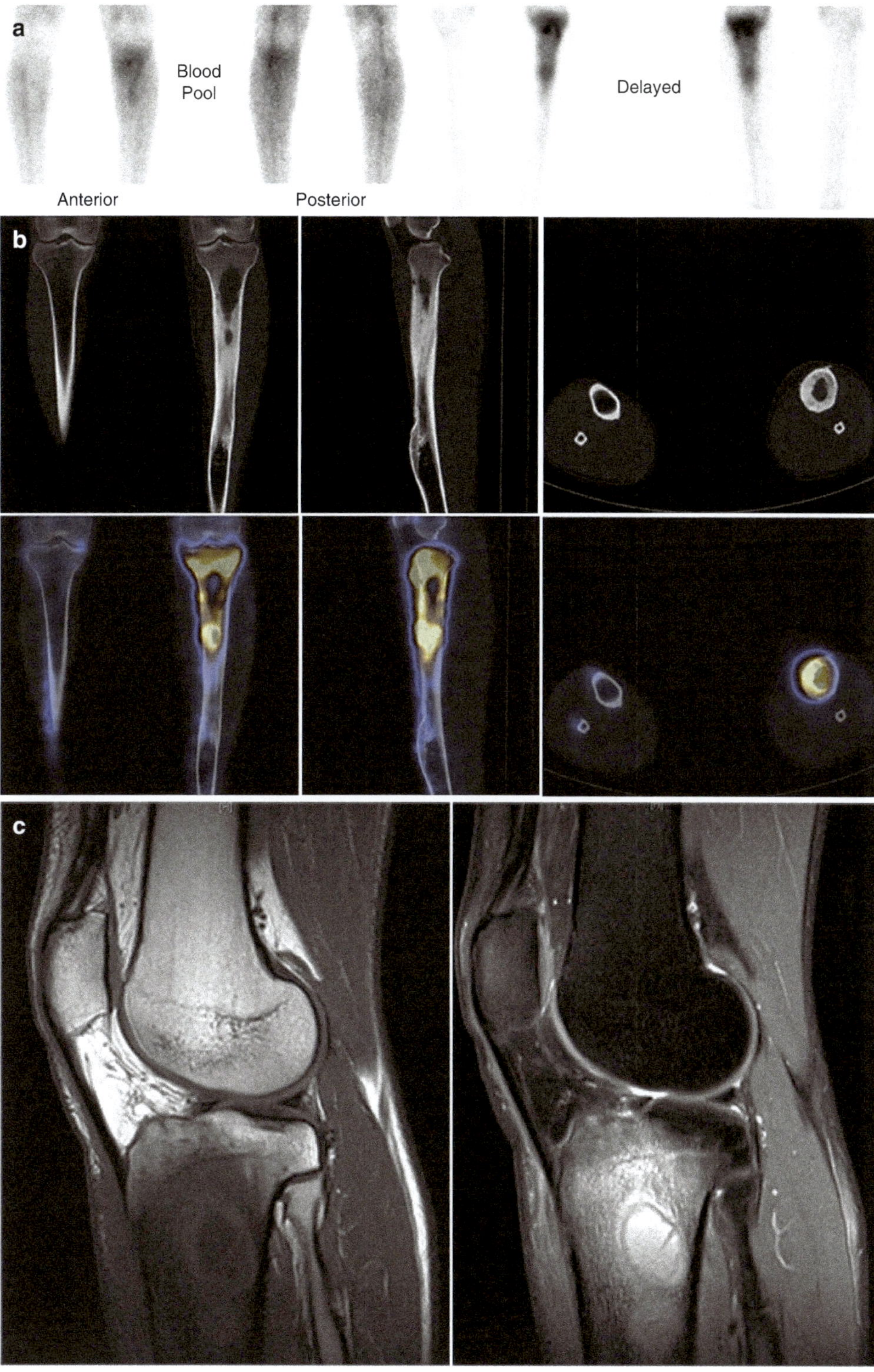
a
Blood
Pool
Delayed
Anterior
Posterior
b
c

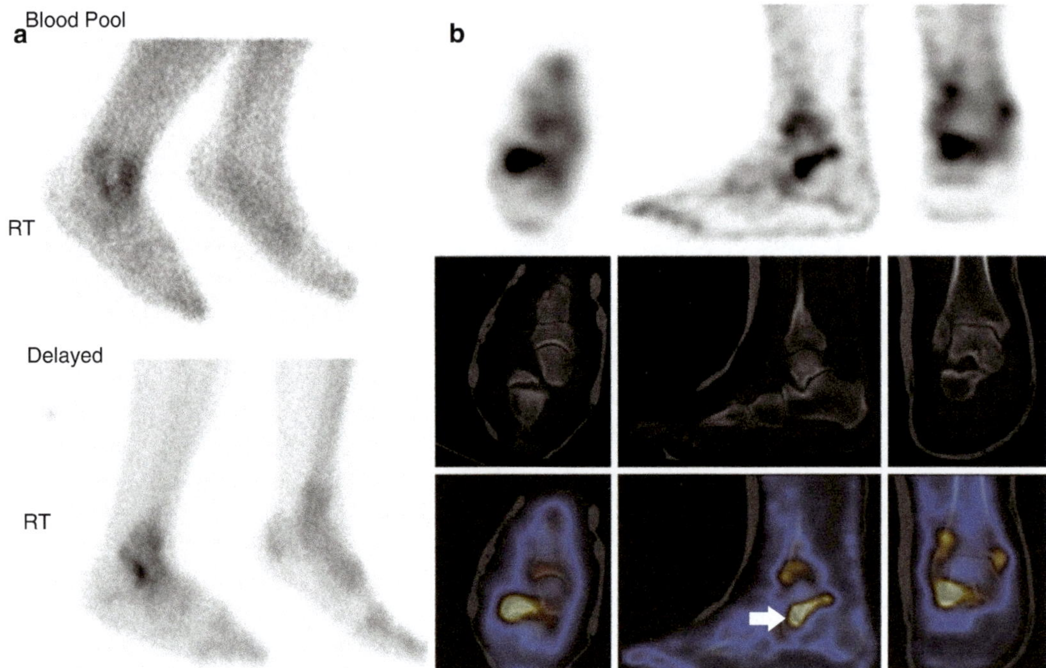

Fig. 9.37 (**a, b**) Past history of the right ankle arthroscopy with persisting sinus and culture proven infection. Bone scan was performed to rule-out deep-seated infection. Increased tracer uptake is noted in the right ankle in both phases of the two-phase bone scan (**a**). SPECT-CT of right foot (**b**) localizes increased tracer uptake in the right ankle to the distal tibiofibular joint and inferolateral talar facet with sclerosis and trabecular coarsening on CT, suggestive of infection (arrow in **b**). Increased tracer uptake is also seen in the anterior tibiotalar joint, which is suggestive of **impingement**

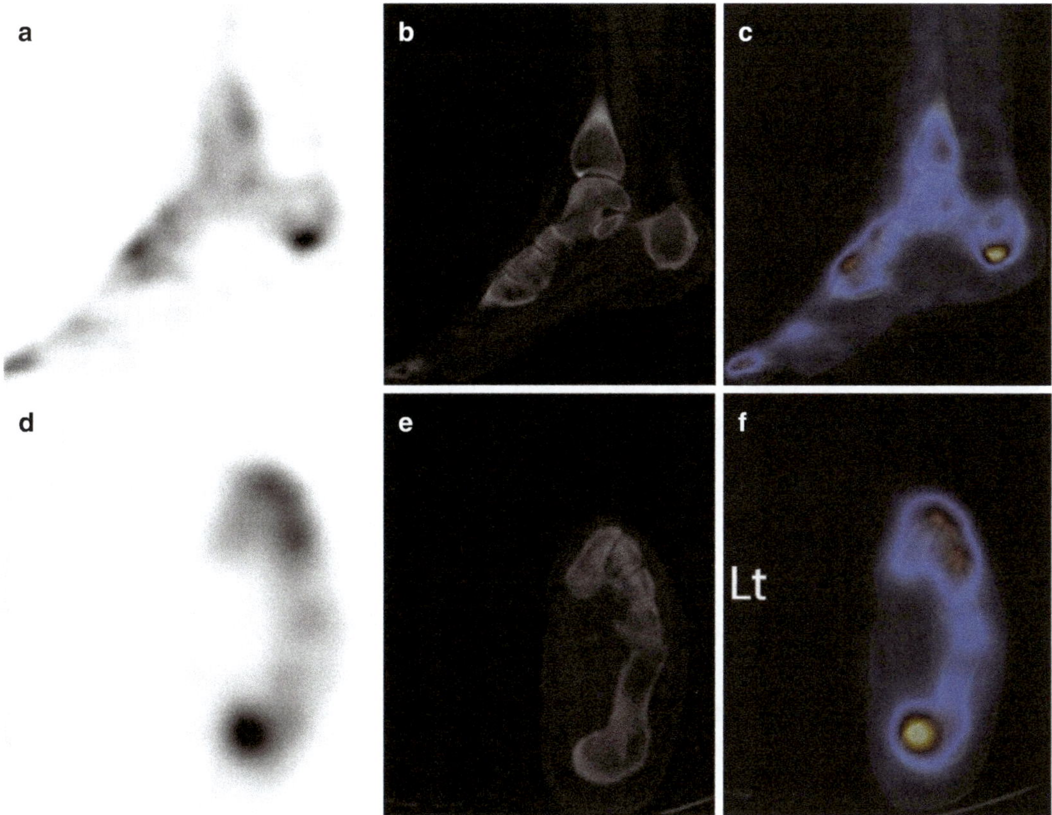

Fig. 9.38 A patient with vague pain in the left hindfoot underwent two-phase ^{99m}Tc-MDP bone scan and SPECT-CT of left foot to determine the pain aetiology. Increased vascularity and tracer uptake were seen in the left calcaneum on two-phase bone scan (not shown), which on SPECT-CT (**a–f**) localizes to inferior aspect of left calcaneum at the site of attachment of planar fascia with adjacent plantar fascia thickening. This is suggestive of **left planar fasciitis**, which is likely the cause of pain

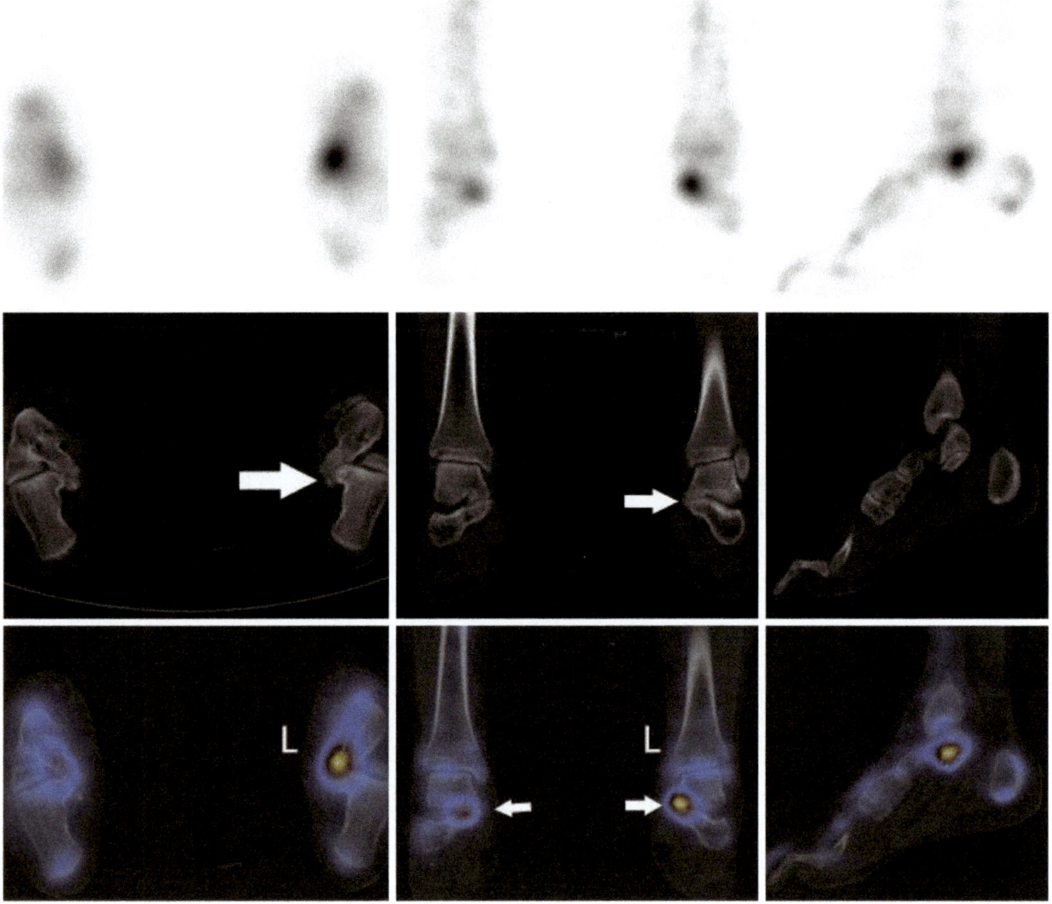

Fig. 9.39 Bilateral medial ankle pain. Two-phase ^{99m}Tc-MDP bone scan showed increased tracer uptake (left > right) with increased vascularity in bilateral ankles (not shown). SPECT-CT of ankles and feet localizes increased tracer uptake to the medial aspect of bilateral talo-calcaneal articulations showing cystic changes along the medial facet of the sub-talar joints (arrows). The findings are suggestive of **fibrous coalition of medial facet of the talus** with the calcaneum bilaterally, metabolically active on the left side

References

1. Bartel TB, Kuruva M, Gnanasegaran G, Beheshti M, Cohen EJ, Weissman AF, Yarbrough TL. SNMMI procedure standard for bone scintigraphy 4.0. J Nucl Med Technol. 2018;46(4):398–404. PMID: 30518604.
2. Erba PA, Israel O. SPECT/CT in infection and inflammation. Clin Transl Imaging. 2014;2:519–35.
3. Gnanasegaran G, Barwick T, Adamson K, Mohan H, Sharp D, Fogelman I. Multislice SPECT/CT in benign and malignant bone disease: when the ordinary turns into the extraordinary. Semin Nucl Med. 2009;39(6):431–42.
4. Brien EW, Mirra JM, Kerr R. Benign and malignant cartilage tumors of bone and joint: their anatomic and theoretical basis with an emphasis on radiology, pathology and clinical biology. I. The intramedullary cartilage tumors. Skelet Radiol. 1997;26(6):325–53.
5. Lichtenstein L, Jaffe HL. Chondrosarcoma of bone. Am J Pathol. 1943;19(4):553–89.
6. Devas MB. Stress fractures of the tibia in athletes or shin soreness. J Bone Joint Surg Br. 1958;40-B(2):227–39.
7. Slocum DB. The shin splint syndrome. Medical aspects and differential diagnosis. Am J Surg. 1967;114(6):875–81.
8. Reshef N, Guelich DR. Medial tibial stress syndrome. Clin Sports Med. 2012;31(2):273–90. https://doi.org/10.1016/j.csm.2011.09.008.
9. Holder LE, Michael RH. The specific scintigraphic pattern of "shin splints in the lower leg": concise communication. J Nucl Med. 1984;25(8):865–9.
10. Lieberman CM, Hemingway DL. Scintigraphy of shin splints. Clin Nucl Med. 1980;5(1):31.

11. Lafforgue P. Pathophysiology and natural history of avascular necrosis of bone. Joint Bone Spine. 2006;73(5):500–7. https://doi.org/10.1016/j.jbspin.2006.01.025.

12. Hernigou P, Voisin MC, Marichez M, Despres E, Goutallier D. Comparison of nuclear magnetic resonance and histology in necrosis of the femoral head. Rev Rhum Mal Osteoartic. 1989;56(11):741–4.

13. Glimcher MJ, Kenzora JE. Nicolas Andry award. The biology of osteonecrosis of the human femoral head and its clinical implications: 1. Tissue biology. Clin Orthop Relat Res. 1979;138:284–309.

14. Gardeniers J. A new international classification of osteonecrosis of the ARCO (Association Research Circulation Osseous) Committee. ARCO News. 1992;4:41–6.

15. McGonagle D, Gibbon W, Emery P. Classification of inflammatory arthritis by enthesitis. Lancet. 1998;352(9134):1137–40. https://doi.org/10.1016/S0140-6736(97)12004-9.

16. Soames R. Skeletal system. In: Williams P, editor. Grays anatomy. 38th ed. Edinburgh: Churchill Livingstone; 1995. p. 674–6.

17. Bennet P, Wood P, editors. Population studies of the rheumatic diseases. 1966 1968; New York. Amsterdam: Excerpta Medica Foundation; 1968.

18. Fam AG, Rubenstein JD, Chin-Sang H, Leung FY. Computed tomography in the diagnosis of early ankylosing spondylitis. Arthritis Rheum. 1985;28(8):930–7.

19. Scharf S. SPECT/CT imaging in general orthopedic practice. Semin Nucl Med. 2009;39(5):293–307. https://doi.org/10.1053/j.semnuclmed.2009.06.002.

20. Altman RD, Bloch DA, Hochberg MC, et al. Prevalence of pelvic Paget's disease of bone in the United States. J Bone Miner Res. 2000;15:461–5.

21. Guyer PB, Clough PW. Paget's diseases of bone: some observations on the relation of the skeletal distribution to pathogenesis. Clin Radiol. 1978;29:421–6.

22. Cortis K, Micalleg K, Mizzi A. Imaging Paget's disease of bone—from head to toe. Clin Radiol. 2011;66:662–72.

23. Gumà M, Rotés D, Holgado S, et al. Paget's disease of bone: study of 314 patients. Med Clin (Barc). 2002;119:537–40.

24. Horvai AE, Boyce BF. Metabolic bone diseases. Semin Diagn Pathol. 2011;28:13–25.

25. Wittenberg K. The blade of grass sign. Radiology. 2001;221:199–200.

26. Fogelman I, Carr D. A comparison of bone scanning and radiology in the assessment of patients with symptomatic Paget's disease. Eur J Nucl Med. 1980;5:417–21.

27. Lichtenstein L. Polyostotic fibrous dysplasia. Arch Surg. 1938;36:874–98.

28. Campanacci M. Bone and soft-tissue tumors: clinical features, imaging, pathology abd treatment. 2nd ed. New York: Springer; 1999.

29. DiCaprio MR, Enneking WF. Fibrous dysplasia. Pathophysiology, evaluation, and treatment. J Bone Joint Surg Am. 2005;87(8):1848–64. https://doi.org/10.2106/JBJS.D.02942.

30. Ito T, Goto K, Yoh K, Niho S, Ohmatsu H, Kubota K, et al. Hypertrophic pulmonary osteoarthropathy as a paraneoplastic manifestation of lung cancer. J Thorac Oncol. 2010;5(7):976–80. https://doi.org/10.1097/JTO.0b013e3181dc1f3c.

31. Shih WJ. Pulmonary hypertrophic osteoarthropathy and its resolution. Semin Nucl Med. 2004;34(2):159–63.

32. Sainani NI, Lawande MA, Parikh VP, Pungavkar SA, Patkar DP, Sase KS. MRI diagnosis of hypertrophic osteoarthropathy from a remote childhood malignancy. Skelet Radiol. 2007;36(Suppl 1):S63–6. https://doi.org/10.1007/s00256-006-0186-1.

33. Buckwalter KA, Farber JM. Application of multidetector CT in skeletal trauma. Semin Musculoskelet Radiol. 2004;8(2):147–56. https://doi.org/10.1055/s-2004-829486.

34. Querellou S, Arnaud L, Williams T, Breton S, Colin D, Le Roux PY, et al. Role of SPECT/CT compared with MRI in the diagnosis and management of patients with wrist trauma occult fractures. Clin Nucl Med. 2014;39(1):8–13.

35. Love C, Marwin SE, Palestro CJ. Nuclear medicine and the infected joint replacement. Semin Nucl Med. 2009;39:66–78. [PubMed] [Google Scholar].

36. Wooley PH, Nasser S, Fitzgerald RH. The immune response to implant materials in humans. Clin Orthop Relat Res. 1996;326:63–70. [PubMed] [Google Scholar].

37. Toumbis CA, Kronick JL, Wooley PH, Nasser S. Total joint arthroplasty and the immune response. Semin Arthritis Rheum. 1997;27:44–7. [PubMed] [Google Scholar].

38. Spector M, Shortkroff S, Hsu HP, Lane N, Sledge CB, Thornhill TS. Tissue changes around loose prostheses. A canine model to investigate the effects of an antiinflammatory agent. Clin Orthop Relat Res. 1990;(261):140–52. [PubMed] [Google Scholar].

39. Pandey R, Drakoulakis E, Athanasou NA. An assessment of the histological criteria used to diagnose infection in hip revision arthroplasty tissues. J Clin Pathol. 1999;52:118–23. [PMC free article] [PubMed] [Google Scholar].

40. Del Arco A, Bertrand ML. The diagnosis of periprosthetic infection. Open Orthop J. 2013;7:178–83. [PMC free article] [PubMed] [Google Scholar].

41. Tomas X, Bori G, Garcia S, Garcia-Diez AI, Pomes J, Soriano A, Ríos J, Almela M, Mensa J, Gallart X, et al. Accuracy of CT-guided joint aspiration in patients with suspected infection status post-total hip arthroplasty. Skeletal Radiol. 2011;40:57–64. [PubMed] [Google Scholar].

42. Gelman MI, Coleman RE, Stevens PM, Davey BW. Radiography, radionuclide imaging, and arthrography in the evaluation of total hip and

knee replacement. Radiology. 1978;128:677–82. [PubMed] [Google Scholar].

43. Ostlere S. How to image metal-on-metal prostheses and their complications. AJR. 2011;197:558–67.

44. Mulcahy H, Chew FS. Current concepts of hip arthroplasty for radiologists: part I, features and radiographic assessment. AJR. 2012;199:559–69.

45. Oswald SJ, et al. Three-phase bone scan and indium white blood cell scintigraphy following porous coated hip arthroplasty: a prospective study of the prosthetic tip. J Nucl Med. 1989;30(8):1321–31.

46. Oswald SG, et al. The acetabulum: a prospective study of three-phase bone and indium white blood cell scintigraphy following porous-coated hip arthroplasty. J Nucl Med. 1990;31:274–80.

47. Gnansegaran G, Cook GJ. Nuclear medicine imaging techniques of musculoskeletal system. In: Ahmadzadehfar H, et al., editors. Clinical nuclear medicine. 2nd ed. Springer; 2020. p. 381–430.

48. Van den Wyngaert T, Strobel K, Kampen WU, Kuwert T, et al. The EANM practice guidelines for bone scintigraphy. Eur J Nucl Med Mol Imaging. 2016;43(9):1723–38.

49. Rager O, Schaller K, Payer M, Tchernin D, Ratib O, Tessitore E. SPECT/CT in differentiation of pseudarthrosis from other causes of back pain in lumbar spinal fusion: report on 10 consecutive cases. Clin Nucl Med. 2012;37(4):339–43.

50. Russo VM, Dhawan RT, Baudracco I, Dharmarajah N, Lazzarino AI. Casey AT hybrid bone SPECT/CT imaging in evaluation of chronic low back pain: correlation with facet joint arthropathy. World Neurosurg. 2017;107:732–8.

51. Sumer J, Schmidt D, Ritt P, Lell M, Forst R, Kuwert T, Richter R. SPECT/CT in patients with lower back pain after lumbar fusion surgery. Nucl Med Commun. 2013;34(10):964–70.

52. Al-Nabhani K, Michopoulou S, Allie R, Alkalbani J Saad Z, Sajjan R, Syed R, Bomanji J. Painful knee prosthesis: can we help with bone SPECT/CT? Nucl Med Commun. 2014;35(2):182–8.

53. Cew CG, Lewis P, Middleton F, van den Wijngaard R, Deshaies A. Radionuclide arthrogram with SPECT/CT for the evaluation of mechanical loosening of hip and knee prostheses. Ann Nucl Med. 2010;24(10):735–43.

54. Hirschmann A, Hirschmann MT. Chronic knee pain: clinical value of MRI versus SPECT/CT. Semin Musculoskelet Radiol. 2016;20(1):3–11.

55. Hirschmann MT, Amsler F, Rasch H. Clinical value of SPECT/CT in the painful total knee arthroplasty (TKA): a prospective study in a consecutive series of 100 TKA. Eur J Nucl Med Mol Imaging. 2015;42(12):1869–82.

56. Slevin O, Schmid FA, Schiapparelli F, Rasch H, Hirschmann MT. Knee Surg Increased in vivo patellofemoral loading after total knee arthroplasty in resurfaced patellae. Sports Traumatol Arthrosc. 2017:4803–4.

57. Anesthetic blocks, Clin J Pain. 2015;31(12):1054–9.

58. Lee I, Budiawan H, Moon JY, Cheon GJ, Kim YC, Paeng JC, Kang KW, Chung JK, Lee DS. The value of SPECT/CT in localizing pain site and prediction of treatment response in patients with chronic low back pain. J Korean Med Sci. 2014;29(12):1711–6.

59. Hudyana H, Maes A, Vandenberghe T, Fidlers L, Sathekge M, Nicolai D, Van de Wiele C. Accuracy of bone SPECT/CT for identifying hardware loosening in patients who underwent lumbar fusion with pedicle screws. Eur J Nucl Med Mol Imaging. 2016;43(2):349–54.

60. Schleich FS, Schürch M, Huellner MW, Hug U, von Wartburg U, Strobel K, Veit-Haibach P. Diagnostic and therapeutic impact of SPECT/CT in patients with unspecific pain of the hand and wrist. EJNMMI Res. 2012;2(1):53.

61. Huellner MW, Bürkert A, Schleich FS, Schürch M, Hug U, von Wartburg U, Strobel K, Veit-Haibach P. SPECT/CT versus MRI in patients with nonspecific pain of the hand and wrist—a pilot study. Eur J Nucl Med Mol Imaging. 2012;39(5):750–9.

62. Huellner MW, Strobel K. Clinical applications of SPECT/CT in imaging the extremities. Eur J Nucl Med Mol Imaging. 2014;41(Suppl 1):S50–8.

63. Barthassat E, Afifi F, Konala P, Rasch H, Hirschmann MT. Evaluation of patients with painful total hip arthroplasty using combined single photon emission tomography and conventional computerized tomography (SPECT/CT)—a comparison of semi-quantitative versus 3D volumetric quantitative measurements. BMC Med Imaging. 2017;17(1):31.

64. Biersack HJ, Wingenfeld C, Hinterthaner B, Frank D, Sabet A. SPECT-CT of the foot. Nuklearmedizin. 2012;51(1):26–31.

65. Singh VK, Javed S, Parthipun A, Sott AH. The diagnostic value of single photon-emission computed tomography bone scans combined with CT (SPECT-CT) in diseases of the foot and ankle. Foot Ankle Surg. 2013;19(2):80–3.

66. Gnanasegaran G, Paycha F, Strobel K, van der Bruggen W, Kampen WU, Kuwert T, Van den Wyngaert T. Bone SPECT/CT in postoperative spine. Semin Nucl Med. 2018;48(5):410–24.

67. van der Bruggen W, Hirschmann MT, Strobel K, Kampen WU, Kuwert T, Gnanasegaran G, Van den Wyngaert T, Paycha F. SPECT/CT in the postoperative painful knee. Semin Nucl Med. 2018;48(5):439–53.

68. Van den Wyngaert T, Paycha F, Strobel K, Kampen WU, Kuwert T, van der Bruggen W, Gnanasegaran G. SPECT/CT in postoperative painful hip arthroplasty. Semin Nucl Med. 2018;48(5):425–38.

69. Strobel K, van der Bruggen W, Hug U, Gnanasegaran G, Kampen WU, Kuwert T, Paycha F, van den Wyngaert T. SPECT/CT in postoperative hand and wrist pain. Semin Nucl Med. 2018;48(5):396–409.

70. Kampen WU, Westphal F, Van den Wyngaert T, Strobel K, Kuwert T, Van der Bruggen W,

Gnanasegaran G, Jens JH, Paycha F. SPECT/CT in postoperative foot and ankle pain. Semin Nucl Med. 2018;48(5):454–68.

71. Love C, et al. Role of nuclear medicine in diagnosis of the infected joint replacement. Radiographics. 2001;21:122901238.

72. Classification of chronic pain. Descriptions of chronic pain syndromes and definitions of pain terms. Prepared by the International Association for the Study of Pain, Subcommittee on Taxonomy. Pain Suppl. 1986;3:S1–226. [PubMed] [Google Scholar].

73. Fischer SG, Perez RS. Complex regional pain syndrome-diagnosis, treatment and future perspectives. Eur Neurol Rev. 2011;6:270–5. [Google Scholar].

74. Goh EL, Chidambaram S, Ma D. Complex regional pain syndrome: a recent update. Burns Trauma. 2017;5:2. [PMC free article] [PubMed] [Google Scholar].

75. Birklein F, O'Neill D, Schlereth T. Complex regional pain syndrome: an optimistic perspective. Neurology. 2015;84:89–96. [PubMed] [Google Scholar].

76. Stanton-Hicks M, Jänig W, Hassenbusch S, Haddox JD, Boas R, Wilson P. Reflex sympathetic dystrophy: changing concepts and taxonomy. Pain. 1995;63:127–33.

77. Harden RN, Bruehl S, Stanton-Hicks M, Wilson PR. Proposed new diagnostic criteria for complex regional pain syndrome. Pain Med. 2007;8: 326–31.

78. Cappello ZJ, Kasdan ML, Louis DS. Meta-analysis of imaging techniques for the diagnosis of complex regional pain syndrome type I. J Hand Surg Am. 2012;37:288–96.

79. Wasner G, Schattschneider J, Binder A, Baron R. Complex regional pain syndrome—diagnostic, mechanisms, CNS involvement and therapy. Spinal Cord. 2003;41:61–75.

80. Schürmann M, Zaspel J, Löhr P, Wizgall I, Tutic M, Manthey N, et al. Imaging in early posttraumatic complex regional pain syndrome: a comparison of diagnostic methods. Clin J Pain. 2007;23:449–57. [PubMed] [Google Scholar].

81. Baroudi M, Derome P, Malo M. Severe heterotopic ossification and stiffness after revision knee surgery for a periprosthetic fracture. Arthroplasty Today. 2017;3:147–50.

82. Choi Y, Kim K, Lim S, Lim J. Early presentation of heterotopic ossification mimicking pyomyositis—two case reports. Ann Rehabil Med. 2012;36:713–8.

83. Nagaraj N, Elgazzar A, Fernandez-Ulloa M. Heterotopic ossification mimicking infection: scintigraphic evaluation. Clin Nucl Med. 1995;20:763–6.

84. Elgazzar AH. Orthopedic nuclear medicine. 2nd ed. New York: Springer; 2017.

85. Shehab D, Elgazzar H, Collier B. Heterotopic ossification. J Nucl Med. 2002;43:346–53.

86. Nitzan DW, Katsnelson A, Bermanis I, Brin I, Casap N. The clinical characteristics of condylar hyperplasia: experience with 61 patients. J Oral Maxillofac Surg. 2008;66(2):312–8.

87. Raijmakers PG, Karssemakers LH, Tuinzing DB. Female predominance and effect of gender on unilateral condylar hyperplasia: a review and meta-analysis. J Oral Maxillofac Surg. 2012;70(1):e72–6.

88. Olate S, Almeida A, Alister JP, et al. Facial asymmetry and condylar hyperplasia: considerations for diagnosis in 27 consecutives patients. Int J Clin Exp Med. 2013;6(10):937–41.

89. Karssemakers LH, Nolte JW, Saridin CP, Raijmakers PG, Becking AG. Unilateral condylar hyperactivity. Ned Tijdschr Tandheelkd. 2012;119(10):500–4.

90. Walters M, Claes P, Kakulas E, et al. Robust and regional 3D facial asymmetry assessment in hemimandibular hyperplasia and hemimandibular elongation anomalies. Int J Oral Maxillofac Surg. 2013;42(1):36–42.

91. Jones RH, Tier GA. Correction of facial asymmetry as a result of unilateral condylar hyperplasia. Int J Oral Maxillofac Surg. 2012;70(6):1413–25.

92. Karssemakers LH, Raijmakers PG, Nolte JW, Tuinzing DB, Becking AG. Interobserver variation of single-photon emission computed tomography bone scans in patients evaluated for unilateral condylar hyperactivity. Oral Surg Oral Med Oral Pathol Oral Radiol. 2013;115(3):399–405.

93. Nishimura M, Okamoto Y, Tokoro T, et al. Clinical potential of oral nicorandil to improve myocardial Fatty Acid metabolism after percutaneous coronary intervention in hemodialysis patients. Nephron Clin Pract. 2014;126(1):24–32.

94. Du C, Ying H, Zhou J, et al. Prediction of the response to docetaxel-based chemotherapy for locoregionally advanced nasopharyngeal carcinoma: the role of double-phase 99mTC-MIBI SPECT/CT. Med Oncol. 2014;31(2):833, 8 p.

95. Ventura M, Franssen GM, Oosterwijk E, Boerman OC, Jansen JA, Walboomers XF. SPECT vs. PET monitoring of bone defect healing and biomaterial performance in vivo. J Tissue Eng Regen Med. 2016;10(10):843–54.

96. Derlin T, Busch JD, Habermann CR. 99Tcm-MDP SPECT/CT for assessment of condylar hyperplasia. Clin Nucl Med. 2013;38(1):e48–9.

97. Alyamani A, Abuzinada S. Management of patients with condylar hyperplasia: a diverse experience with 18 patients. Ann Maxillofac Surg. 2012;2(1):17–23.

98. Sittitavornwong S, Gutta R. Bone graft harvesting from regional sites. Oral Maxillofac Surg Clin. 2010;22(3):317–30.

99. Berding G, Bothe K, Gratz KF, Schmelzeisen R, Neukam FW, Hundeshagen H. Bone scintigraphy in the evaluation of bone grafts used for mandibular reconstruction. Eur J Nucl Med. 1994;21(2):113–7.

100. Kirschner MH, Manthey N, Tatsch K, Nerlich A, Hahn K, Hofmann GO. Use of three-phase bone scans and SPET in the follow-up of patients with allogenic vascularized femur transplants. Nucl Med Commun. 1999;20:517–24. [PubMed] [Google Scholar].

101. Buyukdereli G, Guney IB, Ozerdem G, Kesiktas E. Evaluation of vascularized graft reconstruction of

the mandible with Tc-99m MDP bone scintigraphy. Ann Nucl Med. 2006;20:89–93. [PubMed] [Google Scholar].

102. Porter BA, Shields AF, Olson DO. Magnetic resonance imaging of bone marrow disorders. Radiol Clin North Am. 1986;24:269–89.

103. Fornasier VL, Czitrom AA. Collapsed vertebrae: a review of 659 autopsies. Clin Orthop. 1978;131:261–5.

104. Jung HS, Jee WH, McCauley TR, et al. Discrimination of metastatic from acute osteoporotic compression spinal fractures with MR imaging. Radiographics. 2003;23:179–87.

105. Fuster D, Tomás X, Mayoral M, Soriano A, Manchón F, Cardenal C, Monegal A, Granados U, Garcia S, Pons F. Prospective comparison of whole-body (18) F-FDG PET/CT and MRI of the spine in the diagnosis of haematogenous spondylodiscitis. Eur J Nucl Med Mol Imaging. 2015;42(2):264–71.

106. Jutte P, Lazzeri E, Sconfienza LM, Cassar-Pullicino V, Trampuz A, Petrosillo N, Signore A. Diagnostic flowcharts in osteomyelitis, spondylodiscitis and prosthetic joint infection. Q J Nucl Med Mol Imaging. 2014;58(1):2–19.

107. De Winter F, Gemmel F, Van De Wiele C, Poffijn B, Uyttendaele D, Dierckx R. 18-Fluorine fluorodeoxyglucose positron emission tomography for the diagnosis of infection in the postoperative spine. Spine (Phila Pa 1976). 2003;28(12):1314–9.

108. Fuster D, Solà O, Soriano A, Monegal A, Setoain X, Tomás X, Garcia S, Mensa J, Rubello D, Pons F. A prospective study comparing whole-body FDG PET/CT to combined planar bone scan with 67Ga SPECT/CT in the Diagnosis of Spondylodiskitis. Clin Nucl Med. 2012;37(9):827–32.

109. McCall IW, Park WM, O'Brien JP, Seal V. Acute traumatic intraosseous disc herniation. Spine (Phila Pa 1976). 1985;10(2):134–7.

110. Seymour R, Williams LA, Rees JI, Lyons K, Lloyd DC. Magnetic resonance imaging of acute intraosseous disc herniation. Clin Radiol. 1998;53(5):363–8.

111. Stabler A, Bellan M, Weiss M, Gartner C, Brossmann J, Reiser MF. MR imaging of enhancing intraosseous disk herniation (Schmorl's nodes). AJR Am J Roentgenol. 1997;168(4):933–8. https://doi.org/10.2214/ajr.168.4.9124143.

112. Trout AT, Sharp SE, Anton CG, Gelfand MJ, Mehlman CT. Spondylolysis and beyond: value of SPECT/CT in evaluation of low back pain in children and young adults. Radiographics. 2015;35(3):819–34. https://doi.org/10.1148/rg.2015140092.

113. Yagan R. CT diagnosis of limbus vertebra. J Comput Assist Tomogr. 1984;8(1):149–51.

114. Khashaba A. Acute intraosseous disc herniation. Injury. 2000;31(4):271–2.

115. Crawford BA, Van der Wall H. Bone scintigraphy in acute intraosseous disc herniation. Clin Nucl Med. 2007;32(10):790–2.

116. Elgazzar AH, Abdel-Dayem HM, Clark JD, et al. Multimodality imaging of osteomyelitis. Eur J Nucl Med. 1995;22:1043–63.

117. Hakim SG, Bruecker CW, Jacobsen H, et al. The value of FDG-PET and bone scintigraphy with SPECT in the primary diagnosis and follow-up of patients with chronic osteomyelitis of the mandible. Int J Oral Maxillofac Surg. 2006;35:809–16.

118. Horger M, Eschmann SM, Pfannenberg C, et al. Added value of SPECT/CT in patients suspected of having bone infection: preliminary results. Arch Orthop Trauma Surg. 2007;127:211–21.

119. Palestro CJ, Love C, Tronco GG, et al. Combined labeled leukocyte and technetium 99m sulfur colloid bone marrow imaging for diagnosing musculoskeletal infection. Radiographics. 2006;26:859–70.

120. Palestro CJ, Kim CK, Swyer AJ, et al. Total-hip arthroplasty: periprosthetic indium-111-labeled leukocyte activity and complementary technetium-99m-sulfur colloid imaging in suspected infection. J Nucl Med. 1990;31:1950–5.

121. Horger M, Eschmann SM, Pfannenberg C, et al. The value of SPET/CT in chronic osteomyelitis. Eur J Nucl Med Mol Imaging. 2003;30:1665–73.

Jan Bucerius

10.1 Introduction

Based on the data from National Health and Nutrition Examination Survey (NHANES) 2013 to 2016, an estimated 18.2 million Americans ≥20 years of age suffer from coronary heart disease (CHD) [1, 2]. In 2017, CHD caused approximately 365.914 deaths in the United States [1, 2].

It is well known, that the risk of patients with stable coronary artery disease (CAD) varies considerably based on the extent of anatomical involvement and of myocardial ischemia [3]. In addition, it is also known, that, unfortunately, a disagreement exists between the angiographic severity of CAD and myocardial perfusion abnormalities [4–6].

Hemodynamically significant CAD, which is defined as a coronary stenosis >50%, causes a narrowing of the lumen in one or several coronary arteries and, consequently, an impaired maximum perfusion to the myocardium. As a consequence, myocardial ischemia or infarction may occur in the respective territory of the left ventricle of the heart. Myocardial infarction depicts an irreversible condition, whereas myocardial ischemia is a reversible process which reflects a misbalance between the demand and the supply of oxygen to the myocardium. Under healthy conditions, the coronary artery dilates in response to this misbalance and an increased blood flow due to this vascular dilation leads to a delivery of additional oxygen. With pathological altered and narrowed vessels in the context of CAD, the response to the increased oxygen demand is limited due to the limited blood flow (classical angina) [7, 8]. As a less common cause of decreased myocardial perfusion, spasm of a coronary artery can mimic the clinical findings of CAD (Prinzmetal angina) [7, 8].

In general, the combination of two factors is usually responsible for the lack of blood supply to the myocardium: Firstly, a total or near-total occlusion of a coronary artery as described above, and, secondly, an insufficient flow through collateral vessels to meet the metabolic demands of tissue [7].

CAD usually develops over decades even though myocardial infarction can occur without any warning or signs of disease and can cause sudden death. Progression of coronary atheroma is accelerated in patients with diabetes, hypercholesterolemia, uremia, elevated homocysteine levels, and diets rich in saturated and trans fats. As already mentioned above, coronary stenosis >50% of the lumen diameter limit the maximum blood flow through the vessel, but still may not be accompanied by symptoms. In contrast, patients with stenoses >70% of the coronary lumen

J. Bucerius (✉)
Department of Nuclear Medicine, University Medicine Göttingen, Georg-August-University Göttingen, Göttingen, Germany
e-mail: jan.bucerius@med.uni-goettingen.de

frequently depict symptoms such as dyspnea and or chest pain during exertion. The vascular lumen must be narrowed by >90% to decrease myocardial perfusion at rest [7].

10.2 Myocardial Perfusion Imaging

Myocardial perfusion imaging (MPI) with single photon computed tomography (SPECT) offers a robust approach for diagnosing obstructive CAD, quantifying the magnitude of myocardium at risk, assessing the extent of tissue viability, and guiding therapeutic management with regard to patient selection for revascularization [9]. For further information about the methodic of MPI please refer to respective textbooks, reviews, and the respective guidelines of MPI of the Society of Nuclear Medicine and Molecular Imaging (SNMMI), the American Society of Nuclear Cardiology (ASNC), and the European Association of Nuclear Medicine (EANM) [10–12].

The reported average sensitivity of the myocardial perfusion SPECT for detecting >50% angiographic stenosis is 87% (range: 71–97%), whereas the average specificity is 73% (range: 36–100%) [9, 13]. It was shown, that by using attenuation correction methods especially the specificity of MPI might be improved, mainly among patients undergoing exercise stress testing [9, 13]. The very high negative predictive value (NPV) of a normal MPI of 99% has been proven among decades by a countless number of studies. Patients with CAD and a normal result of the MPI have an excellent prognosis with a cumulative cardiac event rate (cardiac-related death and non-fatal myocardial infarction) of less than 1% per year [13–21]. In a meta-analysis comprising 39 studies with almost 70,000 patients a normal myocardial perfusion SPECT was associated with a cumulative cardiac event rate of 0.85% per year [19]. In contrast, patients with a pathological result of the MPI were identified with a cardiac event rate of 5.9% per year [19].

However, despite its widespread use and acceptance, a recognized limitation of MPI is that frequently only coronary territories supplied by the most severe stenosis are identified. Consequently, MPI is relatively insensitive to accurately delineate the extent of obstructive angiographic CAD, especially in the setting of multivessel CAD. In a recent study of 101 patients with significant angiographic left main coronary stenosis, Berman et al. reported that by perfusion assessment alone, even with gated-SPECT, high-risk disease with moderate to severe perfusion defects (involving >10% myocardium at stress) was identified in only 59% by quantitative analysis. Conversely, absence of significant perfusion defect ($\geq$5% myocardium) was seen in 15% of patients [22]. Gated-SPECT, for which data are recorded with synchronization to the patient's cardiac cycle, further improves the diagnostic performance of MPI as it is processed to show regional wall motion and ejection fraction in addition to myocardial perfusion data [7].

As another limitation, based on the nature of MPI SPECT, it can only detect coronary lesions that induce perfusion defects, i.e., flow-limiting stenosis. Obviously, MPI is therefore not able to exclude the presence of subclinical nonobstructive coronary atherosclerosis [19, 23–25]. This is potentially important, especially in patient subgroups with an intermediate-high clinical risk in whom extensive subclinical CAD may be observed and may explain, at least in part, the limitations of perfusion imaging alone to identify low-risk patients among those with high clinical risk (e.g., diabetes, end-stage renal disease) [9, 19, 26].

To further strengthen this limitation, it has to be pointed out that approximately 70% of plaque ruptures leading to myocardial infarctions occur in lesions that are nonobstructive and therefore may be missed by SPECT [27]. Indeed, large longitudinal studies in patients undergoing myocardial perfusion SPECT have shown that a substantial proportion of patients suffering from cardiac events (43% of patients suffering an acute MI and 31% succumbing to cardiac death) have normal or near-normal perfusion scans prior to their event [28, 29].

10.3 Cardiac CT

10.3.1 Coronary Artery Calcium CT

Coronary artery calcium (CAC) is a constituent of atherosclerosis detected almost exclusively in atherosclerotic arteries and CAC detection has become an established method for cardiovascular risk assessment, which is particularly useful in asymptomatic intermediate risk individuals [30, 31].

The Agatston score is one of the most common methods used for CAC scoring that is calculated by multiplying the lesion area by a density factor [32]. However, one major drawback of the Agatston score is related to the fact, that the increase of that score over time might just represent an increase in plaque attenuation (density) rather than plaque size over time [33]. Additionally, only a small percentage of patients with coronary calcifications are also identified with a coronary stenosis [34].

Evaluation of CAC is nowadays supported by current guidelines, systemic reviews and large scaled population studies reporting high major adverse cardiac events (MACE) rates in patients with high CAC scores [35–38]. It is well known that the risk of MACE increases with the extent of CAC. For patients with high CAC scores (>400) the risk for MACE is up to $\geq 2\%$, which is similar to that of patients with established CAD, for patients. In contrast, patients with no CAC face an annual MACE rate of approximately 0.4% [35, 36].

Even more impressive, in a recent meta-analysis involving 29,312 asymptomatic patients with a zero CAC score with a mean follow-up period of 50 months, only 154 of patients (0.47%) without CAC had a cardiovascular event during follow-up, as compared with 1749 of 42,283 patients (4.14%) with CAC. The cumulative relative risk ratio was 0.15 (95% CI: 0.11–0.21, $p < 0.001$) [39]. Furthermore, it was also shown, that a zero CAC score was more predictive than a negative intima media thickness test or negative stress test of decreased cardiovascular events [40, 41].

As already mentioned above, despite the doubtless advantages of determining CAC in patients suspected for CAD, very high CAC does not necessarily confirm the presence of obstructive CAD. However, according to the Mayo Clinic guidelines, the probability of the presence of a hemodynamically significant stenosis is greater in patients with a calcium score (CS) >400 (Table 10.1) [34, 42].

Table 10.1 Standardized categories for the CAC score

Agatston score	Calcium score categories	Probability of significant CAD	Cardiovascular risk	Recommendations
0	Absent	Very unlikely (<5%)	Very low	Reassure patient. General guidelines for primary prevention of CV diseases
1–10	Minimal	Very unlikely (<10%)	Low	General guidelines for primary prevention of CV diseases
11–100	Mild	Mild or minimal coronary stenosis likely	Moderate	Counsel about risk factors modification, strict adherence with primary prevention goals. Daily ASA
101–400	Moderate	Non obstructive CAD, highly likely, obstructive CAD possible	Moderately high	Institute risk factor modification and secondary prevention goals. Consider exercise testing
>400	Extensive	High likelihood of significant coronary stenosis (>90%)	High	Institute very aggressive risk factor modification. Consider exercise or pharmacological nuclear stress testing for the detection o inducible ischemia

CV cardiovascular; *ASA* acetylsalicylic acid
(Adapted from: Cademartiri F, Casolo G, Midiri M, eds: Calcium score and coronary plaque, In Clinical Applications of Cardiac CT. New York: Springer; 2012:121) [41]
From: Youssef G, Kalia N, Darabian S, Budoff MJ. Coronary Calcium: New Insights, Recent Data, and Clinical Role. Curr Cardiol Rep 2013; 15: 325 (please also refer to cited reference in Table 10.1) [34]

On the other hand, a very low or negative CAC cannot completely exclude obstructive CAD. This is mainly due for patients with non-calcified plaques, which are typically present in younger patients or young smokers [35, 36]. Furthermore, even despite the known correlation between increased calcium burden, atherosclerosis and obstructive CAD, a modest only relationship between calcified plaque burden and obstructive CAD could be found [43–45]. Nevertheless, information about CAC improves the pre-coronary computed tomographic angiography (CCTA) probability of obstructive CAD and can help in the interpretation of CCTA since the non-contrast scan used for CAC determination may be able to better demonstrate calcifications than the contrast study used for CCTA [35].

10.3.2 Coronary Computed Tomographic Angiography

CCTA has advanced over the past years as the most accurate tool for noninvasive coronary angiography. Current multi-slice devices coupled with improved acquisition protocols allow robust and reproducible assessment of coronary morphology with high temporal and spatial resolution at rather low-radiation exposure [46–48]. CCTA was shown to obtain high-quality images of the coronary arteries with an average sensitivity for detecting at least one coronary artery with a >50% stenosis is 94% (range: 75–100%). On the other hand, specificity falls off compared to the sensitivity with an average value of 77% (range: 49–100%) [9, 49]. The corresponding average positive predictive value (PPV) and NPV are 84% (range: 50–100%) and 87% (range: 35–100%), respectively, and the overall diagnostic accuracy is 89% (range: 68–100%) [9, 49].

The robustness of 64-row CCTA for complete visualization of the coronary tree was recently confirmed by two multicenter, single-vendor trials [26, 50].

In the 2008 published Assessment by Coronary Computed Tomographic Angiography of Individuals Undergoing Invasive Coronary Angiography (ACCURACY) trial, 230 chest pain patients without known CAD were included and underwent both CCTA and invasive coronary angiography (ICA). On a patient-based model, the sensitivity, specificity, PPV, and NPV to detect ≥50% or ≥70% coronary stenosis were 95%, 83%, 64%, and 99%, respectively, and 94%, 83%, 48%, 99%, respectively. However, the specificity was found to be significantly reduced in case of calcium scores ≥400 [26]. The authors concluded, that 64-row CCTA possesses a high diagnostic accuracy for the detection of obstructive coronary stenosis at both thresholds of 50 and 70% stenosis. Furthermore, based on the 99% NPV, CCTA might be established as an effective noninvasive alternative to ICA to rule out obstructive coronary artery stenosis.

The Coronary Artery Evaluation Using 64-Row Multidetector Computed Tomography Angiography (CORE-64) trial enrolled 291 patients with a prevalence of obstructive CAD of 56% and CAC scores ≤600. As with in the ACCURACY trial, all patients underwent CCTA and ICA. However, the CORE-64 trial provides additional evidence that is somewhat discordant to the ACCURACY trial and to initial results from single-center studies [26, 50, 51]. On a per-patient basis, a sensitivity for detecting at least 1 coronary artery with ≥50% stenosis of 85% was found, which is considerably lower than in single-center studies and in the ACCURACY trial using similar technology [26, 50, 51]. In contrast, the specificity was 90%, higher than what was previously reported. The corresponding average PPV and NPV were 91% and 83%, respectively, surprisingly different from those in most previous studies [50, 51]. This relatively high PPV and low NPV might be explained by the high prevalence of obstructive CAD in the patients studied.

However, another prospective, multicenter, multi-vendor study with 64-row MDCT CCTA involving 360 symptomatic patients with acute and stable angina and an even higher prevalence of CAD (68%) reported values of sensitivity, specificity, PPV and NPV for detecting ≥50% stenoses, on a patient-based model, of 99%, 64%, 86%, and 97%, respectively [52]. No patients or segments were excluded because of impaired image quality attributable to either coronary motion or calcifications, which may have led to the low specificity reported in this trial [52].

Except for the CORE 64 trial study, these and other single-center studies consistently reported that CCTA has a particularly high NPV and allows the identification of CAD at an early stage, before emergence of ischemia [35]. From a clinical perspective, a normal CCTA is therefore helpful, as it effectively excludes the presence of obstructive CAD and the need for further testing [9]. Furthermore, CCTA with no detectable plaque defines a low clinical risk with an excellent prognosis with an annual event rate of 0.3%, and makes management decisions straight-forward [53].

However, one has to keep in mind, that the results are generally limited to relatively large vessel sizes ($\geq$1.5 mm), excluding the results of smaller or uninterpretable vessels (generally distal vessels and side branches). The inclusion of these "difficult" vessels would lower the sensitivity. Furthermore, based on the anatomical related nature of this imaging technique, CCTA does not provide information on myocardial perfusion or metabolism. This is mainly critical as it was shown that percent narrowing or absolute stenosis lumen area on ICA correlates poorly with the degree of impaired coronary flow reserve [54]. Accordingly, only half of the lesions considered significant on CCTA are linked with abnormal perfusion [23, 55–57]. All of these data clearly indicate, that luminal obstruction of the coronaries seen on CCTA does not necessarily indicate the presence of ischemia. Importantly, although a normal CCTA practically excludes relevant hemodynamic CAD, the inverse is frequently not true [35]. Obviously, there seem to be many factors that might influence the relation between anatomical findings and functional, i. e. hemodynamically, consequences, which cannot in total be clarified by anatomical imaging alone [58].

10.4 Integration of Nuclear MPI and CT

Whereas the superiority of applying dual-modality imaging for improved detection and staging of cancer has been proven over years by the results of hybrid positron emission tomography (PET) and CT (PET/CT) imaging, that concept still needs to be proven to be beneficial in the cardiovascular setting as well. This is mainly due for the relatively new hybrid SPECT/CT technique. The aim of hybrid imaging is to provide an accurate spatial alignment between separate anatomical (CT) and functional (MPI) data sets into one fused image. CT scanners are nowadays able to image cardiac and coronary anatomy with high spatial resolution. On the other hand, nuclear imaging in general and MPI in particular can sensitively and reliably identify functional abnormalities. This information together with imaging of the morphology by means of CT might be able to provide information beyond that achievable with either stand-alone or side-by-side interpretation of the respective data sets [9, 35]. It is obvious, that in hybrid imaging both data sets contribute equally to the image information, which helps to reduce the number of equivocal results [59].

Furthermore, it was shown, that hybrid MPI and CCTA can accurately allocate the culprit lesion in multivessel CAD, which is particularly important because in more than half of the cases, the proposed "standard" distribution of myocardial perfusion territories does not correspond with the individual coronary anatomy [60, 61]. MPI information helps to overcome the drawback of a reduced sensitivity of CCTA in distal coronary segments and side branches as mentioned above. In contrast, one of the main pitfalls of semiquantitative MPI, the diagnosis of multivessel CAD, can be improved by adding CCTA information [35]. Additionally, assessing regional myocardial perfusion with MPI together with information about the coronary artery tree as provided by CCTA eliminates uncertainties in the relationship of perfusion defects, scar regions and diseased coronary arteries in watershed regions, mainly in patients with multiple perfusion abnormalities and multivessel CAD [35].

10.4.1 Integration of CT with MPI for Attenuation Correction

One of the drawbacks of MPI is the non-homogeneous photon attenuation in the thorax which may reduce both, specificity and sensitivity of MPI. Whereas non-uniform regional perfusion defects may be misinterpreted as a perfusion defect and therefore may impact specificity of MPI, sensitivity may be reduced due to improperly scaling of images to regions suppressed by attenuation, potentially masking true perfusion defects [35]. Correcting for these attenuation artifacts in cardiac imaging remains being a challenge because of cardiac and respiratory motion [62, 63]. CT as part of hybrid SPECT/CT imaging technique seems to have the potential to overcome these problems as using the CT component for attenuation correction improved the specificity of SPECT MPI to 80–90% [64]. However, one needs to take into account, that despite the fact, that SPECT/CT studies have shown that low-dose CT acquisition is feasible for attenuation correction in cardiac imaging, a potential misalignment between emission and transmission data might cause incomplete correction and, consequently, artificial perfusion defects [35]. Therefore, careful quality control to avoid reconstruction artifacts is mandatory. It was recently shown, that the frequency of these misalignments is quite high with significant clinical consequences in case they are not corrected [65, 66]. Notably, mainly because of the lower spatial resolution of SPECT, the effect of misalignments is less severe for cardiac SPECT/CT compared to cardiac PET/CT [67]. Usually, the alignment of emission and transmission data is currently performed manually, which may lead to a relevant variability. However, steps toward automated methods for quality control have already been made and might offer a solution to overcome this drawback in the future [35, 68, 69].

10.4.2 MPI and CAC

Detection of CAC was shown to provide incremental value to MPI [70–72]. Recent reports suggest, that CAC may have the potential to improve the diagnostic and prognostic value of MPI. Mainly in case of a normal MPI, CAC was shown to potentially enhance the diagnosis of CAD, which was particularly due in severe multivessel CAD [72, 73]. There is growing evidence

that CAC scores are generally predictive of a higher likelihood of ischemia on MPI, and the available data support the concept of a threshold phenomenon governing this relationship [9]. Indeed, it was seen that myocardial ischemia was significantly more frequently diagnosed with increasing CAC scores. This was especially the fact among patients with CAC >400 [72, 74, 75].

The approach of combining CAC with MPI is promoted by the relative ease to obtain CAC images for which no contrast injection is needed and which is associated with a low overall radiation exposure. Furthermore, an increasing availability of hybrid scanners integrating low- or high-end CT devices with SPECT camera systems is seen and further supportive of implementing combined MPI and CAC imaging into clinical routine [47].

In a study by Schepis et al., a CAC score >709 was found to provide the optimal cutoff to detect patients with obstructive CAD despite normal perfusion in SPECT MPI [73]. In this situation, the normal SPECT imaging most likely reflects balanced ischemia. Using this threshold, the addition of the CAC score to the SPECT MPI data was reported to improve the sensitivity for identifying patients with obstructive CAD over the results of SPECT MPI alone, without a significant decrease in specificity. In contrast, CAC scores >400, especially in symptomatic patients with intermediate likelihood of CAD, may be less effective in excluding CAD. This is mainly the case in young subjects and women [73].

Regarding the added prognostic value of combining CAC with MPI, higher MACE rates are reported for patients with higher CAC scores, even in case of a normal stress MPI [76]. This is mainly due for patients with known CAD or with greater comorbidities [76]. Therefore, CAC as a direct marker of coronary atherosclerosis is helpful in identifying patients requiring a more intensive management of risk factors or follow-up protocol [35]. Furthermore, data suggest, that incremental risk stratification can be obtained by incorporating information about the anatomical extent of atherosclerosis as provided by CAC to conventional MPI without CT [9].

10.4.3 MPI and CCTA

The first clinical results of hybrid MPI and CCTA appear encouraging, as they support that this approach offer superior diagnostic information with regard to identification of the culprit vessels (Fig. 10.1) [9, 55, 77, 78]. This is mainly due to the fact, that MPI provides valuable clinical information regarding the pathophysiological significance of coronary stenoses, especially when the sensitivity of CCTA is substantially reduced, which is the case in more distal segments of the coronary arteries and side branches [9, 49]. Previously published studies indicate, that this benefit of combing CCTA with MPI becomes evident both in low-risk CAD populations as well as in patients with multivessel CAD [77, 79, 80]. In 2009, van Werkhoven et al. published their results about the incremental prognostic value over SPECT MPI alone in patients with suspected CAD [53]. In 541 patients referred for further cardiac evaluation, both multi-slice CCTA and MPI were performed. Both scans were performed with stand-alone CT and SPECT

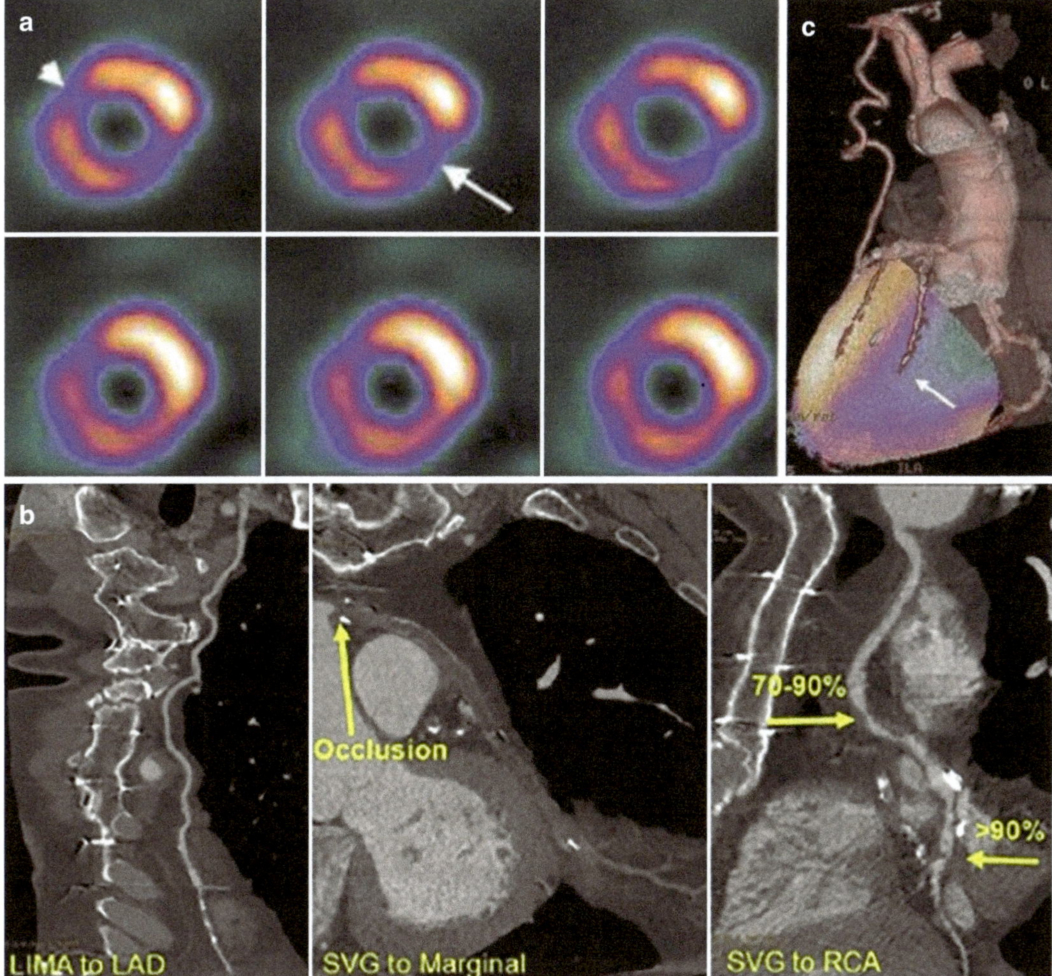

Fig. 10.1 Hybrid SPECT/CCTA. Reprinted with permission from: Rispler S, Aronson D, Abadi S, Roguin A, Engel A, Beyar R, Israel O, Keidar Z. Integrated SPECT/CT for assessment of haemodynamically significant coronary artery lesions in patients with acute coronary syndrome. Eur J Nucl Med Mol Imaging 2011; 38: 1917–1925 [81]

within a time frame of 3 months and therefore not using a "true" hybrid SPECT/CT approach. MACE were recorded over a median follow-up time of 672 days. The median hard event rate in patients with none or mild CAD by CCTA was 1.8% versus 4.8% in patients with significant CAD by CCTA. Accordingly, a normal MPI and abnormal MPI were associated with an annualized hard event rate of 1.1% and 3.8%, respectively. After adjustment for clinical risk factors, obstructive plaque detected by CCTA and an abnormal MPI was independently predictive for late events. This prediction significantly improved when combing the two modalities compared with either modality alone. Concordantly normal CCTA and MPI were associated with an annual event rate of 1%, whereas this rate increased to 9% in case of concordantly abnormal CCTA and MPI results. Importantly, the presence of non-calcified plaques provided incremental prognostic information over baseline clinical variables, MPI, and significant CAD on CCTA [53].

In a study by Rispler et al., published in 2007, 56 patients with angina pectoris underwent single-session SPECT MPI and CCTA with a hybrid SPECT/16-row CT device and coronary angiography within 4 weeks [55]. The ability of fused SPECT/CCTA images to diagnose physiologically significant lesions showing >50% stenosis and reversible perfusion defects in the same territory was determined and compared with CCTA stand-alone. They found a total of 224 coronary segments in the 56 patients included, 12 patients and 54 segments (23%) were excluded from further analysis of CCTA. Therefore, a total of 170 coronary segments were evaluated. The sensitivity, specificity, PPV, and NPV of CCTA were 96%, 63%, 31%, and 99%, respectively, as compared with 96%, 95%, 77%, and 99%, respectively, for combined SPECT/CCTA. Based on these results, it becomes quite obvious, that hybrid SPECT/CCTA imaging mainly results in improved specificity and PPV to detect hemodynamically significant coronary lesions in patients with chest pain [55].

Several other studies underscored the incremental diagnostic accuracy or co-registration and fusion of stand-alone acquired MPI and CCTA over side-by-side interpretation (Table 10.2) [9, 77, 82, 83]. Further strengthen these findings, Rispler et al. found added diagnostic information provided by fused analysis not obtained on side-by-side analysis in almost one-third of patients [55].

In another, well-designed and recently published study by Schaap et al., the diagnostic performance of hybrid SPECT/CCTA versus stand-alone SPECT and CCTA for the diagnosis of significant CAD was evaluated [84]. Ninety-eight patients with stable angina complaints and a median pre-test likelihood of 87% were prospectively included in their study. Hybrid

Table 10.2 Diagnostic value of SPECT/CT or PET/CT software image fusion compared with side-by-side analysis

Technology	N	Benefit by hybrid imaging	Reference
SPECT/64-row MDCT and 3-D image fusion	38 patients with ≥1 SPECT defects	Among equivocal lesions, haemodynamic significance is confirmed in 35% and excluded in 25%	10
16- and 64-row MDCT and MPI (SPECTor ^{82}Rb PET)	50 patients suspected of CAD	Modification of the initial interpretation in 28% of the cases Trend to increase in 17% the sensitivity in patients with multivessel disease	11
Automated SPECT/64-row MDCT registration software	35 patients suspected of CAD	Improved diagnostic performance in the RCA and LCx, not in LAD	79

N number of patients, *RCA* right coronaty artery, *LCx* left circumflex artery, *LAD* left anterior descending artery
Reprinted with permission from: Flotats A, Knuuti J, Gutberlet M, Marcassa C, Bengel FM, Kaufmann PA, Rees MR, Hesse B; Cardiovascular Committee of the EANM, the ESCR and the ECNC. Hybrid cardiac imaging: SPECT/CT and PET/CT. A joint position statement by the European Association of Nuclear Medicine (EANM), the European Society of Cardiac Radiology (ESCR) and the European Council of Nuclear Cardiology (ECNC). Eur J Nucl Med Mol Imaging 2011; 38: 201–212 [35]
Reference [10] (Table) = 77 (manuscript); 11 = 83; 79 = 82

SPECT/CCTA was performed prior to conventional coronary angiography. Hybrid analysis was performed by combined interpretation of SPECT and CCTA images. The diagnostic performance was calculated for hybrid SPECT/CCTA and stand-alone SPECT and CCTA on per patient level. Fractional flow reserve measurements <0.80 served as a reference for significant CAD and was seen in 57.9% of the patients included. Non-conclusive SPECT or CCTA results were found in 32.7% of the patients. Stand-alone SPECT and CCTA had a sensitivity of 93%, specificity 79%, PPV 85%, NPV 89% and a sensitivity of 98%, specificity 62%, PPV 77%, and NPV 96%, respectively. Hybrid analysis of SPECT and CCTA led to an improved overall performance with a sensitivity, specificity, PPV, and NPV for the presence of significant CAD of 96, 95, 96, and 95%, respectively [84]. Based on the results of the study, two highly interesting conclusions can be drawn. First of all, in >40% of the patients with a high pre-test likelihood no significant CAD was demonstrated. This clearly emphasizes the value of accurate pre-treatment cardiovascular imaging. Secondly, by combing SPECT and CCTA, significant CAD can be accurately diagnosed and excluded, surpassing the diagnostic performance of stand-alone myocardial SPECT and CCTA [84].

Whereas CCTA alone tends to overestimate coronary stenosis, the combination with MPI, and therefore with the information about the hemodynamic relevance of the observed stenosis, allows the identification of many false-positive CCTA findings [35]. Mainly in case of motion artifacts or severe coronary calcifications, the specificity and PPV of stand-alone CCTA becomes suboptimal [35]. In this context, it needs to be pointed out, that non-evaluable, severely calcified vessels especially benefit from further testing due to the relatively high likelihood of obstructive disease, whereas non-evaluable vessels with motion artifacts do not usually have hemodynamic relevance. The latter is particularly the case in the right coronary artery (RCA) territory [35, 85]. However, hybrid imaging with CCTA and SPECT MPI is not only of particular value in the RCA, but also in lesions of distal segments, diagonal branches, and the left circumflex artery (LCX) [77, 83]. On the other hand, CCTA improves the detection of multivessel CAD, which is one of the main pitfalls of MPI as already mentioned above, and increases the diagnostic confidence for categorizing intermediate lesions and equivocal perfusion defects [9, 55].

10.5 Radiation Exposure

Both, SPECT and CT are diagnostic modalities that use ionizing radiation to generate images for the functional and morphological evaluation of the heart.

The radiation exposure related to MPI is lower for the nowadays most frequently used ^{99m}Tc(^{99m}technetium-)-labeled agents (like ^{99m}Tc-sestamibi, ^{99m}Tc-tetrofosmin) compared to the use of ^{201}thallium (^{201}Tl). Depending on the applied protocol (1- or 2-day protocol), the injected dose, and the used camera system, the radiation exposure of ^{99m}Tc-sestamibi or ^{99m}Tc-tetrofosmin may differ with an increasing dose by applying a 1-day protocol. The reported effective doses for ^{99m}Tc-sestamibi (rest) are 0.009 mSv/MBq (stress: 0.0079 mSv/MBq) and for ^{99m}Tc-tetrofosmin (rest) 0.0069 mSv/MBq (stress: 0.0069 mSv/MBq), respectively. For ^{201}Tl, one has to consider an effective dose of 0.14 mSv/MBq, which will even increase with a re-injection of ^{201}Tl [10, 86–88]. However, nowadays, SPECT-related radiation exposure can be markedly reduced by the use of new iterative reconstruction methods in combination with dedicated detectors and collimators optimized specifically for MPI [89, 90]. Further emphasizing the necessity of reducing the radiation exposure to the patients in MPI, a statement document was published by Cerqueira et al. in 2010 regarding the best practice methods to further minimize the radiation exposure of MPI by obtaining the highest quality diagnostic images [91].

The effective patient radiation dose from cardiac CT varies widely depending on the protocol, instrumentation, and patient size [35]. For a CAC scan, which can also be used to perform MPI attenuation correction, the radiation exposure of approximately 1 mSv is rather low [92]. However, the dose tends to be higher with lower slice thickness, as in this case, the radiation dosage needs to be increased to obtain the same signal to noise ratio [93]. In a 2009 published cross-sectional, international, multicenter study of 1965 CCTA scans performed at 50 study sites, the estimated mean radiation dose was 12 mSv (interquartile range: 8–18 mSv) [94]. A reduction of the radiation exposure can be achieved by implementation of modern cardiac CT acquisition protocols. Prospective (step-and-shoot) ECG triggering, ECG-controlled current modulation (reduction of the tube current by 80% during systole) and body mass-adapted tube voltage (reduction of the tube voltage to 100 kV in patients <90 kg of weight) allow reduction of the radiation dose from CCTA by 60–80% [79, 95–97]. Along with this, application of the most recent high-pitch scanning protocols using dual-source CT scanners have even further lowered doses into the sub-milli-Sievert range [46, 47].

10.6 Clinical Applications

It is well accepted, that the clinical use of imaging should depend on the pre-test likelihood of CAD [35]. In the 2011 joint position statement by the European Association of Nuclear Medicine (EANM), the European Society of Cardiac Radiology (ESCR) and the European Council of Nuclear Cardiology (ECNC), a proposed clinical algorithm for the use of imaging techniques, including hybrid imaging, in patients with chronic chest pain was published (Fig. 10.2) [35]. Furthermore, it was stated, that for symptomatic patients without known CAD and low to moderate pre-test (i. e. <50%-) likelihood of disease, which is typically seen in young and middle-aged patients, CCTA would probably be essential to (virtually) exclude CAD [35]. Whereas in case of a normal result, further diagnostic tests are avoided, abnormal or equivocal findings need to be confirmed or rejected by MPI or ICA [35]. Especially in these patients, hybrid imaging would lead to a more rapid diagnosis. Today, when initial tests yield equivocal results and fur-

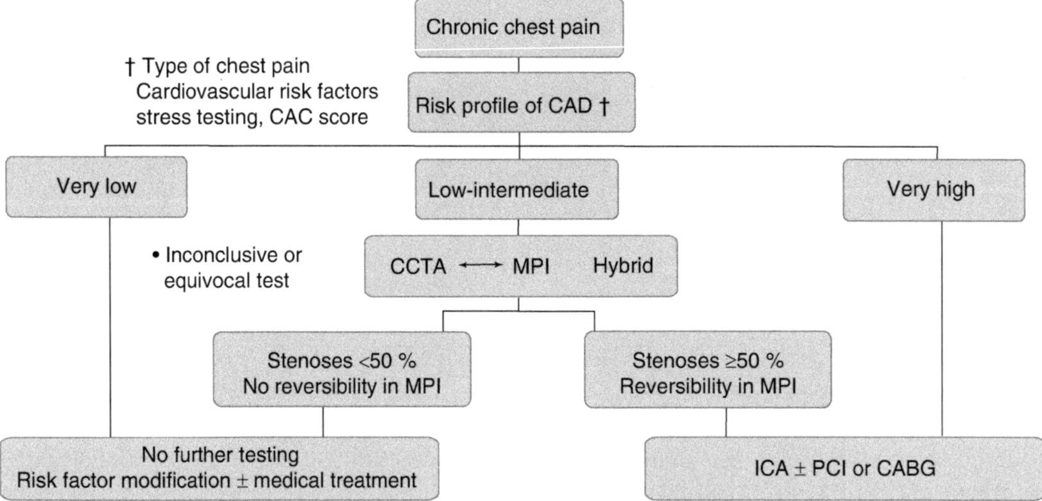

Fig. 10.2 Proposed algorithm for the clinical use of different imaging modalities. From: Flotats A, Knuuti J, Gutberlet M, Marcassa C, Bengel FM, Kaufmann PA, Rees MR, Hesse B; Cardiovascular Committee of the EANM, the ESCR and the ECNC. Hybrid cardiac imaging: SPECT/CT and PET/CT. A joint position statement by the European Association of Nuclear Medicine (EANM), the European Society of Cardiac Radiology (ESCR) and the European Council of Nuclear Cardiology (ECNC). Eur J Nucl Med Mol Imaging 2011; 38: 201–212 [35]

ther assessment to exclude CAD with final certainty is needed, many of these patients are referred for ICA. Hybrid cardiac imaging offers a substantially improved diagnostic confidence and the more frequent use of these techniques would therefore result in a reduction of the number of patients, which are currently unnecessarily exposed to ICA [35].

In patients with higher pre-test likelihood of disease (i.e., >50% likelihood), which are characteristically those with known CAD or older age, MPI might be a better first-line test compared to CCTA [35]. This group of patients is more likely to have extensive CAC and also includes patients with known or suspected microvascular endothelial dysfunction, e.g., diabetics [35, 85, 98]. In case of equivocal MPI findings, suggestive of artifacts, microvascular- or multivessel disease, CCTA can be added. In these patients, the hybrid imaging approach would lead to an improved diagnostic accuracy and would also allow for a complete evaluation of the hemodynamic relevance of coronary stenosis and the assessment of the viability in myocardial territories supplied by occluded arteries [35]. The accurate co-registration of CCTA- and MPI data, would allow to gain information about coronary stenoses and perfusion defects and therefore would also improve the evaluation of hemodynamic properties of even fairly small coronary branches [35]. By confirming the hemodynamic relevance of given lesions, hybrid cardiac imaging might help to avoid potentially harmful revascularization attempts and also provides a platform for multidisciplinary coronary teams including an interventional cardiologist and a cardiac surgeon to discuss the most appropriate treatment strategy (medical conservative vs. percutaneous vs. surgical revascularization) [47]. In this context, Schaap et al. prospectively evaluated, to what extent treatment decisions for patients with stable angina pectoris can be made based on hybrid MPI SPECT and CCTA as the question remains whether these imaging results lead to similar treatment decisions as compared to stand-alone SPECT and ICA [99]. They included 107 patients with stable anginal complaints and an intermediate to high pre-test likelihood for CAD. The

study outcome was the treatment decision categorized as: no revascularization, percutaneous coronary intervention (PCI) or coronary artery bypass grafting (CABG). Treatment decisions were made in two steps. Firstly, based on the results of hybrid SPECT/CCTA and, secondly, based on SPECT and ICA. Based on the latter approach, revascularization (PCI or CABG) was indicated in 50% of the patients. Percentage agreement of treatment decisions in all patients based on hybrid SPECT/CCTA versus SPECT and conventional angiography on the necessity of revascularization was 92%. Percentage agreement of treatment decisions in patients with matched, unmatched and normal hybrid SPECT/CCTA findings was 95%, 84% and 100%, respectively. Therefore, combining functional data from SPECT and anatomical information from CCTA was be able to accurately indicate for and defer patients from revascularization [99].

In asymptomatic patients with moderate pre-test likelihood of disease CAC imaging is recommended as a reasonable choice for refining the risk stratification [35, 100].

Besides the named joint EANM, ESCR, and ECNC position statement about hybrid imaging, a SNMMI (Society of Nuclear Medicine and Molecular Imaging)/ASNC (American Society of Nuclear Cardiology)/SCCT (Society of Cardiovascular CT) guideline for cardiac SPECT/CT and PET/CT (version 1.0) was published in 2013 and can be referred for further information [10, 35].

10.7 Future Perspective of Cardiac SPECT/CT

Even though several studies indicated the usefulness of cardiac SPECT/CT in terms of impact on treatment strategy and consequently on outcome, confirmation of those promising results of the relevance of functional and anatomical cardiac imaging by prospective, well-powered multicenter trials including appropriate follow-up periods was clearly needed. In such an attempt several studies such as the SPARC-, EVINCI- and PROMISE trial had been set up several years ago and, in the meanwhile, provided new data regarding the benefit of hybrid cardiac imaging [6, 47, 101–107].

In 2012, the results of the SPARC (Study of Myocardial Perfusion and Coronary Anatomy Imaging Roles in Coronary Artery Disease) trial on 1.709 patients without a documented history of CAD and an intermediate to high likelihood of CAD undergoing cardiac SPECT, PET, or 64-slice CCTA were published by Hachamovitch et al. [105]. Based on the assessment of the 90-day post-test rates of coronary catheterization and medication changes, they found noninvasive studies with only a modest impact on the clinical management of patients referred for clinical testing. Not surprisingly, the post-imaging use of cardiac catheterization and medical therapy increased in proportion to the degree of abnormal study results, however, the frequency of catheterization and medication use suggested possible undertreatment of higher-risk patients. Interestingly, compared with functional imaging with stress MPI, catheterization referral rates and subsequent need for revascularization were greater after CCTA together with similar rates of medication use in patients after normal/nonobstructive and mildly abnormal study findings [105]. However, the main results of the SPARC trial are discussed controversially and concluding, that noninvasive testing has only a modest impact in clinical management of patients referred for clinical testing seem to be rather preliminary [108]. In this context, the 2015 published PROMISE (PROspective Multicenter Imaging Study for Evaluation of chest pain) trial including 10.003 symptomatic patients referred to a strategy of initial anatomical testing with the use of CCTA or to functional testing (exercise electrocardiography, nuclear stress testing, or stress echocardiography) revealed that CCTA was associated with fewer catheterizations showing no obstructive CAD than was functional testing (3.4% vs. 4.3%, $p = 0.02$), although more patients in the CCTA group underwent catheterization within 90 days after randomization (12.2% vs. 8.1%). The results of this trial strengthen the impact of functional testing in symptomatic patients with suspected CAD who required noninvasive testing and revealed that an initial strategy of CCTA was not associated with better clinical outcomes than functional testing over a median follow-up of 2 years [106]. Based on those two well-designed prospective trials one could at least assume, that combining functional MPI with anatomical information by CCTA might pave the way for a higher impact of noninvasive cardiac imaging on post-test clinical management of the patients and might overcome drawbacks of each imaging modality by combing their benefits. With that regard, the results of the EVINCI trial as well as of a meta-analysis published by Rizvi et al. in 2018 are quite elucidating [6, 107].

The ENVICI-(EValuation of INtegrated Cardiac Imaging for the Detection and Characterization of Ischaemic Heart Disease) trial included 252 patients with stable angina and intermediate (i.e. 20–90%) pre-test likelihood of CAD who underwent myocardial perfusion scintigraphy (MPS), CCTA, and quantitative coronary angiography (QCA) with fractional flow reserve (FFR) and aimed to evaluate the added value of hybrid (i.e. MPS/CCTA) cardiac imaging in diagnosing hemodynamically significant CAD [6]. QCA revealed an overall prevalence of significant CAD (>70% stenosis or 30–70% with FFR $\leq$ 0.80) in the included patients of 37%. MPS identified 1004 pathological myocardial segments of which 246 (25%) had to be reclassified from their standard coronary distribution to another territory by hybrid imaging [6]. Accordingly, hybrid imaging reassigned an entire perfusion defect to another coronary territory in 45 of the 252 (18%) patients, leading to a change of the final diagnosis in 42% of cases. Furthermore, hybrid imaging led to a noninvasive CAD rule-out (41% of patients) and to a rule-in (24% of patients) in two-thirds of the included patients. Consequently, hybrid imaging was associated with negative and positive predictive values of 88% and 87%, respectively and with a more reliable co-localization of myocardial perfusion defects with subtending coronary arteries than standardized myocardial segmentation models accounting for variations in individual coronary anatomy [6]. Underscoring the beneficial effects of combining functional and anatomical cardiac imaging, data of a meta-analysis published by Rizvi et al. in 2018 demonstrated different hybrid cardiac imaging approaches (SPECT/CCTA, PET/CCTA, CMR/CCTA) in general to improve diagnostic specificity for the detection of obstructive CAD compared with stand-alone CCTA [107]. Among the three distinct hybrid imaging modalities as mentioned above, hybrid SPECT/CCTA demonstrated the highest sensitivity at both a per-patient and per-vessel level for assessment of obstructive CAD and PET/CCTA the highest specificity also on a per-patient as well as per-vessel level [107].

From a more technical point of view, at this point it still remains uncertain to some degree whether hybrid scanners offer advantages over software fusion of data sets obtained from different scanners, as by either way one can obtain hybrid images [109]. The scan time discrepancy between emission from nuclear and CT transmission determines that high-end CT facilities constituting the CT component of hybrid cardiac scanners will be blocked by long emission scan time and is therefore forced to operate at low capacity. Furthermore, the integrated scanner also makes it more difficult and expensive to integrate the rapid changes in technology, especially CT [9]. On the other hand, a combined device may fit into one room and needs one operating team and does not require positioning of the patient into two different scanners. The development of ultrafast SPECT scanners allowing substantially shorter acquisition time may shift the balance toward hybrid scanners in the future [9].

The potential diagnostic benefit of hybrid cardiac SPECT/CT needs to be weighed against the potential drawbacks, especially with regard to the added radiation dose to the patients. However, new low-dose CCTA acquisition protocols with prospective ECG triggering have recently been introduced and shown to offer a tremendous reduction in radiation dose to an average of 2.1 mSv at maintained accuracy [95, 110–112].

Finally, moderate to severe cardiac mismatch between MPI and CT might impact the quality of the fused images and therefore the diagnostic performance of the hybrid imaging approach (Fig. 10.3a) [113]. With current SPECT/CT systems, the low-dose CT obtained for attenuation correction and the SPECT data are acquired sequentially, and patient movement may occur between the two types of acquisition (Fig. 10.3b) [113]. Misregistration may occur if care is not taken in the acquisition and processing of the datasets and may lead to new and unexpected kinds of artifacts. Importantly, even a registration error of as little as 7 mm can lead to a substantial

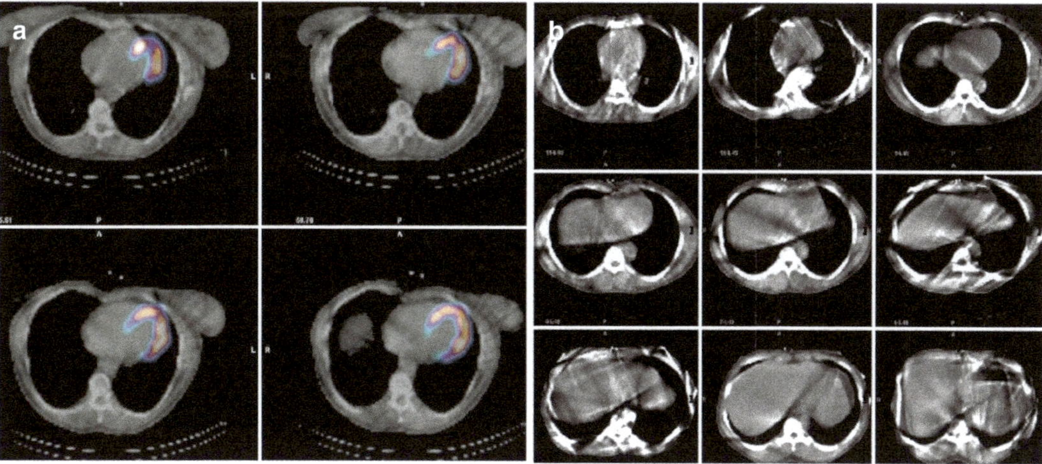

Fig. 10.3 (**a**, **b**) Examples of sources of artifacts in hybrid cardiac SPECT/CT imaging. From: Goetze S, Wahl RL. Prevalence of misregistration between SPECT and CT for attenuation-corrected myocardial perfusion SPECT. J Nucl Cardiol 2007; 14: 200–206 [113]

degradation in the quality of attenuation corrected images [65, 114]. A careful review of the raw SPECT and CT images as well as the attenuation corrected maps and registration is therefore mandatory to avoid reconstruction artifacts due to misregistration.

References

1. Virani SS, Alonso A, Benjamin EJ, Bittencourt MS, Callaway CW, Carson AP, Chamberlain AM, Chang AR, Cheng S, Delling FN, Djousse L, Elkind MSV, Ferguson JF, Fornage M, Khan SS, Kissela BM, Knutson KL, Kwan TW, Lackland DT, Lewis TT, Lichtman JH, Longenecker CT, Loop MS, Lutsey PL, Martin SS, Matsushita K, Moran AE, Mussolino ME, Perak AM, Rosamond WD, Roth GA, Sampson UKA, Satou GM, Schroeder EB, Shah SH, Shay CM, Spartano NL, Stokes A, Tirschwell DL, VanWagner LB, Tsao CW, American Heart Association Council on Epidemiology and Prevention Statistics Committee and Stroke Statistics Subcommittee. Heart Disease and Stroke Statistics-2020 update: a report from the American Heart Association. Circulation. 2020;141:e139–e596.
2. National Center for Health Statistics. National Health and Nutrition Examination Survey (NHANES) public use data files. Centers for Disease Control and Prevention website. https://www.cdc.gov/nchs/nhanes/. Accessed 1 Apr 2019.
3. Task Force Members. 2013 ESC guidelines on the management of stable coronary artery disease: the Task Force on the management of stable coronary artery disease of the European Society of Cardiology. Eur Heart J. 2013;34:2949–3003.
4. Gaemperli O, Schepis T, Valenta I, Koepfli P, Husmann L, Scheffel H, et al. Functionally relevant coronary artery disease: comparison of 64-section CT angiography with myocardial perfusion SPECT. Radiology. 2008;248:414–23.
5. Tonino PA, Fearon WF, De Bruyne B, Oldroyd KG, Leesar MA, Ver Lee PN, et al. Angiographic versus functional severity of coronary artery stenoses in the FAME study fractional flow reserve versus angiography in multivessel evaluation. J Am Coll Cardiol. 2010;55:2816–21.
6. Liga R, Vontobel J, Rovai D, Marinelli M, Caselli C, Pietila M, Teresinska A, Aguadé-Bruix S, Pizzi MN, Todiere G, Gimelli A, Chiappino D, Marraccini P, Schroeder S, Drosch T, Poddighe R, Casolo G, Anagnostopoulos C, Pugliese F, Rouzet F, Le Guludec D, Cappelli F, Valente S, Gensini GF, Zawaideh C, Capitanio S, Sambuceti G, Marsico F, Filardi PP, Fernández-Golfín C, Rincón LM, Graner FP, de Graaf MA, Stehli J, Reyes E, Nkomo S, Mäki M, Lorenzoni V, Turchetti G, Carpeggiani C, Puzzuoli S, Mangione M, Marcheschi P, Giannessi D, Nekolla S, Lombardi M, Sicari R, Scholte AJ, Zamorano JL, Underwood SR, Knuuti J, Kaufmann PA, Neglia D, Gaemperli O, EVINCI Study Investigators. Multicentre multi-device hybrid imaging study of coronary artery disease: results from the EValuation of INtegrated Cardiac Imaging for the Detection and Characterization of Ischaemic Heart Disease (EVINCI) hybrid imaging population. Eur Heart J Cardiovasc Imaging. 2016;17:951–60.
7. Fox J, Pandit-Taskar N, Strauss HW. Cardiac anatomy and pathophysiology of coronary circulation as a basis for imaging. In: Marzullo P, Mariani G, editors. From basic cardiac imaging to image fusion. Milan, Heidelberg, New York, Dordrecht, London: Springer; 2013.
8. Prinzmetal M, Kennamer R, Merliss R, Wada T, Bor N. Angina pectoris. I. A variant from angina pectoris: preliminary report. Am J Med. 1959;27:375–88.
9. Kaufmann PA, Di Carli MF. Hybrid SPECT/CT and PET/CT imaging: the next step in noninvasive cardiac imaging. Semin Nucl Med. 2009;39:341–7.
10. Dorbala S, Di Carli MF, Delbeke D, Abbara S, DePuey EG, Dilsizian V, Forrester J, Janowitz W, Kaufmann PA, Mahmarian J, Moore SC, Stabin MG, Shreve P. SNMMI/ASNC/SCCT guideline for cardiac SPECT/CT and PET/CT 1.0. J Nucl Med. 2013;54:1485–507.
11. Dorbala S, Ananthasubramaniam K, Armstrong IS, Chareonthaitawee P, DePuey EG, Einstein AJ, Gropler RJ, Holly TA, Mahmarian JJ, Park MA, Polk DM, Russell R 3rd, Slomka PJ, Thompson RC, Wells RG. Single Photon Emission Computed Tomography (SPECT) myocardial perfusion imaging guidelines: instrumentation, acquisition, processing, and interpretation. J Nucl Cardiol. 2018;25:1784–846.
12. Verberne HJ, Acampa W, Anagnostopoulos C, Ballinger J, Bengel F, De Bondt P, Buechel RR, Cuocolo A, van Eck-Smit BL, Flotats A, Hacker M, Hindorf C, Kaufmann PA, Lindner O, Ljungberg M, Lonsdale M, Manrique A, Minarik D, Scholte AJ, Slart RH, Trägårdh E, de Wit TC, Hesse B, European Association of Nuclear Medicine (EANM). EANM procedural guidelines for radionuclide myocardial perfusion imaging with SPECT and SPECT/CT: 2015 revision. Eur J Nucl Med Mol Imaging. 2015;42:1929–40.
13. Klocke FJ, Baird MG, Lorell BH, Bateman TM, Messer JV, Berman DS, O'Gara PT, Carabello BA, Russell RO Jr, Cerqueira MD, St John Sutton MG, DeMaria AN, Udelson JE, Kennedy JW, Verani MS, Williams KA, Antman EM, Smith SC Jr, Alpert JS, Gregoratos G, Anderson JL, Hiratzka LF, Faxon DP, Hunt SA, Fuster V, Jacobs AK, Gibbons RJ, Russell RO, American College of Cardiology, American Heart Association, American Society for Nuclear Cardiology. ACC:/AHA/ASNC guidelines for the clinical use of cardiac radionuclide imaging—executive summary: a report of the American College of Cardiology/American Heart Association Task

Force on Practice Guidelines (ACC/AHA/ASNC Committee to revise the 1995 guidelines for the clinical use of cardiac radionuclide imaging). J Am Coll Cardiol. 2003;42:1318–33.

14. Bateman TM. Clinical relevance of a normal myocardial perfusion scintigraphic study. J Nucl Cardiol. 1997;4:172–3.

15. Berman DS, Germano G, Shaw LJ. The role of nuclear cardiology in clinical decision making. Semin Nucl Med. 1999;29:280–97.

16. Des Prez RD, Shaw LJ, Gillespie RL, Jaber WA, Noble GL, Soman P, Wolinsky DG, Williams KA. Cost-effectiveness of myocardial perfusion imaging: a summary of the currently available literature. J Nucl Cardiol. 2005;12:750–9.

17. Sabharwal NK, Lahiri A. Role of myocardial perfusion imaging for risk stratification in suspected or known coronary artery. Heart. 2003;89:1291–7.

18. Schuijf JD, Shaw LJ, Wijns W, Lamb HJ, Poldermans D, de Roos A, van der Wall EE, Bax JJ. Cardiac imaging in coronary artery disease: differing modalities. Heart. 2005;91:1110–7.

19. Shaw LJ, Iskandrian AE. Prognostic value of gated myocardial perfusion SPECT. J Nucl Cardiol. 2004;11:171–85.

20. Underwood SR, Anagnostopoulos C, Cerqueira M, Ell PJ, Flint EJ, Harbinson M, Kelion AD, Al-Mohammad A, Prvulovich EM, Shaw LJ, Tweddel AC. Myocardial perfusion scintigraphy: the evidence. Eur J Nucl Med Mol Imaging. 2004;31:261–91.

21. Zimmermann R, vom Dahl J, Schäfers M, Schwaiger M. Positionsbericht nuklearkardiologische Diagnostik—update. Z Kardiol. 2002;91:88–92.

22. Berman DS, Kang X, Slomka PJ, Gerlach J, de Yang L, Hayes SW, Friedman JD, Thomson LE, Germano G. Underestimation of extent of ischemia by gated SPECT myocardial perfusion imaging in patients with left main coronary artery disease. J Nucl Cardiol. 2007;14:521–8.

23. Di Carli MF, Dorbala S, Curillova Z, Kwong RJ, Goldhaber SZ, Rybicki FJ, Hachamovitch R. Relationship between CT coronary angiography and stress perfusion imaging in patients with suspected ischemic heart disease assessed by integrated PET-CT imaging. J Nucl Cardiol. 2007;14:799–809.

24. Gaemperli O, Schepis T, Koepfli P, Valenta I, Soyka J, Leschka S, Desbiolles L, Husmann L, Alkadhi H, Kaufmann PA. Accuracy of 64-slice CT angiography for the detection of functionally relevant coronary stenoses as assessed with myocardial perfusion SPECT. Eur J Nucl Med Mol Imaging. 2007;34:1162–71.

25. Schuijf JD, Wijns W, Jukema JW, Atsma DE, de Roos A, Lamb HJ, Stokkel MP, Dibbets-Schneider P, Decramer I, De Bondt P, van der Wall EE, Vanhoenacker PK, Bax JJ. Relationship between noninvasive coronary angiography with multi-slice computed tomography and myocardial perfusion imaging. J Am Coll Cardiol. 2006;48:2508–14.

26. Budoff MJ, Dowe D, Jollis JG, Gitter M, Sutherland J, Halamert E, Scherer M, Bellinger R, Martin A, Benton R, Delago A, Min JK. Diagnostic performance of 64-multidetector row coronary computed tomographic angiography for evaluation of coronary artery stenosis in individuals without known coronary artery disease: results from the prospective multicenter ACCURACY (Assessment by Coronary Computed Tomographic Angiography of Individuals Undergoing Invasive Coronary Angiography) trial. J Am Coll Cardiol. 2008;52:1724–32.

27. Falk E, Shah PK, Fuster V. Coronary plaque disruption. Circulation. 1995;92:657–71.

28. Berman DS, Kang X, Hayes SW, Friedman JD, Cohen I, Abidov A, Shaw LJ, Amanullah AM, Germano G, Hachamovitch R. Adenosine myocardial perfusion single-photon emission computed tomography in women compared with men. Impact of diabetes mellitus on incremental prognostic value and effect on patient management. J Am Coll Cardiol. 2003;41:1125–33.

29. Hachamovitch R, Berman DS, Shaw LJ, Kiat H, Cohen I, Cabico JA, Friedman J, Diamond GA. Incremental prognostic value of myocardial perfusion single photon emission computed tomography for the prediction of cardiac death: differential stratification for risk of cardiac death and myocardial infarction. Circulation. 1998;97:535–43.

30. Ross R. The pathogenesis of atherosclerosis: a perspective for the 1990s. Nature. 1993;362:801–9.

31. Greenland P, Alpert JS, Beller GA, Benjamin EJ, Budoff MJ, Fayad ZA, Foster E, Hlatky MA, Hodgson JM, Kushner FG, Lauer MS, Shaw LJ, Smith SC Jr, Taylor AJ, Weintraub WS, Wenger NK, Jacobs AK, American College of Cardiology Foundation/American Heart Association Task Force on Practice Guidelines. ACCF/AHA guideline for assessment of cardiovascular risk in asymptomatic adults: executive summary: a report of the American College of Cardiology Foundation/American Heart Association Task Force on Practice Guidelines. Circulation. 2010;122:2748–64.

32. Agatston AS, Janowitz WR, Hildner FJ, Zusmer NR, Viamonte M Jr, Detrano R. Quantification of coronary artery calcium using ultrafast computed tomography. J Am Coll Cardiol. 1990;15:827–32.

33. Callister TQ, Cooil B, Raya SP, Lippolis NJ, Russo DJ, Raggi P. Coronary artery disease: improved reproducibility of calcium scoring with an electron-beam CT volumetric method. Radiology. 1998;208:807–14.

34. Youssef G, Kalia N, Darabian S, Budoff MJ. Coronary calcium: new insights, recent data, and clinical role. Curr Cardiol Rep. 2013;15:325–32.

35. Flotats A, Knuuti J, Gutberlet M, Marcassa C, Bengel FM, Kaufmann PA, Rees MR, Hesse B, Cardiovascular Committee of the EANM, the ESCR and the ECNC. Hybrid cardiac imaging: SPECT/CT and PET/CT. A joint position statement by the European Association of Nuclear

Medicine (EANM), the European Society of Cardiac Radiology (ESCR) and the European Council of Nuclear Cardiology (ECNC). Eur J Nucl Med Mol Imaging. 2011;38:201–12.

36. Greenland P, Bonow RO, Brundage BH, Budoff MJ, Eisenberg MJ, Grundy SM, Lauer MS, Post WS, Raggi P, Redberg RF, Rodgers GP, Shaw LJ, Taylor AJ, Weintraub WS, American College of Cardiology Foundation Clinical Expert Consensus Task Force (ACCF/AHA Writing Committee to Update the 2000 Expert Consensus Document on Electron Beam Computed Tomography), Society of Atherosclerosis Imaging and Prevention; Society of Cardiovascular Computed Tomography. ACCF/AHA 2007 clinical expert consensus document on coronary artery calcium scoring by computed tomography in global cardiovascular risk assessment and in evaluation of patients with chest pain: a report of the American College of Cardiology Foundation Clinical Expert Consensus Task Force (ACCF/AHA Writing Committee to Update the 2000 Expert Consensus Document on Electron Beam Computed Tomography) developed in collaboration with the Society of Atherosclerosis Imaging and Prevention and the Society of Cardiovascular Computed Tomography. J Am Coll Cardiol. 2007;49:378–402.

37. Bellasi A, Lacey C, Taylor AJ, Raggi P, Wilson PW, Budoff MJ, Vaccarino V, Shaw LJ. Comparison of prognostic usefulness of coronary artery calcium in men versus women (results from a meta- and pooled analysis estimating all-cause mortality and coronary heart disease death or myocardial infarction). Am J Cardiol. 2007;100:409–14.

38. Detrano R, Guerci AD, Carr JJ, Bild DE, Burke G, Folsom AR, Liu K, Shea S, Szklo M, Bluemke DA, O'Leary DH, Tracy R, Watson K, Wong ND, Kronmal RA. Coronary calcium as a predictor of coronary events in four racial or ethnic groups. N Engl J Med. 2008;358:1336–45.

39. Sarwar A, Shaw LJ, Shapiro MD, Blankstein R, Hoffmann U, Cury RC, Abbara S, Brady TJ, Budoff MJ, Blumenthal RS, Nasir K. Diagnostic and prognostic value of absence of coronary artery calcification. JACC Cardiovasc Imaging. 2009;2:675–88.

40. Folsom AR, Kronmal RA, Detrano RC, O'Leary DH, Bild DE, Bluemke DA, Budoff MJ, Liu K, Shea S, Szklo M, Tracy RP, Watson KE, Burke GL. Coronary artery calcification compared with carotid intima-media thickness in the prediction of cardiovascular disease incidence: the Multi-Ethnic Study of Atherosclerosis (MESA). Arch Intern Med. 2008;168:1333–9.

41. Gottlieb I, Sara L, Brinker JA, Lima JA, Rochitte CE. CT coronary calcification: what does a score of "0" mean? Curr Cardiol Rep. 2011;13:49–56.

42. Rumberger JA, Brundage BH, Rader DJ, Kondos G. Electron beam computed tomographic coronary calcium scanning: a review and guidelines for use in asymptomatic persons. Mayo Clin Proc. 1999;74:243–52.

43. Budoff MJ, Diamond GA, Raggi P, Arad Y, Guerci AD, Callister TQ, Berman D. Continuous probabilistic prediction of angiographically significant coronary artery disease using electron beam tomography. Circulation. 2002;105:1791–6.

44. Rumberger JA, Schwartz RS, Simons DB, Sheedy PF 3rd, Edwards WD, Fitzpatrick LA. Relation of coronary calcium determined by electron beam computed tomography and lumen narrowing determined at autopsy. Am J Cardiol. 1994;73:1169–73.

45. Rumberger JA, Simons DB, Fitzpatrick LA, Sheedy PF, Schwartz RS. Coronary artery calcium area by electron-beam computed tomography and coronary atherosclerotic plaque area. A histopathologic correlative study. Circulation. 1995;92:2157–62.

46. Achenbach S, Marwan M, Ropers D, Schepis T, Pflederer T, Anders K, Kuettner A, Daniel WG, Uder M, Lell MM. Coronary computed tomography angiography with a consistent dose below 1 mSv using prospectively electrocardiogram-triggered high-pitch spiral acquisition. Eur Heart J. 2010;31:340–6.

47. Gaemperli O, Bengel FM, Kaufmann PA. Cardiac hybrid imaging. Eur Heart J. 2011;32:2100–8.

48. Stein PD, Yaekoub AY, Matta F, Sostman HD. 64-slice CT for diagnosis of coronary artery disease: a systematic review. Am J Med. 2008;121:715–25.

49. Di Carli MF, Hachamovitch R. New technology for noninvasive evaluation of coronary artery disease. Circulation. 2007;115:1464–80.

50. Miller JM, Rochitte CE, Dewey M, Arbab-Zadeh A, Niinuma H, Gottlieb I, Paul N, Clouse ME, Shapiro EP, Hoe J, Lardo AC, Bush DE, de Roos A, Cox C, Brinker J, Lima JA. Diagnostic performance of coronary angiography by 64-row CT. N Engl J Med. 2008;359:2324–36.

51. Miller JM, Dewey M, Vavere AL, Rochitte CE, Niinuma H, Arbab-Zadeh A, Paul N, Hoe J, de Roos A, Yoshioka K, Lemos PA, Bush DE, Lardo AC, Texter J, Brinker J, Cox C, Clouse ME, Lima JA. Coronary CT angiography using 64 detector rows: methods and design of the multi-centre trial CORE-64. Eur Radiol. 2009;19:816–28.

52. Meijboom WB, Meijs MF, Schuijf JD, Cramer MJ, Mollet NR, van Mieghem CA, Nieman K, van Werkhoven JM, Pundziute G, Weustink AC, de Vos AM, Pugliese F, Rensing B, Jukema JW, Bax JJ, Prokop M, Doevendans PA, Hunink MG, Krestin GP, de Feyter PJ. Diagnostic accuracy of 64-slice computed tomography coronary angiography: a prospective, multicenter, multivendor study. J Am Coll Cardiol. 2008;52:2135–44.

53. van Werkhoven JM, Schuijf JD, Gaemperli O, Jukema JW, Boersma E, Wijns W, Stolzmann P, Alkadhi H, Valenta I, Stokkel MP, Kroft LJ, de Roos A, Pundziute G, Scholte A, van der Wall EE, Kaufmann PA, Bax JJ. Prognostic value of multislice computed tomography and gated single-photon emission computed tomography in patients with suspected coronary artery disease. J Am Coll Cardiol. 2009;53:623–32.

54. Gould KL. Identifying and measuring severity of coronary artery stenosis. Quantitative coronary arteriography and positron emission tomography. Circulation. 1988;78:237–45.

55. Rispler S, Keidar Z, Ghersin E, Roguin A, Soil A, Dragu R, Litmanovich D, Frenkel A, Aronson D, Engel A, Beyar R, Israel O. Integrated single-photon emission computed tomography and computed tomography coronary angiography for the assessment of hemodynamically significant coronary artery lesions. J Am Coll Cardiol. 2007;49:1059–67.

56. Machac J. Cardiac positron emission tomography imaging. Semin Nucl Med. 2005;35:17–36.

57. Hacker M, Jakobs T, Hack N, Nikolaou K, Becker C, von Ziegler F, Knez A, König A, Klauss V, Reiser M, Hahn K, Tiling R. Sixty-four slice spiral CT angiography does not predict the functional relevance of coronary artery stenoses in patients with stable angina. Eur J Nucl Med Mol Imaging. 2007;34:4–10.

58. Schelbert HR. Anatomy and physiology of coronary blood flow. J Nucl Cardiol. 2010;17:545–54.

59. Kaufmann PA. Cardiac hybrid imaging: state-of-the-art. Ann Nucl Med. 2009;23:325–31.

60. Schindler TH, Magosaki N, Jeserich M, Oser U, Krause T, Fischer R, Moser E, Nitzsche E, Zehender M, Just H, Solzbach U. Fusion imaging: combined visualization of 3D reconstructed coronary artery tree and 3D myocardial scintigraphic image in coronary artery disease. Int J Card Imaging. 1999;15:357–68.

61. Javadi MS, Lautamäki R, Merrill J, Voicu C, Epley W, McBride G, Bengel FM. Definition of vascular territories on myocardial perfusion images by integration with true coronary anatomy: a hybrid PET/CT analysis. J Nucl Med. 2010;51:198–203.

62. O'Connor MK, Kemp BJ. Single-photon emission computed tomography/computed tomography: basic instrumentation and innovations. Semin Nucl Med. 2006;36:258–66.

63. Madsen MT. Recent advances in SPECT imaging. J Nucl Med. 2007;48:661–73.

64. Masood Y, Liu YH, Depuey G, Taillefer R, Araujo LI, Allen S, Delbeke D, Anstett F, Peretz A, Zito MJ, Tsatkin V, Wackers FJ. Clinical validation of SPECT attenuation correction using x-ray computed tomography-derived attenuation maps: multi-center clinical trial with angiographic correlation. J Nucl Cardiol. 2005;12:676–86.

65. Goetze S, Brown TL, Lavely WC, Zhang Z, Bengel FM. Attenuation correction in myocardial perfusion SPECT/CT: effects of misregistration and value of reregistration. J Nucl Med. 2007;48:1090–5.

66. Kennedy JA, Israel O, Frenkel A. Directions and magnitudes of misregistration of CT attenuation-corrected myocardial perfusion studies: incidence, impact on image quality, and guidance for reregistration. J Nucl Med. 2009;50:1471–8.

67. McQuaid SJ, Hutton BF. Sources of attenuation-correction artefacts in cardiac PET/CT and SPECT/CT. Eur J Nucl Med Mol Imaging. 2008;35:1117–23.

68. Chen J, Caputlu-Wilson SF, Shi H, Galt JR, Faber TL, Garcia EV. Automated quality control of emission-transmission misalignment for attenuation correction in myocardial perfusion imaging with SPECT-CT systems. J Nucl Cardiol. 2006;13:43–9.

69. Kovalski G, Israel O, Keidar Z, Frenkel A, Sachs J, Azhari H. Correction of heart motion due to respiration in clinical myocardial perfusion SPECT scans using respiratory gating. J Nucl Med. 2007;48:630–6.

70. Scholte AJ, Schuijf JD, Kharagjitsingh AV, Dibbets-Schneider P, Stokkel MP, Jukema JW, van der Wall EE, Bax JJ, Wackers FJ. Different manifestations of coronary artery disease by stress SPECT myocardial perfusion imaging, coronary calcium scoring, and multislice CT coronary angiography in asymptomatic patients with type 2 diabetes mellitus. J Nucl Cardiol. 2008;15:503–9.

71. Haramati LB, Levsky JM, Jain VR, Altman EJ, Spindola-Franco H, Bobra S, Doddamani S, Travin MI. CT angiography for evaluation of coronary artery disease in inner-city outpatients: an initial prospective comparison with stress myocardial perfusion imaging. Int J Cardiovasc Imaging. 2009;25:303–13.

72. Schenker MP, Dorbala S, Hong EC, Rybicki FJ, Hachamovitch R, Kwong RY, Di Carli MF. Interrelation of coronary calcification, myocardial ischemia, and outcomes in patients with intermediate likelihood of coronary artery disease: a combined positron emission tomography/computed tomography study. Circulation. 2008;117:1693–700.

73. Schepis T, Gaemperli O, Koepfli P, Namdar M, Valenta I, Scheffel H, Leschka S, Husmann L, Eberli FR, Luscher TF, Alkadhi H, Kaufmann PA. Added value of coronary artery calcium score as an adjunct to gated SPECT for the evaluation of coronary artery disease in an intermediate-risk population. J Nucl Med. 2007;48:1424–30.

74. He ZX, Hedrick TD, Pratt CM, Verani MS, Aquino V, Roberts R, Mahmarian JJ. Severity of coronary artery calcification by electron beam computed tomography predicts silent myocardial ischemia. Circulation. 2000;101:244–51.

75. Berman DS, Wong ND, Gransar H, Miranda-Peats R, Dahlbeck J, Hayes SW, Friedman JD, Kang X, Polk D, Hachamovitch R, Shaw L, Rozanski A. Relationship between stress-induced myocardial ischemia and atherosclerosis measured by coronary calcium tomography. J Am Coll Cardiol. 2004;44:923–30.

76. Shaw LJ, Narula J. Risk assessment and predictive value of coronary artery disease testing. J Nucl Med. 2009;50:1296–306.

77. Gaemperli O, Schepis T, Valenta I, Husmann L, Scheffel H, Duerst V, Eberli FR, Luscher TF, Alkadhi H, Kaufmann PA. Cardiac image fusion from stand-alone SPECT and CT: clinical experience. J Nucl Med. 2007;48:696–703.

78. Namdar M, Hany TF, Koepfli P, Siegrist PT, Burger C, Wyss CA, Luscher TF, von Schulthess GK, Kaufmann PA. Integrated PET/CT for the assess-

ment of coronary artery disease: a feasibility study. J Nucl Med. 2005;46:930–5.

79. Husmann L, Herzog BA, Gaemperli O, Tatsugami F, Burkhard N, Valenta I, Veit-Haibach P, Wyss CA, Landmesser U, Kaufmann PA. Diagnostic accuracy of computed tomography coronary angiography and evaluation of stress-only single-photon emission computed tomography/computed tomography hybrid imaging: comparison of prospective electrocardiogram-triggering vs. retrospective gating. Eur Heart J. 2009;30:600–7.

80. Gaemperli O, Schepis T, Kalff V, Namdar M, Valenta I, Stefani L, Desbiolles L, Leschka S, Husmann L, Alkadhi H, Kaufmann PA. Validation of a new cardiac image fusion software for three-dimensional integration of myocardial perfusion SPECT and stand-alone 64-slice CT angiography. Eur J Nucl Med Mol Imaging. 2007;34:1097–106.

81. Rispler S, Aronson D, Abadi S, Roguin A, Engel A, Beyar R, Israel O, Keidar Z. Integrated SPECT/CT for assessment of haemodynamically significant coronary artery lesions in patients with acute coronary syndrome. Eur J Nucl Med Mol Imaging. 2011;38:1917–25.

82. Slomka PJ, Cheng VY, Dey D, Woo J, Ramesh A, Van Kriekinge S, Suzuki Y, Elad Y, Karlsberg R, Berman DS, Germano G. Quantitative analysis of myocardial perfusion SPECT anatomically guided by coregistered 64-slice coronary CT angiography. J Nucl Med. 2009;50:1621–30.

83. Santana CA, Garcia EV, Faber TL, Sirineni GK, Esteves FP, Sanyal R, Halkar R, Ornelas M, Verdes L, Lerakis S, Ramos JJ, Aguadé-Bruix S, Cuéllar H, Candell-Riera J, Raggi P. Diagnostic performance of fusion of myocardial perfusion imaging (MPI) and computed tomography coronary angiography. J Nucl Cardiol. 2009;16:201–11.

84. Schaap J, Kauling RM, Boekholdt SM, Nieman K, Meijboom WB, Post MC, Van der Heyden JA, de Kroon TL, van Es HW, Rensing BJ, Verzijlbergen JF. Incremental diagnostic accuracy of hybrid SPECT/CT coronary angiography in a population with an intermediate to high pre-test likelihood of coronary artery disease. Eur Heart J Cardiovasc Imaging. 2013;14:642–9.

85. Sato A, Nozato T, Hikita H, Miyazaki S, Takahashi Y, Kuwahara T, Takahashi A, Hiroe M, Aonuma K. Incremental value of combining 64-slice computed tomography angiography with stress nuclear myocardial perfusion imaging to improve noninvasive detection of coronary artery disease. J Nucl Cardiol. 2010;17:19–26.

86. International Commission on Radiological Protection. Radiation dose to patients from radiopharmaceuticals: addendum 2 to ICRP publication 53. Ann ICRP. 1998;28:1–126.

87. International Commission on Radiological Protection. Radiation dose to patients from radiopharmaceuticals: a third addendum to ICRP publication 53, ICRP publication 106—approved by the Commission in October 2007. Ann ICRP. 2008;38:1–197.

88. Hesse B, Tägil K, Cuocolo A, Anagnostopoulos C, Bardiés M, Bax J, Bengel F, Busemann Sokole E, Davies G, Dondi M, Edenbrandt L, Franken P, Kjaer A, Knuuti J, Lassmann M, Ljungberg M, Marcassa C, Marie PY, McKiddie F, O'Connor M, Prvulovich E, Underwood R, van Eck-Smit B. EANM/ESC procedural guidelines for myocardial perfusion imaging in nuclear cardiology. Eur J Nucl Med Mol Imaging. 2005;32:855–97.

89. Slomka PJ, Patton JA, Berman DS, Germano G. Advances in technical aspects of myocardial perfusion SPECT imaging. J Nucl Cardiol. 2009;16:255–76.

90. Esteves FP, Raggi P, Folks RD, Keidar Z, Askew JW, Rispler S, O'Connor MK, Verdes L, Garcia EV. Novel solid-state-detector dedicated cardiac camera for fast myocardial perfusion imaging: multicenter comparison with standard dual detector cameras. J Nucl Cardiol. 2009;16:927–34.

91. Cerqueira MD, Allman KC, Ficaro EP, Hansen CL, Nichols KJ, Thompson RC, Van Decker WA, Yakovlevitch M. Recommendations for reducing radiation exposure in myocardial perfusion imaging. J Nucl Cardiol. 2010;17:709–18.

92. Schepis T, Gaemperli O, Koepfli P, Rüegg C, Burger C, Leschka S, Desbiolles L, Husmann L, Alkadhi H, Kaufmann PA. Use of coronary calcium score scans from stand-alone multislice computed tomography for attenuation correction of myocardial perfusion SPECT. Eur J Nucl Med Mol Imaging. 2007;34:11–9.

93. Einstein AJ, Henzlova MJ, Rajagopalan S. Estimating risk of cancer associated with radiation exposure from 64-slice computed tomography coronary angiography. JAMA. 2007;298:317–23.

94. Hausleiter J, Meyer T, Hermann F, Hadamitzky M, Krebs M, Gerber TC, McCollough C, Martinoff S, Kastrati A, Schömig A, Achenbach S. Estimated radiation dose associated with cardiac CT angiography. JAMA. 2009;301:500–7.

95. Husmann L, Valenta I, Gaemperli O, Adda O, Treyer V, Wyss CA, Veit-Haibach P, Tatsugami F, von Schulthess GK, Kaufmann PA. Feasibility of low-dose coronary CT angiography: first experience with prospective ECG-gating. Eur Heart J. 2008;29:191–7.

96. Lehmkuhl L, Gosch D, Nagel HD, Stumpp P, Kahn T, Gutberlet M. Quantification of radiation dose savings in cardiac computed tomography using prospectively triggered mode and ECG pulsing: a phantom study. Eur Radiol. 2010;20:2116–25.

97. Hoffmann U, Ferencik M, Cury RC, Pena AJ. Coronary CT angiography. J Nucl Med. 2006;47:797–806.

98. Berman DS, Hachamovitch R, Shaw LJ, Friedman JD, Hayes SW, Thomson LE, Fieno DS, Germano G, Slomka P, Wong ND, Kang X, Rozanski A. Roles of nuclear cardiology, cardiac computed tomography, and cardiac magnetic resonance: assessment of patients with suspected coronary artery disease. J Nucl Med. 2006;47:74–82.

99. Schaap J, de Groot JA, Nieman K, Meijboom WB, Boekholdt SM, Post MC, Van der Heyden JA, de Kroon TL, Rensing BJ, Moons KG, Verzijlbergen JF. Hybrid myocardial perfusion SPECT/CT coronary angiography and invasive coronary angiography in patients with stable angina pectoris lead to similar treatment decisions. Heart. 2013;99:188–94.

100. Greenland P, Bonow RO, Brundage BH, Budoff MJ, Eisenberg MJ, Grundy SM, Lauer MS, Post WS, Raggi P, Redberg RF, Rodgers GP, Shaw LJ, Taylor AJ, Weintraub WS, Harrington RA, Abrams J, Anderson JL, Bates ER, Grines CL, Hlatky MA, Lichtenberg RC, Lindner JR, Pohost GM, Schofield RS, Shubrooks SJ Jr, Stein JH, Tracy CM, Vogel RA, Wesley DJ, American College of Cardiology Foundation Clinical Expert Consensus Task Force (ACCF/AHA Writing Committee to Update the 2000 Expert Consensus Document on Electron Beam Computed Tomography), Society of Atherosclerosis Imaging and Prevention; Society of Cardiovascular Computed Tomography. ACCF/AHA 2007 clinical expert consensus document on coronary artery calcium scoring by computed tomography in global cardiovascular risk assessment and in evaluation of patients with chest pain: a report of the American College of Cardiology Foundation Clinical Expert Consensus Task Force (ACCF/AHA Writing Committee to Update the 2000 Expert Consensus Document on Electron Beam Computed Tomography). Circulation. 2007;115:402–26.

101. Hachamovitch R, Johnson JR, Hlatky MA, Cantagallo L, Johnson BH, Coughlan M, Hainer J, Gierbolini J, Di Carli MF. The study of myocardial perfusion and coronary anatomy imaging roles in CAD (SPARC): design, rationale, and baseline patient characteristics of a prospective, multicenter observational registry comparing PET, SPECT, and CTA for resource utilization and clinical outcomes. J Nucl Cardiol. 2009;16:935–48.

102. PROspective Multicenter Imaging Study for Evaluation of Chest Pain (PROMISE). Funded by the National Heart, Lung, and Blood Institute. https://www.promisetrail.org. Accessed 29 July 2013.

103. Douglas PS, Hoffmann U, Lee KL, Mark DB, Al-Khalidi HR, Anstrom K, Dolor RJ, Kosinski A, Krucoff MW, Mudrick DW, Patel MR, Picard MH, Udelson JE, Velazquez EJ, Cooper L, PROMISE Investigators. PROspective Multicenter Imaging Study for Evaluation of chest pain: rationale and design of the PROMISE trial. Am Heart J. 2014;167:796–803.

104. EVINCI (Evaluation of Integrated Cardiac Imaging). A European multi-centre, multi-modality cardiac imaging project funded by the European Commission within the Seventh Framework Program Number HEALTH-F2-2009-222915. http://www.escardio.org/communities/Working-Groups/EVINCI/Pages/EVINCI-home.aspx. Accessed 29 July 2013.

105. Hachamovitch R, Nutter B, Hlatky MA, Shaw LJ, Ridner ML, Dorbala S, Beanlands RS, Chow BJ, Branscomb E, Chareonthaitawee P, Weigold WG, Voros S, Abbara S, Yasuda T, Jacobs JE, Lesser J, Berman DS, Thomson LE, Raman S, Heller GV, Schussheim A, Brunken R, Williams KA, Farkas S, Delbeke D, Schoepf UJ, Reichek N, Rabinowitz S, Sigman SR, Patterson R, Corn CR, White R, Kazerooni E, Corbett J, Bokhari S, Machac J, Guarneri E, Borges-Neto S, Millstine JW, Caldwell J, Arrighi J, Hoffmann U, Budoff M, Lima J, Johnson JR, Johnson B, Gaber M, Williams JA, Foster C, Hainer J, Di Carli MF; SPARC Investigators. Patient management after noninvasive cardiac imaging results from SPARC (Study of myocardial perfusion and coronary anatomy imaging roles in coronary artery disease). J Am Coll Cardiol. 2012;59:462–74.

106. Douglas PS, Hoffmann U, Patel MR, Mark DB, Al-Khalidi HR, Cavanaugh B, Cole J, Dolor RJ, Fordyce CB, Huang M, Khan MA, Kosinski AS, Krucoff MW, Malhotra V, Picard MH, Udelson JE, Velazquez EJ, Yow E, Cooper LS, Lee KL, PROMISE Investigators. Outcomes of anatomical versus functional testing for coronary artery disease. N Engl J Med. 2015;372:1291–300.

107. Rizvi A, Han D, Danad I, Ó Hartaigh B, Lee JH, Gransar H, Stuijfzand WJ, Roudsari HM, Park MW, Szymonifka J, Chang HJ, Jones EC, Knaapen P, Lin FY, Min JK, Peña JM. Diagnostic performance of hybrid cardiac imaging methods for assessment of obstructive coronary artery disease compared with stand-alone coronary computed tomography angiography: a meta-analysis. JACC Cardiovasc Imaging. 2018;11:589–99.

108. Beller GA. Patient management after noninvasive cardiac imaging: a commentary on the reported results from SPARC. J Nucl Cardiol. 2012;19:182–4.

109. Gaemperli O, Kaufmann PA. Hybrid cardiac imaging: more than the sum of its parts? J Nucl Cardiol. 2008;15:123–6.

110. Husmann L, Valenta I, Kaufmann PA. Coronary angiography with low-dose computed tomography at 1.4 mSv. Herz. 2008;33:75.

111. Herzog BA, Husmann L, Burkhard N, Gaemperli O, Valenta I, Tatsugami F, Wyss CA, Landmesser U, Kaufmann PA. Accuracy of low-dose computed tomography coronary angiography using prospective electrocardiogram-triggering: first clinical experience. Eur Heart J. 2008;29:3037–42.

112. Herzog BA, Husmann L, Landmesser U, Kaufmann PA. Low-dose computed tomography coronary angiography and myocardial perfusion imaging: cardiac hybrid imaging below 3mSv. Eur Heart J. 2009;30:644.

113. Goetze S, Wahl RL. Prevalence of misregistration between SPECT and CT for attenuation-corrected myocardial perfusion SPECT. J Nucl Cardiol. 2007;14:200–6.

114. Dvorak RA, Brown RKJ, Corbett JR. Interpretation of SPECT/CT myocardial perfusion images: common artifacts and quality control techniques. Radiographics. 2011;31:2041–57.

SPECT/CT in Sentinel Node Scintigraphy

11

Renato A. Valdés Olmos and Sergi Vidal-Sicart

11.1 Introduction

Since the introduction of the sentinel node (SN) procedure almost 30 years ago SN imaging became an essential component for lymphatic mapping and preoperative SN identification in melanoma, breast cancer and other malignancies.

In the footsteps of lymphoscintigraphy a new generation of large field gamma cameras facilitated the incorporation of SPECT/CT to the SN procedure in various malignancies. The functional information from SPECT can be combined with the morphological information from CT by applying both techniques in one session. The resulting SPECT/CT fused images are able to depict SNs in an anatomical landscape providing a helpful roadmap for surgeons with information concerning the location of SNs with respect to blood vessels, muscles and lymph node basins.

SPECT/CT has been useful in melanoma and breast cancer patients with unusual or complex drainage as observed in melanoma of the neck or the upper part of the trunk and in breast cancer with drainage outside of the axilla. SPECT/CT can also visualize SNs in the axilla when lymph nodes are not depicted on planar images or when lymph nodes are masked by the overlying injection site. Furthermore, in areas such as the pelvis, retroperitoneum and upper abdomen in gastrointestinal, gynaecological and urological malignancies, SPECT-CT is considered to be essential to localize SNs. SPECT/CT and planar lymphoscintigraphy, performed in a single acquisition session, are complementary for SN identification and a combined interpretation of both modalities is necessary. On the other hand, the preoperative information obtained by SPECT/CT and reported by nuclear physicians is being used by surgeons in the operating room to recognize anatomical landmarks, thus resulting in a more effective handling of portable devices for SN localization.

11.2 Clinical Background

Resting on the hypothesis of the existence of an orderly and predictable pattern of lymphatic drainage to a regional lymph node basin, the SN concept concerns functioning of lymph nodes on a direct drainage pathway as effective filters for tumour cells [1]. In practical terms, all lymph

R. A. Valdés Olmos (✉)
Department of Radiology, Interventional Molecular Imaging Laboratory and Section of Nuclear Medicine, Leiden University Medical Centre, Leiden, Netherlands
e-mail: R.A.Valdes_Olmos@lumc.nl

S. Vidal-Sicart
Nuclear Medicine Department, University Hospital Clinic, Barcelona, Spain

Institut d'Investigacions Biomèdiques, August Pi Sunyer (IDIBAPS), Barcelona, Spain
e-mail: SVIDAL@clinic.cat

© The Author(s), under exclusive license to Springer Nature Switzerland AG 2022
H. Ahmadzadehfar et al. (eds.), *Clinical Applications of SPECT-CT*,
https://doi.org/10.1007/978-3-030-65850-2_11

"

nodes with direct drainage from the primary tumour must be considered as SNs.

Another concept important to emphasize is that the SN procedure is a multidisciplinary modality based on the combination of preoperative imaging, intraoperative detection and refined histopathological analysis.

For preoperative SN imaging colloid particles labelled with ^{99m}Tc are usually used. Radioactive colloid particles are incorporated into the macrophages by phagocytosis enabling prolonged lymph node retention and an adequate detection window. This enables not just the acquisition of delayed planar images and SPECT/CT but also intraoperative SN localization using portable devices based on gamma ray detection.

Furthermore, the SN procedure is oriented to the detection of lymph node metastases in patients without clinical evidence of regional metastases [2]. Today preoperative selection makes it possible to identify patients with palpable lymph nodes at clinical examination, suspected lymph nodes at ultrasound or CT, or tumour-positive lymph nodes at aspiration cytology. In clinical practice this leads to consider the SN biopsy as a procedure principally oriented to the detection of subclinical metastases. This category includes submicrometastases ($\leq$0.2 mm), micrometastases (>0.2 mm and $\leq$2 mm), and small macrometastases (between >2 mm and <5 mm) [3].

11.3 Technical SPECT-CT Aspects for SN Imaging

Protocols for SPECT/CT are determined by the objectives of the SN procedure. SPECT/CT is essentially oriented to the anatomical localization of SNs. This explains why SPECT/CT is acquired using a low dose CT. Acquisition of a diagnostic high dose CT, with or without intravenous contrast, is not really necessary because the SN procedure primarily aims to identify subclinical metastases in lymph nodes that are not enlarged.

For SN localisation the CT component of SPECT/CT must be of sufficient quality to provide optimal anatomical information. All modern SPECT/CT cameras enable the evaluation of the lymph nodes corresponding with the radioactive nodes on fused SPECT/CT images by acquiring a low dose (40 mAs) CT. In superficial areas such as the groin and the axilla, slides of at least 5 mm are recommended. For more complex anatomical areas (head/neck, pelvis, abdomen) 2 mm slides may be necessary. With this approach SPECT/CT can accurately localize SNs in relation to the vascular structures and muscles in deep anatomical areas.

The CT component is also used to correct the SPECT signal for tissue attenuation and scattering. After these corrections SPECT can be fused with CT [4]. A grey scale is used to display the morphology in the background image (CT), whereas a colour scale is used to display the SN in the foreground image (SPECT).

To read images SPECT/CT is mostly displayed in a similar manner as that of conventional tomography [5]. Multiplanar reconstruction (MPR) enables a two-dimensional display of fused images in relation to CT and SPECT. The use of cross-reference lines allows for the navigation between axial, coronal and sagittal views. At the same time this tool leads to correlate radioactive SNs seen on fused SPECT/CT with lymph nodes seen on CT (Fig. 11.1a–c). Most frequently, a radioactive SN corresponds with a single lymph node on CT, but in some cases it correlates with a cluster of lymph nodes. This information may be helpful for the intraoperative procedure and the post-excision control using portable gamma cameras or probes as more radioactive SNs may be harvested at the same location.

Fused SPECT/CT images may also be displayed using Maximum Intensity Projection (MIP). MIP is a specific type of rendering in which the brightest voxels are projected into a three-dimensional image allowing improved anatomical SN localisation and recognition by the

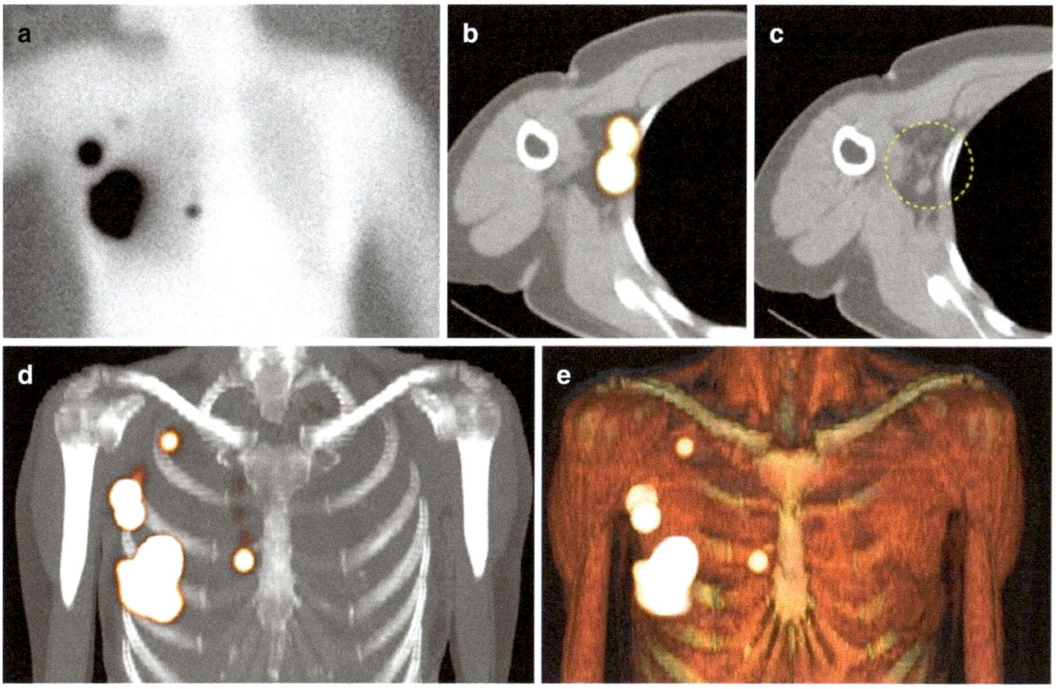

Fig. 11.1 Planar anterior lymphoscintigraphy (**a**) showing drainage from the injection site in the right breast to the axilla and the internal mammary chain. Multiplanar reconstruction (MPR) with display of similar planes for axial fused SPECT/CT (**b**) and CT (**c**) images enables identification of the axillary sentinel nodes (circle). On images generated with maximum intensity projection (MIP) (**d**) and volume rendering (**e**) the sentinel nodes are displayed in an anatomical 3D landscape

surgeon (Fig. 11.1d). One limitation of MIP is that the presence of other high-attenuation voxels on CT can complicate the recognition of the vasculature and other anatomical structures. Another limitation of MIP is that it concerns a two-dimensional representation, which is not able to accurately depict the actual relationships of the vessels and other structures [6].

Another possibility to support SN localization is a three-dimensional display using volume rendering. In this modality different colours are assigned to anatomical structures such as vessels, muscle, bone and skin (Fig. 11.1e). This results in better anatomical reference points and incorporates an additional dimension in the recognition of SNs, for instance in relation to the vasculature. By incorporating a colour display, volume rendering improves visualization of complex anatomy and 3D relationships.

11.4 Comprehensive Interpretation of Lymphoscintigraphy and SPECT/CT

SPECT/CT and lymphoscintigraphy are complementary modalities acquired in a single session with the same equipment. SPECT/CT provides landmarks to anatomically localize SNs already visualized on planar images. However, SPECT/CT can detect additional SNs principally in areas with a high number of lymph nodes such as the neck, or with complex anatomy such as the pelvis and abdomen. SPECT/CT is also useful to detect SNs in the vicinity of the injection site. To understand the combined use of lymphoscintigraphy and SPECT/CT it is necessary to elucidate some aspects related to image interpretation [7]. First of all by acquiring early and delayed planar images lymphoscintigraphy can identify SNs in a majority of cases. In current protocols SPECT/CT is performed following delayed planar images (mostly 2–4 h after tracer administration). This sequential acquisition helps to clarify the role of both modalities. However, it is necessary to specify some criteria for SN identification on preoperative images. Based on lymphoscintigraphy, the main criteria to identify lymph nodes as SNs are the visualization of lymphatic ducts, the time of appearance, the lymph node basin, and the intensity of lymph node uptake [8]. Following

these criteria visualized radioactive lymph nodes may be classified as:

1. Definitely SNs: this category includes all lymph nodes draining from the site of the primary tumour through its own lymphatic vessel (Fig. 11.2a), or a single radioactive lymph node in a lymph node basin [9].
2. Highly probable SNs: this category includes lymph nodes appearing between the injection site and a first draining node (Fig. 11.2b), or nodes with increasing uptake appearing in other lymph node stations.

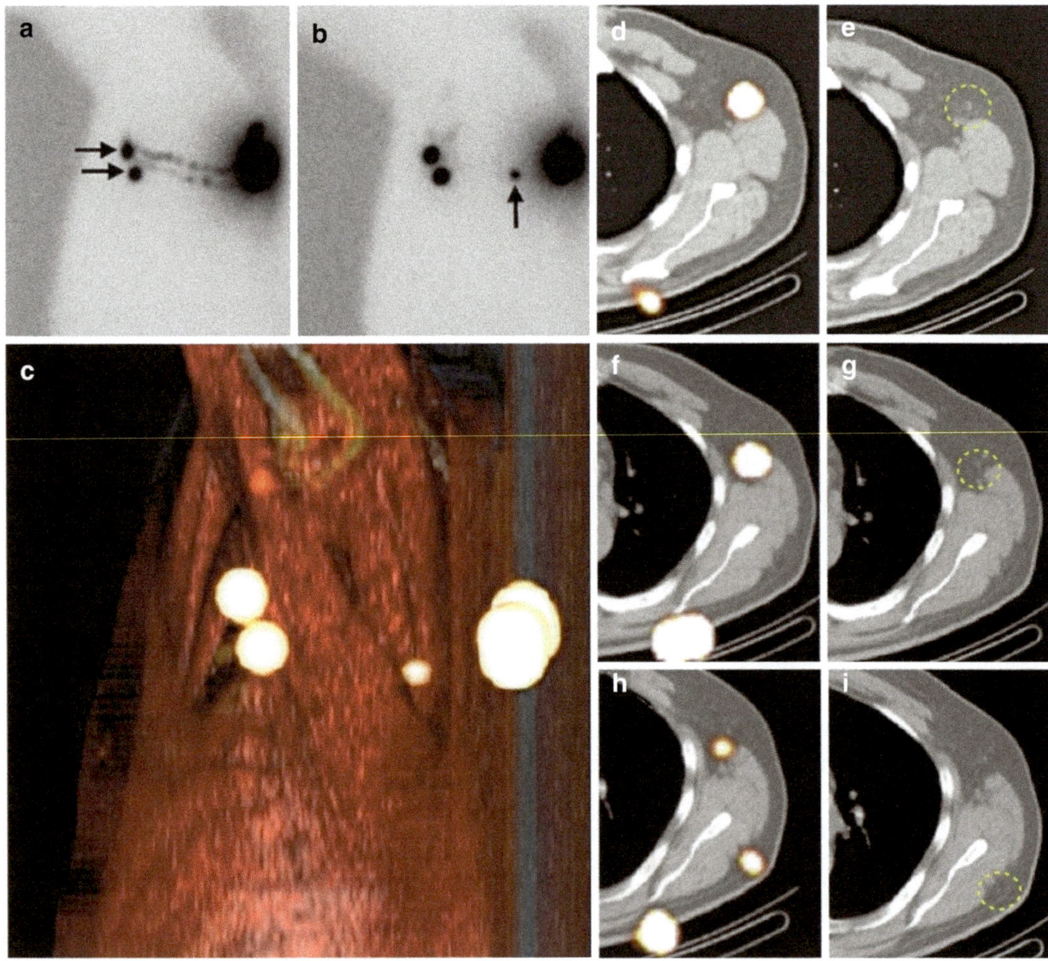

Fig. 11.2 Lateral early planar lymphoscintigraphy (**a**) in a patient with a melanoma of the back showing lymphatic ducts from the injection site to two lymph nodes (horizontal arrows) in the left axilla. These nodes are considered as definitely sentinel nodes. On delayed lateral planar image (**b**) an additional node (vertical arrow) is seen in the vicinity of the injection site; this node is highly probable a sentinel node too. Sentinel nodes are anatomically localized using volume rendering (**c**) and SPECT/CT (**d, f, h**). On CT (**e, g, i**) not enlarged sentinel nodes (circles) are seen

3. Less probable SNs: all higher echelon nodes (in trunk and extremities) or lower echelon nodes (head and neck) may be included in this category.

Early planar images are essential to identify first draining lymph nodes as SNs by visualization of their lymphatic ducts. These nodes (category 1) can be distinguished from secondary lymph nodes (category 3) mostly appearing on delayed planar images and showing less uptake.

In other cases a single lymph node is seen on early and/or delayed images. This node is also considered as a definite SN (category 1). However, in some cases SPECT/CT leads to detect additional lymph nodes in other basins. This may occur for instance in the pelvis when two basins are located at the same level and there is superposition of the radioactive nodes on planar images (Fig. 11.3). These nodes can be considered as definite (category 1) or highly probable sentinel nodes (category 2). Less frequently a radioactive lymph node may appear between the injection site and a first draining node; its increasing uptake can confirm this node as a highly probable SN (category 2) and it helps to differentiate this node from prolonged valve activity in a lymphatic duct, which mostly decreases in intensity on delayed images.

11.5 Clinical Relevance of SPECT/ CT

11.5.1 Cutaneous Melanoma

In a prospective multicentre study including 262 melanoma patients SPECT/CT demonstrated to have clinical value by revealing 70 additional SNs in 53 patients with 25% additional nodes in head and neck melanoma, 25.5% in upper limb melanoma, 20.5% in trunk melanoma and 12.9% in lower limb melanoma [10]. In the same study SPECT/CT did modify the surgical approach in 97 patients (37%).

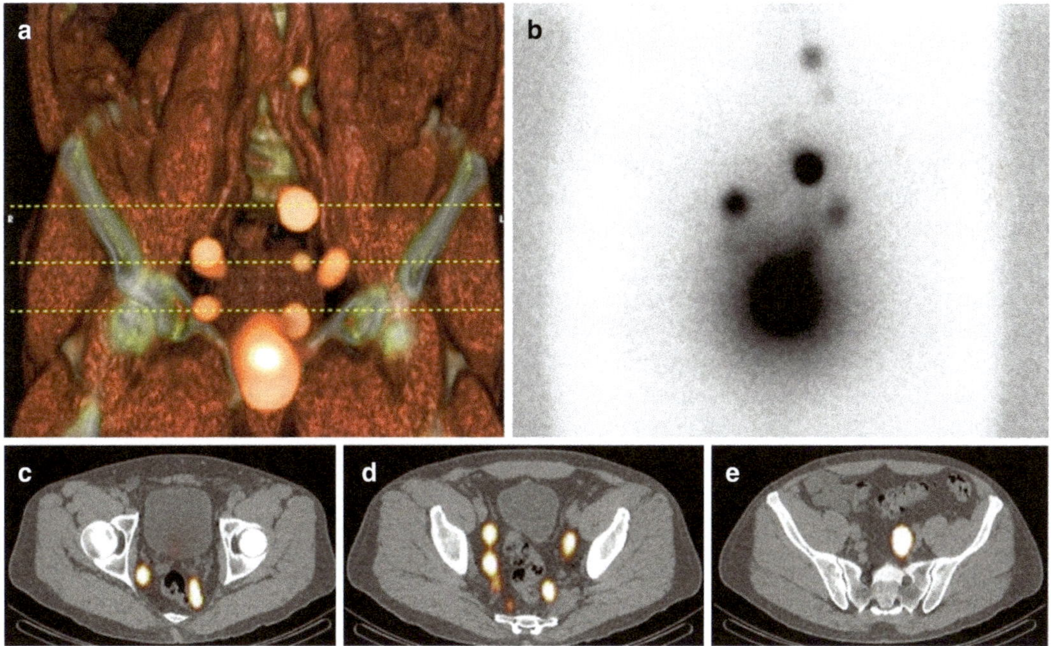

Fig. 11.3 Volume rendering SPECT/CT (**a**) obtained 2 h after tracer injection into the prostate showing drainage to lymph nodes along the iliac vessels. Horizontal stripped lines indicate from inferior to superior the levels of display of the axial fused SPECT/CT images (**c–e**). Note that at these levels SPECT/CT is able to display more sentinel nodes than planar images (**b**)

In concordance with these results SPECT/CT revealed almost 19% more SNs than planar lymphoscintigraphy concerning 255 patients with trunk melanoma; in 40 out of these patients lymphatic drainage to additional basins required surgical adjustment [11].

The additional value of SPECT/CT in melanoma was confirmed in another study comparing the results of 149 patients for whom a SPECT/CT was performed with a group of 254 patients without SPECT/CT. SPECT/CT detected more SNs (average 2.4 against 1.87 without SPECT/CT) and more metastatic SNs (average 0.34 against 0.21). The use of SPECT/CT was associated with a significant higher rate of the 4-year disease-free interval (93.9%) when compared with the group of patients without SPECT/CT (79.2%) [12]. The same group of investigators described higher frequency of metastatic involvement and higher rate of disease-free survival in patients with SPECT/CT assisted SN biopsy compared with patients without SPECT/CT [13].

In a meta-analysis concerning 17 studies and 1438 melanoma patients, average SN detection rate was 98.28% for SPECT/CT and 95.53% for planar lymphoscintigraphy. The average impact of SPECT/CT on surgery resulted in 37.43% of cases [14].

The use of SPECT/CT has gained relevance after the results of the second Multicenter Selective Lymphadenectomy Trial (MSLT-2) and other randomized controlled trials where, following tumour-positive SN, completion lymph node dissection versus observation was evaluated [15, 16]. Patients with SN metastases larger than 1 mm might benefit more from observation than from immediate lymph node dissection. In this context surveillance of the draining lymph node basin(s) assessed by SN mapping during staging and particularly the findings of SPECT/CT may constitute a diagnostic baseline for further control with ultrasonography [17].

11.5.2 Breast Cancer

In a study involving 114 patients, SPECT/CT was detected in 81 patients with 151 additional SNs, of which 19 are tumour-positive. Of overall 61 tumour-positive SNs in 52 patients SPECT/CT detected all nodes, whereas planar images detected only 42 [18].

In a series including 741 patients SPECT/CT allowed the exact position of SNs in the axilla: just under 50% was located in the mid or posterior group of axillary level I and not exclusively in the antero-pectoral group as generally assumed [19].

In 1182 breast cancer patients SPECT/CT detected more SNs than planar lymphoscintigraphy (2165 vs. 1892) with a drainage basin mismatch of 16.5% leading to a surgical adjustment in 17% of the cases [10].

The role of SPECT/CT to clarify lymphatic drainage outside the axilla was assessed in 56 patients with 81 internal mammary nodes depicted by lymphoscintigraphy. SPECT/CT showed 74 of these nodes in the internal mammary territory and 14 in the mediastinal basins [20]. SPECT/CT represents a diagnostic solution to increase identification of internal mammary SNs and consequently reduces false negative rate of SN biopsy [21].

Lymphatic drainage outside the axilla is particularly relevant in patients with previous breast surgery scheduled for SN biopsy due to local relapse. In this context SPECT/CT was useful to localize SNs in 122 evaluated patients with ipsilateral breast cancer relapse showing a higher visualization rate than planar scintigraphy. Territory mismatch between SPECT/CT and planar scintigraphy was found in 60% of patients with SN visualization leading to surgical adjustment in 21.3% of them [22].

SPECT/CT is also useful to identify SNs in patients with overweight. In a study including 122 patients SPECT/CT was performed in 49 of them who had no SN visualization on planar images. SPECT/CT led to the detection of SN in 29 of these obese patients (59%) [23]. In a recent study in 59 patients with overweight/obese patients (BMI > 25 kg/m^2) planar scintigraphy failed to identify SNs in 49 whereas SPECT/CT failed in only 18 [24].

In general, SPECT/CT has been indicated in breast cancer patients without SN visualization on planar scintigraphy. In a recent evaluation

SPECT/CT localized SNs in 66 out of 284 patients (23.2%) without SN visualization on planar scintigraphy. In the case of persistent non-visualization despite SPECT/CT, radiocolloid reinjection resulted in approximately 62% success rate (36/58) suggesting the possibility to perform reinjection before SPECT/CT [25].

11.5.3 Head and Neck Malignancies

The lymphatic system of the head and neck includes approximately 250–300 lymph nodes divided into various nodal groups. Further, there are marked variations in the lymphatic drainage depending on the primary lesion site. For instance, scalp melanomas of the frontal zone can drain to different lymph nodes when compared with melanomas of the parietal or occipital areas. Also, for the face and the forehead drainage to different basins may occur. In the oral cavity, malignancies of the lingual apex may drain to other groups in comparison with well-lateralized lesions in the tongue or floor of the mouth. Due to this high lymph node density and variability in drainage patterns SPECT/CT appears to be essential not only to accurately identify SNs in an anatomical landscape, but also to detect additional SNs in the vicinity of the primary lesions or in patients with aberrant drainage to different lymph node basins. SPECT/CT is also helpful for the localization of SNs in relation to the surgical neck dissections levels [26]. In a study including 66 consecutive patients with early stage oral cancer and a clinically negative neck carcinoma, SPECT/CT identified a 22% additional SNs in the neck, and in 20% of the patients with at least one positive SN the only positive node was detected by SPECT/CT [27]. In another series including 34 patients additional SNs were found by SPECT/CT in 15, and in 7 patients the anatomical level of SN location was reclassified [28].

Also in head/neck melanoma SPECT/CT has been found to be useful with visualization of 29% additional SNs in the parotid/preauricular region and 44% in level Vb in comparison with planar imaging acquired during lymphoscitigraphy [29].

SPECT/CT detected additional SNs in 6 out of 38 (16%) patients with head and neck melanoma and led to an adjustment of the surgical approach in 11 patients [30].

In another study SPECT/CT modified the surgical approach (more superficial incision or incision at another site) in 9 out of 34 (27%) patients with head and neck malignancies [31].

Recently, SPECT/CT is being used in an ongoing trial to tailor elective nodal irradiation in head and neck squamous cell carcinoma patients. Using lymph drainage mapping by SPECT/CT following radiocolloid injections around the tumour site patients with a minimal risk of contralateral nodal failure are selected for unilateral elective nodal irradiation. The trial aims to minimize the proportion of patients that undergo bilateral irradiation [32].

11.5.4 Pelvic and Retroperitoneal Malignancies

The lymphatic system of the pelvis is the expected area of drainage of various male and female urogenital malignancies. There are different nodal groups receiving lymphatic drainage from the pelvic structures: the external iliac nodes which medial subgroup includes the obturator nodes, the internal iliac lymph nodes and the nodes in the trajectory of the common iliac vessels. SNs from malignancies of the prostate, bladder, cervix and endometrial have been found in these iliac basins. However, aberrant drainage to the para-aortic and interaortocaval nodes as well as to SNs in the proximity of the anterior abdominal wall is also possible. In 68 patients with pelvic cancers SPECT/CT detected not only more SNs than planar imaging (195 vs. 138) but it did also correct the localization in 51.6% with a surgical adjustment of 65.6% [10].

Particularly for prostate cancer there is consensus today that SPECT/CT is becoming an essential tool for SN identifications [33].

In 46 prostate cancer patients, SN visualization rate increased from 91% for planar scintigraphy to 98% when SPECT/CT was performed. SPECT/CT also depicted more SNs than planar images (average 4.3 vs. 2.2 SNs). Forty-four percent of the SNs containing metastases were only visualized by SPECT/CT [34].

In 37 out of 121 prostate cancer patients (31%) SPECT/CT localized SNs outside the area of extended pelvic lymph node dissection which is often used to stage the pelvis; these SNs were found in different locations: presacral, Cloquet's node, inguinal, para-aortic, abdominal wall, pararectal, behind the common iliac artery, and lateral to the external iliac artery [35]. SPECT/CT showed draining SNs outside the territory of the extended pelvic lymphadenectomy in 76% of 84 patients scheduled for SN biopsy by laparoscopy [36].

In treated prostate cancer patients SPECT/CT revealed a higher percentage of SNs (80% vs. 34%) outside the pelvic para-iliac region in comparison to untreated patients [37]. In another study SPECT/CT findings led to a 25% impact of lymphatic drainage on conformal pelvic irradiation in 23 prostate cancer patients [38]. Furthermore, SPECT/CT contributed to personalize pelvic lymph node irradiation in a series including 57 intermediate and high-risk prostate cancer patients [39].

In testicular cancer drainage to nodes along the abdominal aorta and cava is usually found, but in some cases SNs are also found in the trajectory of the funicular vessels. SPECT/CT identified interaortocaval or paracaval SNs in five patients with right-sided testicular cancer and para-aortic SNs in five patients with left-sided tumours; in three patients SNs along the funicular vessels were detected [40].

In renal cell carcinoma lymphatic drainage was seen in 14/20 patients (70%) and SPECT/CT detected 26 SNs. Most frequent SNs were located para-aortic but also drainage to retrocaval, hilar, celiac trunk and thoracic (internal mammary chain, mediastinal and pleural) SNs was seen [41]. SPECT/CT was useful to depict lymphatic drainage outside the locoregional retroperitoneal templates in 14 out of 40 patients (35%) with renal tumours [42]. Non-visualization of SNs in renal tumours as established by means of SPECT/CT in 27 out of 73 patients (37%) was significantly associated with patient age and further

with high vascularization of kidney and tumours which might cause a wash-out effect of the injected radiotracer with decreased migration to lymph nodes [43].

In a series of 41 patients with cervical cancer SPECT/CT did increase the SN detection rate to 95% and was useful to depict unilateral drainage in 19 patients [44]. In another study SPECT/CT identified SNs in 51 out of 55 patients (93%) with stage IAB-IIA cervical cancer. High sensitivity and negative predictive value were found for patients with SPECT/CT SN visualization on both sides of the pelvis, but not for patients with unilateral lymphatic drainage [45]. In a meta-analysis evaluating eight studies the median overall SN detection rate was 98.6% for SPECT/CT and 85.3% for planar lymphoscintigraphy [46].

Concerning endometrial cancer in 44 high-risk patients SPECT/CT identified SNs in 34 of them (77%) with a total of 110 depicted SNs. The most frequent location was the external iliac chain (71%) but drainage to para-aortic SNs was also usual (44%). SPECT/CT was able to localize the only pelvic metastatic lymph node that was not depicted on planar images [47]. In another evaluation, SPECT/CT SN detection rate was 90% in 40 stage-I endometrial cancer patients and achieved bilateral detection in 26 of them [48]. Recently, in 151 patients with endometrial cancer, SPECT/CT detected SNs in external iliac (45%), obturator (30%), common iliac (14%), internal iliac (9%), para-aortic (1%), parametrium (1%) and presacral (1%). The overall pelvic SN detection was 77% for SPECT/CT and 68% for planar lymphoscintigraphy [49].

11.5.5 Other Malignancies

In stage Ia non-small lung cancer SPECT/CT visualized SNs in 39/63 patients (62%) and was useful to anatomically depict SNs in hilar and mediastinal lymph node basins [50]. In another series SPECT/CT identified SN in 12 out of 24 patients (50%) with early stage non-small cell lung cancer. Drainage was seen to ipsilateral hilar and mediastinal lymph node basins as well as to distant locations (internal mammary chain, retrocrural space and gastrohepatic ligament) [51].

In vulvar cancer, SPECT/CT detected more SNs than planar lymphoscintigraphy (mean 8.7 vs. mean 5.9) in 40 patients scheduled for biopsy; SPECT/CT identified aberrant drainage in 7 patients (17.5%) [52]. In another study, SPECT/CT established that in the groin 93% of the SNs are localized in the medial and central Daseler's zones which can be of importance for the extent of inguinal lymph node dissection [53].

In penile cancer, SPECT/CT contributed to zonal mapping of lymphatic drainage by depicting approximately 96% of SNs in the central and superior quadrants and only less than 4% in the inferior Daseler's zones [54]. Out of 52 groins corresponding to 26 penile cancer patients SPECT/CT identified 19 SNs in 16 groins that were overlooked by planar imaging [55].

11.6   General Indications of SPECT/CT

Indications for SPECT/CT in the SN procedure depend on the kind of malignancy and the complexity of lymphatic drainage. They will also depend on the multidisciplinary criteria adopted by surgeons and nuclear physicians in the different hospitals.

Generally speaking, indications for SPECT/CT for imaging in the SN procedure are as follows [5]:

1. Detection of SNs in cases without visualization at planar lymphoscintigraphy [30]. Due to the correction for tissue attenuation SPECT/CT is usually more sensitive than planar images (Fig. 11.4) and may be particularly useful in obese patients [23].

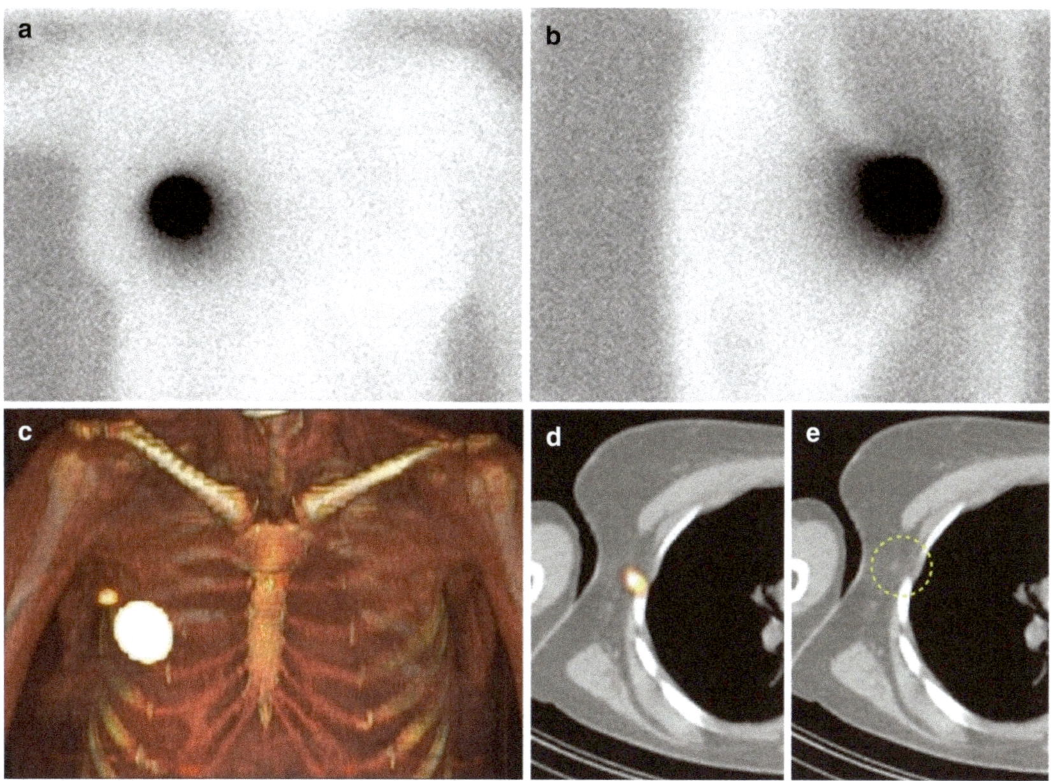

Fig. 11.4 Anterior (**a**) and lateral (**b**) delayed planar images showing no tracer migration from the injection site in the right breast. By contrast on both volume rendering (**c**) and axial SPECT/CT (**d**) a sentinel node is visualized in level I of the right axilla. Note on CT (**e**) that the sentinel node is not enlarged (circle)

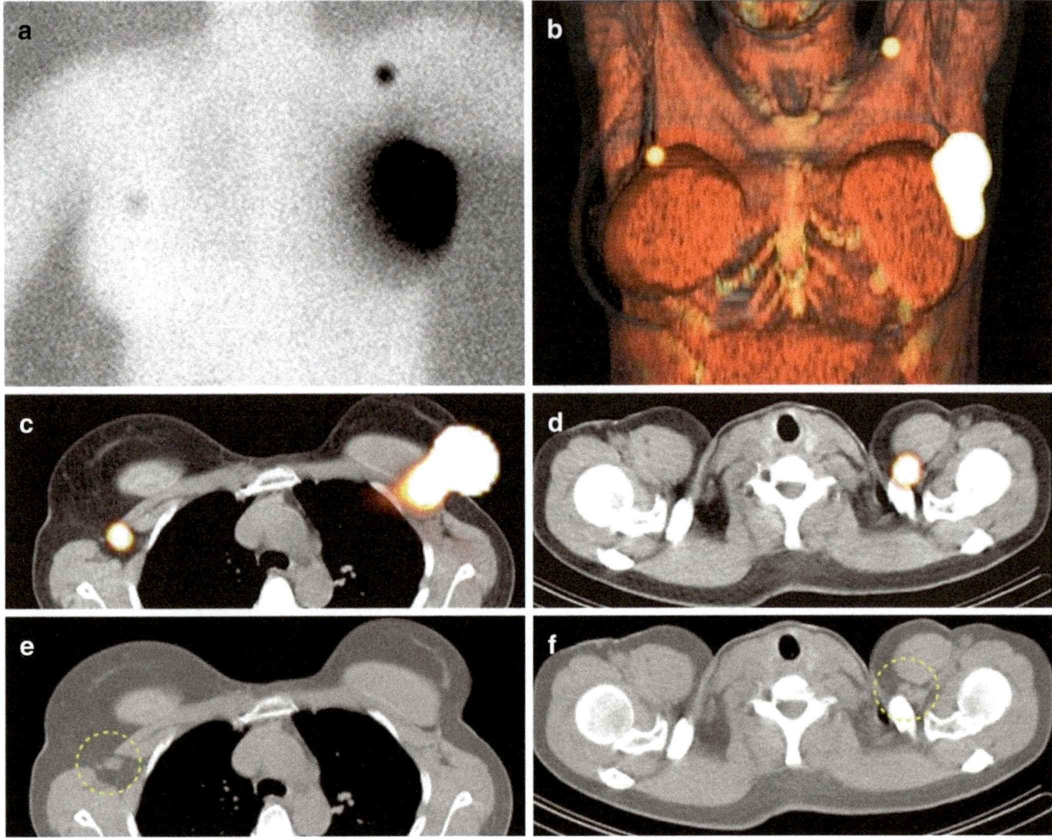

Fig. 11.5 Planar delayed scintigraphy (**a**) showing aberrant drainage from the injection site in the left breast to lymph nodes in the upper area of the left axilla and to the contralateral axilla in a patient with a left breast cancer recurrence. Patient had bilateral breast prostheses and in the past had undergone a left axillary lymph node dissection. Note on volume rendering (**b**) and axial SPECT/CT (**c**, **d**) that the sentinel nodes are localized in the top of level II/III of the left axilla and in level I of the right axilla. Both nodes are also seen (circles) on CT (**e**, **f**)

2. Localisation of SNs in areas with complex anatomy and a high number of lymph nodes such as the head and neck, or in cases with unexpected lymphatic drainage (e.g. between the pectoral muscles, internal mammary chain, level II or III of the axilla, in the vicinity of the scapula) at planar lymphoscintigraphy (Fig. 11.5). SPECT/CT is also helpful in cases with aberrant lymphatic drainage as, for instance, seen in patients who had undergone breast surgery in the past (Fig. 11.6).

3. Anatomical localisation and detection of additional sentinel nodes in areas of deep lymphatic drainage such as the pelvis (Fig. 11.2), abdomen or mediastinum.

4. Detection of SNs in near-the-injection-site areas of drainage as observed for neck nodes in periauricular melanomas (Fig. 11.7), sub-

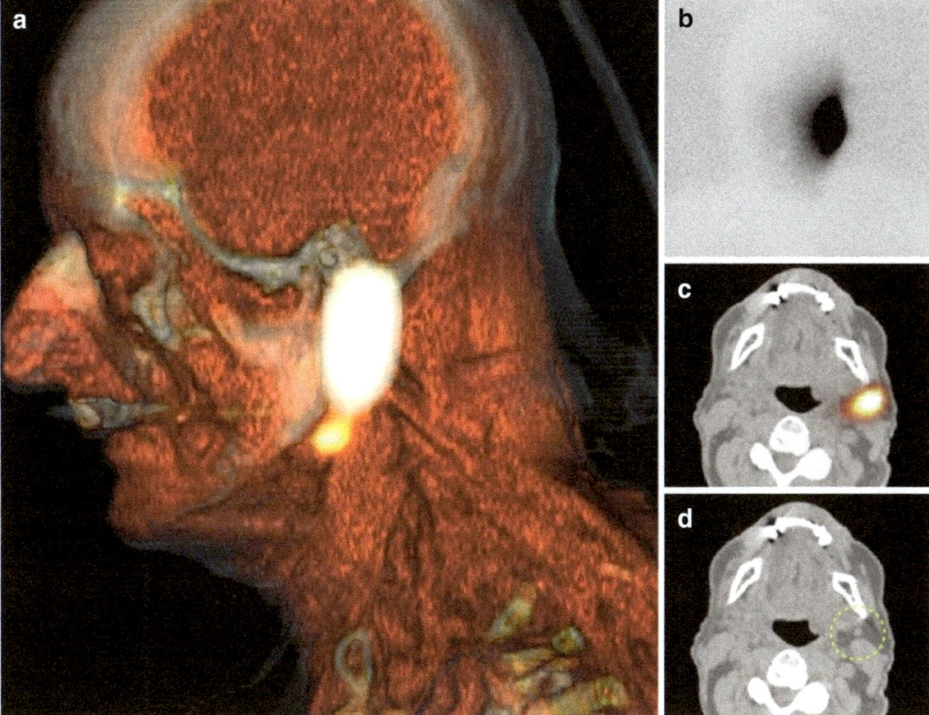

Fig. 11.6 Planar delayed scintigraphy (**a**) and volume rendering SPECT/CT (**b**) showing drainage from the injection in the right breast to the ipsilateral axilla. On axial SPECT/CT (**c**) and CT (**d**) the most cranial sentinel nodes are seen in level II of the axilla. By contrast the lower radioactive lymph node (**e**) corresponds with an interpectoral (circle) sentinel node on CT (**f**)

Fig. 11.7 In a patient with periauricular melanoma, lateral SPECT/CT imaging generated with volume rendering (**a**) showing drainage from the injection site to a left subman-dibular sentinel node. No drainage was depicted on planar image (**b**). The submandibular sentinel node seen on axial SPECT/CT (**c**) is not enlarged (circle) on CT (**d**)

mental and submaxillary nodes in oral cavity cancer and melanomas of the lower part of the face, periscapular and supraclavicular nodes in melanomas of the upper part of the trunk, intercostal and retroperitoneal nodes in melanomas of the back, and intramammary nodes in breast cancer.

An overview of SPECT/CT indications in various malignancies is shown in Table 11.1.

11.7 SPECT/CT as a Roadmap for Intraoperative Detection of Sentinel Nodes

The use of the above mentioned scintigraphic categories to characterize radioactive lymph nodes is also attributing to surgical decision making. Lymph nodes of the first two categories (definitely or highly probable SNs) are the nodes recognized by the nuclear physician and those that must be removed

Table 11.1 Overview of indications and additional clinical value of SPECT/CT for sentinel node imaging

Malignancy	Spect/CT indication	Additional value SPECT/CT
Breast cancer	No SN visualization on planar images Anatomical localisation atypical SNs	*Axilla*: SN detection (obese patients), SN localization in levels II/III *Non-axillary:* SN localisation internal mammary chain, intramammary, interpectoral
Melanoma	Localization of SNs depicted on planar images Detecting SNs in basins of aberrant drainage Detection occult near-the-injection-site SNs	SN localization in usual (axilla, groin) and aberrant basins (popliteal, epitrochlear, retroperitoneal, intercostal, intermuscular) SN detection in basins in the vicinity of primary lesions (parotid, periauricular, periscapular)
Oral cavity cancer	SN localization in neck surgical levels Detection of occult near-the-injection-site SNs	SNs localized in relation to anatomical structures Detection of submental and submaxillary SNs in floor of mouth malignancies
Penile cancer	Localisation of SNs in the groin	Differentiation inguinal SNs from secondary iliac lymph nodes
Vulvar cancer	Localisation of SNs in the groin	Differentiation inguinal SNs from secondary iliac lymph nodes
Prostate cancer	SN localisation in iliac areas SN detection outside area of extended pelvic lymph node dissection	Differentiation between external and internal iliac SNs Detection of SNs presacral, Cloquet's node, inguinal, para-aortic, abdominal wall, paravesical, pararectal, behind the common iliac artery, and lateral to the external iliac artery
Testicular cancer	Localisation of retroperitoneal SNs	Differentiation between para-aortic and aortocaval SNs Detection of SNs along funicular vessels
Renal cell carcinoma	Localisation of retroperitoneal SNs Aberrant lymphatic drainage detection	Differentiation between para-aortic and aortocaval SNs Detection atypical located SNs (mediastinal, intercostal)
Cervix cancer	Localisation of SNs in iliac areas Aberrant lymphatic drainage detection	SN localisation in iliac basins including obturator fossa Detection of presacral and para-aortic SNs
Endometrial cancer	Localization SNs in iliac areas Aberrant lymphatic drainage detection	SN localization in iliac basins including obturator fossa Often detection of para-aortic SNs
Lung cancer	Anatomical localization SNs	Localisation of hilar SNs Detection of mediastinal SNs (paratracheal, subcarinal)

in the operation room by the surgeon. Less probable SNs may sometimes be removed depending on the degree of remaining radioactivity measured by the gamma probe or the portable gamma camera during the control of the excision fossa.

A crucial role to guide surgical SN resection is reserved to nuclear physicians in charge of generating the imaging reports. Practical guidelines to achieve this process have been recently described for oral cavity cancer [26]. This approach is applicable for the various SN procedures and includes the description of the different components of the lymphatic mapping study and in particular of SPECT/CT. Important SPECT/CT aspects to be included in the nuclear medicine report are the following:

1. Localization of SNs already depicted on lymphoscintigraphy, with description of lymph node stations and clear reference to specific landmarks as blood vessels, muscles and other anatomical structures which can guide surgeons to recognize SN locations in the operation room.
2. Identification and anatomical localization of additional SNs not depicted on planar lymphoscintigraphy.
3. Correlation of findings of fused SPECT/CT with those of CT. In many cases radioactive SNs correspond with single lymph nodes. However, in some cases radioactivity on SPECT/CT corresponds with multiple lymph nodes on CT [26]. The observation of these clusters of SNs on low dose CT (Fig. 11.8) is important preoperative information that may predict the presence of multiple radioactive SNs at the same site and may facilitate an accurate post-excision control after removal of the first radioactive node by the surgeon

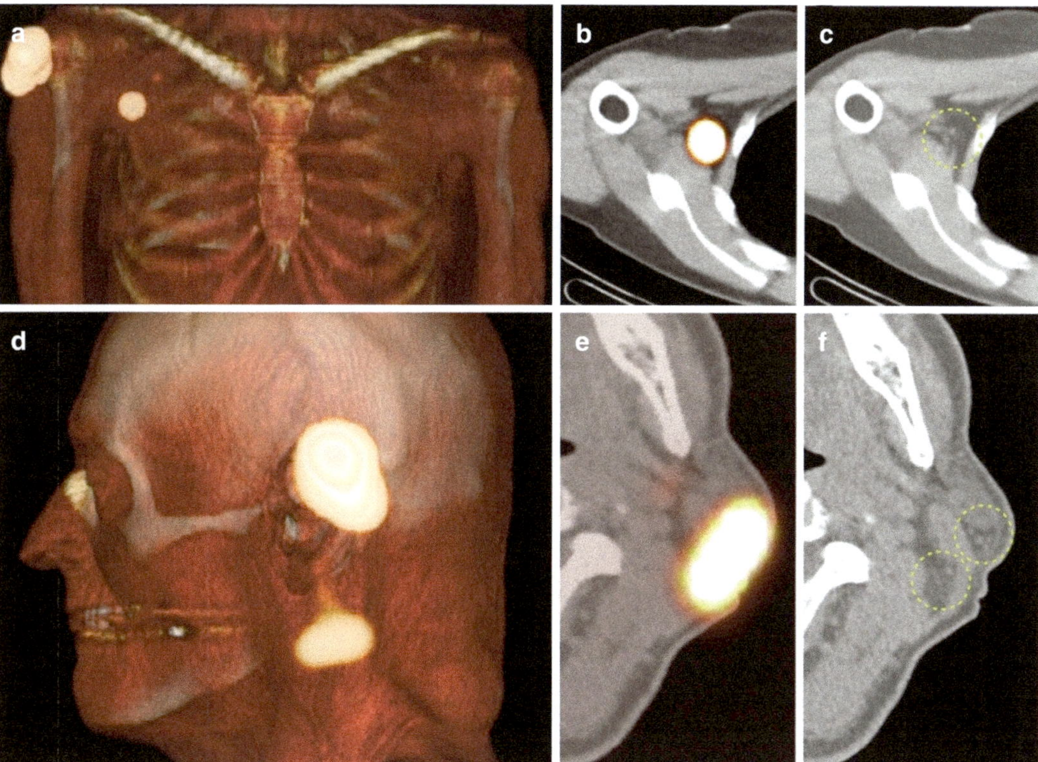

Fig. 11.8 In a patient with a melanoma of the right shoulder, volume rendering (**a**) and axial (**b**) SPECT/CT show drainage from the injection site to a sentinel node in level I of the right axilla. The radioactive hot spot seen of SPECT/CT corresponds on CT (**c**) with a cluster of lymph nodes (circle). In another patient with a left retroauricular melanoma, drainage to the left side of the neck is seen on volume rendering (**d**) and axial (**e**) SPECT/CT. At the same level, clusters of lymph nodes (circles) behind the left parotid and the sternocleidomastoid muscle are seen on CT (**f**)

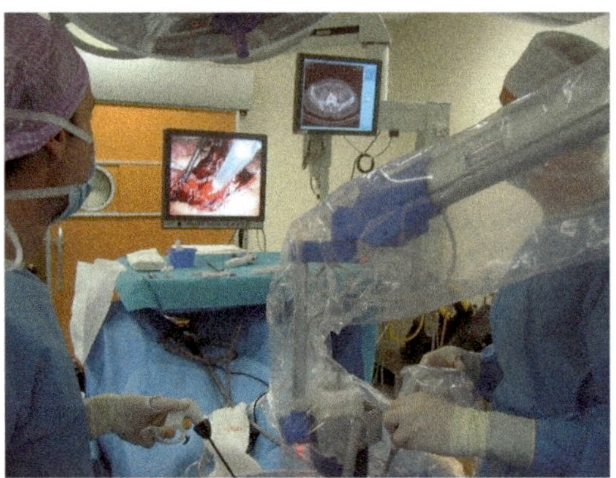

Fig. 11.9 Display of SPECT/CT during a laparoscopic procedure aimed to remove a sentinel node along the iliac vessels in a prostate cancer patient. Intraoperative sentinel node localization was also guided by a portable gamma camera as seen in the foreground

particularly for areas such as the pelvis and head/neck.

4. Clear description of secondary findings on low dose non-enhanced CT including enlarged lymph nodes, incidental findings and abnormalities.

5. Nuclear physicians need to select SPECT/CT slices preparing specific key images to be uploaded to the PACS (or printed if PACS is not readily available in the operating theatre)

and linked to the imaging reports. Also, the continuous display of SPECT/CT images on a screen in the operating room (Fig. 11.9) can help surgeons in the intraoperative search by recognition of anatomical structures adjacent to the sentinel node.

A summary of the points to be included in SPECT/CT reports is given in Fig. 11.10.

11.8 New Strategies Combining SPECT/CT and PET/CT

The extended experience with SN biopsy has become the basis to expand interventional nuclear medicine approaches in recent years [56]. A concrete example concerns the combined use of the SN procedure, including SPECT/CT, and PSMA PET/CT to stage the pelvis in clinically N0 intermediate or high-risk prostate cancer patients. In an attempt to find an alternative to extended pelvic lymph node dissection this approach led to 100% sensitivity in the identification of N1 patients with a correct pelvic regional staging in 94% of the cases [57]. PSMA PET/CT was first used in all patients and SPECT/CT-based SN biopsy only in patients with a negative PSMA.

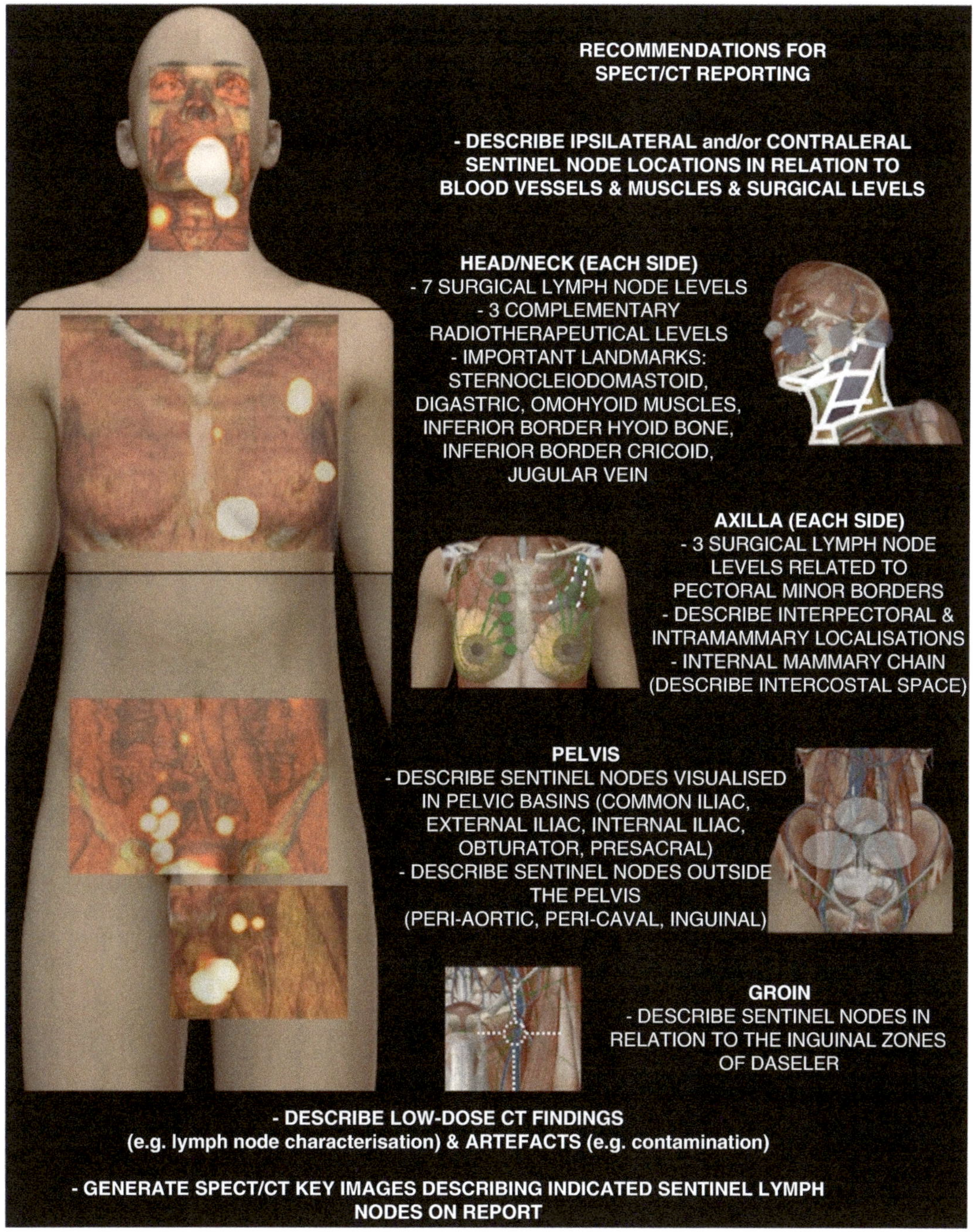

Fig. 11.10 Summary of the points recommended to be included in reports of SPECT/CT concerning sentinel node locations in head/neck, axilla, pelvis and groin

References

1. Morton DL, Wen DR, Wong JH, Economou JS, Cagle LA, Storm FK, et al. Technical details of intraoperative lymphatic mapping for early stage melanoma. Arch Surg. 1992;127:392–9.
2. Giuliano AE, Conolly JL, Edge SB, Mittendorf EA, Rugo HS, Solin LJ, et al. Breast Cancer-Major changes in the American Joint Committee on Cancer eight edition cancer staging manual. CA Cancer J Clin. 2017;67:290–303.
3. Brierly JD, Gospodarowicz MK, Wittekind C, editors. TNM classification of malignant tumours. 8th ed. Hoboken: Wiley-Blackwell; 2017.
4. Delbeke D, Coleman RE, Guiberteau MJ, Brown ML, Royal HD, Siegel BA, et al. Procedure guidelines for SPECT/CT imaging. J Nucl Med. 2006;47:1227–34.
5. Valdés Olmos RA, Rietbergen DD, Vidal-Sicart S, Manca G, Giammarile F, Mariani G. Contribution of SPECT/CT imaging to radioguided sentinel lymph node biopsy in breast cancer, melanoma, and other solid cancers: from "open and see" to "see and open". Q J Nucl Med Mol Imaging. 2014;58:127–39.
6. Fishman EK, Ney DR, Heath DG, Corl FM, Horton KM, Johnson PT. Volume rendering versus maximum intensity projection in CT angiography: what works best, when, and why. Radiographics. 2006;26:905–22.
7. Vidal-Sicart S, Brouwer OR, Valdés Olmos RA. Evaluation of the sentinel lymph node combining SPECT/CT with the planar images and its importance for the surgical act. Rev Esp Med Nucl. 2011;30:331–7.
8. Nieweg OE, Estourgie S, Valdés Olmos RA. Lymphatic mapping and sentinel node biopsy. In: Ell PJ, Gambhir SS, editors. Nuclear medicine in clinical diagnosis and treatment. 3rd ed. Edinburgh: Churchill Livingstone; 2004. p. 229–60.
9. Bluemel C, Herrmann K, Giammarile F, Nieweg OE, Dubreuil J, Testori A, et al. EANM practice guidelines for lymphoscintigraphy and sentinel lymph node biopsy in melanoma. Eur J Nucl Med Mol Imaging. 2015;42:1750–66.
10. Jimenez-Hefferman A, Ellmann A, Sado H, Huiç D, Bal C, Parameswaram R, et al. Results of a prospective multicenter International Atomic Energy Agency sentinel node trial on the value of SPECT/CT over planar imaging in various malignancies. J Nucl Med. 2015;56:1338–44.
11. Benk M, Wocial K, Lewandowska W, Rutkowski P, Teterycz P, Jarek P, et al. Value of planar lymphoscintigraphy (PL) versus SPECT/CT in evaluation of sentinel lymph node in trunk melanoma—one center, large series retrospective study. Nucl Med Rev Cent East Eur. 2018;21:79–84.
12. Stoffels I, Boy C, Pöppel T, Kuhn J, Klötgen K, Dissemond J, et al. Association between lymph node excision with or without preoperative SPECT/CT and metastatic node detection and disease-free survival in melanoma. JAMA. 2012;308:1007–14.
13. Stoffels I, Herrmann K, Rekowski J, Jansen P, Schadendorf DStang A, et al. Sentinel lymph node excision with or without preoperative hybrid single-photon emission computed tomography/computed tomography (SPECT/CT) in melanoma: study protocol for a multicentric randomized controlled trial. Trials. 2019;20:99.
14. Quartuccio N, Garau LM, Arnone A, Pappalardo M, Rubello D, Arnone G, et al. Comparison of 99mTc-labeled colloid SPECT/CT and planar lymphoscintigraphy in sentinel lymph node detection in patients with melanoma: a meta-analysis. J Clin Med. 2020;9:1680.
15. Faries MB, Thompson JF, Cochran AJ, Andtbacka RH, Mozzillo N, Zager JS, et al. Complete dissection or observation for sentinel node metastasis in melanoma. N Engl J Med. 2017;376:2211–22.
16. Leiter U, Stadler R, Mauch C, Hohenberger W, Brockmeyer N, Berking C, et al. Complete lymph node dissection versus no dissection in patients with sentinel lymph node biopsy positive melanoma (DeCOG-SLT): a multicentre, randomized, phase 3 trial. Lancet Oncol. 2016;17:757–67.
17. Perissinoti A, Rietbergen DDD, Vidal-Sicart S, Riera AA, Valdés Olmos RA. Melanoma & nuclear medicine: new insights & advances. Melanoma Manag. 2018;5:MMT06.
18. Stanzel S, Pernthaler B, Schwarz T, Bjelic-Radisic V, Kerschbaumer S, Aigner RM. Diagnostic and prognostic value of additional SPECT/CT in sentinel lymph node mapping in breast cancer patients. Nuklearmedizin. 2018;57:92–9.
19. Uren RF, Howman-Giles R, Chung DJ, Spillane AJ, Noushi FGillet D, et al. SPECT/CT scans allow precise anatomical location of sentinel lymph nodes in breast cancer and redefine lymphatic drainage from the breast to the axilla. Breast. 2012;21:480–6.
20. Serrano-Vicente J, Rayo-Madrid JI, Dominguez-Grande ML, Infante-Torre JR, García-Bernardo L, Moreno-Caballero M, et al. Role of SPECT/CT in breast cancer sentinel node biopsy when internal mammary chain drainage is observed. Clin Transl Oncol. 2016;18:418–25.
21. Manca G, Volterrani D, Mazzarri S, Duce V, Svirydenka A, Giuliano A, et al. Sentinel lymph node mapping in breast cancer; a critical reappraisal of the internal mammary chain issue. Q J Nucl Med Mol Imaging. 2014;58:114–26.
22. Borrelli P, Donswijk ML, Stokkel MP, Teixeira SC, van Tinteren H, Rutgers EJ, et al. Contribution of SPECT/CT for sentinel node localization in patients with ipsilateral breast cancer relapse. Eur J Nucl Med Mol Imaging. 2017;44:630–7.
23. Lerman H, Lievshitz G, Zak O, Metser U, Schneebaum S, Even-Sapir E. Improved sentinel node identification by SPECT/CT in overweight patients with breast cancer. J Nucl Med. 2007;28:201–6.
24. Siddique M, Khalid Nawaz M, Bashir H. The usefulness of SPECT/CT in sentinel node mapping of early stage breast cancer patients showing negative or equivocal findings on planar scintigraphy. Asia Ocean J Nucl Med Biol. 2018;6:80–9.

25. Pouw B, Hellingman D, Kieft M, Vogel WV, van Os KJ, Rutgers EJT, et al. The hidden sentinel node in breast cancer: reevaluating the role of SPECT/CT and tracer reinjection. Eur J Surg Oncol. 2016;42:497–503.
26. Giammarile F, Schilling C, Gnanasegaran G, Bal C, Oyen WJG, Rubello D, et al. The EANM practical guidelines for sentinel lymph node localization in oral cavity squamous cell carcinoma. Eur J Nucl Med Mol Imaging. 2019;46:623–37.
27. Den Toom IJ, van Schie A, van Weert S, Karagozoglu KH, Bloemena E, Hoekstra OS, et al. The added value of SPECT/CT for the identification of sentinel lymph nodes in early stage oral cancer. Eur J Nucl Med Mol Imaging. 2017;44:9998–1004.
28. Haerle SK, Hany TF, Strobel K, Sidler D, Stoeckli SJ. Is there an additional value of SPECT/CT over planar lymphoscintigraphy for sentinel node mapping in oral/oropharyngeal squamous cell carcinoma? Ann Surg Oncol. 2009;16:3118–24.
29. Trinh BB, Chapman BC, Gleisner A, Kwak JJ, Morgan R, McCarter MD, et al. SPECT/CT adds distinct lymph node basins and influences radiologic findings and surgical approach for sentinel lymph node biopsy in head and neck melanoma. Ann Surg Oncol. 2018;25:1716–22.
30. Vermeeren L, Valdés Olmos RA, Klop MC, van der Ploeg IMC, Nieweg OE, Balm AJM, et al. SPECT/CT for sentinel lymph node mapping in head and neck melanoma. Head Neck. 2011;33:1–6.
31. Klode J, Poeppel T, Boy C, Mueller S, Schadendorf D, Korber A, et al. Advantages of preoperative hybrid SPECT/CT in detection of sentinel lymph nodes in cutaneous head and neck malignancies. J Eur Acad Dermatol Venereol. 2011;25:1213–21.
32. De Veij Mestdagh PD, Schreuder WH, Vogel WV, Donswijk ML, van Werkhoven E, van der Wal JE, et al. Mapping of sentinel lymph node drainage using SPECT/CT to tailor elective nodal irradiation in head and neck cancer patients (SUSPECT-2): a single-center prospective trial. BMC Cancer. 2019;19:1110.
33. Van der Poel HG, Wit EM, Acar C, van den Berg NS, van Leeuwen FWB, Valdes Olmos RA, et al. Sentinel node biopsy for prostate cancer: report from a consensus panel meeting. BJU Int. 2017;120:204–11.
34. Vermeeren L, Valdés Olmos RA, Meinhardt W, Bex A, van der Poel HG, Vogel WW, et al. Value of SPECT/CT for detection and anatomic localization of sentinel lymph nodes before laparoscopic sentinel node lymphadenectomy in prostate cancer. J Nucl Med. 2009;50:865–70.
35. Meinhardt W, van der Poel HG, Valdés Olmos RA, Bex A, Brouwer OR, Horenblas S. Laparoscopic sentinel lymph node biopsy for prostate cancer: the relevance of locations outside the extended dissection area. Prostate Cancer. 2012;2012:751753.
36. Martínez-Sarmiento M, Pérez-Ardavin J, Monserrat-Monfort JJ, Sánchez-González JP, Sopena-Novales P, Bello-Arqués P, et al. Sentinel lymph node selective biopsy in prostate cancer. Arch Esp Urol. 2019;72:842–50.
37. Vermeeren L, Meinhardt W, van der Poel HG, Valdés Olmos RA. Lymphatic drainage from the treated versus untreated prostate: feasibility of sentinel node biopsy in recurrent cancer. Eur J Nucl Med Mol Imaging. 2010;37:2012–26.
38. Krengli M, Ballare A, Cannillo B, Rudoni M, Kocjancic E, Loi G, et al. Potential advantage of studying the lymphatic drainage by sentinel node technique and SPECT/CT image fusion for pelvic irradiation of prostate cancer. Int J Radiat Oncol Biol Phys. 2006;66:1100–4.
39. Michaud AV, Samain B, Ferrer L, Fleury V, Dore M, Colombie M, et al. Haute couture or ready-to-wear? Tailored pelvic radiotherapy for prostate cancer based on individualized sentinel lymph node detection. Cancers. 2020;12:944.
40. Brouwer OR, Valdés Olmos RA, Vermeeren L, Hoefnagel CA, Nieweg OE, Horenblas S. SPECT/CT and a portable γ-camera for image-guided laparoscopic sentinel node biopsy in testicular cancer. J Nucl Med. 2011;52:5551–4.
41. Bex A, Vermeeren L, Meinhardt W, Prevoo W, Horenblas S, Valdés Olmos RA. Intraoperative sentinel node identification and sampling in clinically node-negative renal cell carcinoma: initial experience in 20 patients. World J Urol. 2011;29:793–9.
42. Kuusk T, De Bruijn R, Brouwer OR, De Jong J, Donswijk ML, Grivas N, et al. Lymphatic drainage from renal tumours in vivo: a prospective sentinel node study using SPECT/CT imaging. J Urol. 2018;199:1426–32.
43. Kuusk T, Donswijk ML, Valdés Olmos RA, De Bruijn RE, Brouwer OR, Hendricksen K, et al. An analysis of SPECT/CT non-visualization of sentinel lymph nodes in renal tumours. EJNMMI Res. 2018;8:105.
44. Martinez A, Zerdoud S, Mery E, Bouissou E, Ferron G, Querleu D. Hybrid imaging by SPECT/CT for sentinel lymph node detection in patients with cancer of the uterine cervix. Gynecol Oncol. 2010;119:431–5.
45. Novikov SN, Krzhivitskii PI, Kanaev SV, Berlev IV, Bisyarin MI, Artemyeva AS. SPECT-CT visualization and biopsy of sentinel lymph nodes in patients with stage IAB-IIA cervical cancer. Ann Nucl Med. 2020;34(10):781–6. https://doi.org/10.1007/s12149-020-01503-5.
46. Hoogendam JP, Veldhuis WB, Hobbelink M, Verheijen RH, van den Bosch MA, Zweemer RP. 99mTc SPECT/CT versus planar lymphoscintigraphy for preoperative sentinel lymph node detection in cervical cancer: a systemic review and metaanalysis. J Nucl Med. 2015;56:675–80.
47. Perissinotti A, Paredes P, Vidal-Sicart S, Torné A, Albela S, Navales I, et al. Use of SPECT/CT for improved sentinel lymph node localization in endometrial cancer. Gynecol Oncol. 2013;129:42–8.
48. Elisei F, Crivellaro C, Giuliani D, Dolci C, De Ponti E, Montanelli L, et al. Sentinel-node mapping in endometrial cancer patients: comparing SPECT/CT, gamma probe and dye. Ann Nucl Med. 2017;31:93–9.

49. Togami S, Kawamura T, Yanazume S, Kamio M, Kobayashi H. Comparison of lymphoscintigraphy and single photon emission computed tomography with computed tomography (SPECT/CT) for sentinel lymph node detection in endometrial cancer. Int J Gynecol Cancer. 2020;30:626–30.

50. Nomori H, Ikeda K, Mori T, Shiraishi S, Kobayashi H, Kawanaka K, et al. Sentinel node identification in clinical stage Ia non-small lung cancer by a combined single photon emission computed tomography/computed tomography system. J Thorac Cardiovasc Surg. 2007;134:182–7.

51. Abele JT, Allred K, Clare T, Bédard ELR. Lymphoscintigraphy in early-stage non-small cell lung cancer with technetium-99m nanocolloids and hybrid SPECT/CT: a pilot project. Ann Nucl Med. 2014;28:477–83.

52. Klapdor R, Länger F, Gratz KF, Hillemans P, Hertel H. SPECT/CT for SLN dissection in vulvar cancer: improved SLN detection and dissection by preoperative three-dimensional anatomical localisation. Gynecol Oncol. 2015;138:590–6.

53. Collarino A, Donswijk ML, van Driel WJ, Stokkel MP, Valdés Olmos RA. The use of SPECT/CT for anatomical mapping of lymphatic drainage in vulvar cancer: possible implications for the extent of inguinal lymph node dissection. Eur J Nucl Med Mol Imaging. 2015;42:2064–71.

54. Omorphos S, Saad Z, Kirkham A, Nigam R, Malone P, Bomanji J, et al. Zonal mapping of sentinel lymph nodes in penile cancer patients using fused SPECT/CT imaging and lymphoscintigraphy. Urol Oncol. 2018;36:530.e1–530.e6.

55. Naumann CM, Colberg C, Jüptner M, Marx M, Zhao Y, Jiang P, et al. Evaluation of the diagnostic value of preoperative sentinel lymph node (SLN) imaging in penile carcinoma patients without palpable inguinal lymph nodes via single photon emission computed tomography/computed tomography (SPECT/CT) as compared to planar scintigraphy. Urol Oncol. 2018;36:92.e17–24.

56. Valdés Olmos RA, Rietbergen DDD, Rubello D, Pereira Arias-Bouda LM, Collarino A, Colletti PM, et al. Sentinel node imaging and radioguided surgery in the era of SPECT/CT and PET/CT. Toward new interventional nuclear medicine strategies. Clin Nucl Med. 2020;45(10):771–7. https://doi.org/10.1097/RLU.0000000000003206.

57. Hinsenveld FJ, Wit EWK, van Leeuwen PJ, Brouwer OR, Donswijk ML, Tillier CN, et al. Prostate-specific membrane antigen PET/CT combined with sentinel node biopsy for primary lymph node staging in prostate cancer. J Nucl Med. 2020;61:540–5.

Lung SPECT/CT

12

Paul J. Roach

12.1 Introduction

The accurate diagnosis of pulmonary embolism (PE) is challenging for both clinicians and imaging specialists. Misdiagnosis must be avoided because untreated PE has a mortality rate reported to be up to 30%, and unnecessary treatment with anticoagulation places patients at risk of bleeding [1–3].

For many years, the ventilation/perfusion (*V/Q*) lung scan was the primary imaging test to assess patients with suspected PE [4]. More recently, radiographic computed tomography pulmonary angiography (CTPA) is used preferentially in most patients [4–6]. These two imaging studies have largely replaced invasive pulmonary angiography and digital subtraction angiography in the assessment of patients with PE, and both are utilised widely in hospitals and imaging centres worldwide.

Experience with *V/Q* scintigraphy spans over 50 years, with its use first described by Wagner et al. in 1964 [7]. The principle of the test is that in patients with PE, lung perfusion is compromised secondary to occlusive thrombi in the pulmonary arterial tree, whereas ventilation to these areas is generally unaffected [8]. This results in the so-called ventilation/perfusion (*V/Q*) mis-

match, i.e. where ventilation is normal but perfusion is reduced or absent [8, 9].

12.2 Limitations of Planar Lung Scintigraphy

Although widely used over many decades, the planar lung scan is a test that is widely recognised as having limitations [5, 10–13].

When the lungs are imaged in only two dimensions (2D), as occurs with planar imaging, there is significant overlap of anatomical segments, and as a result, it is frequently difficult to assign defects to specific lung segments. Accurately determining the extent of embolic involvement in each individual segment can also be problematic as the size and shape of each lung segment varies [12]. In addition, embolic defects may not be detected if there is 'shine through' occurring from underlying lung segments with normal perfusion. This can result in an underestimation of the extent of perfusion loss in patients with PE [14]. Furthermore, not all segments of the lungs are visualised on conventional planar lung scintigraphy. Specifically, the medial basal segment of the right lower lobe is not routinely seen on planar scintigraphy [12, 15].

In addition to these inherent technical limitations of planar (2D) lung scintigraphy, there are the problems posed by the widely used probabilistic criteria generally used to report these studies [16–20]. The use of probabilities for lung scan

P. J. Roach (✉)
Department of Nuclear Medicine, Royal North Shore Hospital, Sydney, NSW, Australia
e-mail: paul.roach@sydney.edu.au

reporting became widespread following the publication of the large multicentre PIOPED study in 1990 [21]. This landmark study highlighted some of the limitations of planar lung scanning, particularly in relation to specificity. Given the management implementations, if a patient is diagnosed with PE, this is a condition in which clinicians prefer binary (i.e. positive or negative) reports whenever possible, rather than inconclusive, 'indeterminate' or even probabilistic reports [22].

12.3 Advantages of SPECT Imaging

SPECT (single-photon emission computed tomography) is widely used in many areas of radionuclide imaging today because of its ability to image in three dimensions (3D). It has been shown to be superior to planar imaging in the evaluation of many conditions, such as assessing myocardial perfusion as well as brain and liver imaging [23, 24]. In contrast to planar imaging, SPECT avoids the problems introduced by segmental overlap and 'shine through' of the adjacent lung, making it better able to image all segments of the lungs and more accurately define the size and location of perfusion defects [12]. Hence, it would be expected that SPECT V/Q scintigraphy would be superior to planar imaging. Furthermore, with the widespread availability today of multi-detector gamma cameras (and increasingly SPECT/CT scanners) as well as improved computing power allowing faster processing, lung scintigraphy is ideally suited to SPECT acquisition.

The advantages of SPECT over planar lung imaging have been demonstrated in numerous published manuscripts over many years, both in animals and in humans. In a study performed in which subsegmental and segmental clots were induced in dogs, SPECT was shown to be more sensitive than planar imaging [25]. Similar results were described by Bajc and co-workers in a study that compared SPECT with planar imaging using

^{99m}Tc-DTPA aerosols and ^{99m}Tc-MAA in pigs [26]. Artificial emboli labelled with ^{201}Tl were induced and SPECT was found to have an increased sensitivity (91% versus 64%) and specificity (87% versus 79%) compared with planar imaging. In a study using Monte Carlo simulation of lungs containing defects to mimic PE, Magnussen and co-workers also demonstrated that SPECT was more sensitive than planar imaging (97% versus 77%) [15].

The advantage of SPECT imaging over planar lung scintigraphy has also been consistently demonstrated in human studies. In a series of 53 patients with suspected PE, Bajc and co-workers found SPECT to be more sensitive than planar imaging (100% versus 85%) in the detection of PE [27]. In addition, the authors concluded that SPECT demonstrated less interobserver variation and better delineation of mismatched defects compared with planar imaging. Collart and co-workers, in a study of 114 patients, also demonstrated that SPECT was more specific than planar imaging (96% versus 78%) and had better intra-observer reproducibility (94% versus 91%) and interobserver reproducibility (88% versus 79%) [28]. In a pivotal study of 83 patients with suspected PE, Reinartz et al. demonstrated that SPECT was superior to planar imaging in terms of sensitivity (97% versus 76%), specificity (91% versus 85%) and accuracy (94% versus 81%) [29]. In this paper, SPECT increased the number of detectable defects at the segmental level by 12.8% and at the subsegmental level by 82.6%.

Another advantage of V/Q SPECT imaging is that it has been consistently shown to have a much lower indeterminate rate than planar imaging, typically less than 5% [8, 30, 31]. In one large series from Canada, V/Q SPECT was shown to have a very high negative predictive value (98.5%) for PE with only 3% of studies being reported as indeterminate for PE [32].

The published data to date is consistent and taken together indicates that SPECT has a greater sensitivity and specificity and improved reproducibility compared with planar lung imaging.

12.4 Need for Correlation with Anatomical Imaging

From the viewpoint of the lung scan, ventilation/perfusion mismatch would ideally only be caused by PE, with all other pathological processes producing other scintigraphic appearances. Unfortunately, that is not the case and the reality is that many different pathological processes can affect pulmonary ventilation and perfusion. Ventilation/perfusion mismatch can be seen in other conditions, including congenital pulmonary vascular abnormalities, veno-occlusive disease, vasculitis, emphysema, radiation therapy-induced changes and extrinsic vascular compression from conditions such as neoplasm and mediastinal adenopathy [8, 33] (Fig. 12.1). To further complicate the issue, the classic V/Q 'mismatch' pattern is sometimes not seen in patients with PE. Subsequent to the acute embolic event, clots often become partly resolved or the process of recanalisation occurs, resulting in mismatch becoming less distinct. Furthermore, in some patients, pulmonary infarction occurs subsequent to PE resulting in a matched reduction (or loss) of both ventilation and perfusion on V/Q scintigraphy, an appearance typically seen with non-embolic pathologies [8]. Hence, it should be remembered that not all patients with PE will have V/Q mismatch, and not all patients with V/Q mismatch on lung scanning will have PE. For this reason, the chest X-ray appearances have been considered pivotal by many to aid in the interpretation of the V/Q scan, and the findings are often used to improve the accuracy and specificity of V/Q reporting [8, 21, 34]. At some centres, including my own at Royal North Shore Hospital, Sydney, the chest X-ray has often been used to triage individual patients prior to deciding which imaging test would be the most appropriate to perform. Patients with normal, or near-normal, radiographic appearances may be referred for V/Q scintigraphy, whereas those patients with abnormal radiographic appearances may preferentially be referred for CTPA [35]. The ability of CTPA to image the lung parenchyma gives it a definite advantage over lung scintigraphy as it can more readily identify conditions which may mimic PE clinically, such as pneumonia, abscess, pleural or pericardial effusions, aortic dissection, oesophageal rupture and malignancy [5, 6, 36, 37]. While the benefits of adding anatomical information to V/Q scans are well recognised, until recently, the only option

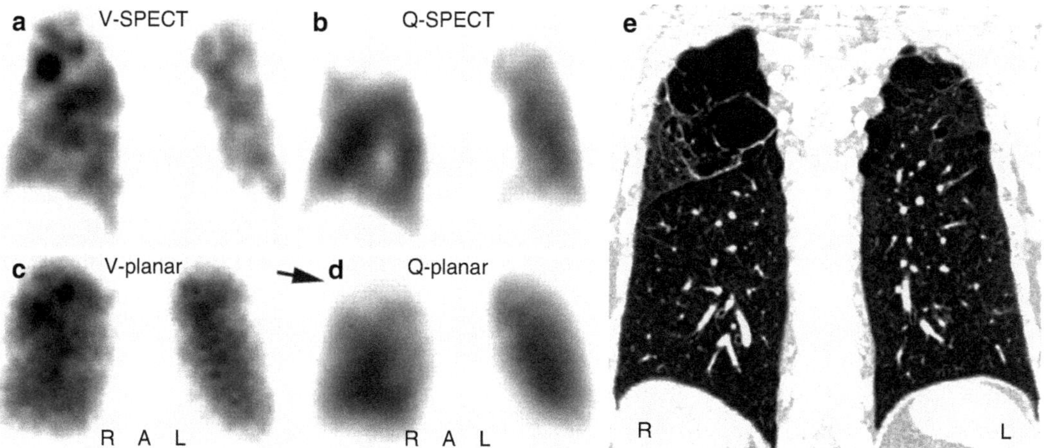

Fig. 12.1 Ventilation (V) and perfusion (Q) SPECT images in a patient with severe chronic obstructive pulmonary disease (COPD) and pulmonary emphysema. A large emphysematic bullae in the right upper lobe (**e**) seen on CT led to a false-positive diagnosis on V/Q scintigraphy (**b, d**, mismatch perfusion defects marked by *arrows*). The patient did not have PE. Technegas can ventilate into emphysematous bullae (**a, c**). In this case, the CT would have demonstrated the cause of the perfusion reduction evident on SPECT imaging and would have avoided the false-positive V/Q scan (R right, A anterior, L left). (Reprinted with permission from Reinartz et al. [29])

for reporting specialists has been to view a chest X-ray or a diagnostic CT scan performed non-contemporaneously [38].

12.5 Combining Functional and Anatomical Images

12.5.1 Visual and Software Fusion

Recent years have witnessed an increasing emphasis on combining the structural information provided by anatomical techniques, such as CT scanning, with the functional information provided by nuclear medicine imaging [39]. While reporting specialists have been able to visually compare different images placed side by side (the so-called visual fusion) for many years, the accuracy of such an approach is frequently limited [39, 40]. A more robust approach is to fuse SPECT or PET images with CT or MRI using sophisticated data-matching algorithms. This so-called software fusion has been used since the early 1990s with great success in many applications, such as brain imaging [39]. However, the 'deformable' and flexible nature of much of the body, as well as differences in the scanning bed shapes, arm positioning and breathing protocols can make accurate registration of a SPECT study and a diagnostic CT scan acquired on a separate scanner problematic [38]. Despite these limitations, our group has demonstrated the feasibility of the software fusion approach with lung scintigraphy. In a pilot study of 30 patients with suspected PE, SPECT perfusion data were fused with CTPA using commercial software which was based on an iterative approach employing an automated mutual information algorithm [38]. We demonstrated that all nine patients with positive CTPA studies performed as the initial investigation for PE had co-localised perfusion defects on the subsequent fused CTPA/ SPECT images (Fig. 12.2). Of the 11 *V/Q* scans initially reported as intermediate probability, 27% were able to be reinterpreted as low probability due to co-localisation of defects with parenchymal or pleural pathology. While we

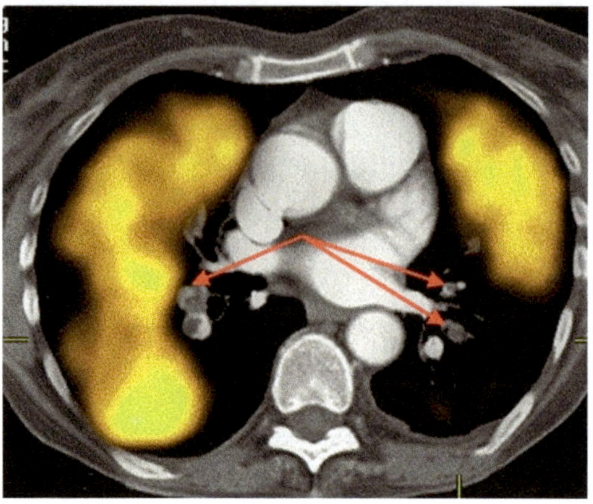

Fig. 12.2 Co-registered CTPA/perfusion SPECT (transverse slice) demonstrating extensive perfusion defects on SPECT corresponding with proximal bilateral PE shown on CTPA (*arrowed*). (Reprinted with permission from Roach et al. [41])

have demonstrated that the approach of using software fusion is technically feasible and can improve the diagnostic accuracy of the lung SPECT, it may not be practical in all centres, particularly if the required software programs or operator experience is lacking.

12.5.2 Hardware Fusion

With the increasing availability of integrated SPECT/CT and PET/CT scanners, 'hardware fusion' is now routinely employed in many areas of nuclear medicine practice [39]. As the two data-sets are acquired on the same scanning bed in the same imaging session, much greater registration accuracy is seen with hybrid SPECT/CT scanners compared with software fusion techniques [39, 42–44]. At my own hospital campus in Sydney, where we have three SPECT/CT scanners, we routinely perform SPECT/CT scanning in most areas of nuclear medicine, including bone scans, gallium (infection) scans, myocardial perfusion studies as well as scans of the liver, parathyroid and adrenal glands. As well, irtually all lung scans are now done using SPECT/CT scanning. This is in addition to all of our PET scans which are performed on a hybrid PET/CT scanner.

12.6 *V/Q* Lung SPECT/CT

In the case of lung scanning, the emergence of hybrid SPECT/CT scanners gives reporting specialists two options to combine structural and functional data and potentially to improve overall diagnostic accuracy of the modality.

Firstly, SPECT perfusion can be co-registered with diagnostic CTPA studies. By combining the 3D scintigraphic perfusion data with a CTPA demonstrating the actual clot location, the advantages of each imaging test are realised. This may be of particular benefit if either study is inconclusive. However, as either study will be diagnostic in most patients, the value of this approach may be limited and, given the software and operator skill required, may not be feasible in many imaging centres.

Secondly, a *V/Q* SPECT can be performed concurrently with a 'low dose' CT done concurrently, or more typically sequentially, on the same scanning device. This technique is feasible in any imaging facility equipped with a SPECT/CT scanner. Several studies have shown a significant improvement in the diagnostic accuracy of the lung scan using this approach.

These two approaches are discussed in more detail below.

12.6.1 SPECT and CTPA Fusion

Co-registering the perfusion SPECT data with a diagnostic CTPA study is an approach which may be of particular value in cases of an inconclusive CTPA study. The concept of this approach is that the combined images may help to characterise the perfusion pattern seen scintigraphically in any area distal to a potential clot on the angiographic study [38] (Fig. 12.2). By combining the demonstrated very high sensitivity of perfusion SPECT with the high specificity of CTPA, an overall improved diagnostic accuracy of the combined investigation would be expected compared with either study alone. New generation hybrid devices are equipped with diagnostic multi-slice

CT scanners, and hence it is possible to perform both *V/Q* SPECT and CTPA if required in a single imaging session. While this may not be feasible in all institutions or in all patients, it is an option with current generation scanner technology. An alternative way of fusing perfusion SPECT data with CTPA is to use commercial software programs to co-register the data which may have been acquired on different scanning devices. Such software programs can generate displays of ventilation, perfusion, lung CT, fusion images and CTPA. This approach may be of value in difficult or complex cases where a conclusive result cannot be made based on either study alone. In the case of CTPA, which is being used more frequently in many centres as the initial imaging study to evaluate suspected PE, one of the challenges faced by reporting radiologists is the increasing amount of data to review with each patient study [45]. In a study at my institution, we assessed whether the fusion of SPECT perfusion data could improve the accuracy of CTPA by guiding the attention of the reporting radiologist to the relevant pulmonary artery [46]. Of the 35 patients studied, there was an 8% increase in the sensitivity of CTPA when fused with SPECT perfusion data. This led to a change in final diagnosis (from PE negative to PE positive) in 6% of patients (Fig. 12.3). Provided adequate software is available to perform the fusion of perfusion SPECT and CTPA, this approach could be readily utilised in imaging departments and might potentially allow clots to be detected more accurately in difficult or inconclusive CTPA studies, thus improving the overall utility of the test. One approach might be to refer discordant SPECT *V/Q* and CTPA results for co-registration and consensus review with all data available. While either a CTPA or *V/Q* SPECT will be able to provide a diagnosis in most patients, there may be some instances where performing both studies on the same patient may be required to more confidently diagnose (or exclude) PE. This approach could be considered in patients where an accurate diagnosis is critical if either study yields an inconclusive result or is technically suboptimal.

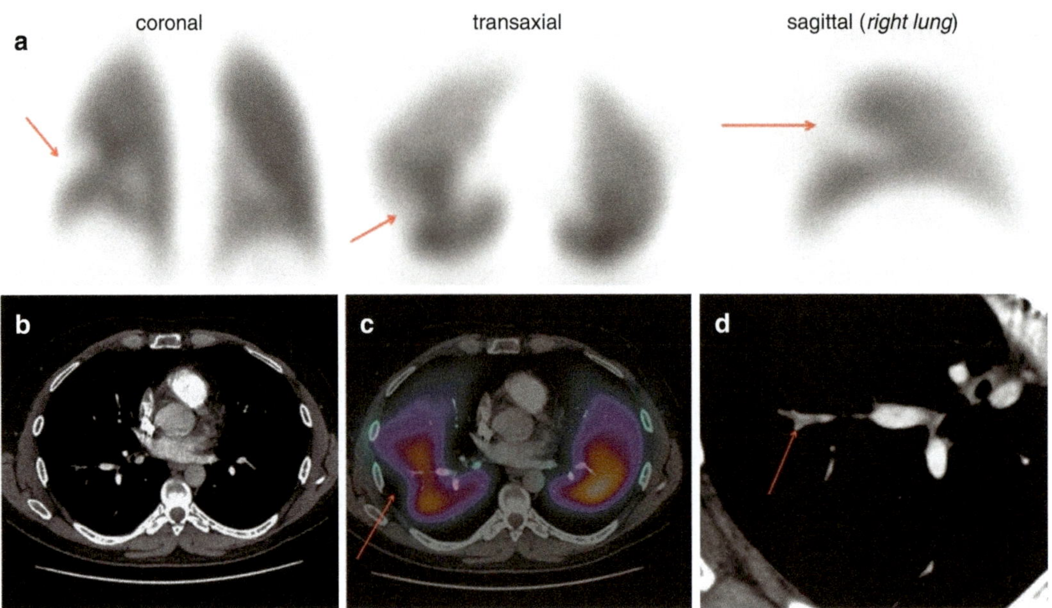

Fig. 12.3 Images of a 43-year-old male with suspected PE. Representative perfusion images of the *V/Q* SPECT (**a**) show a (mismatched) perfusion defect in the superior segment of the right lower lobe (*arrowed*). A CTPA (**b**) was reported as normal. A fused image of the CTPA and perfusion SPECT (**c**) was generated, and following a more targeted review by the radiologist of the vascular tree on the CTPA (**d**), an embolus was evident (*arrowed*). Fusion of SPECT and CTPA may help guide radiologists to the relevant part of the pulmonary vascular tree to review more carefully, thereby increasing the sensitivity of CTPA

12.6.2 Combined *V/Q* SPECT with Low-Dose CT

12.6.2.1 Overview

The second option is to perform a 'low dose' CT in conjunction with the *V/Q* SPECT study. In this case, the study is generally done without intravenous contrast and using a much lower beam current than diagnostic CT scanning. Typically, this is in the order of 20–80 mA s. This approach has the advantage of providing anatomical information, such as vascular, parenchymal and pleural abnormalities, which may explain the cause of perfusion defects seen on the *V/Q* SPECT scan. While *V/Q* SPECT has been shown to be highly sensitive, this approach may better characterise the case of any perfusion reductions, thus altering the final SPECT interpretation and improving overall specificity [47–49]. With the increasingly availability of hybrid SPECT/CT scanners, this approach can be easily performed in most nuclear medicine departments. The CT scan is typically done on the same scanning device, without the need to move the patient, usually immediately after the SPECT acquisitions have been done.

12.6.2.2 Protocols

In general, patients undergoing *V/Q* SPECT/CT studies have the ventilation SPECT study acquired first, followed in most cases by the perfusion SPECT and then the low-dose CT. Each of the acquisitions is detailed below.

Ventilation

For imaging ventilation, several alternatives exist. These include inert radioactive gases such as ^{81m}Kr and ^{133}Xe, radiolabelled aerosols such as ^{99m}Tc-diethylene triamine penta-acetic acid (^{99m}Tc-DTPA) and the ultrafine carbon suspension $^{99mTc\text{-}Technegas}$ [50]. Although the gases are considered to most accurately represent regional ventilation, these are typically not used due to the requirement for continuous administration during the acquisition and the high cost of the ^{81m}Kr generator [51]. Although ^{133}Xe gas has the advantage of a longer half-life, its use is complicated by errors resulting from its recirculation due to clearance into the pulmonary circulation [52, 53]. Combined with its poor spatial resolution, it is a less than ideal agent to image ventilation [51].

Given these limitations, ^{99m}Tc-labelled particulate aerosols such as ^{99m}Tc-DTPA or the carbon-labelled nanoparticle ^{99m}Tc-Technegas are much more widely used due to their greater availability, low cost and good image quality [51]. Although the choice of agent depends on factors such as local availability and cost, both have been reported to produce SPECT ventilation scans of good diagnostic quality. The most widely available is ^{99m}Tc-DTPA, which can be used with doses of just 0.8 mCi (30 MBq) [27]. However, because of the relatively larger mean particle mass, problems may arise from central airway deposition, particularly in patients with chronic obstructive pulmonary disease (COPD) [54]. Technegas, with a smaller particle size, generally has greater alveolar penetration than ^{99m}Tc-DTPA. This results in less impaction in the central airways, with Technegas being demonstrated to have a similar distribution to that of an inert gas [55–59]. Together with its lack of lung clearance during image acquisition, Technegas is an ideal agent for ventilation SPECT. Typically, the doses of ^{99m}Tc-based imaging agents administered are identical to those used in conventional planar imaging. The EANM procedure guidelines for *V/Q* SPECT recommend an inhaled dose of 30 MBq Technegas [8]; however, some authors have proposed a slight increase in the administered dose in an attempt to improve image quality [29, 32]. At our institution, 13.5 mCi (500 MBq) of ^{99m}Tc is added to a Technegas generator, with the aim of delivering a dose of approximately 1.35 mCi (50 MBq) to the patient. This equates to a posterior count rate of approximately 2.0–2.5 kcps. The ventilation agent is usually administered with the patient lying supine so as to facilitate uniform distribution of activity throughout the lung fields [60]. Acquisition parameters for the ventilation study are described below in the section on "SPECT: gamma camera hardware, image acquisition and processing".

Perfusion

As with planar imaging, ^{99m}Tc-macroaggregated albumin (^{99m}Tc-MAA) is generally used to assess perfusion [8]. The distribution of MAA, which is proportional to regional blood flow, will be reduced distal to vascular occlusions in the pulmonary arteries. Thus, it can be considered that perfusion imaging performed in this fashion has an inherent 'amplification' as even a small embolus can cause a large section of lung to be hypo-perfused. The dose of ^{99m}Tc-MAA used is dependent on the ventilation agent and dose used. If a radioactive gas is used, the dose of perfusion agent is typically lower than if a technetium-based ventilation agent is used. This is because the signal from the radioactive gas can be separated from that of the perfusion agent based on the energy level of the emitted photons. Additionally, in the case of ^{81m}Kr, the short half-life results in negligible gas remaining in the lungs during perfusion imaging. If a technetium-based agent is used for both ventilation and perfusion imaging, the typical approach is to 'drown out' the underlying ventilation signal by administering a substantially greater dose of perfusion agent. A perfusion-ventilation dose ratio of at least 3:1 is generally required [8, 60]. At my institution, the standard administered activity of ^{99m}Tc-MAA is 6 mCi (220 MBq). This results in an effective radiation dose for the combined ventilation and perfusion scan of approximately 2.5 mSv. Other authors have proposed the use of lower administered activities, including the EANM procedure guidelines for *V/Q* SPECT which recommend an inhaled dose of 30 MBq Technegas and 120 MBq of ^{99m}Tc-MAA [8]. It is advised that each site should review the image quality being acquired on their own local scanners and ensure that studies are optimised. The dose used by each department should be based on factors such as the collimator used, gamma camera sensitivity, processing parameters and the local radiation protection guidelines [60]. Some adjustment to acquisition times and/or administered doses may be required depending on the quality of images being generated.

In the case of pregnant patients, a dose reduction is usually implemented. This can be achieved by omitting the ventilation scan or by reducing the administered dose of both the ventilation and perfusion agents, usually by half [60]. This will necessitate a longer acquisition time so as to maintain adequate count density thereby generating images of good quality. The CT scan may also be omitted in pregnant patients to reduce breast radiation exposure.

SPECT: Gamma Camera Hardware, Image Acquisition and Processing

To perform SPECT and SPECT/CT imaging, multiheaded hybrid gamma cameras are required [50]. A typical protocol that uses a modern SPECT/CT camera requires 25–30 min of total acquisition time for a ventilation and perfusion dataset and a CT scan of the thorax. At Royal North Shore Hospital, Sydney, our acquisition protocol uses 3° radial steps over 360° with the ventilation study acquired for 12 s per projection and the perfusion study acquired for 8 s per projection [60]. Other centres have reported adequate SPECT quality in as little as 6 min [32]. Although it is possible to perform SPECT with a single-head camera, the acquisition time becomes prohibitive for standard clinical practice, and if SPECT/CT imaging is to be performed, only multi-detector SPECT/CT scanners are commercially available. When using ^{99m}Tc radionuclides, low-energy, high-resolution collimators should ideally be used. These optimise image quality, although at the expense of reduced counts compared with low-energy all-purpose collimator [60]. If a higher-energy radionuclide such as ^{81m}Kr is used for ventilation, a medium energy collimator may be required. A matrix size of 128×128 (or greater) is appropriate for today's gamma cameras, although some reports have described using a 64×64 matrix with acceptable image quality [29, 50]. With image reconstruction, iterative techniques, such as the ordered-subset expectation-maximisation algorithm (OSEM), are increasingly replacing filtered back projection in many areas of image reconstruction in nuclear medicine [61]. These algorithms permit the inclusion of many physical aspects of the imaging process in the system model, such as attenuation, Compton scattering and resolution

degradation. Consequently, they offer better control of signal-to-noise in the event that a study is low in counts [62].

For *V/Q* SPECT reconstruction, we use an ordered-subset expectation-maximisation algorithm (eight iterations, four subsets) smoothed with a post-reconstruction 3D Butterworth filter using a cut-off of 0.8 cycles/cm with an order of 9 [60]. Traditionally, corrections for photon attenuation and scatter are not routinely applied to *V/Q* SPECT, although they would be required for any quantitative analysis (e.g. individual lobar function, as discussed below).

CT Protocols for Use with SPECT *V/Q* Scans

Clinical SPECT/CT systems currently available from manufacturers typically have dual-head scintillation cameras positioned in front of the CT scanner and sharing a common imaging table. The CT scanner quality varies, and the commercial vendors have used two different approaches in recent years with their production of clinical SPECT/CT scanners. The original SPECT/CT imaging approach was to use a low-output, slow-acquisition CT scanner. The Infinia Hawkeye (General Electric Healthcare Systems, Milwaukee, WI) was the first SPECT/CT scanner marketed commercially. Its current iteration comprises a CT scanner consisting of a low-output X-ray tube (2.5 mA) and four linear arrays of detectors which can simultaneously acquire four 5-mm anatomic slices in 13.6 s with a spatial resolution of greater than 3 LP/cm. The slow scan speed (up to 4 min) can be an advantage in regions where there is physiologic motion because the CT image blurring from the motion is comparable to that of the emission scans, resulting in a good match in fused images. This is particularly relevant in lung SPECT/CT where ventilation and perfusion SPECT is acquired during normal tidal breathing [63].

The second approach, which has evolved more recently, has been the development of newer generation hybrid SPECT/CT systems which incorporate diagnostic helical (multi-slice) CT scanners combined with dual-head scintillation cameras. Each of the major commercial equipment vendors now market these devices. Various configurations are available, with the number of slices ranging from 1 to, the ability to utilise variable tube currents (20–500 mA s), slice thicknesses (0.6–12 mm) and rotation speeds of 0.5–1.5 s [63]. These systems exhibit high contrast spatial resolution with approximately four to five times the patient radiation dose of that from the Infinia Hawkeye system. However, these systems can be used for diagnostic quality CT as well as for attenuation correction and anatomical localisation using low-dose parameters [64]. Given these advantages, these systems now account for most of the SPECT/CT scanners sold commercially today.

While breath holding is typically employed for diagnostic CT studies, this is not feasible during *V/Q* SPECT acquisitions, which typically take up to 15 min for each of the ventilation and perfusion scans. Hence, respiratory motion misregistration is a potential problem, and the ideal breathing protocol used for CT in *V/Q* SPECT/CT should ensure that the position of the diaphragm on the SPECT scans matches as closely as possible that of the CT images. To reduce misregistration between the SPECT and CT data as much as possible, it has been recommended that CT scans should be acquired during breath holding at mid-inspiration volume, or with the patient continuing shallow breathing during the CT acquisition [65].

The CT scan is typically acquired either between, or after, the two SPECT study acquisitions. The same principles of maintaining identical patient positioning throughout the study applies. It is preferable that the CT scan is not acquired prior to ventilation SPECT as the patient may move significantly during the ventilation procedure thus introducing misregistration artefact when co-registering the SPECT and CT data [63]. Acquisition parameters will vary between manufacturers and CT design.

Image Display and Reviewing

After co-registration of the ventilation, perfusion and CT datasets, the data are best viewed simultaneously in transverse, coronal and sagittal planes on a workstation. Each of the commercial vendors marketing SPECT/CT scanners provide software which can display SPECT/CT images across the range of typical clinical studies performed. There are also third-party solutions available, independent of the commercial SPECT/CT manufacturers. The software programs vary with some allowing for one dataset to be manually aligned with the others, whereas others allow for automatic registration of the studies to each other [66]. As noted above, image registration is best facilitated by reducing, or preferably eliminating, any patient motion between the ventilation SPECT, perfusion SPECT and low-dose CT studies. However, if significant patient motion has occurred between any of the three datasets, some image manipulation and adjustment will be required.

Although images can be printed to film, given the amount of data to be considered, SPECT/CT data are generally best reviewed directly on a workstation. This allows the reporter to interactively examine the linked ventilation and perfusion SPECT studies as well as the CT in each of the three orthogonal imaging planes and to adjust the relative image intensities, especially of fused images. The ability to triangulate defects should be an essential component of any software used to review and report *V/Q* SPECT/CT studies. Review of images on a workstation also facilitates the viewing of CT data in different windows so that the lungs, soft tissue and bones can all be reviewed as appropriate. An example of a typical *V/Q* SPECT/CT displays in a patient with PE is shown in Fig. 12.4.

In addition to tomographic display of *V/Q* SPECT images, further data processing can also be performed. In the case in which ^{99m}Tc is used for both ventilation and perfusion imaging, perfusion data can be corrected for the background activity of the preceding ventilation scan using image subtraction of co-registered datasets [27, 67]. Although this ventilation subtraction enhances perfusion defect contrast, it is not currently in widespread use. The use of SPECT also facilitates novel ways of displaying *V:Q* quotient data to assist image reporting. Palmer and co-workers have described a technique where these images can be presented as either 3D surface-shaded images or as tomographic sections in

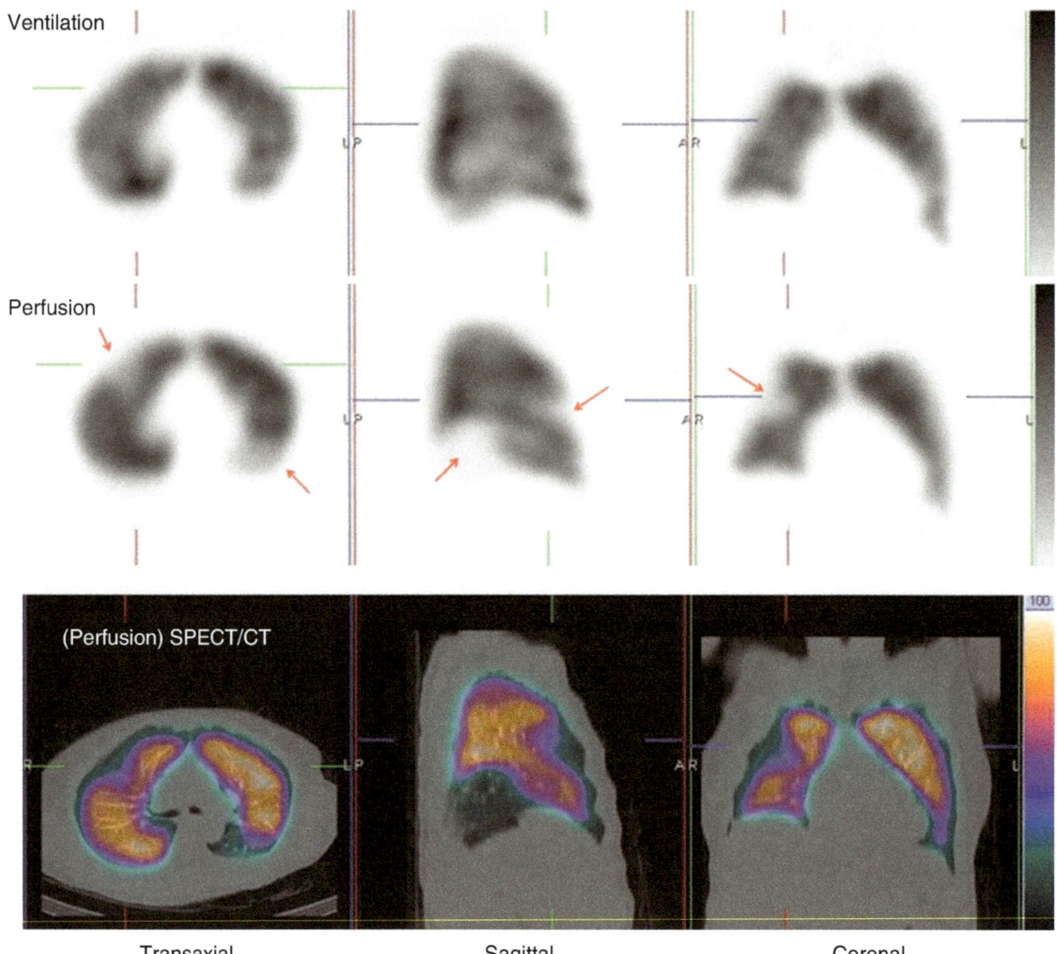

Fig. 12.4 Representative ventilation, perfusion and fused SPECT/CT images in a patient with multiple PE. Several mismatched defects are evident (*arrowed*). There are no underlying structural abnormalities on the CT to account for the perfusion reductions

each of the orthogonal planes [67]. These so-called quotient images can be helpful in facilitating image reporting and are a useful way of demonstrating the location and extent of mismatched defects. Figure 12.5 shows an example of an abnormal SPECT study and corresponding selected $V:Q$ quotient images in a patient with multiple PE. SPECT imaging facilitates other novel ways of interpreting image data, such as objective analysis by examining the pixel-based $V:Q$ ratio. Our group has described such an approach, and while not routinely available in commercial processing and display programs, such techniques have the potential to decrease the number of non-diagnostic or indeterminate scans [68, 69].

While there are several ways that V/Q SPECT studies can be reported, most reporting specialists would use the EANM reporting guidelines for V/Q SPECT. Originally published in 2009, these guidelines recommend that studies are reported as positive for PE if there is V/Q mismatch of at least one segment or two subsegments that conforms to the pulmonary vascular

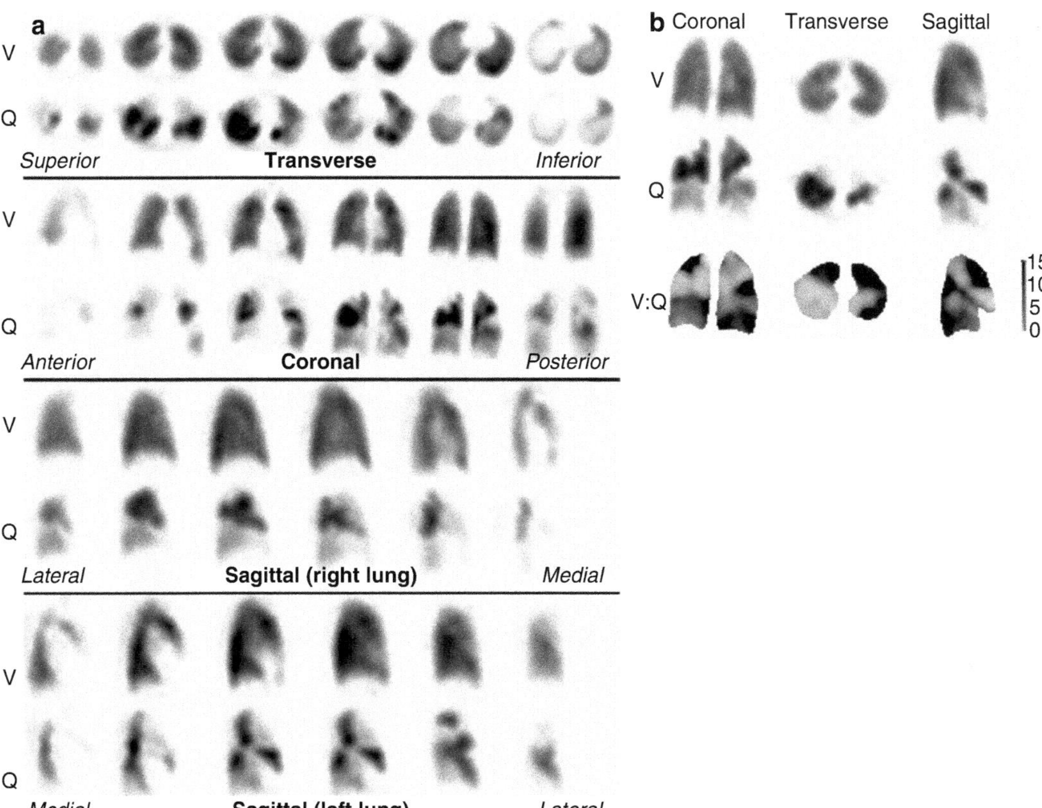

Fig. 12.5 (**a**) Example of a patient with multiple bilateral PE. Ventilation (*V*) and perfusion (*Q*) images are aligned and displayed in transverse, coronal and sagittal planes. Multiple perfusion defects in areas with normal ventilation can be seen. (**b**) Representative coronal, transverse and sagittal ventilation (*V*), perfusion (*Q*) and *V:Q* quotient images from the patient shown in (a). Areas of pulmonary embolism correspond to dark areas on the *V:Q* quotient images, indicating a high *V:Q* ratio value. (Reprinted with permission from Roach et al. [50])

anatomy [8]. These guidelines recommend that the study is considered negative for PE if there is either a normal perfusion pattern conforming to the anatomic boundaries of the lungs; matched or reversed mismatch *V/Q* defects of any size, shape or number in the absence of mismatch; or mismatch that does not have a lobar, segmental or subsegmental pattern. Studies are considered to be non-diagnostic for PE if there are multiple *V/Q* abnormalities not typical of specific diseases. While these guidelines do not specifically address *V/Q* SPECT/CT, the addition of the CT component is likely to help classify the *V/Q* SPECT pattern more appropriately, particularly given the information that the CT provides on the anatomy of each individual patient, particularly in relation to the borders of the lungs and segments, the location of the fissures and major vessels and the presence of any associated parenchymal disease. At my institution, we pay particular note of the location of the fissures, as a reduction in perfusion (and to a lesser degree ventilation) corresponding with the fissures is often noted on SPECT imaging. This seems most evident in the posterior aspects of the oblique fissures and is more noticeable on perfusion than ventilation SPECT images. We hypothesise that this is due to fact that alveoli predominate at the pleural surface and there is a relative paucity of pulmonary vessels, with the pleura supplied by the bronchial circulation. Therefore, when SPECT imaging is performed, there is good distribution of Technegas (which has good peripheral penetration), whereas relatively little ^{99m}Tc MAA accumulates. We consider any linear perfusion reduction seen on SPECT corresponding to the fissures to be artefactual (Fig. 12.6).

While other reporting schema have been proposed for *V/Q* SPECT, it is certainly recommended

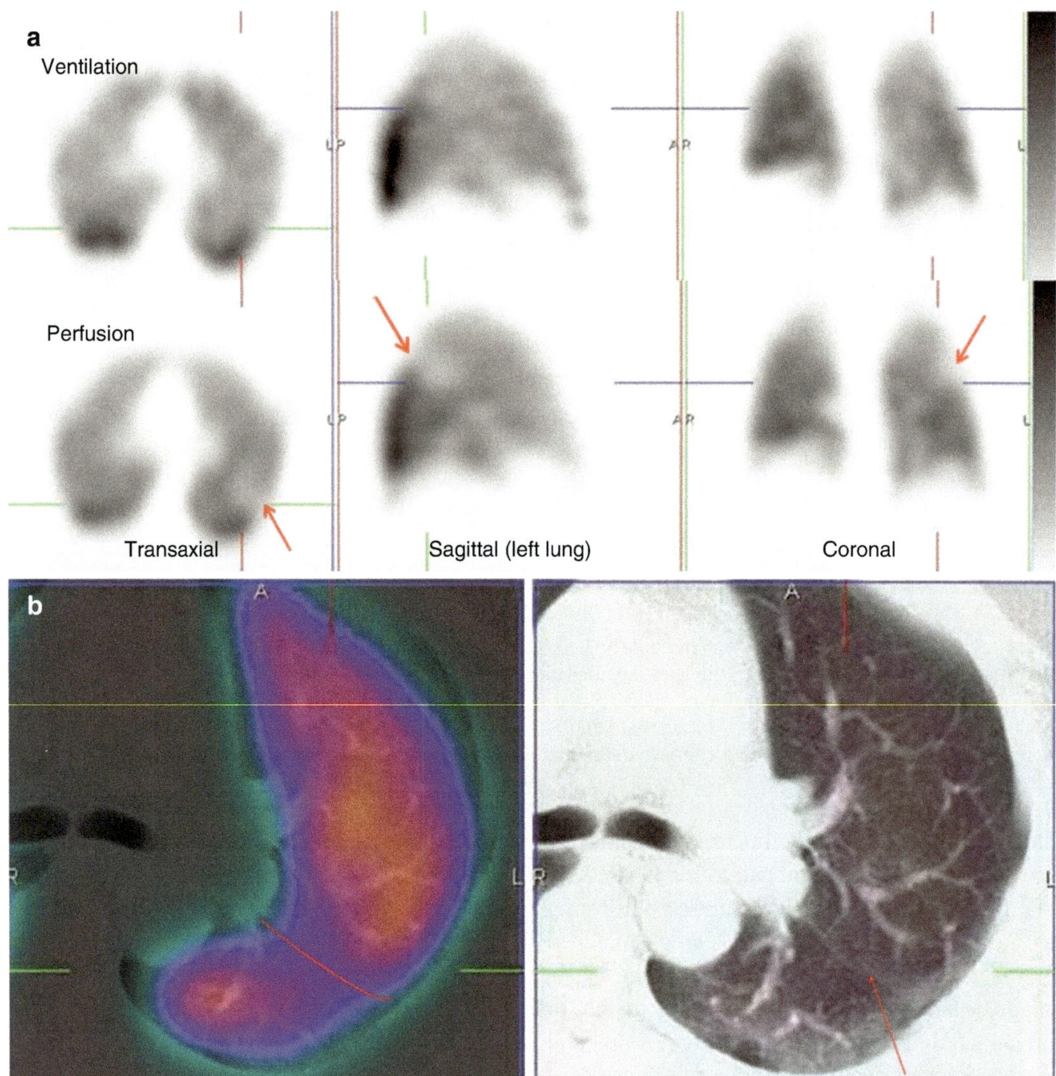

Fig. 12.6 (**a**) Representative ventilation and perfusion SPECT images in a patient with suspected PE show a linear mismatch in the left upper/mid-zone (*arrowed*). This is non-segmental in appearance. (**b**) Fused perfusion SPECT/CT (*left*) and the (unfused) CT (*right*) of the left lung show the perfusion reduction to correspond with the oblique fissure (marked and *arrowed* in *red*). SPECT/CT helps to characterise the cause of SPECT perfusion defects, thereby increasing the specificity of *V/Q* scintigraphy. EANM reporting guidelines for *V/Q* SPECT recommend that studies are reported as positive for PE if there is *V/Q* mismatch of at least one segment or two subsegments provided that it conforms to the pulmonary vascular anatomy. In this case, the defect does not conform to pulmonary vascular anatomy

that the probabilistic reporting used for many years with planar scintigraphy should not be used for *V/Q* SPECT/CT [29, 70]. Given the typical binary reporting approach to CTPA reporting, it is important that definitive reports be given for *V/Q* SPECT (and *V/Q* SPECT/CT) whenever possible so as to keep the test relevant as a primary screening test for patients with suspected PE.

12.7 Clinical Value of *V/Q* SPECT/ CT

Several studies have shown that combined SPECT/CT lung scanning improves specificity and overall diagnostic accuracy of lung scintigraphy.

In a preliminary study from my own institution, we performed ventilation (using Technegas) and perfusion SPECT studies as well as a low-dose (30–50 mA s) CT scan in 48 patients with suspected PE [71]. In this series, 16 patients were considered to have had PE based on clinical and imaging findings and follow-up, and of these, 15 patients (94%) had a positive *V/Q* SPECT scan. Of the remaining 32 patients without PE, six (19%) had false-positive *V/Q* SPECT scans; however, three of these patients (50%) were correctly reclassified as PE negative when the SPECT/CT scan was viewed. Hence the addition of a low-dose CT to *V/Q* SPECT improved the diagnostic accuracy of lung scintigraphy by reducing false-positive scan results by 50% in this pilot study. In particular, it was noted that low-dose CT could characterise physiological features such as pulmonary vessels and fissures, as well as pathological features such as consolidation and emphysema that can result in defects on perfusion scintigraphy.

More recently, the improvement in diagnostic accuracy by combining *V/Q* SPECT with low-dose CT has been confirmed in a prospective study by a group from Copenhagen, Denmark [31]. In this series of 81 consecutive patients, ^{81m}Kr gas was used as the ventilation agent, and the final diagnosis was based on a composite reference standard comprising ECG, lower limb ultrasound, D-dimer result and 6 months of clini-

cal follow-up. They found that the sensitivities of *V/Q* SPECT alone and *V/Q* SPECT combined with low-dose CT were identical at 97%. However, the addition of low-dose CT imaging increased the specificity of SPECT scintigraphy from 88% to 100%. The addition of anatomical data demonstrated that mismatched perfusion defects could be attributed to structures such as fissures as well as pathological conditions such as emphysema, pneumonia, atelectasis and pleural fluid. The inconclusive rate for *V/Q* SPECT alone was only 5% (four patients); however, this fell to zero when SPECT was combined with low-dose CT imaging. These data do indicate that the combination of *V/Q* SPECT can yield very high sensitivity, specificity and overall accuracy in the diagnosis of PE.

These studies have also shown that concurrent low-dose CT is feasible to do in most Nuclear Medicine departments today, is well tolerated by patients (even those that were critically ill) and adds little overall imaging time to the acquisition (typically less than 1–2 min).

Some case examples from my institution showing the value of hybrid SPECT/CT imaging are shown in Figs. 12.7 and 12.8.

12.8 Is the Ventilation Scan Necessary?

Given that fused CT and perfusion SPECT can be readily performed, the need for a ventilation study may be questioned as the information from the CT may be adequate on its own to provide information on structural or airways abnormalities (CTPA + Q study). Several studies have assessed whether a CT scan can replace the need for a scintigraphic ventilation scan in patients with suspected PE. In a study of 30 patients from my own department, we found that 87% of the 96 mismatched perfusion defects seen on *V/Q* SPECT occurred in areas where there was no underlying parenchymal abnormality detected on CTPA to account for the perfusion reduction [72]. In the remaining 13% of mismatched *V/Q* defects, CTPA revealed corresponding parenchymal abnormalities, mostly subsegmental atelecta-

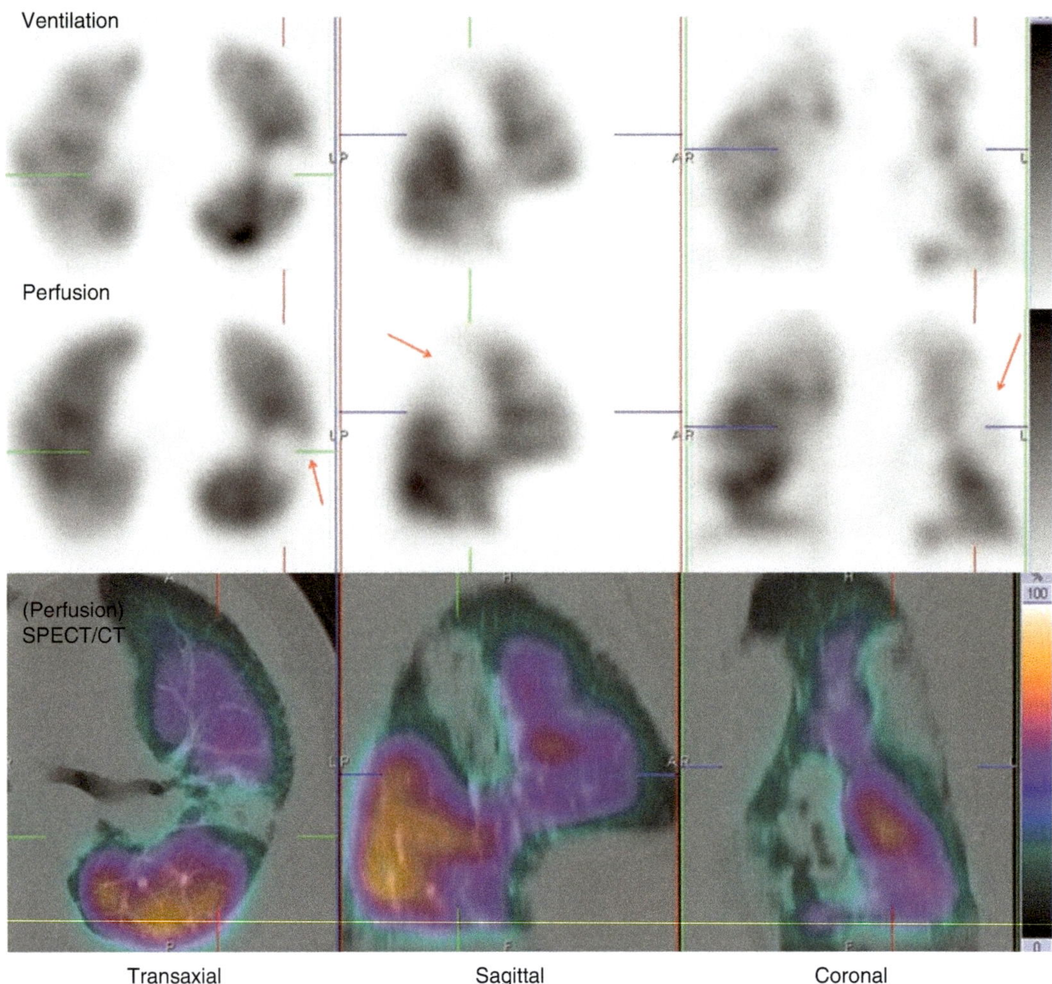

Fig. 12.7 Representative ventilation, perfusion and SPECT/CT images in an 84-year-old male with dyspnea. A large matched defect is evident on SPECT in the left upper and mid-zone (*arrowed*). This corresponds with extensive consolidation demonstrated on the SPECT/CT images. This is seen to lie anterior to the oblique fissure

sis, which correlated with the areas of perfusion reduction on the SPECT study. Of note, the extent of the parenchymal abnormality on CT in these mismatched *V/Q* defects was significantly smaller than the extent of perfusion reduction. Twelve mismatched perfusion defects on CTPA/Q were identified as false positives with matched defects evident on the *V/Q* images. These defects were seen in two asthmatic patients, presumably related to air trapping which has a similar CT appearance to hypo-attenuation from hypo-perfused lung distal to PE.

In the Danish study described above, results were also reported for the use of perfusion SPECT alone (i.e. ventilation omitted) combined with low-dose CT [31]. In this series, the sensitivity of this approach was high (93%), but the specificity fell to only 51% with the accuracy reported at 68%. In addition to the high false-positive rate, there was also a high non-diagnostic rate using this approach (17%).

Thus, while the literature remains limited, it does appear that omitting the ventilation component of the SPECT study will compromise accuracy, and, in particular, the specificity of *V/Q* SPECT scintigraphy, by producing a higher false-positive rate. The question of whether ventilation scans can be omitted in the evaluation of

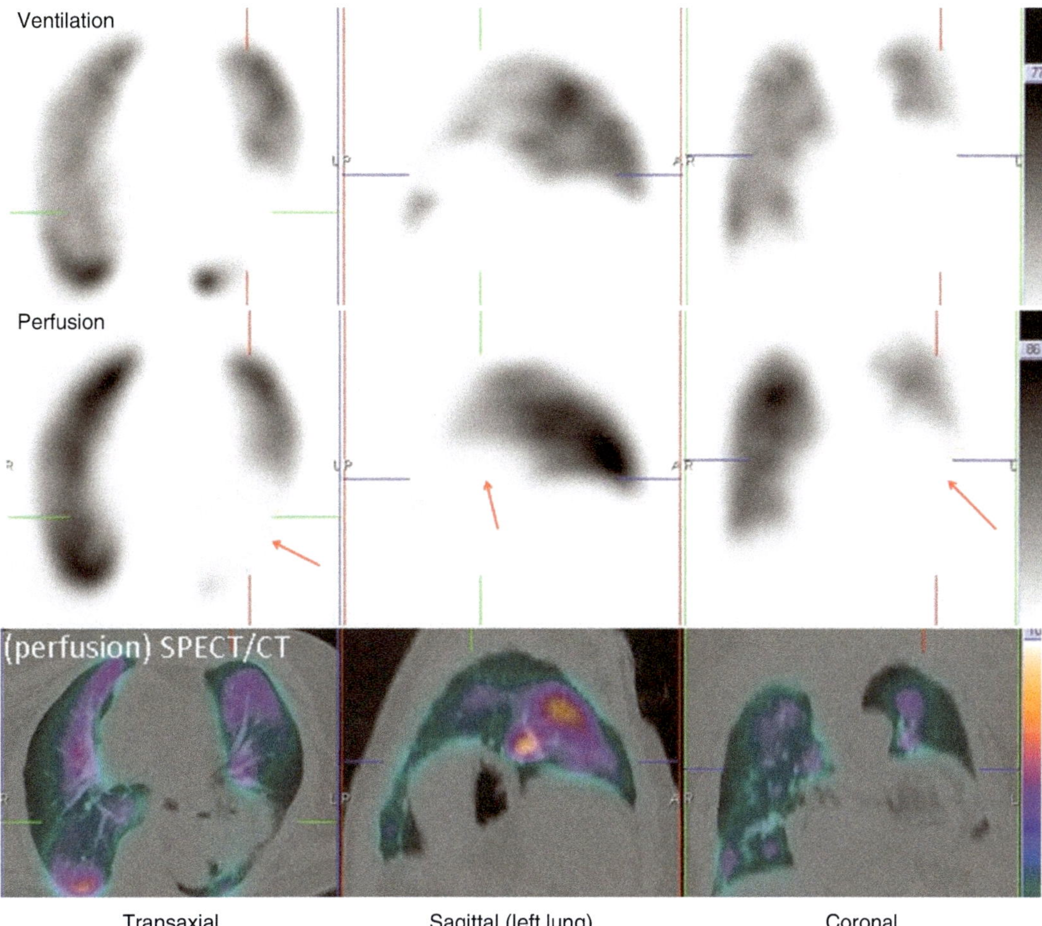

Fig. 12.8 Representative ventilation, perfusion and SPECT/CT images in a 63-year-old male with chest pain. A large matched defect is evident on SPECT in the left lower zone (*arrowed*). This corresponds with a large hiatus hernia on the SPECT/CT images

patients with suspected PE, has come under particular focus during the COVID-19 pandemic. Many centers, and professional associations, advised against the use of ventilation studies in patients with known, or suspected, COVID 19 due to the potential staff infection risks from the aerosol generating procedure [73–75]. While some centers ceased performing ventilation scans altogether, others (including our own) opted for a more selective approach. In patients in whom COVID-19 was not confidently excluded, we and others would perform a perfusion SPECT scan. If normal, PE is confidently ruled out. If there were perfusion abnormalities seen, a low dose CT would be done. If this showed physiological or

pathological findings that could account for the areas of perfusion reduction, then PE could be confidently excluded. If not, a ventilation scan would generally then be required, with the operators taking appropriate safety precautions, including full PPE. Due to the requirement for decay of the perfusion scan, a delay of several hours at least would generally be required before the ventilation scan could be attempted. Some groups advocated a reversal of the usual order of scanning, i.e. a low dose perfusion followed by a higher dose ventilation scan to obviate the need for any delay [76]. However in our center, we found that image quality was adversely impacted by this approach, hence would recall the patients several hours later, or the next day, for the ventilation component when it was required. The downside of this approach overall however is a delay in diagnosis in some patients. Nevertheless, we found that the combination of perfusion SPECT +/- low dose CT could rule out PE in the majority of patients referred to our department with suspected PE.

12.9 How Does *V/Q* SPECT/CT Compare with CTPA?

Multi-detector CTPA has evolved to the point where it is now widely used as the primary imaging investigation in patients with potential PE [4, 22]. While highly specific, its sensitivity is not perfect [77]. With the multi-detector CT scanners used in the large PIOPED II study, CTPA had a reported sensitivity of 83%, indicating that emboli were missed in one of every six patients [77]. Although the accuracy of CTPA appears to be high in cases in which the scan result is in keeping with the pretest clinical suspicion, this is not true of cases in which there is discordance between scan results and clinical likelihood.

CTPA, because of its anatomical nature, has an advantage of potentially diagnosing other pathologies, such as pneumonia or aortic dissection. However, this is at the expense of exposing the patient to increased radiation (something that is particularly concerning in the case of young women) and to the potential risks of contrast administration, such as allergy or nephrotoxicity [78, 79]. *V/Q* SPECT has been shown to be better able to quantify the extent of perfusion abnormalities (which may be valuable in guiding treatment decisions) and can assess reperfusion after PE, something not easily done with CTPA [70].

Overall, there is relatively little literature directly comparing SPECT *V/Q* and CTPA. In 2004, Reinartz and co-workers compared the performance of *V/Q* SPECT (using Technegas) with multi-detector (4-slice) CTPA [29]. In their series of 83 patients, they determined that SPECT was more sensitive (97% versus 86%) but less specific (91% versus 98%) than CTPA. Both modalities

had comparable overall accuracy (94% versus 93%). In another series from Australia, Miles and co-workers prospectively compared *V/Q* SPECT with CTPA performed using a 16-slice scanner in 100 patients with suspected PE [80]. They also concluded that the overall accuracy of both examinations was comparable, suggesting that SPECT *V/Q* and CTPA could be used interchangeably. They concluded that SPECT *V/Q* has potential advantages over CTPA in that it was feasible to perform in more patients and had fewer contraindications, a lower patient radiation dose and fewer non-diagnostic findings. This study supports the notion that each of these studies has its advantages over the other. In the case of *V/Q* SPECT, its advantage is a high sensitivity, whereas CTPA has the advantage of a high specificity. Given that the literature directly comparing *V/Q* SPECT (and *V/Q* SPECT/CT) is limited, it would be desirable to perform a prospective multicentre trial to answer the question. However, this would be difficult for several reasons [70]. Firstly, evaluating the clinical effectiveness of rapidly evolving health technologies is problematic. In this case, both CT and *V/Q* SPECT technology continue to develop, and therefore, any published direct comparison inevitably reports on previous-generation technology. Secondly, a robust 'gold standard' is lacking for the diagnosis of PE resulting in the *V/Q* scan and/or CTPA being pivotal in determining the presence or absence of disease [27, 36]. Thirdly, ethics committees may, quite correctly, question the need to subject individuals to the radiation exposure from both *V/Q* SPECT and CTPA, especially in individuals without PE. Lastly, the time interval between the two studies being performed could result in embolus fragmentation, movement or lysis, thus affecting the perceived accuracy of each modality.

As stated above, the challenge for the *V/Q* scan is that ventilation/perfusion mismatch is not specific for PE, and in some cases of PE (e.g. in the case of pulmonary infarction), matched patterns can occur. For this reason, the anatomical information provided by a chest X-ray has been considered essential in the interpretation of *V/Q* scans. With the advent of SPECT/CT scanners, the integration of anatomical information from the CT with the functional information from SPECT is now feasible and should increase the specificity of *V/Q* scanning. Other than PE, *V/Q* mismatch can be seen with conditions such as radiation therapy-induced changes and extrinsic vascular compression from conditions such as neoplasm and mediastinal adenopathy [8, 33]. Each of these can be detected with low-dose CT. Furthermore, matched changes can be seen with non-embolic aetiologies such as pneumonia, abscess, pleural or pericardial effusions, malignancy and pulmonary infarction [5, 6, 36, 37]. Once again, each of these should be evident if a CT, even if done at a 'low' diagnostic dose, is performed.

In the Danish study of *V/Q* SPECT/CT mentioned earlier, the authors directly compared the accuracy of current generation CTPA with *V/Q* SPECT/CT [31]. They found that SPECT and SPECT/CT both had higher sensitivity for the detection of PE than CTPA (done on the same hybrid machine equipped with a 16 slice CT scanner). Although CTPA had a specificity of 100%, its sensitivity was only 68%. The superior sensitivity of *V/Q* SPECT compared with CTPA has been demonstrated in other studies and raised questions about the use of CTPA as the primary imaging study for the detection of PE in clinical practice. The sensitivity of CTPA in this study is lower than the 83% noted in the large multicentre PIOPED II study, a figure that led the investigators of that study to conclude that additional information would be required to exclude PE due to the significant false-negative rate of CTPA [77].

Other concerns with the use of CTPA noted by the Danish authors include the risk of complications related to intravenous contrast (a factor which accounted for 50% of the 96 patients excluded from the study) and its high thoracic radiation dose. The use of iodinated contrast administration is a significant disadvantage of CTPA with reports of about 3% of patients experiencing some type of immediate contrast reaction and 0.06% requiring treatment [81]. Contrast-induced nephropathy is reported in 1–3% of patients with CTPA [82]. This compares with scintigraphy where side effects are all but non-existent [83].

High radiation exposure is another limitation of CTPA. Breast radiation dose from CTPA, which has been estimated between 10 and 70 mSv, is a particular concern in younger women [84–86]. By comparison, the breast radiation dose from the *V/Q* scan is in the order of 0.28–1 mSv [87]. While CTPA has overall radiation doses reported in the order of 8–20 mSv, the levels received from a low-dose CT study performed in conjunction with a lung SPECT study is much lower [35, 83–85]. Gutte and co-workers estimated that the radiation dose from their 20 mAs CT studies was approximately 1 mSv [31]. In my institution, using similar CT parameters (20–50 mA s), we have estimated radiation doses from the CT in the order of 1–2 mSv. This compares favourably with the 2–2.5 mSv from the *V/Q* scan itself and is well below the levels received from a diagnostic CTPA [83].

A further issue for CTPA is the rate of technical artefacts that can occur, primarily due to poor contrast opacification of the pulmonary arteries and motion artefacts, but also body habitus of some patients which can affect image noise [88]. Indeterminate study rates due to technical factors have been estimated at between 5% and 11% [30, 89, 90]. In pregnant patients, the rate is even higher, and it has been shown that as many as one-third of CTPA procedures performed during pregnancy are technically inadequate, even with 64-slice CT scanners [22, 91]. This is thought to be attributable to a greater pressure in the inferior vena cava during pregnancy. As a result, repeat studies are not infrequently performed to try to optimise the diagnostic accuracy of the study, resulting in doubling of the radiation dose. By comparison, technical artefacts should not impact *V/Q* SPECT/CT, and literature suggests that the test has a very high sensitivity and specificity; hence additional imaging should only rarely be required [31].

Both CTPA and *V/Q* SPECT have their strengths and weaknesses (listed in Table 12.1), and the test selected for any individual patient will vary according to patient factors (especially age and gender but also the presence of coexisting lung disease) as well as institution factors, including availability and local expertise. Given its excellent sensitivity and superior safety and radiation exposure profile, there is a strong argument that *V/Q* SPECT should be favoured as the initial screening test for PE [22]. The addition of a low-

Table 12.1 Summary of the advantages and limitations of CTPA and *V/Q* SPECT/CT

	CTPA	*V/Q* SPECT/CT
Sensitivity	Moderate	High
Specificity	Very high	Slightly lower
Accuracy with abnormal radiograph	Unaffected	Sometimes affected
Provides other diagnoses	Frequent	Frequent
Incidental findings require follow-up	Frequent	Less frequent
Radiation dose	High	Lower
Possible allergic reaction	Yes	No
Risk of contrast nephropathy	Yes	No
Technical failure rate	Higher	Rare
Availability (especially out of routine hours)	High	Usually lower
Accuracy in pregnancy	Lower	High
Accuracy in chronic PE	Lower	High
Performance in obstructive lung disease	Unaffected	May be affected
Role and accuracy in follow-up	Limited	Very good

dose CT further strengthens this argument as it addresses many of the advantages cited for CTPA (i.e. ruling out other conditions, such as pneumonia, abscess, pleural or pericardial effusions, malignancy). While diagnostic CT with intravenous contrast is needed to evaluate certain conditions, such as aortic dissection or coronary artery disease, the advent of *V/Q* SPECT/CT further enhances the overall diagnostic ability of *V/Q* scintigraphy, thus allowing centres to choose either CTPA or V/Q SPECT to assess suspected PE with either study being of generally high sensitivity and specificity. In the choice of which one to choose in specific patients, could be based on factors such as patient age, sex, contrast risk and local availability as well as operator and reporter expertise.

12.10 Clot Localisation

The addition of the CT data to SPECT *V/Q* also provides interesting insights into the accuracy of clot localisation on *V/Q* SPECT. As anatomical information is sparse when *V/Q* SPECT data is interpreted, assumptions must be made about the lung anatomy in each patient. Segmental lung maps (based on normal anatomical references) are typically utilised to assist reporting specialists in localisation of perfusion defects; however, individual anatomy varies, and in the case of PE, the lungs are frequently abnormal, with coexistent lung patholo-

gies, such as atelectasis and pleural effusions, often seen [50, 92]. SPECT/CT imaging allows for segmental anatomy to be accurately determined in each individual patient, and this may facilitate more accurate localisation of clots into the correct lung segments. In a study from my centre of 30 patients with positive *V/Q* SPECT studies in which a normal lung tomographic segmental lung chart was used as a guide to localise segments, 20% of defects were assigned to the incorrect anatomical lung segment [93]. Inaccurate localisations were most commonly seen in the mid-zone segments and were most noticeable in patients with evidence of lower lobe volume loss on CT (Fig. 12.9). The fact that anatomical localisation of perfusion abnormalities on *V/Q* SPECT can be improved by adding CT data in a significant number of patients may be relevant in patients with non-diagnostic *V/Q* SPECT studies, many of whom would have a CTPA done subsequently to confirm the findings of the SPECT study. If the reporting radiologist is directed to specifically analyse the incorrect lung segment based on the assumptions of the patient's likely anatomy using the *V/Q* SPECT appearances, the sensitivity and accuracy of the study are reduced.

12.11 Consolidative Opacities

While *V/Q* mismatch is the well-described hallmark of PE, pulmonary infarction can result in matched changes of ventilation and perfusion, a

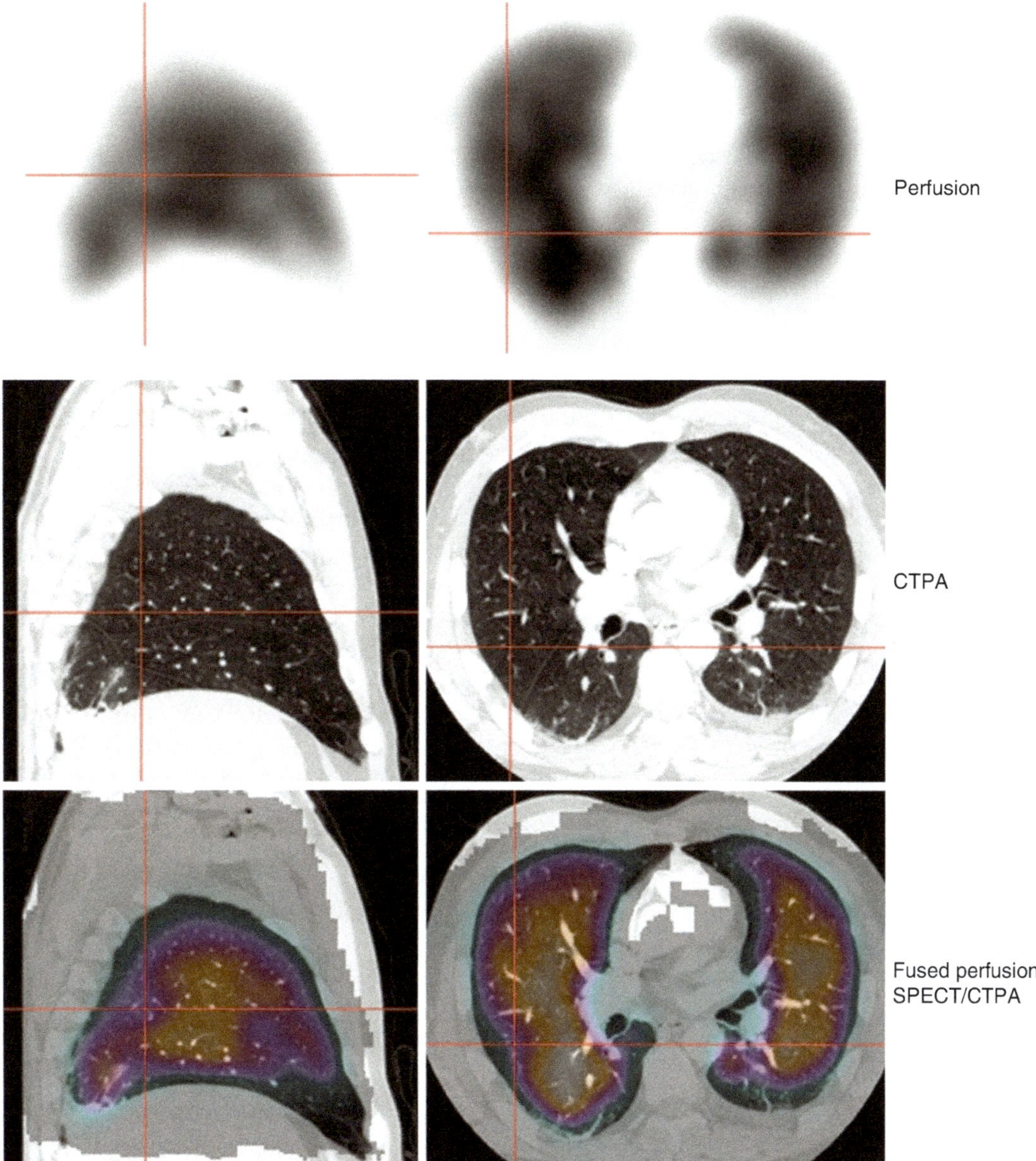

Fig. 12.9 Sagittal and transaxial perfusion, CTPA and fused perfusion SPECT/CTPA slices in a patient with PE. Based on normal lung charts, the defect shown (*red cross hair*) was localised to the superior segment of the right lower lobe. The CTPA demonstrates volume loss in the lower lobe due to atelectasis. The oblique fissure is displaced posteroinferiorly. When the two studies are fused, the perfusion defect localises to the posterior segment of the right upper lobe in this patient. Combining the SPECT study with the patient's CT can improve the accuracy of segmental localisation. (Reprinted with permission from Roach et al. [41])

pattern not usually associated with the diagnosis of PE. While determining the aetiology of pulmonary consolidation can be difficult, *V/Q* SPECT/CT may provide useful information which may help to characterise the underlying pathological process.

In a study of 38 patients in which gated SPECT was performed, Zaki et al. found that consolidative opacities secondary to PE preferentially occur peripherally, whereas inflammatory disease-induced lesions tend to be seen preferentially at the proximal portion of defects [94]. This study supports the premise that PE, and its sequelae including pulmonary infarction, typically affects the peripheral aspects of the lungs. When *V/Q* SPECT/CT demonstrates matched reductions more proximally, non-embolic causes may be more likely.

12.12 Barriers to Implementation of *V/Q* SPECT/CT

While the advantages of *V/Q* SPECT/CT studies compared with traditional planar imaging, SPECT-only scintigraphy and CTPA have been detailed above, the technique is still not routinely performed in many nuclear medicine departments. Surprisingly, in an era where SPECT (and now SPECT/CT) are routinely used in many areas of nuclear medicine, lung scintigraphy is still done using planar imaging in many part of the world, including in much of the United States [41]. There are several reasons why the transition to *V/Q* SPECT and hence *V/Q* SPECT/CT has not occurred.

Firstly, there is the lack of an ideal ventilation agent in some countries. As detailed above, Technegas is well suited to *V/Q* SPECT, and while it would ideally be used for *V/Q* SPECT/CT studies, it is not commercially available in some countries, including the United States. An alternative is to use ^{99m}Tc DTPA aerosols. In a direct comparison of Technegas and ^{99m}Tc DTPA aerosol in 63 patients, Jogi et al. showed that the SPECT images obtained using either ventilation agent were comparable, although in patients with obstructive lung disease, Technegas was clearly superior due to its better peripheral penetration [54]. While Technegas ideally would be used for ventilation SPECT imaging, this study does support the use of aerosols as an alternative should Technegas not be available locally.

Secondly, there is a wide body of literature describing the accuracy as well as the strengths and limitations of planar *V/Q* imaging [21, 34, 95]. Several large multicentre trials have been performed in numerous countries and the various reporting criteria used have been well established and periodically refined to help optimise the overall accuracy of the test [35, 96, 97]. A normal planar lung scan has a very high negative predictive value, and for reporting specialists with many years of experience, there may be the belief that there is little to be gained by making the transition to SPECT imaging. It should, however, be remembered that the published literature, as detailed above, consistently demonstrates improvements in sensitivity, specificity and reproducibility with SPECT imaging [8, 29, 70]. This is important in the era of CTPA which has increasingly supplanted the planar *V/Q* scan as the diagnostic imaging test of choice in many centres around the world, most noticeably in the United States [4, 6]. To restrict *V/Q* scintigraphy to a 2D methodology is, in many ways, analogous to a radiologist persisting with a chest X-ray for imaging the thorax and lungs, rather than transitioning to CT scanning. While reporting specialists, especially during the transition period, may prefer to acquire both planar and SPECT images on the same patient, this is problematic due to the amount of imaging time that would be required. As many patients would be unable to tolerate the time required (over 60 min), this is not feasible for many patients, especially those that are ill, dyspneic or elderly. Fortunately, planar images can be generated from SPECT data using several approaches. While we have described a technique using a reprojection method [98], many of the commercial vendors offer a simpler approach using an 'angular summing' method [29]. For those used to viewing planar images, this can be useful in the transition from planar imaging to SPECT-only imaging and may prove useful even beyond this point to give a general, familiar and rapid view of the lungs for quick evaluation.

Thirdly, For Nuclear Medicine specialists, particularly those not trained in cross-sectional anatomy, visualisation of the lungs in 3D is a challenge compared with the 2D approach of planar *V/Q* imaging. This requires knowledge of the cross-sectional anatomy of the lungs as well as the 3D appearances of lung segments, fissures, major vessels and airways as well as other intrathoracic structures. However, with the diffusion of PET/CT and SPECT/CT worldwide, nearly all specialists reporting Nuclear Medicine studies would increasingly be visualising the thorax in 3D, thus a shift to

V/Q SPECT, and *V/Q* SPECT/CT imaging should be less of a challenge to most specialists today than previously. In addition, cross-sectional imaging atlases and computerised programs are now commonly located in most Nuclear Medicine reporting rooms to further aid in this transition.

Finally, some reporters may be under the misconception that SPECT, and SPECT/CT, imaging takes significantly longer to perform than traditional planar imaging or is more difficult for technologists to perform. This is not the case. Many centres perform SPECT imaging faster than can be done with traditional six or eight view planar imaging [29, 32]. At my institution, where dual-headed SPECT/CT scanners are used, a typical acquisition protocol takes about 25–30 min [50]. Other centres report slightly faster image acquisition times with images produced of high diagnostic quality. For instance, the group from University Hospital in Lund, Sweden, acquired ventilation studies (using ^{99m}Tc-DTPA) in just under 11 min and perfusion images in just under 6 min [27]. The group from Centre Hospitalier Universitaire de Sherbrooke in Quebec, Canada, acquired their data in similar times having published studies using 12 min acquisition times for ventilation (using Technegas) and 6 min for perfusion utilising a dual-head scanner [32]. With current generation multi-slice CT scanners, the addition of a 'low dose' CT scan adds only 1–2 min to these times. Thus, image acquisition times in the range of 20–30 min are routine today with *V/Q* SPECT/CT. For technologists used to performing planar *V/Q* scans, the transition to SPECT is welcomed. The multiple repositioning of the detectors and patient arms required with planar imaging is no longer required, resulting in easier data acquisitions for the technologists. At Royal North Shore Hospital, the technologists now much prefer SPECT (and SPECT/CT) imaging for *V/Q* scintigraphy and would only choose to perform a planar study in unusual circumstances, such as for a patient who could not undergo SPECT imaging, e.g. if they were unable to lie supine on the scanning bed. With SPECT/CT scanning now standard in many areas of nuclear medicine, *V/Q* SPECT/CT acquisitions should be a quite routine procedure for nuclear medicine technologists.

12.13 Thrombus Imaging

Over the last few decades, there have been numerous attempts to develop radiolabelled thrombus imaging agents to assess deep venous thrombosis and PE. While none are yet in routine clinical practice, these agents allow differentiation of old clots from new and allow imaging of acute thrombus in any part of the body, most commonly in the legs and the lungs. While thoracic SPECT imaging has been performed using such agents in recent years, the lack of background activity complicates exact localisation of clot within the pulmonary vascular tree [99]. Hybrid SPECT/CT would be ideally suited for use with such agents, and this is another

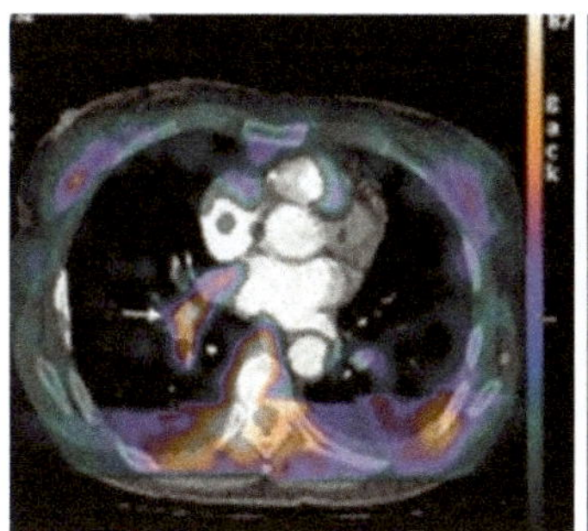
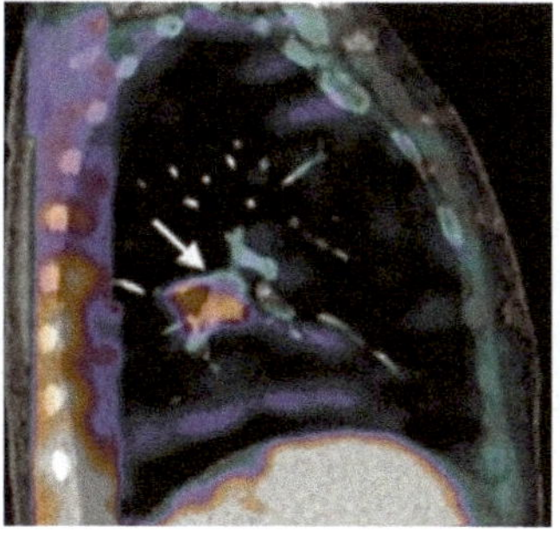
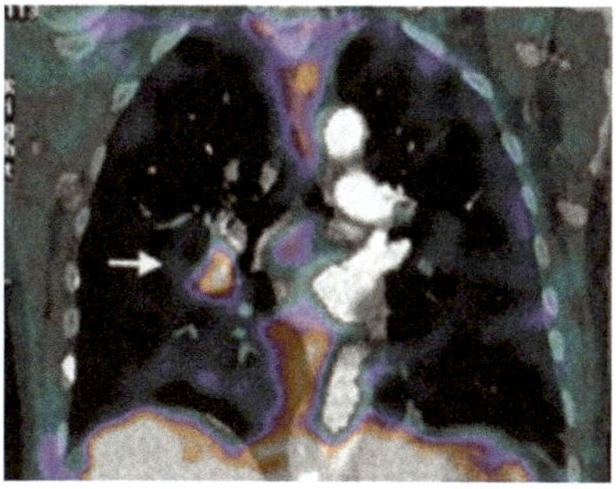

Fig. 12.10 Fused SPECT/CT images of acute PE after administration of ^{99m}Tc-labelled anti-d-dimer antibody fragments. The thrombus (*arrowed*) corresponds to an intravascular contrast-filling defect on the CTPA. (Reprinted with permission from Morris [99])

promising application in patients with suspected PE which may develop in the future (Fig. 12.10).

12.14 *V/Q* SPECT/CT: Role in Applications Other than PE

V/Q SPECT/CT is finding increased utility in a number of other conditions beyond its use in the diagnosis and management of PE. These include allowing optimal selection of radiotherapy fields for lung cancer therapy and the preoperative quantification of lung function prior to resection [63].

12.14.1 Radiotherapy Treatment Planning

In the treatment of patients with lung cancer, literature suggests that administering a higher dose of external beam radiotherapy is associated with improved survival [100, 101]. However, the dose is limited due to the sensitivity of normal lung and the development of radiation pneumonitis and fibrosis [102–105].

Patients with lung cancer requiring radiotherapy may have areas of healthy lung included in the radiotherapy fields. Considering that most of these patients will have a significant cigarette smoking history, they often begin treatment with marked impairment of their respiratory function and can ill afford further reductions in their lung function. Acute radiation toxicity occurs in up to 10% of patients receiving radiotherapy to the lungs. Long-term reductions also occur due to the development of radiation fibrosis. These two pathologies often overlap but both may progress independently of each other. Following radiotherapy, a decline in lung function has been demonstrated on respiratory function testing and on long-term sequential perfusion scanning. These changes peak in the period approximately 12–18 months after the radiotherapy and are dose dependent [106, 107]. Baseline perfusion scans can be used to identify which portions of the lungs have the most preserved function. It

has been shown that perfusion scans can be used to modify radiotherapy fields in patients thereby affecting the total dose patient received by sparing perfused lung [108–111]. McGuire and co-workers report on an approach that reduced the $F_{(20)}$ and $F_{(30)}$ (the amount of lung receiving 20 Gy or 30 Gy, respectively) values by 16.5% and 6.1% compared to traditional therapy planning [112]. Ventilation SPECT can also be used to plan therapy (Fig. 12.11) [113]. Evidence that these manoeuvres alter long-term lung function remains sparse.

12.14.2 Lung Reduction Surgery Planning

In patients being considered for lung reduction surgery, perfusion imaging is often used to assess lobar function and to estimate the impact of lung surgery on the patient's pulmonary status. Using planar *V/Q* scintigraphy, an assessment of relative regional lung function can be made by dividing the lungs into various zones (typically upper, middle and lower thirds) and determining the relative contribution of each region to overall ventilation and perfusion. Due to overlap of pulmonary lobes and segments and differences in individual patient lung anatomy, such an approach is crude at best and lacks accuracy. The advent of hybrid SPECT/CT allows a similar approach being undertaken in 3D, and when combined with each individual patient's segmental anatomy (determined from their CT scan), a much more accurate assessment of lobar or segmental lung function can be derived (Fig. 12.12). In patients with non-small cell lung cancer, this approach has been shown to play a valuable role in predicting postoperative lung function following lung resection and is highly accurate as a predictor of postoperative FEV1 [114, 115].

One series reported a perfusion ratio of upper to lower lung and demonstrated that poor perfusion to the upper lobes was correlated with the decision to perform lung reduction surgery based on CT assessment [116]. In the US National Emphysema Treatment Trial, perfusion imaging was discontinued in 2001 as it did not add further prognostic

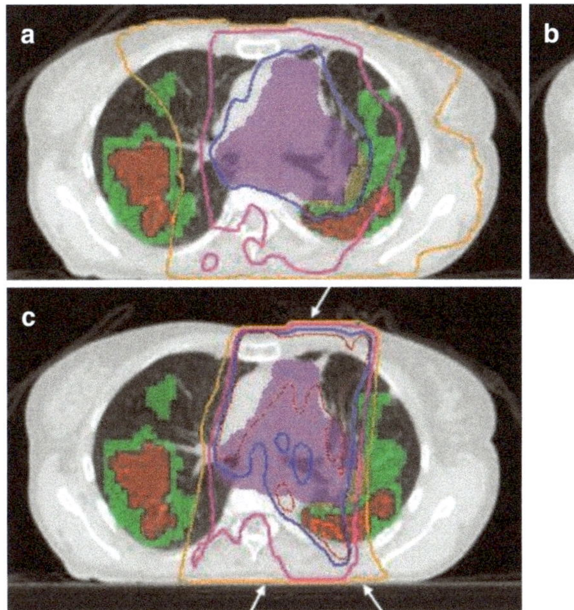
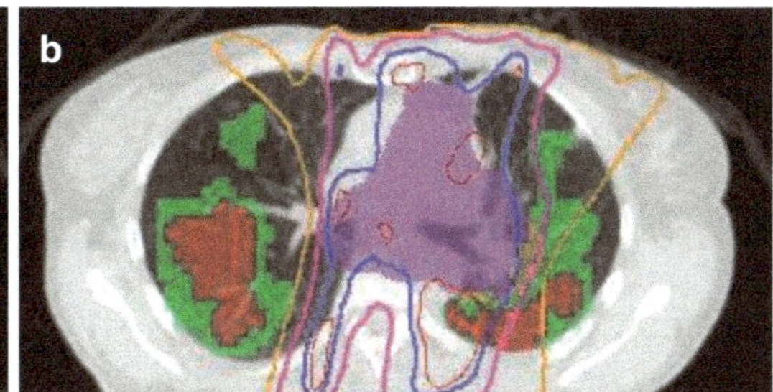

Fig. 12.11 These three transaxial images demonstrate ventilation as a percentage of maximum ventilation with green representing 50% (vv50) of maximum and red 70% or more (vv70). Isodoses of 66.5 Gy, 45 Gy and 20 Gy are shown as blue, pink and orange lines, respectively (white arrows). Image (**a**) has been calculated without reference to *V/Q* data, (**b**) using nine equally spaced beams to avoid vv50 and vv70 regions and (**c**) using a subset of three beam angles also avoiding vv50 and vv70. In this example, there is considerable reduction in the amount of well-ventilated lung being irradiated in both (**b**) and (**c**). The central *purple area* represents the planning target volume (PTV). (Reprinted with permission from Munawar et al. [113])

information to that obtained by other measures. There were a number of limitations to the original technique, specifically, overlap of the anatomic structures being analysed. SPECT scintigraphy, particularly with CT co-registration, allows for accurate segmentation of the lungs with lobar estimates of function made possible [42]. Whether this is of any additional benefit remains to be assessed.

12.15 Further Uses

V/Q SPECT/CT has further potential in assessing the physiologic basis of lung disease, both as a clinical and research tool. *V/Q* SPECT scintigraphy has been used to assess changes in ventilation after lung reduction surgery [117, 118], inhomogeneity of ventilation in emphysema patients [119], regional changes of ventilation and perfusion in asthma [120, 121] and the

degree of lung perfusion impairment in patients with pulmonary arteriovenous fistulae [122] and in estimating regional lung function in patients with interstitial pulmonary disease [123]. Technegas SPECT has been analysed using three-dimensional fractal analysis to quantify heterogenous distribution of tracer [124]. The use of ventilation and perfusion imaging as an investigative tool for lung physiology is of increasing interest, particularly in evaluating the extent of airways closure in patients with airways disease [115] (Fig. 12.13). *V/Q* SPECT/ CT would be well suited to identifying and quantifying the location and extent of non-ventilation in patients with airways disease. By comparing ventilation SPECT with a low-dose CT, it can be determined which areas of lung have non-ventilation (or malventilation) due to underlying emphysema as opposed to airways constriction [115].

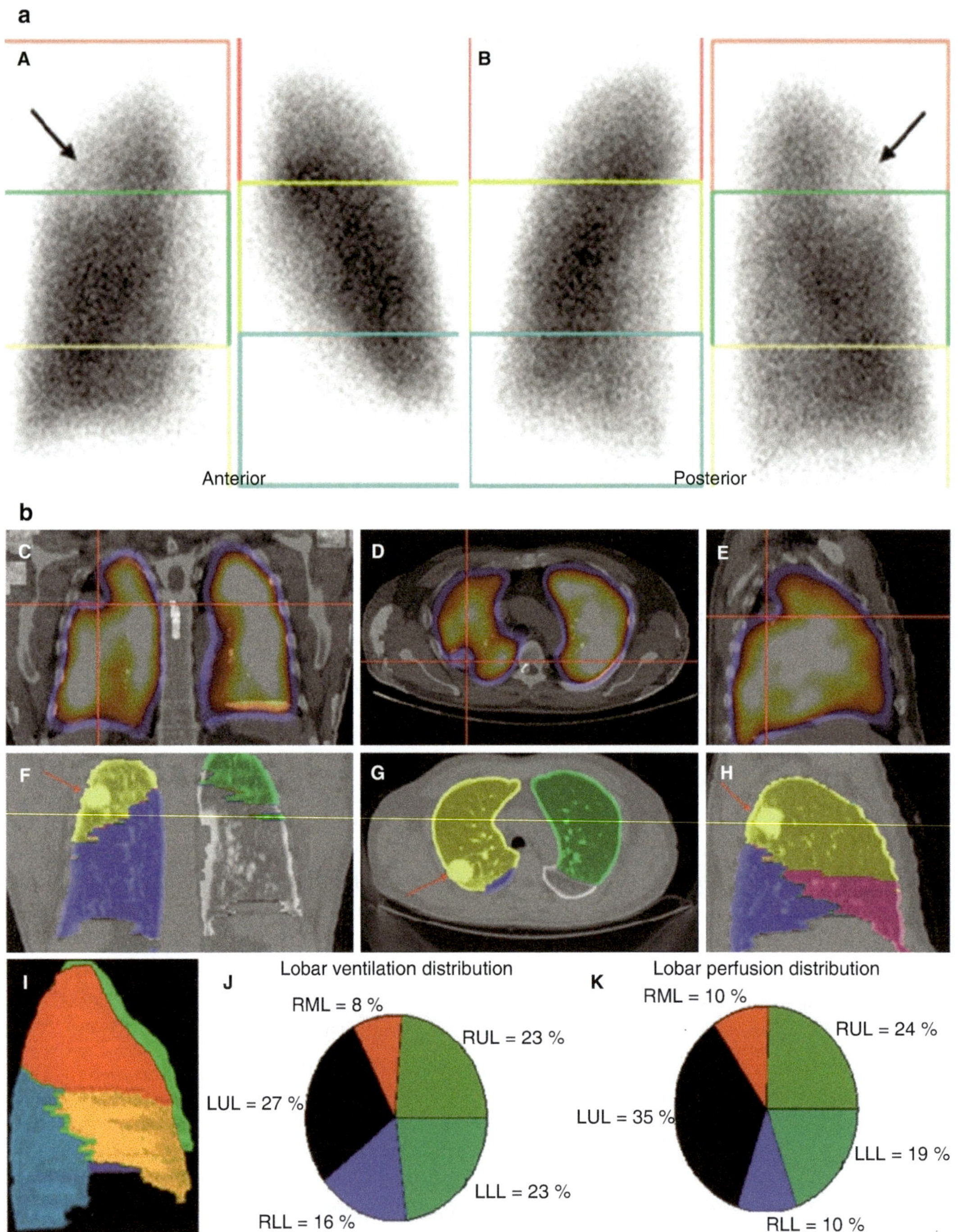

Fig. 12.12 (**a**) Anterior (*A*) and posterior (*B*) planar images in a patient with a right lung carcinoma (*arrowed*). The exact lobar location of the tumour cannot be determined on the planar imaging. (**b**) Fused SPECT/CT perfusion images in the coronal (*C*), transverse (*D*) and sagittal (*E*) planes show the tumour and corresponding perfusion defect (indicated by *cursors*). Corresponding CT scan slices in the coronal (*F*), transverse (*G*) and sagittal (*H*) planes (with patient-specific lobar region-of-interest derived from the CT) show the lesion to be located in the right upper lobe (*arrowed*). 3D patient-specific lobar region-of-interest images (*I*) can be generated and viewed as a rotating MIP image. The SPECT/CT allowed accurate determination of each lobe's relative contribution to overall ventilation (*J*) and perfusion (*K*)

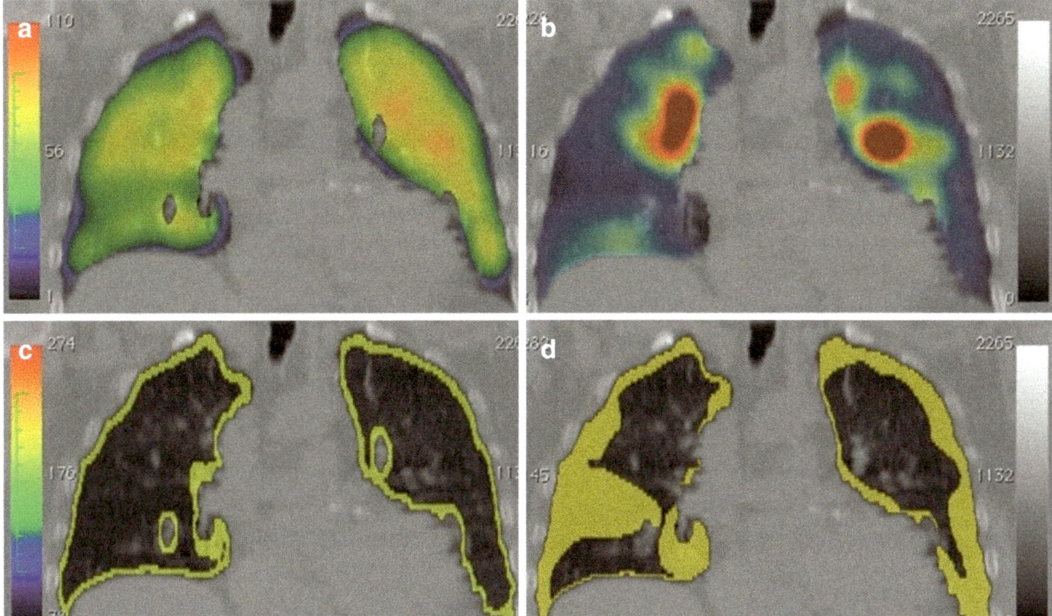

Fig. 12.13 (**a**) Ventilation SPECT/CT fusion image (coronal view) of an asthmatic subject who had severe airway hyperresponsiveness. (**b**) Ventilation SPECT/CT fusion after methacholine challenge when FEV1 had decreased by around 25%. (**c**) and (**d**) are processed images showing non-ventilation (in *yellow*) derived from fusion images. The development of large regions affected by airway closure is evident in the lower lung zones. (Reprinted with permission from King et al. [115])

12.16 Quantitative *V/Q* SPECT

As noted by Bailey and Willowson in our review article on *V/Q* SPECT/CT, many of the potential uses for SPECT *V/Q* in respiratory research mentioned above would benefit from quantitatively accurate *V/Q* scanning [63]. Quantitatively accurate image reconstruction is accepted as de facto in PET and PET/CT studies, but quantitatively accurate SPECT/CT is only a relatively recent development [125]. To examine the global quantitative accuracy in lung SPECT scanning, our institution examined the agreement between the calibrated ('true') dose of ^{99m}Tc-MAA administered to patients (assuming 100% trapping in the lungs) undergoing *V/Q* SPECT/CT studies with that estimated by CT-based attenuation corrected (AC) and scatter corrected (SC) reconstructed SPECT perfusion images after subtraction of the residual ventilation (Technegas) contribution [125]. In a series of 12 subjects, the average difference between the estimated and true activities was found to be −1%, with a range of −7 to +4%. A further validation study in the thorax using the same SPECT/CT AC and SC methodology was able to estimate the concentration of ^{99m}Tc-labelled red blood cells in an equilibrium blood pool SPECT image in the left ventricular chamber. It was found that the average difference between the measured and true concentrations was within −1% of the true value with a range of −6 to +5%, further attesting to the robustness of the methodology in a different imaging scenario [126]. To further define the regional accuracy achievable today, my institution has undertaken a study of the impact of CT-based attenuation and scatter correction to examine the effect on lobar quantification in the lungs. The impact of scatter correction in ventilation (*V*) and perfusion with ventilation subtracted (*Q* − *V*) SPECT studies on a global and regional basis was assessed by considering differences in the total lungs, differences in the left and right lungs separately and differences in each of the segments. Analysis of perfusion studies (*Q*) first involved the subtraction of ventilation counts that remained in the lungs $(Q - V)$ to ensure that counts relating to ^{99m}Tc-MAA perfusion only were included. Although scatter correction results in a decrease in overall counts, negative differences on a lobar level are still possible, as this represents the redistribution of counts to different segments. In the study, 21 consecutive subjects undergoing V/Q SPECT/CT scanning demonstrated that scatter correction, in conjunction with attenuation correction, was seen to have a significant impact on regional lung analysis, with an average difference of over 20% for both ventilation and perfusion studies, but this difference is consistently more substantial in the left lung than the right. For both the ventilation and perfusion analysis, the differences introduced by scatter correction, in order from largest to smallest, are in the left lower lobe, the left upper lobe, the right upper lobe, the right middle lobe and the right lower lobe, respectively. In ventilation studies, the average difference in reconstructed activity concentration as a result of scatter correction in the left lower lobe is as large as 30%. Such large variation over the different segments and dominance of scatter in the left lower lobe strongly suggests that a large contributing factor may be Compton scatter from the heart. This would explain the larger differences seen in the left lung as opposed to the right and again highlights the importance of performing patient-specific, nonuniform corrections particularly in regions of variable density, such as the chest. This highlights the importance of scatter correction being used in conjunction with attenuation correction to achieve accurate quantitative data when imaging the lungs with SPECT.

12.17 Conclusion

The addition of CT data to V/Q SPECT is an exciting and potentially invaluable development in the imaging of patients with suspected PE. In a single imaging procedure, patients can benefit from the high sensitivity of V/Q SPECT scintigraphy as well as the additional diagnostic information provided by three-dimensional morphological imaging of the lungs. This com-bination is of particular benefit in increasing the specificity of V/Q SPECT imaging. Clinically, a low-dose CT can help identify alternative causes of both matched and mismatched V/Q deficits, thus further improving the diagnostic utility of the study. Compared with CTPA, V/Q SPECT/CT has several advantages, including a higher sensitivity, a lower radiation dose, no risk of contrast-related allergy or nephrotoxicity and less technically inadequate studies. In some difficult cases, both a CTPA and a SPECT V/Q may be required to ultimately confirm, or exclude, the presence of PE. In these patients, co-registering the CTPA with the perfusion SPECT can help guide the radiologist to more closely examine an area of perfusion deficit and, in the case of discordant CTPA and V/Q SPECT results, may help to reach a consensus imaging diagnosis. In non-PE applications, it has been demonstrated that quantitatively accurate information from SPECT/CT can be obtained for uses such as measuring regional lung function, planning radiotherapy treatment and providing other functional measurements of respiratory physiology.

References

1. Dalen JE. Pulmonary embolism: what have we learned since Virchow?: treatment and prevention. Chest. 2002;122:1801–17.
2. Levine MN, Raskob G, Beyth RJ, Kearon C, Schulman S. Hemorrhagic complications of anticoagulant treatment: the Seventh ACCP Conference on Antithrombotic and Thrombolytic Therapy. Chest. 2004;126:287S–310.
3. Nijkeuter M, Sohne M, Tick LW, Kamphuisen PW, Kramer MH, et al. The natural course of hemodynamically stable pulmonary embolism: clinical outcome and risk factors in a large prospective cohort study. Chest. 2007;131:517–23.
4. British Thoracic Society Standards of Care Committee Pulmonary Embolism Guideline Development Group. British Thoracic Society guidelines for the management of suspected acute pulmonary embolism. Thorax. 2003;58:470–83.
5. Anderson DR, Kahn SR, Rodger MA, Kovacs MJ, Morris T, et al. Computed tomographic pulmonary angiography vs ventilation-perfusion lung scanning in patients with suspected pulmonary embolism: a randomized controlled trial. JAMA. 2007;298:2743–53.

6. Strashun AM. A reduced role of V/Q scintigraphy in the diagnosis of acute pulmonary embolism. J Nucl Med. 2007;48:1405–7.

7. Wagner HN Jr, Sabiston DC Jr, McAfee JG, Tow D, Stern HS. Diagnosis of massive pulmonary embolism in man by radioisotope scanning. N Engl J Med. 1964;271:377–84.

8. Bajc M, Neilly JB, Miniati M, Schuemichen C, Meignan M, et al. EANM guidelines for ventilation/perfusion scintigraphy: part 1. Pulmonary imaging with ventilation/perfusion single photon emission tomography. Eur J Nucl Med Mol Imaging. 2009;36:1356–70.

9. McNeil BJ, Holman BL, Adelstein SJ. The scintigraphic definition of pulmonary embolism. JAMA. 1974;227:753–6.

10. Glassroth J. Imaging of pulmonary embolism: too much of a good thing? JAMA. 2007;298:2788–9.

11. Dalen JE. New PIOPED recommendations for the diagnosis of pulmonary embolism. Am J Med. 2006;119:1001–2.

12. Meignan MA. Lung ventilation/perfusion SPECT: the right technique for hard times. J Nucl Med. 2002;43:648–51.

13. Schumichen C. V/Q-scanning/SPECT for the diagnosis of pulmonary embolism. Respiration. 2003;70:329–42.

14. Morrell NW, Nijran KS, Jones BE, Biggs T, Seed WA. The underestimation of segmental defect size in radionuclide lung scanning. J Nucl Med. 1993;34:370–4.

15. Magnussen JS, Chicco P, Palmer AW, Bush V, Mackey DW, et al. Single-photon emission tomography of a computerised model of pulmonary embolism. Eur J Nucl Med. 1999;26:1430–8.

16. Gray HW, McKillop JH, Bessent RG. Lung scan reporting language: what does it mean? Nucl Med Commun. 1993;14:1084–7.

17. Gray HW, McKillop JH, Bessent RG. Lung scan reports: interpretation by clinicians. Nucl Med Commun. 1993;14:989–94.

18. Goodman LR, Lipchik RJ. Diagnosis of acute pulmonary embolism: time for a new approach. Radiology. 1996;199:25–7.

19. Scott HR, Gillen GJ, Shand J, Bryden F, Milroy R. A structured approach to the interpretation and reporting of ventilation/perfusion scans. Nucl Med Commun. 1998;19:107–12.

20. Kember PG, Euinton HA, Morcos SK. Clinicians' interpretation of the indeterminate ventilation-perfusion scan report. Br J Radiol. 1997;70:1109–11.

21. PIOPED. Value of the ventilation/perfusion scan in acute pulmonary embolism. Results of the prospective investigation of pulmonary embolism diagnosis (PIOPED). The PIOPED Investigators. JAMA. 1990;263:2753–9.

22. Leblanc M, Paul N. V/Q SPECT and computed tomographic pulmonary angiography. Semin Nucl Med. 2010;40:426–41.

23. Carrasquillo JA, Rogers JV, Williams DL, Shuman WP, Olson DO, et al. Single-photon emission computed tomography of the normal liver. AJR Am J Roentgenol. 1983;141:937–41.

24. Hacot JP, Bojovic M, Delonca J, Meier B, Righetti A. Comparison of planar imaging and single-photon emission computed tomography for the detection and localization of coronary artery disease. Int J Card Imaging. 1993;9:113–9.

25. Osborne DR, Jaszczak RJ, Greer K, Roggli V, Lischko M, et al. Detection of pulmonary emboli in dogs: comparison of single photon emission computed tomography, gamma camera imaging, and angiography. Radiology. 1983;146:493–7.

26. Bajc M, Bitzen U, Olsson B, Perez de Sa V, Palmer J, et al. Lung ventilation/perfusion SPECT in the artificially embolized pig. J Nucl Med. 2002;43:640–7.

27. Bajc M, Olsson CG, Olsson B, Palmer J, Jonson B. Diagnostic evaluation of planar and tomographic ventilation/perfusion lung images in patients with suspected pulmonary emboli. Clin Physiol Funct Imaging. 2004;24:249–56.

28. Collart JP, Roelants V, Vanpee D, Lacrosse M, Trigaux JP, et al. Is a lung perfusion scan obtained by using single photon emission computed tomography able to improve the radionuclide diagnosis of pulmonary embolism? Nucl Med Commun. 2002;23:1107–13.

29. Reinartz P, Wildberger JE, Schaefer W, Nowak B, Mahnken AH, et al. Tomographic imaging in the diagnosis of pulmonary embolism: a comparison between V/Q lung scintigraphy in SPECT technique and multislice spiral CT. J Nucl Med. 2004;45:1501–8.

30. Laurence IJ, Redman SL, Corrigan AJ, Graham RN. V/Q SPECT imaging of acute pulmonary embolus – a practical perspective. Clin Radiol. 2012;67:941–8.

31. Gutte H, Mortensen J, Jensen CV, Johnbeck CB, von der Recke P, et al. Detection of pulmonary embolism with combined ventilation-perfusion SPECT and low-dose CT: head-to-head comparison with multidetector CT angiography. J Nucl Med. 2009;50:1987–92.

32. Leblanc M, Leveillee F, Turcotte E. Prospective evaluation of the negative predictive value of V/Q SPECT using 99mTc-Technegas. Nucl Med Commun. 2007;28:667–72.

33. Li DK, Seltzer SE, McNeil BJ. V/Q mismatches unassociated with pulmonary embolism: case report and review of the literature. J Nucl Med. 1978;19:1331–3.

34. Miniati M, Pistolesi M, Marini C, Di Ricco G, Formichi B, et al. Value of perfusion lung scan in the diagnosis of pulmonary embolism: results of the Prospective Investigative Study of Acute Pulmonary Embolism Diagnosis (PISA-PED). Am J Respir Crit Care Med. 1996;154:1387–93.

35. Freeman LM. Don't bury the V/Q scan: it's as good as multidetector CT angiograms with a lot less radiation exposure. J Nucl Med. 2008;49:5–8.
36. Schoepf UJ, Costello P. CT angiography for diagnosis of pulmonary embolism: state of the art. Radiology. 2004;230:329–37.
37. Hall WB, Truitt SG, Scheunemann LP, Shah SA, Rivera MP, et al. The prevalence of clinically relevant incidental findings on chest computed tomographic angiograms ordered to diagnose pulmonary embolism. Arch Intern Med. 2009;169:1961–5.
38. Harris B, Bailey D, Roach P, Bailey E, King G. Fusion imaging of computed tomographic pulmonary angiography and SPECT ventilation/perfusion scintigraphy: initial experience and potential benefit. Eur J Nucl Med Mol Imaging. 2007;34:135–42.
39. Roach PJ, Bailey DL. Combining anatomy and function: the future of medical imaging. Intern Med J. 2005;35:577–9.
40. Vogel WV, Oyen WJ, Barentsz JO, Kaanders JH, Corstens FH. PET/CT: panacea, redundancy, or something in between? J Nucl Med. 2004;45(Suppl 1):15S–24.
41. Roach PJ, Bailey DL, Schembri GP, Thomas PA. Transition from planar to SPECT V/Q scintigraphy: rationale, practicalities, and challenges. Semin Nucl Med. 2010;40:397–407.
42. Bailey DL, Roach PJ, Bailey EA, Hewlett J, Keijzers R. Development of a cost-effective modular SPECT/CT scanner. Eur J Nucl Med Mol Imaging. 2007;34:1415–26.
43. Schillaci O. Hybrid SPECT/CT: a new era for SPECT imaging? Eur J Nucl Med Mol Imaging. 2005;32:521–4.
44. Lardinois D, Weder W, Hany TF, Kamel EM, Korom S, et al. Staging of non-small-cell lung cancer with integrated positron-emission tomography and computed tomography. N Engl J Med. 2003;348:2500–7.
45. Schoepf UJ. Pulmonary artery CTA. Tech Vasc Interv Radiol. 2006;9:180–91.
46. Gradinscak DJ, Roach P, Schembri GP. Can perfusion SPECT improve the accuracy of CTPA? Eur J Nucl Med Mol Imaging. 2009;36:S463.
47. Gutte H, Mortensen J, Jensen C, von der Recke P, Kristoffersen US, et al. Added value of combined simultaneous lung ventilation-perfusion single-photon emission computed tomography/multi-slice-computed tomography angiography in two patients suspected of having acute pulmonary embolism. Clin Respir J. 2007;1:52–5.
48. Gutman F, Hangard G, Gardin I, Varmenot N, Pattyn J, et al. Evaluation of a rigid registration method of lung perfusion SPECT and thoracic CT. AJR Am J Roentgenol. 2005;185:1516–24.
49. Ketai L, Hartshorne M. Potential uses of computed tomography-SPECT and computed tomography-coincidence fusion images of the chest. Clin Nucl Med. 2001;26:433–41.
50. Roach PJ, Bailey DL, Harris BE. Enhancing lung scintigraphy with single-photon emission computed tomography. Semin Nucl Med. 2008;38:441–9.
51. Petersson J, Sanchez-Crespo A, Larsson SA, Mure M. Physiological imaging of the lung: single-photon-emission computed tomography (SPECT). J Appl Physiol. 2007;102:468–76.
52. van Beek EJ, Dahmen AM, Stavngaard T, Gast KK, Heussel CP, et al. Hyperpolarised 3He MRI versus HRCT in COPD and normal volunteers: PHIL trial. Eur Respir J. 2009;34:1311–21.
53. Suga K, Kawakami Y, Zaki M, Yamashita T, Shimizu K, et al. Clinical utility of co-registered respiratory-gated(99m)Tc-Technegas/MAA SPECT-CT images in the assessment of regional lung functional impairment in patients with lung cancer. Eur J Nucl Med Mol Imaging. 2004;31:1280–90.
54. Jogi J, Jonson B, Ekberg M, Bajc M. Ventilation-perfusion SPECT with 99mTc-DTPA versus Technegas: a head-to-head study in obstructive and nonobstructive disease. J Nucl Med. 2010;51:735–41.
55. Crawford AB, Davison A, Amis TC, Engel LA. Intrapulmonary distribution of 99mtechnetium labelled ultrafine carbon aerosol (Technegas) in severe airflow obstruction. Eur Respir J. 1990;3:686–92.
56. Amis TC, Crawford AB, Davison A, Engel LA. Distribution of inhaled 99mtechnetium labelled ultrafine carbon particle aerosol (Technegas) in human lungs. Eur Respir J. 1990;3:679–85.
57. Burch WM, Boyd MM, Crellin DE. Technegas: particle size and distribution. Eur J Nucl Med. 1994;21:365–7.
58. Lemb M, Oei TH, Eifert H, Gunther B. Technegas: a study of particle structure, size and distribution. Eur J Nucl Med. 1993;20:576–9.
59. Peltier P, De Faucal P, Chetanneau A, Chatal JF. Comparison of technetium-99m aerosol and krypton-81m in ventilation studies for the diagnosis of pulmonary embolism. Nucl Med Commun. 1990;11:631–8.
60. Bailey EA, Bailey DL, Roach PJ. V/Q imaging in 2010: a quick start guide. Semin Nucl Med. 2010;40:408–14.
61. Hudson HM, Larkin RS. Accelerated image reconstruction using ordered subsets of projection data. IEEE Trans Med Imaging. 1994;13:601–9.
62. Hutton BF, Hudson HM, Beekman FJ. A clinical perspective of accelerated statistical reconstruction. Eur J Nucl Med. 1997;24:797–808.
63. Roach PJ, Gradinscak DJ, Schembri GP, Bailey EA, Willowson KP, et al. SPECT/CT in V/Q scanning. Semin Nucl Med. 2010;40:455–66.
64. Patton JA, Turkington TG. SPECT/CT physical principles and attenuation correction. J Nucl Med Technol. 2008;36:1–10.
65. Delbeke D, Coleman RE, Guiberteau MJ, Brown ML, Royal HD, et al. Procedure guideline for SPECT/CT imaging 1.0. J Nucl Med. 2006;47:1227–34.

66. Studholme C, Hill DL, Hawkes DJ. Automated three-dimensional registration of magnetic resonance and positron emission tomography brain images by multiresolution optimization of voxel similarity measures. Med Phys. 1997;24:25–35.

67. Palmer J, Bitzen U, Jonson B, Bajc M. Comprehensive ventilation/perfusion SPECT. J Nucl Med. 2001;42:1288–94.

68. Harris B, Bailey D, Miles S, Bailey E, Rogers K, et al. Objective analysis of tomographic ventilation-perfusion scintigraphy in pulmonary embolism. Am J Respir Crit Care Med. 2007;175:1173–80.

69. Harris B, Bailey DL, Chicco P, Bailey EA, Roach PJ, et al. Objective analysis of whole lung and lobar ventilation/perfusion relationships in pulmonary embolism. Clin Physiol Funct Imaging. 2008;28:14–26.

70. Roach PJ, Bailey DL, Schembri GP. Reinventing ventilation/perfusion lung scanning with SPECT. Nucl Med Commun. 2008;29:1023–5.

71. Herald P, Roach P, Schembri GP. Does the addition of low dose CT improve diagnostic accuracy of V/Q SPECT scintigraphy? J Nucl Med. 2008;49:S91.

72. Gradinscak DJ, Roach P, Schembri GP. Lung SPECT perfusion scintigraphy: can CT substitute for ventilation imaging? Eur J Nucl Med Mol Imaging. 2009;36:S300.

73. Buscombe JR, Notghi A, Croasdale J, et al. COVID-19: guidance for infection prevention and control in nuclear medicine. Nucl Med Commun. 2020;41:499–504.

74. COVID-19 and ventilation/perfusion (V/Q) lung studies. J Nucl Med. 2020;61:23N–24N.

75. Zuckier LS, Moadel RM, Haramati LB, Freeman LM. Diagnostic evaluation of pulmonary embolism during the COVID-19 pandemic. J Nucl Med. 2020;61:630–631.

76. Schaefer WM, Knollmann D and Meyer PT. V/Q SPECT/CT in the Time of COVID-19: Changing the Order to Improve Safety Without Sacrificing Accuracy. Journal of Nuclear Medicine. 2021;62(7):1022–24. https://doi.org/10.2967/jnumed.120.261263.

77. Stein PD, Fowler SE, Goodman LR, Gottschalk A, Hales CA, et al. Multidetector computed tomography for acute pulmonary embolism. N Engl J Med. 2006;354:2317–27.

78. Roach PJ, Thomas P, Bajc M, Jonson B. Merits of V/Q SPECT scintigraphy compared with CTPA in imaging of pulmonary embolism. J Nucl Med. 2008;49:167–8; author reply 8.

79. Roach PJ, Bajc M. Acute pulmonary embolism. N Engl J Med. 2010;363:1972–3; author reply 4–5.

80. Miles S, Rogers KM, Thomas P, Soans B, Attia J, et al. A comparison of single-photon emission CT lung scintigraphy and CT pulmonary angiography for the diagnosis of pulmonary embolism. Chest. 2009;136:1546–53.

81. Toney LK, Lewis DH, Richardson ML. Ventilation/perfusion scanning for acute pulmonary embolism: effect of direct communication on patient treatment outcomes. Clin Nucl Med. 2013;38:183–7.

82. Barrett BJ, Parfrey PS. Clinical practice. Preventing nephropathy induced by contrast medium. N Engl J Med. 2006;354:379–86.

83. Schembri GP, Miller AE, Smart R. Radiation dosimetry and safety issues in the investigation of pulmonary embolism. Semin Nucl Med. 2010;40:442–54.

84. Hurwitz LM, Yoshizumi TT, Goodman PC, Nelson RC, Toncheva G, et al. Radiation dose savings for adult pulmonary embolus 64-MDCT using bismuth breast shields, lower peak kilovoltage, and automatic tube current modulation. AJR Am J Roentgenol. 2009;192:244–53.

85. Parker MS, Hui FK, Camacho MA, Chung JK, Broga DW, et al. Female breast radiation exposure during CT pulmonary angiography. AJR Am J Roentgenol. 2005;185:1228–33.

86. Hurwitz LM, Yoshizumi TT, Reiman RE, Paulson EK, Frush DP, et al. Radiation dose to the female breast from 16-MDCT body protocols. AJR Am J Roentgenol. 2006;186:1718–22.

87. ICRP. Radiation dose to patients from radiopharmaceuticals (addendum 2 to ICRP publication 53). Ann ICRP. 1998;28:1–126.

88. Jones SE, Wittram C. The indeterminate CT pulmonary angiogram: imaging characteristics and patient clinical outcome. Radiology. 2005;237:329–37.

89. Ryu JH, Swensen SJ, Olson EJ, Pellikka PA. Diagnosis of pulmonary embolism with use of computed tomographic angiography. Mayo Clin Proc. 2001;76:59–65.

90. U-King-Im JM, Freeman SJ, Boylan T, Cheow HK. Quality of CT pulmonary angiography for suspected pulmonary embolus in pregnancy. Eur Radiol. 2008;18:2709–15.

91. Ridge CA, McDermott S, Freyne BJ, Brennan DJ, Collins CD, et al. Pulmonary embolism in pregnancy: comparison of pulmonary CT angiography and lung scintigraphy. AJR Am J Roentgenol. 2009;193:1223–7.

92. Yap E, Anderson G, Donald J, Wong CA, Lee YC, et al. Pleural effusion in patients with pulmonary embolism. Respirology. 2008;13:832–6.

93. Gradinscak DJ, Roach P, Schembri GP. Can CT coregistration improve the accuracy of segmental localisation on V/Q SPECT? Eur J Nucl Med Mol Imaging. 2009;36:S463.

94. Zaki M, Suga K, Kawakami Y, Yamashita T, Shimizu K, et al. Preferential location of acute pulmonary thromboembolism induced consolidative opacities: assessment with respiratory gated perfusion SPECT-CT fusion images. Nucl Med Commun. 2005;26:465–74.

95. Worsley DF, Alavi A, Palevsky HI, Kundel HL. Comparison of diagnostic performance with ventilation-perfusion lung imaging in different patient populations. Radiology. 1996;199:481–3.

96. Sostman HD, Coleman RE, DeLong DM, Newman GE, Paine S. Evaluation of revised criteria for

ventilation-perfusion scintigraphy in patients with suspected pulmonary embolism. Radiology. 1994;193:103–7.

97. Gottschalk A, Sostman HD, Coleman RE, Juni JE, Thrall J, et al. Ventilation-perfusion scintigraphy in the PIOPED study. Part II. Evaluation of the scintigraphic criteria and interpretations. J Nucl Med. 1993;34:1119–26.

98. Bailey DL, Schembri GP, Harris BE, Bailey EA, Cooper RA, et al. Generation of planar images from lung ventilation/perfusion SPECT. Ann Nucl Med. 2008;22:437–45.

99. Morris TA. SPECT imaging of pulmonary emboli with radiolabeled thrombus-specific imaging agents. Semin Nucl Med. 2010;40:474–9.

100. Bradley J. A review of radiation dose escalation trials for non-small cell lung cancer within the Radiation Therapy Oncology Group. Semin Oncol. 2005;32:S111–3.

101. Belderbos JS, Heemsbergen WD, De Jaeger K, Baas P, Lebesque JV. Final results of a phase I/II dose escalation trial in non-small-cell lung cancer using three-dimensional conformal radiotherapy. Int J Radiat Oncol Biol Phys. 2006;66:126–34.

102. Hernando ML, Marks LB, Bentel GC, Zhou SM, Hollis D, et al. Radiation-induced pulmonary toxicity: a dose-volume histogram analysis in 201 patients with lung cancer. Int J Radiat Oncol Biol Phys. 2001;51:650–9.

103. Kong FM, Hayman JA, Griffith KA, Kalemkerian GP, Arenberg D, et al. Final toxicity results of a radiation-dose escalation study in patients with non-small-cell lung cancer (NSCLC): predictors for radiation pneumonitis and fibrosis. Int J Radiat Oncol Biol Phys. 2006;65:1075–86.

104. Mazeron R, Etienne-Mastroianni B, Perol D, Arpin D, Vincent M, et al. Predictive factors of late radiation fibrosis: a prospective study in non-small cell lung cancer. Int J Radiat Oncol Biol Phys. 2010;77:38–43.

105. Roeder F, Friedrich J, Timke C, Kappes J, Huber P, et al. Correlation of patient-related factors and dose-volume histogram parameters with the onset of radiation pneumonitis in patients with small cell lung cancer. Strahlenther Onkol. 2010;186:149–56.

106. Zhang J, Ma J, Zhou S, Hubbs JL, Wong TZ, et al. Radiation-induced reductions in regional lung perfusion: 0.1-12 year data from a prospective clinical study. Int J Radiat Oncol Biol Phys. 2010;76:425–32.

107. Woel RT, Munley MT, Hollis D, Fan M, Bentel G, et al. The time course of radiation therapy-induced reductions in regional perfusion: a prospective study with >5 years of follow-up. Int J Radiat Oncol Biol Phys. 2002;52:58–67.

108. Christian JA, Partridge M, Nioutsikou E, Cook G, McNair HA, et al. The incorporation of SPECT functional lung imaging into inverse radiotherapy planning for non-small cell lung cancer. Radiother Oncol. 2005;77:271–7.

109. Lavrenkov K, Singh S, Christian JA, Partridge M, Nioutsikou E, et al. Effective avoidance of a functional spect-perfused lung using intensity modulated radiotherapy (IMRT) for non-small cell lung cancer (NSCLC): an update of a planning study. Radiother Oncol. 2009;91:349–52.

110. McGuire SM, Zhou S, Marks LB, Dewhirst M, Yin FF, et al. A methodology for using SPECT to reduce intensity-modulated radiation therapy (IMRT) dose to functioning lung. Int J Radiat Oncol Biol Phys. 2006;66:1543–52.

111. Yin Y, Chen JH, Li BS, Liu TH, Lu J, et al. Protection of lung function by introducing single photon emission computed tomography lung perfusion image into radiotherapy plan of lung cancer. Chin Med J. 2009;122:509–13.

112. McGuire SM, Marks LB, Yin FF, Das SK. A methodology for selecting the beam arrangement to reduce the intensity-modulated radiation therapy (IMRT) dose to the SPECT-defined functioning lung. Phys Med Biol. 2010;55:403–16.

113. Munawar I, Yaremko BP, Craig J, Oliver M, Gaede S, et al. Intensity modulated radiotherapy of non-small-cell lung cancer incorporating SPECT ventilation imaging. Med Phys. 2010;37:1863–72.

114. Ohno Y, Koyama H, Takenaka D, Nogami M, Kotani Y, et al. Coregistered ventilation and perfusion SPECT using krypton-81m and Tc-99m-labeled macroaggregated albumin with multislice CT: utility for prediction of postoperative lung function in non-small cell lung cancer patients. Acad Radiol. 2007;14:830–8.

115. King GG, Harris B, Mahadev S. V/Q SPECT: utility for investigation of pulmonary physiology. Semin Nucl Med. 2010;40:467–73.

116. Jamadar DA, Kazerooni EA, Martinez FJ, Wahl RL. Semi-quantitative ventilation/perfusion scintigraphy and single-photon emission tomography for evaluation of lung volume reduction surgery candidates: description and prediction of clinical outcome. Eur J Nucl Med. 1999;26:734–42.

117. Inmai T, Sasaki Y, Shinkai T, Ohishi H, Nezu K, et al. Clinical evaluation of 99mTc-Technegas SPECT in thoracoscopic lung volume reduction surgery in patients with pulmonary emphysema. Ann Nucl Med. 2000;14:263–9.

118. Komori K, Kamagata S, Hirobe S, Toma M, Okumura K, et al. Radionuclide imaging study of long-term pulmonary function after lobectomy in children with congenital cystic lung disease. J Pediatr Surg. 2009;44:2096–100.

119. Xu J, Moonen M, Johansson A, Gustafsson A, Bake B. Quantitative analysis of inhomogeneity in ventilation SPET. Eur J Nucl Med. 2001;28:1795–800.

120. Pellegrino R, Biggi A, Papaleo A, Camuzzini G, Rodarte JR, et al. Regional expiratory flow limitation studied with Technegas in asthma. J Appl Physiol. 2001;91:2190–8.

121. Fujita J, Takahashi K, Satoh K, Okada H, Momoi A, et al. Tc-99m Technegas scintigraphy to evaluate the

lung ventilation in patients with oral corticosteroid-dependent bronchial asthma. Ann Nucl Med. 1999;13:247–51.

122. Suga K, Kuramitsu T, Yoshimizu T, Nakanishi T, Yamada N, et al. Scintigraphic analysis of hemodynamics in a patient with a single large pulmonary arteriovenous fistula. Clin Nucl Med. 1992;17:110–3.

123. Sasaki Y, Imai T, Shinkai T, Ohishi H, Otsuji H, et al. Estimation of regional lung function in interstitial pulmonary disease using 99mTc-technegas and 99mTc-macroaggregated albumin single-photon emission tomography. Eur J Nucl Med. 1998;25:1623–9.

124. Nagao M, Murase K. Measurement of heterogeneous distribution on Technegas SPECT images by three-dimensional fractal analysis. Ann Nucl Med. 2002;16:369–76.

125. Willowson K, Bailey DL, Baldock C. Quantitative SPECT reconstruction using CT-derived corrections. Phys Med Biol. 2008;53:3099–112.

126. Willowson K, Bailey DL, Bailey EA, Baldock C, Roach PJ. In vivo validation of quantitative SPECT in the heart. Clin Physiol Funct Imaging. 2010;30:214–9.

Hojjat Ahmadzadehfar and Martha Hoffmann

13.1 Introduction

Radioembolization (RE) with yttrium-90 (^{90}Y) microspheres, also named selective internal radiation therapy (SIRT), is a promising catheter-based liver-directed modality for patients with primary and metastatic liver cancer. RE provides several advantages over traditional treatment methods including its low toxicity profile [1, 2]. Its rationale arises from the anatomic and physiological aspects of hepatic tumours being exploited for the delivery of therapeutic agents. The prominent feature is the dual blood supply of liver tissue from the hepatic artery and the portal vein. Approximately 60–80% of hepatic blood is derived from the gastrointestinal (GI) tract via the portal vein and 20–40% from the systemic circulation via the hepatic artery [3]. Observations on vascular supply to hepatic malignancies have demonstrated that metastatic hepatic tumours measuring >3 mm derive 80–100% of their blood supply from the arterial rather than the portal hepatic circulation [3]. ^{90}Y is a pure β-emitter, produced by neutron bombardment of ^{89}Y in a reactor, with a limited tissue penetration (mean

2.5 mm, max 11 mm) and a short half-life of 64.2 h, making it an ideal transarterial liver-directed agent [4]. Two ^{90}Y microsphere products are commercially available: TheraSphere® (glass microspheres) and Sir-sphere® (resin microspheres). There are some distinct differences in properties between the two products discussed in detail elsewhere [4]. In the selection process of patients referred for RE, several aspects should be considered. Patients selected for RE should have (1) unresectable hepatic primary or metastatic cancer, (2) liver-dominant disease, (3) a life expectancy of at least 3 months and (4) an ECOG performance score of ≤2 as well as a preserved liver function [5]. Overall, the incidence of complications of RE of the liver malignancies for appropriately selected patients and accurately targeted delivery is very low [6]. Serious complications have been reported when microspheres were inadvertently deposited in excessive amounts in organs other than liver or when the liver received more radiation than its tolerance, which is called radioembolization-induced liver disease (REILD) [7]. Radiation and diminished blood supply due to embolisation by the spheres and subsequent hypoxia may result in ulceration and even perforation of the stomach and duodenum [7, 8]. ^{90}Y-induced ulceration of the stomach or duodenum can be resistant to medical therapy and surgery may be required [9]. Reported complications include gastrointestinal ulceration/bleeding, gastritis/duodenitis, cholecystitis, pan-

H. Ahmadzadehfar (✉)
Department of Nuclear Medicine, Klinikum Westfalen, Dortmund, Germany
e-mail: hojjat.ahmadzadehfar@ruhr-uni-bochum.de

M. Hoffmann
Department of Nuclear Medicine, Wiener Privatklinik, Vienna, Austria

creatitis, radiation pneumonitis and hepatic decompensation [2, 5, 7–13].

It is well known that the anatomy of the mesenteric system and the hepatic arterial bed has a high degree of variation, with "normal vascular anatomy" being present in 60% of cases [14].

To avoid the above-mentioned side effects, as well as for detection of the tumour blood supplying vessels, for any candidate selected for RE, an angiographic evaluation combined with ^{99m}Tc-macroaggregated albumin (^{99m}Tc-MAA) scanning precedes the therapy (test angiogram). ^{99m}Tc-MAA has been primarily used to identify lung shunts; however, with the development of single-photon emission tomography/computed tomography (SPECT/CT) imaging, ^{99m}Tc-MAA scintigraphy is now increasingly being used to detect GI shunts [15–19]. SPECT/CT imaging allows direct correlation of anatomic and functional information that provides a better localisation and definition of scintigraphic findings. In addition to anatomic referencing, attenuation correction capabilities of CT are the other benefit of CT co-registration [20]. In this chapter, we address the usefulness and significance of SPECT/CT imaging in the therapy planning of the RE of the liver metastases/tumours divided into the following two main sections:

- ^{99m}Tc-MAA SPECT/CT in the evaluation of extrahepatic abdominal shunting
- ^{99m}Tc-MAA SPECT/CT in the evaluation of intrahepatic tracer distribution

13.2 The Significance of ^{99m}Tc-MAA SPECT/CT Liver Perfusion Imaging in the Treatment Planning of RE

In the test angiogram session, according to the liver vascular anatomy and especially tumoural blood supplying vessels, 150–200 MBq of ^{99m}Tc-MAA should be injected preferably selectively in the right and/or left hepatic artery; however, in some cases regarding the tumoural site(s), it can be injected not selectively in the proper artery or super selectively in the segmental arteries. To avoid non-specific tracer uptake in the abdomen due to free ^{99m}Tc-pertechnetate, 600 mg of perchlorate should be administered orally about 30 min before ^{99m}Tc-MAA application [21]. This procedure should be followed by whole-body scintigraphy and SPECT/CT of the abdomen. The ^{99m}Tc-MAA syringe should be gently tilted before injection to agitate and resuspend the ^{99m}Tc-MAA particles [22].

13.3 Image Acquisition

First, a whole-body scan in anterior and posterior projections should be obtained to calculate the percentage of liver-to-lung shunting and, consequently, the possibility of pulmonary side effects. Determining possible lung damage due to liver-to-lung shunting is relatively simple, as described by Lau et al. [23]. Furthermore, a planar scintigraphic image of the upper abdomen (optionally) followed by SPECT/CT images should be obtained using a hybrid SPECT/CT camera. To date there are no definitive instructions for the ^{99m}Tc-MAA SPECT/CT acquisition and reconstruction and consequently each centre has its own protocol. For ^{99m}Tc-MAA acquisition, a low-energy high-resolution (LEHR) collimator should be used with the energy window set at 140 keV ± 10%. Planar images should be done in a 256 × 256 matrix with 5-min acquisition time. SPECT acquisition should be performed with a 128 × 128 matrix with 60–64 projections per detector (20–30 s/projection); however, there are some centres that perform the acquisition faster [24]. The CT scan should be normally done at a low dose (not diagnostic) with 5-mm slices. If required, there is the possibility of fusing SPECT images with diagnostic CT with contrast agent or magnetic resonance imaging (MRI) images with the help of low-dose CT of SPECT/CT images. SPECT data should be reconstructed with iterative methods following attenuation and scatter correction.

13.4 ^{99m}Tc-MAA SPECT/CT in the Evaluation of Extrahepatic Deposition of Tracer

Detecting hotspots in other organs besides the liver with planar images is not always possible and problems arise when these two-dimensional images are used for more precise evaluations. Extrahepatic spots indirectly mark the possible locations of microspheres misplaced during therapy; however, planar image analysis can be difficult and lead to misinterpretation of possible extrahepatic locations because of the low spatial resolution of planar scintigraphic images. Furthermore, especially in the upper abdomen, the localisation of several different organs within a relatively small region demands the analysis of tomographic images in order to accurately distinguish whether the ^{99m}Tc-MAA has accumulated in the liver or in some adjacent organ [15]. Planar images cannot always make this distinction due to organ superposition. In this setting, ^{99m}Tc-MAA SPECT/CT imaging has been shown to provide valuable additional information compared to planar and SPECT images and is the imaging modality of choice [15–18, 25]. Ahmadzadehfar et al. showed that the sensitivity, specificity, positive predictive value (PPV) and negative predictive value (NPV) of SPECT/CT in the diagnosis of abdominal extrahepatic shunting is 100%, 93%, 89% and 100%, respectively [15]. In this study, in light of the results of ^{99m}Tc-MAA SPECT/CT, the therapy planning changed in 29% of cases compared to 7.8% and 8.9% with planar imaging and SPECT, respectively [15]. In another study from Hamami et al., they reported similar results with the sensitivity and specificity of 100% and 94% for SPECT/CT, respectively, compared to 56% and 78% for SPECT, and 25% and 87% for planar imaging, respectively [17]. Thus, SPECT/CT significantly increases the sensitivity and NPV of ^{99m}Tc-MAA scans compared to planar and SPECT alone [15, 17].

The extrahepatic tracer accumulations in different abdominal regions have different relevancy and should be considered in the therapy planning as follows:

13.4.1 Tracer Accumulation in Gastroduodenal Region as Well as the Intestine

The incidence of GI ulcers following RE is usually between 2.9% and 4.8% [26]. Radiation-induced ulcers have proven to be extremely difficult to treat [26]. The two major causes thought to be responsible for gastroduodenal ulcers are (1) digestive shunting via an aberrant gastroduodenal vessel that is subjected to microsphere injection and (2) microsphere reflux occurring during the injection [16], which is especially the case when using resin microspheres.

Although a diffuse intestinal uptake can often be detected by planar scintigraphy, focal hotspots in the gastroduodenal region, especially in stomach and duodenum, are a very important issue and may frequently be overlooked with planar and SPECT imaging (Figs. 13.1, 13.2, and 13.3). A focally increased GI uptake detected with SPECT/CT has been reported as being between 3.6% and 31% [15–19]. This broad difference of detected GI uptake could be because of the different levels of experience of the interventional radiologist. In such cases, after reviewing the angiograms to find the aberrant vessel(s), the test angiogram should be repeated and RE can be performed only if no more extrahepatic tracer accumulation in the GI region is detectable. In such cases the aberrant vessels should be found and coil embolised. Alternatively, when an embolisation is not technically possible, a superselective or lobar therapy may be performed after an unremarkable repeated superselective or lobar test angiogram. Some centres do not use perchlorate to avoid free ^{99m}Tc uptake of the abdomen, which normally can be detected with SPECT/CT as low to moderately diffuse gastric uptake; however, it can hinder an accurate evaluation of the gastric region. In such cases, a visual distinction between gastric concentration of free ^{99m}Tc and true gastric ^{99m}Tc-MAA shunting could be difficult and concentration of free ^{99m}Tc may be mistaken for nontarget administration of the radionuclide, which considerably reduces the diagnostic confidence. On the other hand, gastric accumulation of

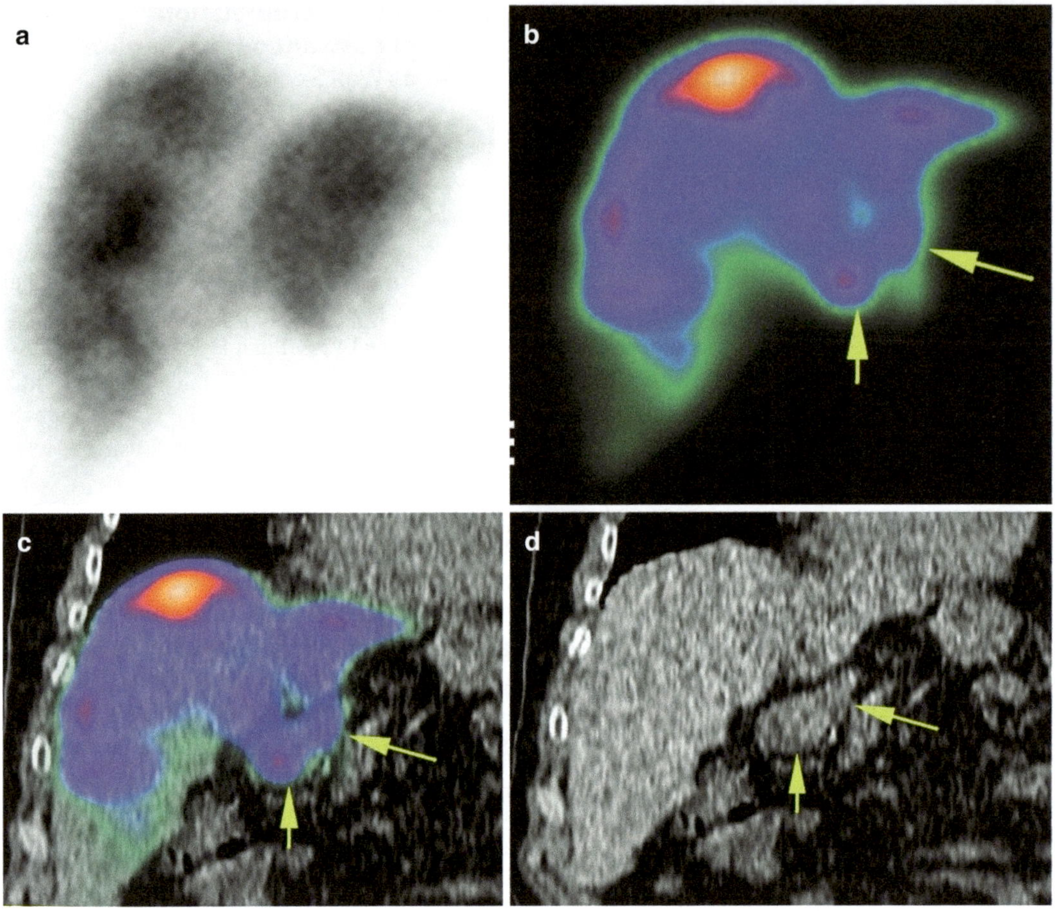

Fig. 13.1 Gastroduodenal accumulation of ^{99m}Tc-MAA (*yellow arrows*, **b–d**) in a patient with colorectal carcinoma, not definable on planar image (**a**)

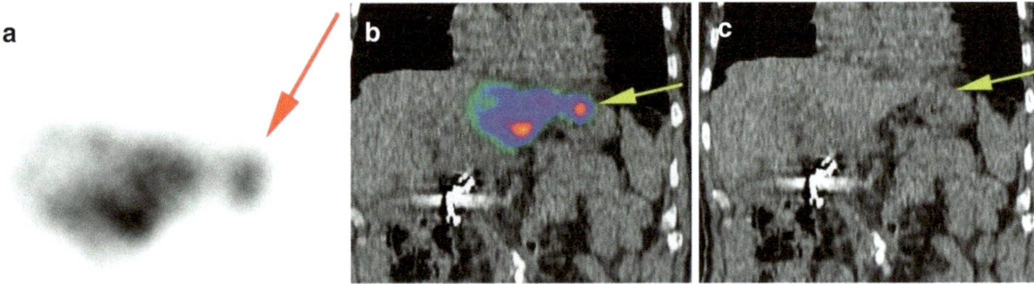

Fig. 13.2 Focally increased gastric uptake of ^{99m}Tc-MAA after injection into the left hepatic artery in a 67 years-old patient with colorectal carcinoma (*yellow*; **b** and **c**), not differentiable from a liver uptake on planar image (*red arrow*; **a**)

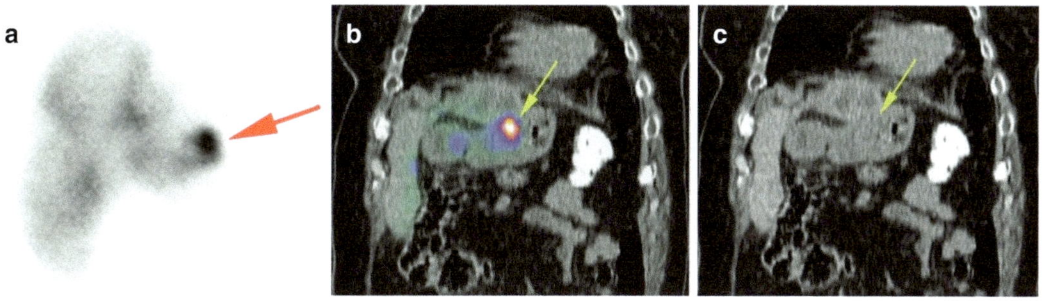

Fig. 13.3 Focally increased gastric uptake of ^{99m}Tc-MAA after injection into the right and left hepatic arteries in a 66 years-old patient with cholangiocellular carcinoma (*yellow*; **b** and **c**), not exactly differentiable from a liver uptake on planar image (*red arrow*; **a**)

^{99m}Tc-MAA can remain unrecognised in the presence of gastric-free ^{99m}Tc [21]. Therefore, we recommend using perchlorate prior to the test angiogram avoiding any misinterpretation of the gastric region.

13.4.2 ^{99m}Tc-MAA Accumulation in the Gallbladder

Radiation cholecystitis is usually subclinical but it is associated with post-procedure morbidity requiring surgical intervention in about 1% of patients [27]. The gallbladder can be evaluated more precisely with SPECT/CT compared to SPECT. In 8–12% of patients, a ^{99m}Tc-MAA accumulation in the gallbladder can be detected by SPECT/CT [15–17]. The approach in cases showing ^{99m}Tc-MAA accumulation in the gallbladder is controversial from no therapy plan changing and prophylactic antibiotic therapy to cholecystectomy prior to RE [15–17]. One strategy to prevent the spheres from reaching the gallbladder and the resulting radiation-induced cholecystitis may be the placement of the catheter distal to the cystic artery. However, this method is only reasonable if it does not result in an inadequate in target distribution of microspheres. The alternative approach could be the prophylactic embolisation of the proximal cystic artery with either absorbable gelatine sponge pledgets or fibred microcoils immediately before radioembolization, which has been shown to be safe and feasible [28]. The intensity of tracer uptake in the gallbladder could also be a helpful guide for making the decision, however, without established consensus [16].

13.4.3 ^{99m}Tc-MAA Accumulation in the Anterior Abdominal Wall (AAW)

Tc-MAA uptake in the anterior abdominal wall (AAW) has been described as a sign of patent hepatic falciform artery (HFA) [29] with a reported incidence of up to 13% [16, 30–33]. The HFA arises as a terminal branch of the middle or left hepatic artery. It runs within the hepatic falciform ligament with the umbilical vein, provides partial blood supply around the umbilicus and communicates with branches of the internal thoracic and superior epigastric arteries [34]. It is known that influx of chemoembolic agents into the HFA can cause supraumbilical skin rash, epigastric pain and skin necrosis. Normally, a patent HFA appears on planar ^{99m}Tc-MAA scans as an elongated tracer accumulation in the mid-abdomen, which could be anatomically better localised with SPECT. SPECT/CT can increase the detection rate of such uptake (Fig. 13.4) [16, 31] and can additionally detect the falciform ligament, especially after multiplanar reconstruction in the coronal view, which increases diagnostic accuracy [31]. Generally, ^{99m}Tc-MAA uptake via the HFA does not result in diagnostic problems except for patients with umbilical hernia [16]. As for all other extrahepatic arteries, we recommend the prophylactic embolisation of HFA in

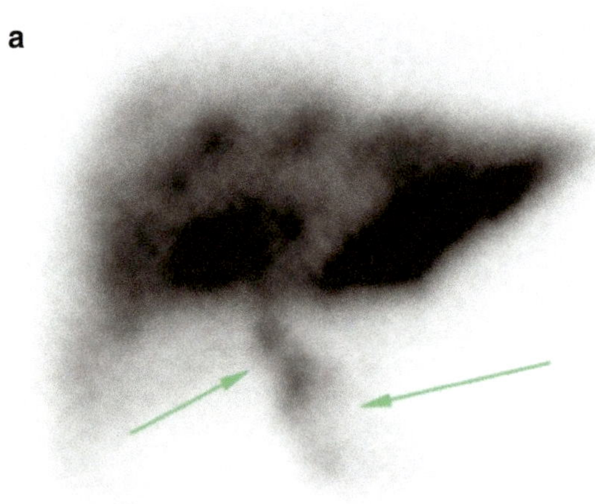
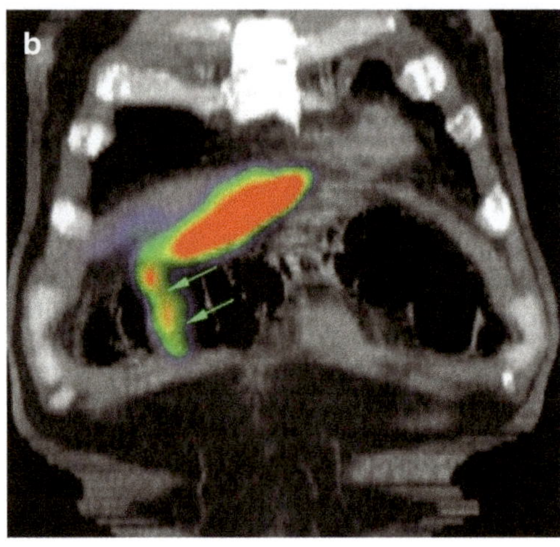

Fig. 13.4 (**a**) Planar scan showing ^{99m}Tc-MAA accumulation in the anterior abdominal wall (*yellow arrows*), indicating a patent hepatic falciform artery. (**b**) Coronal ^{99m}Tc-MAA SPECT/CT image in the same patient

the test angiogram as well as an angiographic reassessment in the patients with ^{99m}Tc-MAA accumulation in AAW prior to the application of ^{90}Y microspheres (Figs. 13.5 and 13.6). However, the post-selective internal radiotherapy side effects in patients with tracer accumulation in AAW on ^{99m}Tc-MAA scan are neither common nor severe [16, 31, 33]. Leong et al. reported one case of self-limiting radiation dermatitis caused by shunting of ^{90}Y microspheres to the AAW via a patent HFA [37]. In a recently published study, a HFA was identified in ^{99m}Tc-MAA SPECT/CT in 16 patients who did not undergo coil embolisation during treatment; only one patient complained of abdominal pain for 48 h, without presenting skin lesions [31]. Thus, there is no absolute need for prophylactic embolisation of the HFA or a treatment plan modification if the HFA is not detectable in an angiography session. Otherwise, being informed about such accumulations can avoid performing multiple and unnecessary endoscopies to detect GI ulcers in patients with unexpected abdominal pain [16] without any detectable gastroduodenal ^{90}Y uptake in post-therapeutic BS scan.

13.4.4 Other Types of Extrahepatic ^{99m}Tc-MAA Uptake

Recently, Lenoir et al. reported tracer uptake in the hepatic artery in 6.6% of patients [16], which had no impact on patient management.

This arterial uptake is likely due to the impaction or aggregation of MAA by arterial microlesions caused by long and complicated angiography procedures or when arteries are weakened by previous procedures [16]. Tracer accumulation in the coil embolisation site can be detected only by SPECT/CT and the detection rate has been reported to be less than 7% [15, 16]. Two reasons for this type of accumulation were described [15]. First, small aberrant vessels ending in this region, which should be found and coil embolised before RE or injection of microspheres, should be performed distal to the vessel; a second possible reason is an incompletely embolised vessel. Knowledge of the anatomic region of extrahepatic perfusion may help the radiologist to estimate the origin of the aberrant vessel. The incomplete coil embolised vessels should be embolised immediately before RE [15].

A light focally increased tracer uptake in the spleen has been reported by Ahmadzadehfar et al. in two cases (2.2%) [15], who also showed ^{90}Y microsphere uptake on BS SPECT/CT [38] without any complications. It seems such tracer accumulations are not harmful. Nevertheless, in such cases the patients should be informed about possible unknown side effects prior to RE. There are also some unusual sites of extrahepatic shunts that seldom occur, such as tracer uptake in the left side of the diaphragm [15, 22], distal of the oesophagus [22], in the paracaval lymph nodes

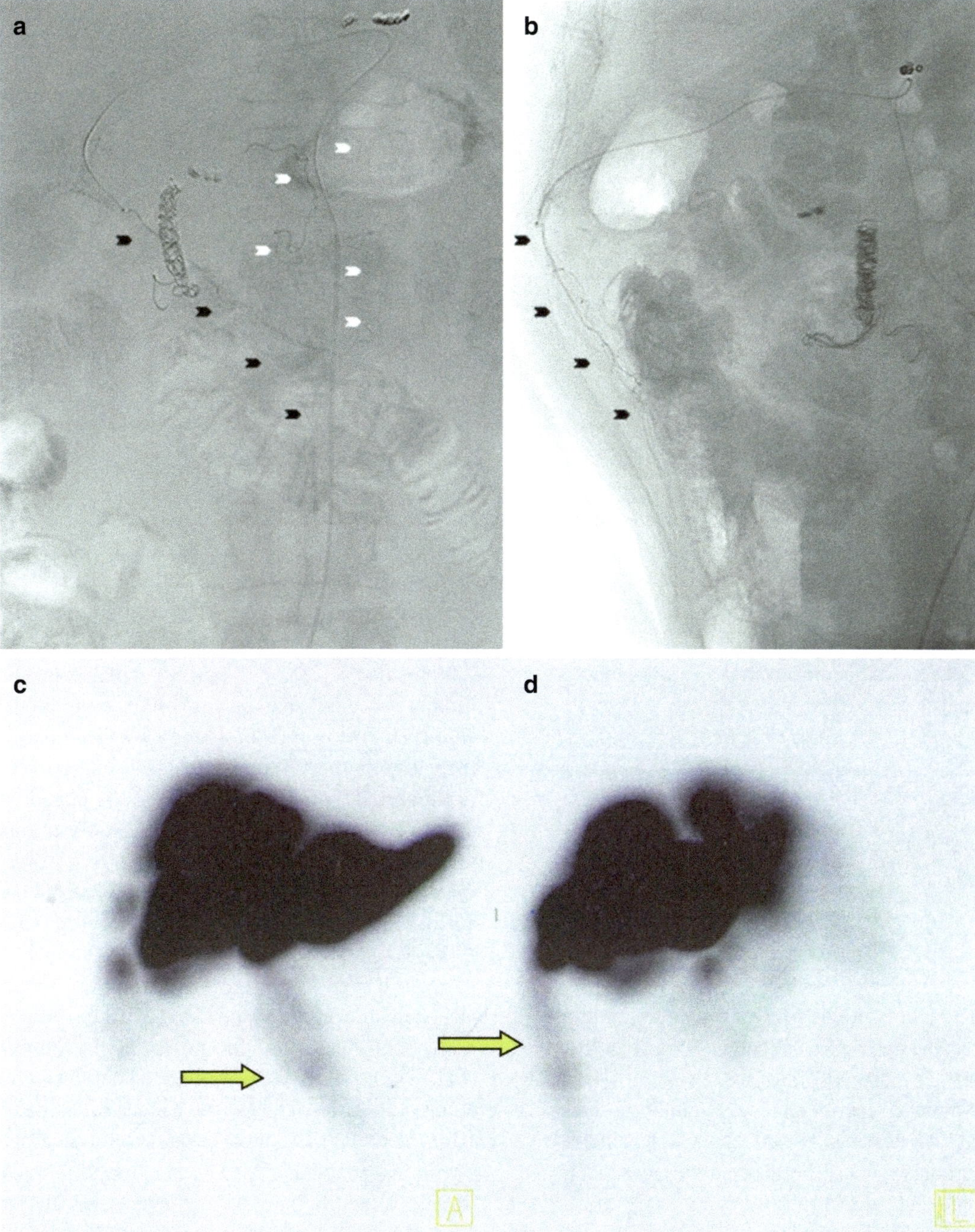

Fig. 13.5 Selective catheterisation of hepatic falciform artery (*black arrowheads*) in posterior-anterior (**a**) and lateral view (**b**) demonstrating the characteristic filling as it travels through the falciform ligament, terminates in the anterior abdominal wall, and anastomoses via collaterals (*white arrowheads*) with the superior epigastric vessels (**c**, **d**). Correspondent ^{99m}Tc-MAA SPECT scan maximum intensity projection coronal view (**c**) and sagittal view (**d**) show a tracer accumulation in anterior abdominal wall (*yellow arrow*). (With kind permission from Springer Science + Business Media, [35], Fig. 2)

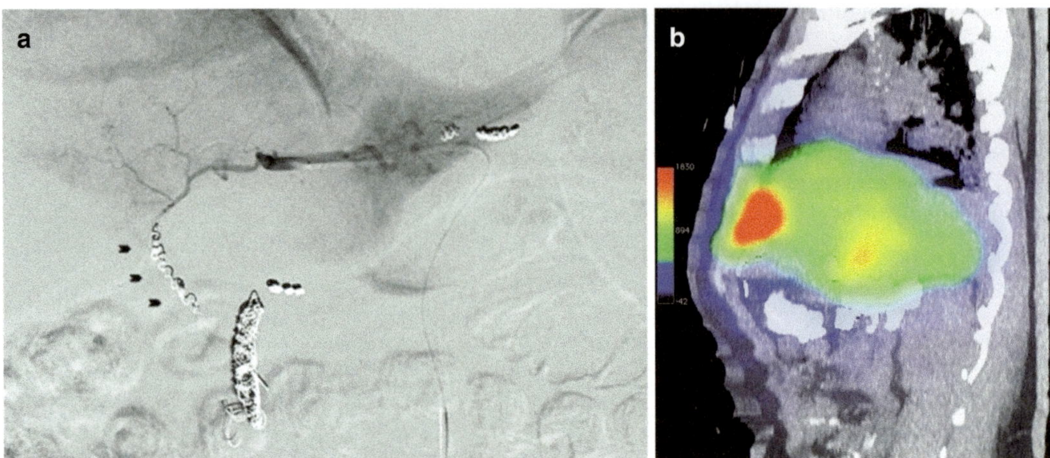

Fig. 13.6 (**a**) Injection in the left hepatic artery after selective embolisation of hepatic falciform artery (*black arrowheads*) of the same patient showed in Fig. 13.5. (**b**) Multiplanar reconstructed sagittal bremsstrahlung SPECT/CT 24 h after radioembolization showed no extra-hepatic tracer accumulation in anterior abdominal wall (With kind permission from Springer Science + Business Media: Ahmadzadehfar et al. [36], Fig. 3)

[22], in the pericardium or focally increased uptake in the pulmonary left lower lobe. In such cases, it is recommended to coil embolise the aberrant vessels.

13.5 ^{99m}Tc-MAA SPECT/CT in the Evaluation of Intrahepatic Tracer Distribution and Its Significance in Therapy Planning

The aim of RE is to treat the complete tumoural area and to avoid, as much as possible, the delivery of particles into the healthy liver tissue. Although intrahepatic accumulation of ^{99m}Tc-MAA—especially in cases of single liver tumours—could be acceptably assessed by planar scan and SPECT imaging, only SPECT/CT can provide a precise evaluation of tracer distribution in the patients with multiple liver tumours and metastases, e.g. ^{99m}Tc-MAA uptake in the tumour thrombus of the portal vein, which is more commonly seen with HCC [22], can be detected only by SPECT/CT. A portal tumour thrombus may be seen on SPECT/CT as a continuous area of activity extending from the tumoural lesion in the liver parenchyma into the portal system [22] and it suggests that the tumour

thrombus is supplied with blood through neovascularisation from the hepatic arteries, as is the tumour itself [22]. ^{99m}Tc-MAA uptake in the tumour thrombus may be a predictor of a favourable response to RE. In a study by Garin et al. [35], 92% of responding patients with portal vein thrombosis (PVT) showed ^{99m}Tc-MAA uptake in the PVT on SPECT/CT images and only in one non-responder with a large tumour was tracer uptake seen in the PVT [35]. Although a positive correlation between the amount of tumoural ^{99m}Tc-MAA uptake and treatment response and its significance in the pre-therapeutic dosimetry has been shown, this issue should still be studied with more patients in prospective settings (Fig. 13.7). Flamen et al. treated ten patients with colorectal cancer. They showed a cut-off value of 1 for the ^{99m}Tc-MAA uptake ratio could predict a significant metabolic response with a sensitivity of 89%, a specificity of 65%, a positive predictive value of 71% and a negative predictive value of 87% [39]. Garin et al. in a study of 36 patients with HCC using ^{90}Y-glass microspheres showed that quantitative ^{99m}Tc-MAA SPECT/CT is predictive of response, progression-free survival and overall survival. They suggested that using tumour dosimetry based on ^{99m}Tc-MAA SPECT/CT imaging could allow an adaption of the therapeutic planning and the activity to be administered [35, 40]. In a recently published paper by

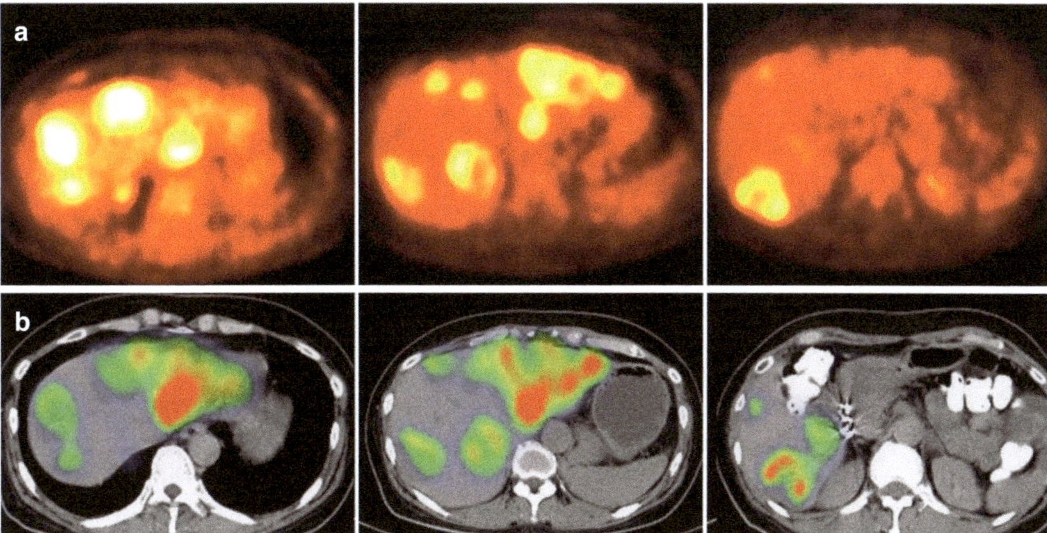

Fig. 13.7 (a) Liver ^{18}F-FDG PET of a patient with liver metastases of colorectal carcinoma shows high FDG accumulation in multiple metastases. (b) ^{99m}Tc-MAA SPECT/CT of the same patient shows high tumour accentuated tracer accumulation without any relevant uptake in the healthy liver tissue. The patient showed a near complete response after treatment with resin microspheres

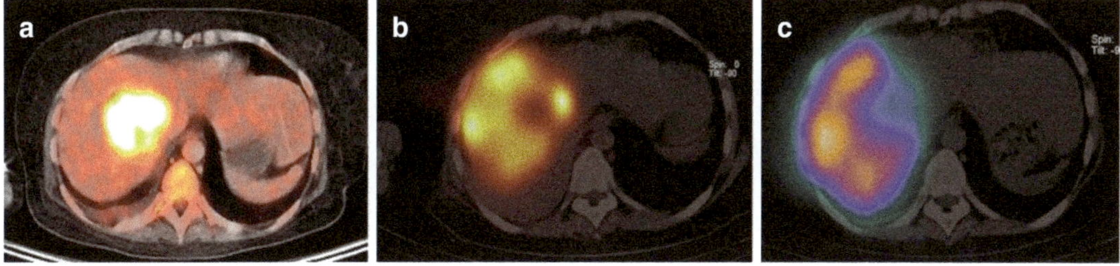

Fig. 13.8 (a) High FDG uptake in a single liver metastasis in a patient with sarcoma. (b) ^{99m}Tc-MAA SPECT/CT showed no tracer uptake in the metastasis. (c) Bremsstrahlung SPECT/CT after therapy with resin microspheres showed also no ^{90}Y microsphere uptake in the metastasis. A progression disease in follow-up confirmed these imagings

the same group, they reported that ^{99m}Tc-MAA SPECT/CT predicted response with a sensitivity of 100% and overall accuracy of 90% in 71 HCC patients [41]. In contrast, Van de Wiele et al. reported in a study of 13 patients with liver metastases from different origins that the percentage of ^{99m}Tc-MAA uptake by lesions was not significantly different between responding and non-responding lesions [24].

Nevertheless, an absence of ^{99m}Tc-MAA uptake in one part of a tumour or one or more liver segments with metastases, detected on SPECT/CT images, is an important issue (Fig. 13.8). A tumour may have an unidentified accessory arterial blood supply or may have parasitised nearby arteries [22]. The liver segments that do not show any ^{99m}Tc-MAA uptake because of accessory arterial blood supply or parasitised arteries normally cannot also be a target for ^{90}Y microspheres. A high and diffuse accumulation of ^{99m}Tc-MAA in the healthy liver tissue is also an important issue. A high radiation dose to the healthy liver tissue can increase the probability of developing a REAILD. The liver vascular mapping with ^{99m}Tc-MAA SPECT/CT imaging makes it possible to evaluate the tumoural and non-tumoural blood supplying vessels, which is of importance for avoiding unnecessary radiation exposure to the nontarget liver tissue and for achieving the tumoural area as much as possible. Sometimes it just needs a tracer application more distally; however, it is not always a straightforward issue and needs special interventional approaches for better targeting.

13.5.1 Detecting Blood Vessels Feeding the Tumour and Selective Administration into These Vessels

In the case of a discrepancy between the segmental distribution of ^{99m}Tc-MAA and the intended vascular territory to be treated, the angiograms should be carefully reviewed trying to find the reason for such discrepancies. It could be because of a tracer injection distal to a branching point that excludes part of the tumoural area [22], but sometimes the accessory arterial blood supplying vessels or parasitised arteries are the cause of such discrepancies [22]. In such cases, the test angiogram should be repeated and ^{99m}Tc-MAA should be injected selectively into the tumour-feeding arteries followed by SPECT/CT imaging for confirmation of exact targeting.

13.5.2 Flow Redistribution

Accessory or replaced hepatic arterial branches are a relatively frequent finding. The occlusion of accessory or aberrant arteries is supposed to result in flow redistribution from two (or multiple) arteries to a single artery. Thus, the infusion of ^{90}Y microspheres for one liver lobe can be accomplished via one artery (rather than by two or several arteries). In 89–95% of cases after occlusion of the accessory or aberrant arteries, a flow redistribution is detectable (angiographic or on ^{99m}Tc-MAA or on BS SPECT/CT) (Fig. 13.9) [27, 42, 43].

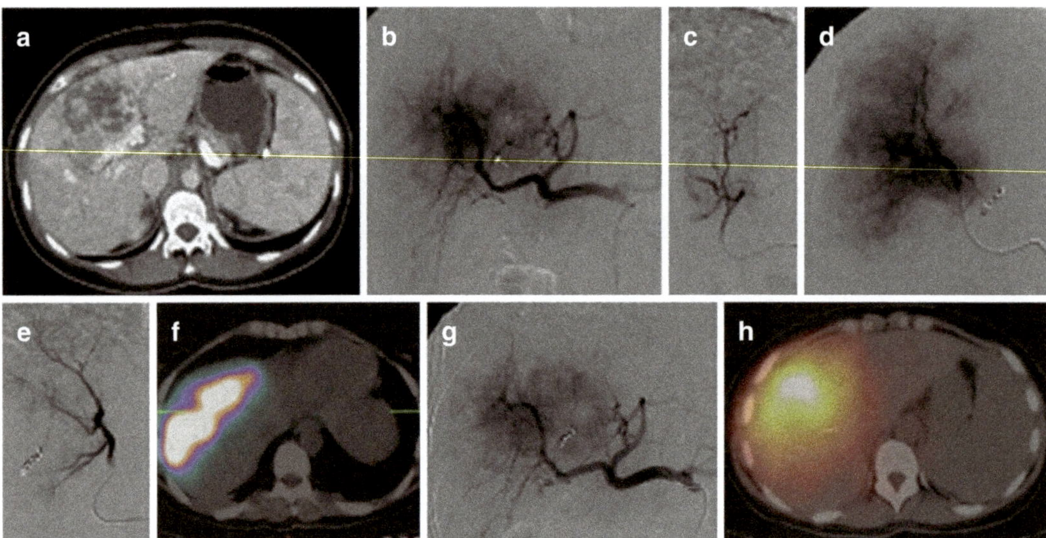

Fig. 13.9 Patient with cholangiocarcinoma. (**a**) CT demonstrates the presence of a mass situated between the right and left liver lobe. (**b**) Common hepatic angiography shows a hypervascular mass that receives vessels from the right and left hepatic arteries. With the aim of avoiding the delivery of the dose to the non-tumoural liver, the selected pedicles to perform the treatment were the artery of segment IV and the right hepatic artery, distal to the origin of the inferior branches. There is an artery (segment VIII) arising from the right hepatic artery that vascularises part of the tumour. (**c**) Selective angiography of the artery of segment VIII. (**d**) Right hepatic angiography after coiling of the segment VIII artery. (**e**) Segment IV angiography after coiling of the segment VIII artery. (**f**) SPECT/CT performed just after the infusion of ^{99m}Tc-MAA. There is homogeneous uptake of the tumour. (**g**) Angiography performed before the delivery of ^{90}Y microspheres. Except for the presence of coils, the angiography is similar to (**b**). Distal branches of the artery of segment VIII are seen. (**h**) Image obtained after radioembolization with ^{90}Y microspheres. There is a homogeneous uptake of all the tumoural volume. The *white dot* within the liver corresponds to the microcoils placed in the artery of segment VIII. (With kind permission from Springer Science + Business Media: Bilbao et al. [42])

13.5.3 Temporary Protective Embolisation of Normal Liver Tissue Using Degradable Starch Microspheres

As mentioned above, catheter position plays an important role in sphere distribution. If the microcatheter is positioned deep in a distal lobar artery, deposition may not be symmetric and homogenous. In general, occlusion of nontarget vessels therefore is an option to facilitate optimal catheter positioning and simple application of the microspheres. Degradable starch microspheres (DSM) are an embolisation material for temporary vascular occlusion and have primarily been used so far in combination with intra-arterial chemotherapy as an alternative to Lipiodol to achieve higher tumoural chemotherapy concentrations with statistically significant better tumour response rates compared to chemotherapy alone [44]. DSM can also be used to achieve blood flow redistribution by embolising normal liver tissue and redirecting blood flow to tumour-affected liver parenchyma. Favourable results of protective embolisation before TACE in cases where the tumour-feeding artery could not be accessed superselectively by microcatheter have been reported in one case series [45, 46]. Such an approach can also be done by using RE and is performed in the University Hospital Bonn [47].

13.6 Conclusion

SPECT/CT adds considerable value to the preprocedural planning of RE by identifying extrahepatic sites at risk for post-RE complications and also is a valuable tool for evaluation of intrahepatic distribution of ^{99m}Tc-MAA which resulted in a more targeted therapy with a better dosimetry.

References

1. Campbell AM, Bailey IH, Burton MA. Analysis of the distribution of intra-arterial microspheres in human liver following hepatic yttrium-90 microsphere therapy. Phys Med Biol. 2000;45:1023–33.

2. Salem R, Thurston KG. Radioembolization with 90Yttrium microspheres: a state-of-the-art brachytherapy treatment for primary and secondary liver malignancies. Part 1: technical and methodologic considerations. J Vasc Interv Radiol. 2006;17:1251–78.

3. Lien WM, Ackerman NB. The blood supply of experimental liver metastases. II. A microcirculatory study of the normal and tumor vessels of the liver with the use of perfused silicone rubber. Surgery. 1970;68:334–40.

4. Ahmadzadehfar H, Biersack HJ, Ezziddin S. Radioembolization of liver tumors with yttrium-90 microspheres. Semin Nucl Med. 2010;40:105–21. https://doi.org/10.1053/j.semnuclmed.2009.11.001. S0001-2998(09)00105-6 [pii].

5. Kennedy A, Nag S, Salem R, Murthy R, McEwan AJ, Nutting C, et al. Recommendations for radioembolization of hepatic malignancies using yttrium-90 microsphere brachytherapy: a consensus panel report from the radioembolization brachytherapy oncology consortium. Int J Radiat Oncol Biol Phys. 2007;68:13–23. https://doi.org/10.1016/j.ijrobp.2006.11.060. S0360-3016(07)00097-1 [pii].

6. Murthy R, Nunez R, Szklaruk J, Erwin W, Madoff DC, Gupta S, et al. Yttrium-90 microsphere therapy for hepatic malignancy: devices, indications, technical considerations, and potential complications. Radiographics. 2005;25(Suppl 1):S41–55. https://doi.org/10.1148/rg.25si055515. 25/suppl_1/S41 [pii].

7. Riaz A, Lewandowski RJ, Kulik LM, Mulcahy MF, Sato KT, Ryu RK, et al. Complications following radioembolization with yttrium-90 microspheres: a comprehensive literature review. J Vasc Interv Radiol. 2009;20:1121–30. https://doi.org/10.1016/j.jvir.2009.05.030, quiz 31.

8. Yip D, Allen R, Ashton C, Jain S. Radiation-induced ulceration of the stomach secondary to hepatic embolization with radioactive yttrium microspheres in the treatment of metastatic colon cancer. J Gastroenterol Hepatol. 2004;19:347–9. 3322 [pii].

9. Carretero C, Munoz-Navas M, Betes M, Angos R, Subtil JC, Fernandez-Urien I, et al. Gastroduodenal injury after radioembolization of hepatic tumors. Am J Gastroenterol. 2007;102:1216–20. https://doi.org/10.1111/j.1572-0241.2007.01172.x. AJG1172 [pii].

10. Leung TW, Lau WY, Ho SK, Ward SC, Chow JH, Chan MS, et al. Radiation pneumonitis after selective internal radiation treatment with intraarterial 90yttrium-microspheres for inoperable hepatic tumors. Int J Radiat Oncol Biol Phys. 1995;33:919–24. 0360301695000393 [pii].

11. Murthy R, Brown DB, Salem R, Meranze SG, Coldwell DM, Krishnan S, et al. Gastrointestinal complications associated with hepatic arterial yttrium-90 microsphere therapy. J Vasc Interv Radiol. 2007;18:553–62. https://doi.org/10.1016/j.jvir.2007.02.002.

12. Salem R, Parikh P, Atassi B, Lewandowski RJ, Ryu RK, Sato KT, et al. Incidence of radiation pneumonitis after hepatic intra-arterial radiotherapy with

yttrium-90 microspheres assuming uniform lung distribution. Am J Clin Oncol. 2008;31:431–8. https://doi.org/10.1097/COC.0b013e318168ef65.

13. Atassi B, Bangash AK, Lewandowski RJ, Ibrahim S, Kulik L, Mulcahy MF, et al. Biliary sequelae following radioembolization with Yttrium-90 microspheres. J Vasc Interv Radiol. 2008;19:691–7. https://doi.org/10.1016/j.jvir.2008.01.003. S1051-0443(08)00092-4 [pii].

14. Covey AM, Brody LA, Maluccio MA, Getrajdman GI, Brown KT. Variant hepatic arterial anatomy revisited: digital subtraction angiography performed in 600 patients. Radiology. 2002;224:542–7.

15. Ahmadzadehfar H, Sabet A, Biermann K, Muckle M, Brockmann H, Kuhl C, et al. The significance of 99mTc-MAA SPECT/CT liver perfusion imaging in treatment planning for 90Y-microsphere selective internal radiation treatment. J Nucl Med. 2010;51:1206–12. https://doi.org/10.2967/jnumed.109.074559.

16. Lenoir L, Edeline J, Rolland Y, Pracht M, Raoul JL, Ardisson V, et al. Usefulness and pitfalls of MAA SPECT/CT in identifying digestive extrahepatic uptake when planning liver radioembolization. Eur J Nucl Med Mol Imaging. 2012;39:872–80. https://doi.org/10.1007/s00259-011-2033-4.

17. Hamami ME, Poeppel TD, Muller S, Heusner T, Bockisch A, Hilgard P, et al. SPECT/CT with 99mTc-MAA in radioembolization with 90Y microspheres in patients with hepatocellular cancer. J Nucl Med. 2009;50:688–92. https://doi.org/10.2967/jnumed.108.058347. jnumed.108.058347 [pii].

18. Denecke T, Ruhl R, Hildebrandt B, Stelter L, Grieser C, Stiepani H, et al. Planning transarterial radioembolization of colorectal liver metastases with Yttrium 90 microspheres: evaluation of a sequential diagnostic approach using radiologic and nuclear medicine imaging techniques. Eur Radiol. 2008;18:892–902. https://doi.org/10.1007/s00330-007-0836-2.

19. Dudeck O, Wilhelmsen S, Ulrich G, Lowenthal D, Pech M, Amthauer H, et al. Effectiveness of repeat angiographic assessment in patients designated for radioembolization using yttrium-90 microspheres with initial extrahepatic accumulation of technitium-99m macroaggregated albumin: a single center's experience. Cardiovasc Intervent Radiol. 2012;35:1083–93. https://doi.org/10.1007/s00270-011-0252-5.

20. Buck AK, Nekolla S, Ziegler S, Beer A, Krause BJ, Herrmann K, et al. SPECT/CT. J Nucl Med. 2008;49:1305–19. https://doi.org/10.2967/jnumed.107.050195. jnumed.107.050195 [pii].

21. Sabet A, Ahmadzadehfar H, Muckle M, Haslerud T, Wilhelm K, Biersack HJ, et al. Significance of oral administration of sodium perchlorate in planning liver-directed radioembolization. J Nucl Med. 2011;52:1063–7.

22. Uliel L, Royal HD, Darcy MD, Zuckerman DA, Sharma A, Saad NE. From the angio suite to the gamma-camera: vascular mapping and 99mTc-MAA hepatic perfusion imaging before liver radioembolization – a comprehensive pictorial review. J Nucl Med. 2012;53:1736–47. https://doi.org/10.2967/jnumed.112.105361.

23. Lau WY, Ho S, Leung TW, Chan M, Ho R, Johnson PJ, et al. Selective internal radiation therapy for nonresectable hepatocellular carcinoma with intraarterial infusion of 90yttrium microspheres. Int J Radiat Oncol Biol Phys. 1998;40:583–92. S0360301697008183 [pii].

24. Van de Wiele C, Stellamans K, Brugman E, Mees G, De Spiegeleer B, D'Asseler Y, et al. Quantitative p retreatment VOI analysis of liver metastases. (99m)Tc-MAA SPECT/CT and FDG PET/CT in relation with treatment response to SIRT. Nuklearmedizin. 2013;52:21–7.

25. Kao YH, Tan EH, Teo TK, Ng CE, Goh SW. Imaging discordance between hepatic angiography versus Tc-99m-MAA SPECT/CT: a case series, technical discussion and clinical implications. Ann Nucl Med. 2011;25:669–76. https://doi.org/10.1007/s12149-011-0516-9.

26. Naymagon S, Warner RR, Patel K, Harpaz N, Machac J, Weintraub JL, et al. Gastroduodenal ulceration associated with radioembolization for the treatment of hepatic tumors: an institutional experience and review of the literature. Dig Dis Sci. 2010;55:2450–8.

27. Lauenstein TC, Heusner TA, Hamami M, Ertle J, Schlaak JF, Gerken G, et al. Radioembolization of hepatic tumors: flow redistribution after the occlusion of intrahepatic arteries. RöFo. 2011;183:1058–64. https://doi.org/10.1055/s-0031-1281767.

28. McWilliams JP, Kee ST, Loh CT, Lee EW, Liu DM. Prophylactic embolization of the cystic artery before radioembolization: feasibility, safety, and outcomes. Cardiovasc Intervent Radiol. 2011;34:786. https://doi.org/10.1007/s00270-010-0021-x.

29. Chernyak I, Bester L, Freund J, Richardson M. Anterior abdominal wall uptake in intrahepatic arterial brachytherapy with yttrium-90 sir spheres for hepatic malignancy. Clin Nucl Med. 2008;33:677–80. https://doi.org/10.1097/RLU.0b013e318184b44f. 00003072-200810000-00004 [pii].

30. Kao YH, Tan AE, Khoo LS, Lo RH, Chow PK, Goh AS. Hepatic falciform ligament Tc-99m-macroaggregated albumin activity on SPECT/CT prior to Yttrium-90 microsphere radioembolization: prophylactic measures to prevent non-target microsphere localization via patent hepatic falciform arteries. Ann Nucl Med. 2011;25:365. https://doi.org/10.1007/s12149-010-0464-9.

31. Ahmadzadehfar H, Mohlenbruch M, Sabet A, Meyer C, Muckle M, Haslerud T, et al. Is prophylactic embolization of the hepatic falciform artery needed before radioembolization in patients with 99mTc-MAA accumulation in the anterior abdominal wall? Eur J Nucl Med Mol Imaging. 2011;38:1477–84. https://doi.org/10.1007/s00259-011-1807-z.

32. Barentsz MW, Vente MA, Lam MG, Smits ML, Nijsen JF, Seinstra BA, et al. Technical solutions to ensure safe yttrium-90 radioembolization in patients with

initial extrahepatic deposition of (99m) technetium-albumin macroaggregates. Cardiovasc Intervent Radiol. 2011;34:1074–9. https://doi.org/10.1007/s00270-010-0088-4.

33. Burgmans MC, Too CW, Kao YH, Goh AS, Chow PK, Tan BS, et al. Computed tomography hepatic arteriography has a hepatic falciform artery detection rate that is much higher than that of digital subtraction angiography and 99mTc-MAA SPECT/CT: implications for planning 90Y radioembolization? Eur J Radiol. 2012;81:3979–84. https://doi.org/10.1016/j.ejrad.2012.08.007.

34. Baba Y, Miyazono N, Ueno K, Kanetsuki I, Nishi H, Inoue H, et al. Hepatic falciform artery. Angiographic findings in 25 patients. Acta Radiol. 2000;41:329–33.

35. Garin E, Lenoir L, Rolland Y, Edeline J, Mesbah H, Laffont S, Porée P, Clément B, Raoul JL, Boucher E. Dosimetry based on 99mTc-macroaggregated albumin SPECT/CT accurately predicts tumor response and survival in hepatocellular carcinoma patients treated with 90Y-loaded glass microspheres: preliminary results. J Nucl Med. 2012;53(2):255–63. https://doi.org/10.2967/jnumed.111.094235.

36. Ahmadzadehfar H, et al. Is prophylactic embolization of the hepatic falciform artery needed before radioembolization in patients with ^{99m}Tc-MAA accumulation in the anterior abdominal wall? Eur J Nucl Med Mol Imaging. 2011;38(8):1477–84.

37. Leong QM, Lai HK, Lo RG, Teo TK, Goh A, Chow PK. Radiation dermatitis following radioembolization for hepatocellular carcinoma: a case for prophylactic embolization of a patent falciform artery. J Vasc Interv Radiol. 2009;20:833. https://doi.org/10.1016/j.jvir.2009.03.011. S1051-0443(09)00220-6 [pii].

38. Ahmadzadehfar H, Muckle M, Sabet A, Wilhelm K, Kuhl C, Biermann K, et al. The significance of bremsstrahlung SPECT/CT after yttrium-90 radioembolization treatment in the prediction of extrahepatic side effects. Eur J Nucl Med Mol Imaging. 2012;39:309. https://doi.org/10.1007/s00259-011-1940-8.

39. Flamen P, Vanderlinden B, Delatte P, Ghanem G, Ameye L, Van Den Eynde M, et al. Multimodality imaging can predict the metabolic response of unresectable colorectal liver metastases to radioembolization therapy with Yttrium-90 labeled resin microspheres. Phys Med Biol. 2008;53:6591–603. https://doi.org/10.1088/0031-9155/53/22/019. S0031-9155(08)89144-0 [pii].

40. Garin E, Lenoir L, Rolland Y, Laffont S, Pracht M, Mesbah H, et al. Effectiveness of quantitative MAA SPECT/CT for the definition of vascularized hepatic volume and dosimetric approach: phantom validation and clinical preliminary results in patients with complex hepatic vascularization treated with yttrium-90-labeled microspheres. Nucl Med Commun. 2011;32:1245–55. https://doi.org/10.1097/MNM.0b013e32834a716b.

41. Garin E, Lenoir L, Edeline J, Laffont S, Mesbah H, Poree P, et al. Boosted selective internal radiation therapy with Y-loaded glass microspheres (B-SIRT) for hepatocellular carcinoma patients: a new personalized promising concept. Eur J Nucl Med Mol Imaging. 2013;40:1057. https://doi.org/10.1007/s00259-013-2395-x.

42. Bilbao JI, Garrastachu P, Herraiz MJ, Rodriguez M, Inarrairaegui M, Rodriguez J, et al. Safety and efficacy assessment of flow redistribution by occlusion of intrahepatic vessels prior to radioembolization in the treatment of liver tumors. Cardiovasc Intervent Radiol. 2010;33:523–31. https://doi.org/10.1007/s00270-009-9717-1.

43. Karunanithy N, Gordon F, Hodolic M, Al-Nahhas A, Wasan HS, Habib N, et al. Embolization of hepatic arterial branches to simplify hepatic blood flow before yttrium 90 radioembolization: a useful technique in the presence of challenging anatomy. Cardiovasc Intervent Radiol. 2011;34:287–94. https://doi.org/10.1007/s00270-010-9951-6.

44. Pohlen U, Rieger H, Mansmann U, Berger G, Buhr HJ. Hepatic arterial infusion (HAI). Comparison of 5-fluorouracil, folinic acid, interferon alpha-2b and degradable starch microspheres versus 5-fluorouracil and folinic acid in patients with non-resectable colorectal liver metastases. Anticancer Res. 2006;26:3957–64.

45. Murata T, Akagi K, Imamura M, Nasu R, Kimura H, Nagata K, et al. Studies on hyperthermia combined with arterial therapeutic blockade for treatment of tumors: (Part III) effectiveness of hyperthermia combined with arterial chemoembolization using degradable starch microspheres on advanced liver cancer. Oncol Rep. 1998;5:709–12.

46. Wang J, Murata S, Kumazaki T. Liver microcirculation after hepatic artery embolization with degradable starch microspheres in vivo. World J Gastroenterol. 2006;12:4214–8.

47. Ahmadzadehfar H, Pieper C, Ezziddin S, Wilhelm K, Schild HH, Meyer C. Feasibility of temporary protective embolization of normal liver tissue using degradable starch microspheres during radioembolization of liver metastases. In: 26th Annual Congress of the EANM, Lyon; 2013.

Bremsstrahlung SPECT/CT 14

Stephan Walrand and Michel Hesse

14.1 Introduction

The first bremsstrahlung imaging was performed early in 1966 by Simon et al. [1, 2] using a rectilinear scanner following a liver radioembolization via the hepatic artery with ^{90}Y loaded 15-μm-diameter microspheres. Although of very low quality, this imaging already provided the main information: the carcinoid tumours were well preferentially targeted (Fig. 14.1).

The first use of an Anger camera for bremsstrahlung imaging was reported by Kaplan et al. in 1985 [3] for [32]P. Since the nineties, bremsstrahlung imaging is widely performed in clinical routine for post-therapy check using beta emitter, such as ^{90}Y synovectomy or ^{90}Y liver radioembolization. While medical publications about bremsstrahlung imaging are sparse up to the first decade of the twenty-first century, they significantly increased during the last decade (Table 14.1). This is to be linked to the expanded amount of performed ^{90}Y liver radioembolizations and developments of (faster) Monte-Carlo (MC) numerical methods to improve bremsstrahlung SPECT reconstructions.

Recently, Lhommel, Walrand et al. showed that the low positron emission of ^{90}Y can be use-

fully imaged by PET after liver radioembolization [4, 5] and after ^{90}Y-DOTATOC therapy as well [6]. Although giving final images a little bit noisier than bremsstrahlung SPECT, pure commercial TOF-PET systems directly provide good spatial resolution and quantification accuracy in ^{90}Y imaging. On the contrary, to achieve similar quality, bremsstrahlung SPECT requires sophisticated reconstruction or acquisition software not yet commercially available [7–9]. Those features explained the increasing use of PET to image ^{90}Y in place of bremsstrahlung SPECT at the begin of last decade (Table 14.1).

However, PET modality is not always easily accessible and as ^{32}P and ^{89}Sr do not own any usable isotope emitting γ rays which could be imaged, bremsstrahlung SPECT remains of paramount importance, as shown by the renewed interest in the last years (Table 14.1).

14.2 Bremsstrahlung SPECT Issues

Accurately imaging ^{90}Y, ^{32}P or ^{89}Sr with a γ camera is one of the most challenging topics in nuclear medicine. The bremsstrahlung X-rays are spread along a continuous spectrum extending to energies up to the maximal beta energy emission, i.e. 2.3 MeV, 1.7 MeV and 1.5 MeV for ^{90}Y, ^{32}P and ^{89}Sr, respectively. The maximal energy usable by γ camera owning a mechanical collimator, such as Anger or CZT cameras, is limited to

S. Walrand (✉) · M. Hesse
Nuclear Medicine, Université Catholique de Louvain, Brussels, Belgium
e-mail: stephan.walrand@uclouvain.be;
michel.hesse@uclouvain.be

© The Author(s), under exclusive license to Springer Nature Switzerland AG 2022
H. Ahmadzadehfar et al. (eds.), *Clinical Applications of SPECT-CT*,
https://doi.org/10.1007/978-3-030-65850-2_14

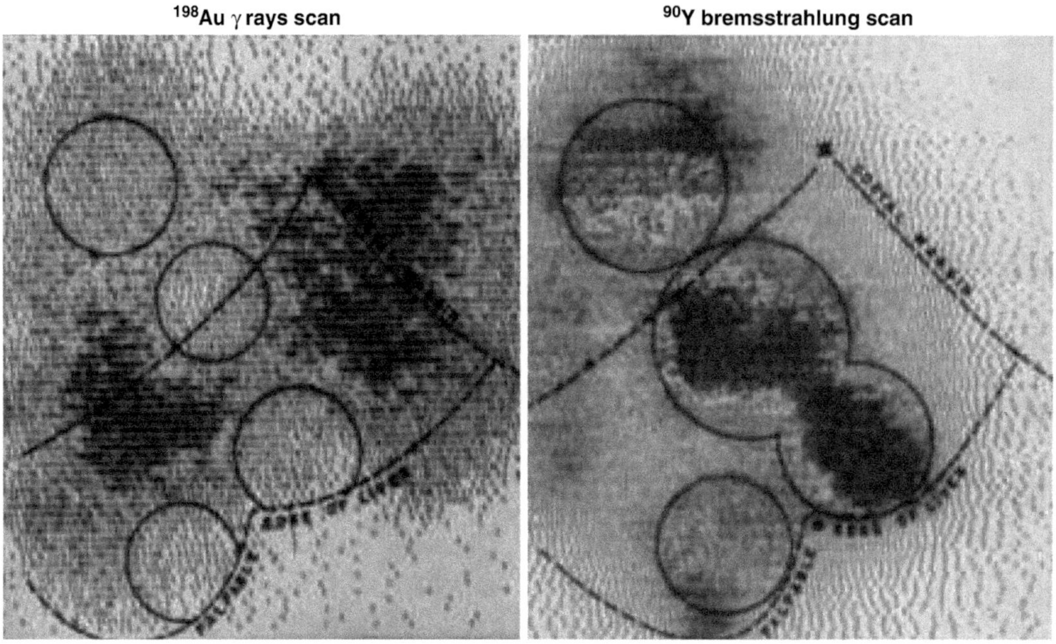

¹⁹⁸Au γ rays scan   ⁹⁰Y bremsstrahlung scan

Fig. 14.1 Tumours appear cold in the diagnostic scan using ¹⁹⁸Au-chloride (1 μm-diameter) injected intravenously and trapped in the reticuloendothelial cells of the liver. (Figure reprinted from [2] with permission of the Radiological Society of North America)

Table 14.1 Sorted articles counts obtained from https://pubmed.ncbi.nlm.nih.gov/ when searching the combination (bremsstrahlung AND (SPECT OR SPET OR PET OR planar OR imaging OR whole-body)) in title/abstract

Year	89Sr	32P		90Y		90Y
		Planar	SPECT	Planar	SPECT	PET
<2007	3	3	3	7		
2007				2	1	
2008					2	
2009				1	3	1
2010	1	1		1	2	3
2011	1			2	4	6
2012	3		2	3	4	7
2012	4		2	3	7	2
2013	3		1	1	11	9
2014	1		1	1	7	7
2015				1	6	3
2016					10	9
2017	1		1	2	3	3
2018			2		11	5
2019				2	6	
2020					8	4

about 0.5 MeV. As a result, all acquisitions using such cameras are inevitably corrupted by high-energy X-rays scattering down into the acquisition energy window.

This high-energy X-rays down scattering contamination includes five different effects (Fig. 14.2): (1) the scattering inside the patient body, (2) the scattering through a collimator septa (usually called penetration), (3) the scattering from a collimator septa, (4) the lead fluorescence K_α and K_β emissions, (5) the back-scattering from the PMT, electronic boards and lead housing of the camera.

Although less frequent, some X-ray paths can include several of the sub-cited effects. Lastly, the β range in the patient also slightly alters the final spatial resolution.

Monte-Carlo simulations allow assessing the individual contributions to the total X-rays producing a photoelectric effect in the camera crystal [10] (Fig. 14.3). Note that contrary to conventional γ emitters, the primary photons rep-resent only a small part of the total detected counts. The most favourable ratio is obtained around 100 keV explaining why the 50 → 150 keV energy window is often chosen [10, 11]. A medium energy general purpose (MEGP) parallel hole collimator is a good choice to reduce the collimator penetration. However, even with this energy window and collimator choice, spatial resolution and quantification accuracy of brems-strahlung SPECT remain low. Different approaches are proposed to improve this situation: physical effects modelling and adapted collimator design.

14.3 Intra-Patient Scatter and Collimator-Detector Response Modelling

With the increasing speed of the computer stations, most tomographic reconstructions in nuclear medicine are nowadays performed using the iterative algorithm OSEM, an accelerated version of the EM-ML. Compared to analytical reconstruction, such as FBP, these iterative algorithms have the benefit to correctly account for the Poisson nature of the statistical noise present in radioactive counts measurement and to avoid apparition of negative voxel artefacts. In addition, iterative algorithms can reconstruct any tomographic acquisition setups, i.e. all physical effects introduced in the projection step of the

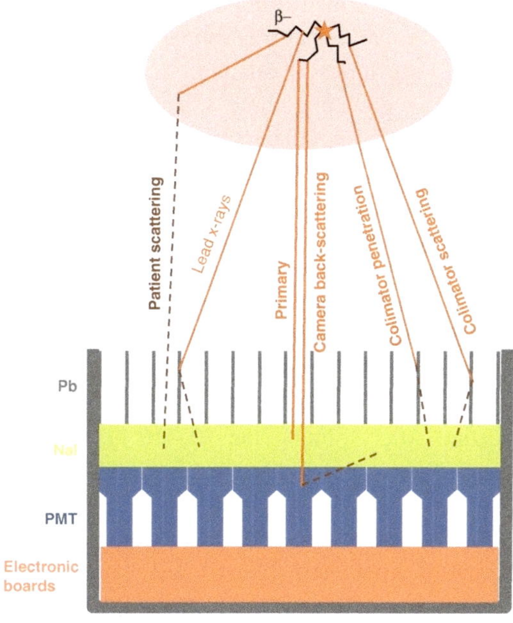

Fig. 14.2 The different X-rays paths producing a photoelectric effect in the camera crystal

Fig. 14.3 ^{90}Y X-ray energy spectra according to photon origin for a point source 5 cm deep in water cube, MEGP collimation, 3/8 in. thick NaI, computed by Monte-Carlo simulation. Courtesy of Dr. S Heard. The primary to total counts curve (dashed black curve) was added by the author of the present chapter

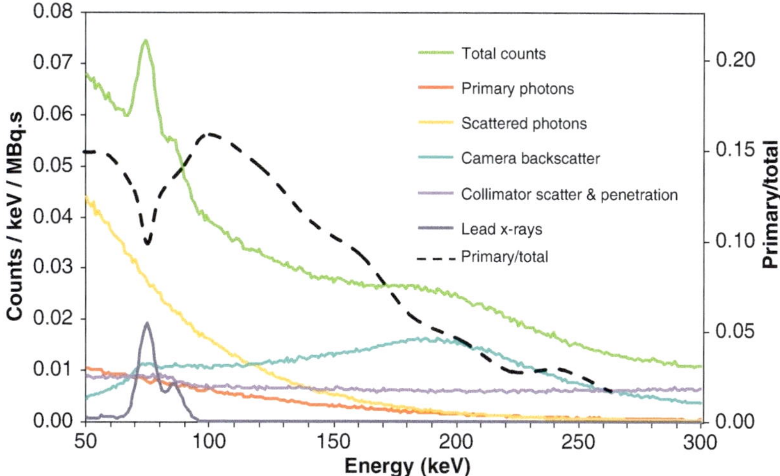

iterative loop will be corrected during the reconstruction process. The state of the art in bremsstrahlung SPECT is thus to model the different X-ray paths during this projection step. However, for the time being an exact modelling of these effects lead to reconstruction time incompatible with the daily SPECT routine.

Minarik et al. [12] built a pre-calculated collimator-detector response (CDR) table by Monte-Carlo simulation and modelled the scatter into the object using the effective source scatter estimation (ESSE) method [13]. The modelling was performed for a 105–195 keV acquisition window in order to avoid the lead fluorescence X-rays contamination. This model was incorporated into the OSEM reconstruction algorithm. Evaluation in an abdominal phantom showed a quantification accuracy of 8.5% for the liver activity. Accuracy in lesions activity measurement was not assessed.

This group applied their correction method in three patients receiving high-dose ^{90}Y radioimmunotherapy [14]. The patients were imaged at 1, 24, 48, 72, 144, 166 h by SPECT/CT after a pre-therapeutic injection of 300 MBq of ^{111}In-ibritumomab. Patients received a ^{90}Y-ibritumomab activity computed to deliver 12 Gy to the liver based on the pharmacokinetics measured with the ^{111}In SPECT/CT and were imaged at the same time points post injection by bremsstrahlung SPECT/CT. The absolute relative differences between organ absorbed dose computed from ^{111}In and ^{90}Y SPECT/CT were 8.8 ± 13.7, 8.9 ± 4.0 and 51.7 ± 18.9 (mean ± std in %), for the liver, kidneys and lungs, respectively. This showed that this bremsstrahlung SPECT/CT correction method can be used for the body region below the lungs: for the time being, the ESSE method does not account for tissues density variation, such as present in the slices crossing the lungs.

Elschot et al. [15] developed a quantitative Monte-Carlo based SPECT reconstruction for ^{90}Y applications. They implemented a Monte-Carlo simulator to model the photon attenuation and scatter for the full ^{90}Y spectrum in the projection step, while pre-calculated convolution kernels were used for the collimator-detector

response. Using a 50–250 keV energy window, they obtained quantification improvements compared to standard clinical SPECT-CT reconstructions for NEMA image quality phantom, and results close to PET-CT for a small set of patients after radioembolization with ^{90}Y resin spheres.

In order to improve the count rate for applications where the activity is modest, such as ^{90}Y radioimmunotherapy, Rong et al. [16] computed by Monte-Carlo the CDR and ESSE for the wide 100–500 keV acquisition window. The computation was performed using separate treatment of photons in various energy ranges and in various logical categories. Evaluation in an elliptical phantom containing three spheres of 5.5 cm, 3.3 cm and 1.5 cm-diameter, with specific activity ten-, ten- and 20-fold that of the surrounding background, showed a quantification accuracy of 7%, 9.7% and 10.2%, respectively.

To better take into account the energy dependence of photon–matter interaction probabilities and to simplify scatter corrections, Siman et al. [17] adapted the standard multi energy window approach to correct ^{90}Y SPECT-CT images for scatter. After splitting the 70–410 keV energy range into six windows whose widths were selected to enable a single attenuation coefficient use per window, they determined from phantoms the 90–125 keV and 310–410 keV ranges to be the best windows for imaging and scatter respectively. The scaling factor to multiply the scatter image was estimated from planar acquisitions of patients. This approach, while improving image quality and quantification, is strongly dependent on the camera and collimator used, and approximate as the scatter factor was averaged over different patients.

Dewaraja et al. [18] made use of Monte-Carlo only to estimate the scatter of photons, that they combined with a 3D OSEM reconstruction with an analytic projector for ^{90}Y SPECT-CT. Using a single energy window of 105–195 keV and a high-energy collimator, they showed that two iterations for the scatter estimation were enough, allowing a reduction of the reconstruction time to about 40 min. They so better recovered the activity in a liver/lung phantom, with values of 86%, 104% and 104% for the recovery in the intrahepatic lesions, normal liver and lungs respectively. They similarly observed an increase of the lesion to liver concentration with their MC reconstruction for patient studies compared to standard SPECT-CT reconstructions.

More recently Chun et al. [19] proposed an interesting approach of joint spectral reconstruction for quantitative ^{90}Y SPECT imaging. They used multiple narrow acquisitions windows with multi-band forward modelling. The latter has the advantage to permit a better modelling of energy dependent physics like using more adequate attenuation coefficients in place of only one corresponding to the mid-range energy. The former allowed the authors to extract and combine activity data from the different energy window acquisitions to improve the reconstructed image. They also presented an accelerated algorithm using energy subsets similarly to the angular subsets in OSEM. MC simulations were used at every five iterations to estimate the scatter components without impacting too much the reconstruction time. With this new algorithm they reached faster convergence of the recovery coefficients in phantom studies than with single spectral/single energy window and multi spectral/single energy window reconstructions. The proposed method has also the advantage to implement matched forward and backward projectors, inducing better convergence stability, unlike most of developed reconstruction algorithms where MC scatter and collimator modelling is only incorporated in the forward projector.

Another physical characteristic seldom considered is the dependence of the bremsstrahlung generation with respect to the tissue types. Lim et al. [20] modelled by Monte-Carlo the bremsstrahlung generation probabilities according to the tissue. With their adapted reconstruction algorithm, they showed on phantom acquisition and simulations improved estimations of ^{90}Y activities in tissues differing from water. Unfortunately that study did not include absolute quantification, nor patient imaging.

Very recently, Xiang et al. [21] made use of latest developments in artificial intelligence to train a deep convolutional neural network from ^{90}Y SPECT projections and CT attenuation maps

to produce scatter projections. The training set was made of simulated numerical phantom data for which actual scatter component is known. With that approach they obtained image quality and contrast recovery similar to MC scatter estimation but in much less time. This still requires developments in training data and quantitative validations, but could pave the way to better bremsstrahlung SPECT-CT reconstructed images in clinical routine.

However, in medical imaging it is always profitable to improve the hardware performance in order to acquire the right events, rather than to correct for the contaminating events afterwards. Indeed, this last solution inevitably results in a higher noise level regarding the statistical nature of primary and contaminating photon. Amazingly, other choices of collimators than MEGP have been considered only very recently.

14.4 Choice of Collimators Better Adapted to Bremsstrahlung Imaging

Van Holen et al. [8] proposed the use of a rotating slat collimator that owns a much higher geometric efficiency than a parallel hole collimator. As a result the relative importance of septal penetration is reduced, resulting in better contrast to noise ratio. Note, that regarding only the primary X-rays, the high geometric efficiency improvement of the rotating slat collimator is counterbalanced by less information provided about the X-ray coming direction. Data publication in a full paper is still pending.

Walrand et al. [9] used a conventional thyroid dedicated medium energy pinhole (MEPH) collimator in bremsstrahlung SPECT in purpose of ^{90}Y liver radioembolization check. Scattering inside the phantom was modelled using an adaptation of an effective scatter model previously developed for ^{99m}Tc [22], similar and anterior to ESSE [13]. Compared to parallel hole collimators, the high-energy X-rays can hit lead material mostly only on the external side of the pinhole collimator housing (Fig. 14.4a). As a result, the lead fluorescence and scattering X-rays cannot

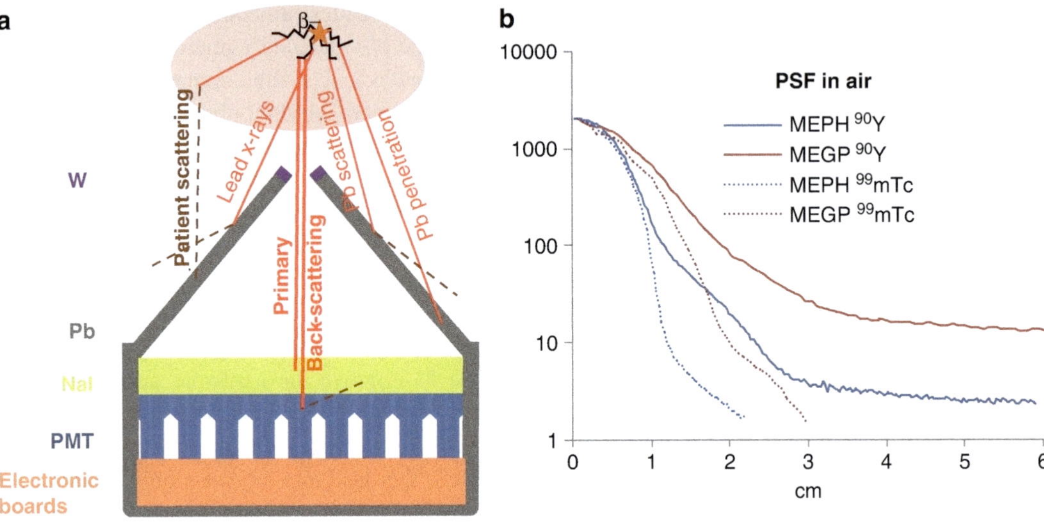

Fig. 14.4 (**a**) reduction of the disturbing X-rays paths contributing to the total crystal photoelectric counts. (**b**) point spread function (PSF) comparison of a ^{90}Y and ^{99m}Tc point source in air with a MEPH and MEGP collimator using a 1/2 in. thick NaI GE 400 AC camera with a 50–150 keV acquisition window. ^{99m}Tc PSF approximates the PSF of the primary photons in the ^{90}Y acquisition

reach the crystal as the collimator housing thickness (2 cm) is sufficient to significantly reduce penetration. Disturbing penetration-scattering can only occur on the small tungsten insert, the fluorescence X-ray emissions of which are located below 10 keV [23]. These features improve the primary to total count ratio (Fig. 14.3). The comparison between ^{90}Y and ^{99m}Tc radial profile in air (Fig. 14.4b) shows that using a 50–150 keV acquisition window the primary photons represent 68% and 31% of the total detected photons for MEPH and MEGP collimators, respectively.

Evaluation in cold and hot spheres phantom [9] showed that MEPH SPECT provided quantification accuracy similar to that of TOF-PET, but with significantly less noise. Helical MEPH SPECTs of a realistic liver radioembolization phantom were also acquired and showed that reproducible accurate activity quantification can be obtained in 1 min acquisition time (relative deviation of healthy liver compartment: $10 \pm 0.1\%$).

Gupta et al. [24] showed the feasibility of real-time visualization of iron-labelled microspheres delivery during liver SIRT in rabbits using MRI. In this paper, cosigned by R. Salem, the authors concluded: "Although quantitative in vivo estimation of microsphere biodistribution may prove technically challenging, the clinical effect could be enormous, thus permitting dose optimization to maximize tumour kill while limiting toxic effects on normal liver tissues." However, human liver SIRT appears quite incompatible with MR: the X-ray angiographic imager will difficultly be implemented around the MR table, and the long duration of liver SIRT, that can overpass 2 h for challenging arterial trees, is not supportable by most of MRI agenda.

14.5 Current Bremsstrahlung SPECT-CT Routine Applications

For the time being, dedicated bremsstrahlung acquisition hardware or reconstruction software are not commercially available, and most bremsstrahlung routine SPECT-CT are performed without any special correction. This is not a major problem as far as they are intended to post-therapy visual check. However, users have to be very cautious when performing quantitative measurement on standard acquisition-reconstruction of bremsstrahlung X-rays.

^{90}Y radio-synovectomy has been the main application of bremsstrahlung routine imaging since 30 years. However, regarding to the small size of the synovial compartment, the higher spatial resolution of PET system is a major benefit to perform an optimal check of this therapy [25]. In addition, as the activity is located into a small volume, noise issues are very limited.

Liver radioembolization with ^{90}Y loaded microspheres by catheterization through the hepatic artery is an emerging treatment for primary and metastatic liver cancer. However selective radioembolization fully confined in the targeted hepatic artery branch is a challenging operation. Microspheres can be spread in the arterial tree along a different pattern than those of the macro-aggregates or of the contrast agent (see "choice of a surrogate" in chapter "SPECT for dosimetry") leading to adverse effects [26].

Until the possibility of tracking the microspheres delivery during the catheterization, it is thus of paramount importance to check the microsphere distribution post therapy in order to take the appropriate cares to reduce the side effects in case of activity delivered in critical tissues. Ahmadzadehfar et al. [27] evaluated the significance of bremsstrahlung SPECT/CT in the prediction of extrahepatic side effects after 188 radioembolizations with ^{90}Y-microspheres. They observed a dramatic improvement of the sensitivity and of the positive predictive value of SPECT/CT (87% and 100%) compared to SPECT alone (13% and 8%), leading to a final accuracy of 99%. The two cases shown in Fig. 14.5 clearly illustrate the benefit of this co-acquisition.

Peptides receptor targeted therapies are usually performed in several cycles in order to limit kidneys toxicity [28]. Fabbri et al. [29, 30] evaluated on anatomical phantom the feasibility to perform organs dosimetry after each ^{90}Y-DOTATOC cycle in order to optimize the

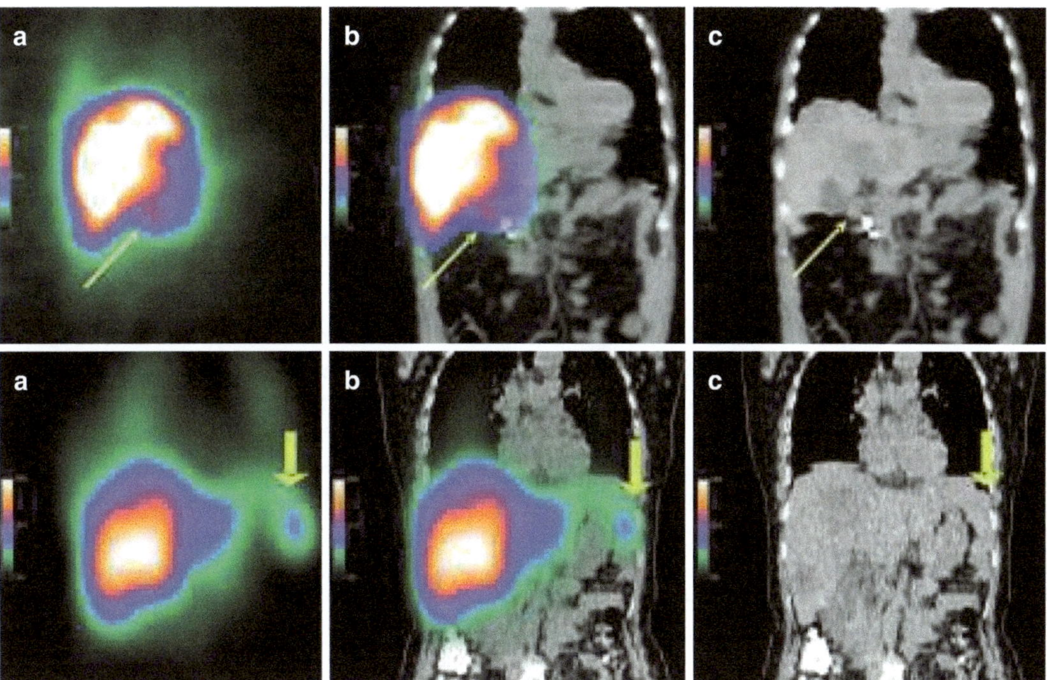

Fig. 14.5 ^{90}Y bremmstrahlung SPECT (**a**)/CT (**c**) co-registration (**b**). Top row: Patient with a focal activity in the duodenum as shown by the SPECT-CT co-registration (thin yellow arrow). Patient received a daily pump inhibitor, but got a duodenal ulcer without active bleeding confirmed by gastroduodenoscopy. Bottom row: Patient with a suspicious focal activity in SPECT (thick yellow arrow), but proved to be hypertrophied left liver lobe in the SPECT-CT co-registration. (Reprinted from [27] with permission of Springer-Verlag)

activity to be injected in the next one. They showed on a phantom that, using the standard reconstruction software of the SPECT/CT system, but with calibration factors depending on the lesion or organ volume measured on the CT, it was possible to access the dosimetry within an accuracy of 10%. Calibration factors ranged from 0.4 to 1.3 for the tissue ranging from 8 to 150 mL. However this method does not correct for the cross scattering organ contamination which can be problematic for the activity quantification in kidneys with close bowel or tumour surrounding activities. Studies on phantom of various sizes and of various activity distributions are thus suitable to further assess its accuracy.

Following a clinical study with ^{90}Y Zevalin to treat lymphomas, Shiba et al. [31] analysed the impact on ^{90}Y bremsstrahlung SPECT images of the presence of residual ^{111}In from pre-therapeutic evaluation. Their results indicated that ^{111}In is still prevalent in the post-therapeutic image 1 week after its injection. Combined with the limited image quality of ^{90}Y bremsstrahlung SPECT, the authors recommend the use of PET/CT imaging for that kind of application.

14.6 Dose–Response Studies Based on Bremsstrahlung SPECT

With the speed-up development in the last decade of computer tools that improve the image quality of bremsstrahlung SPECT/CT, several groups started performing dosimetric studies based on bremsstrahlung and were able to extract dose–response relationships.

Kappadath et al. [32] performed voxel dosimetry based on bremsstrahlung SPECT/CT on patients treated for hepatocellular carcinoma by ^{90}Y-radioembolization with glass microspheres. From SPECT/CT iterative reconstructions including attenuation, scatter and collimator modelling, they obtained a correlation between dose metrics and mRECIST response, with a mean dose of 160 Gy and a mean biological effective dose of 214 Gy for 50% probability of response, giving positive predictive value of 70% and negative predictive value of 62%.

Piasecki et al. [33] studied the dose–response for colorectal liver metastases after ^{90}Y radioembolization. They obtained relationships between predicted tumour doses from ^{99m}Tc-MAA SPECT/CT and responses, but not when looking at the actual ^{90}Y tumour absorbed doses evaluated from ^{90}Y bremsstrahlung SPECT/CT. This may be in part due to the use of standard iterative reconstruction that does not include dedicated scatter or collimator modelling. Using standard manufacturer reconstruction without specific corrections. Schobert et al. [34] were able to obtain dose–response relationship in HCC after ^{90}Y radioembolization, but not for non-HCC lesions, by performing bremsstrahlung SPECT/CT with low energy high resolution collimators and standard iterative reconstruction.

These studies should be looked at as early and promising examples of feasibility of dosimetric analyses, but many developments and validations are still needed before accurate dosimetry can be obtained from bremsstrahlung SPECT/CT imaging.

14.7 Perspectives: New Detectors Better Adapted to Bremsstrahlung Imaging

Cadmium zinc tellurium (CZT) detectors, although still expensive, are emerging in dedicated cardiac SPECT systems [35] where their compactness and absence of dead edge area allows to build area of independent detectors all focussing to the heart. With the future decrease in manufacturing cost, CZT will become more and more used for general purpose γ cameras in order to profit of its better energy resolution [36]. Indeed, for γ emitters, a better energy resolution allows to narrow the acquisition window around the photoelectric peak which reduces the detection of γ rays scattered inside the patient body and results in a better image contrast. These CZT cameras should also be better adapted to bremsstrahlung imaging as the quantity of medium Z material (glass, iron, copper), present between the γ detection area and the detector housing, and which backscatter the high-energy X-rays, will be reduced. The camera housing should prefera-

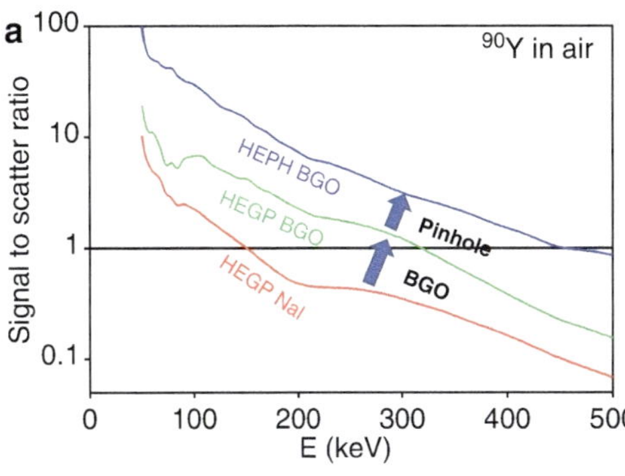

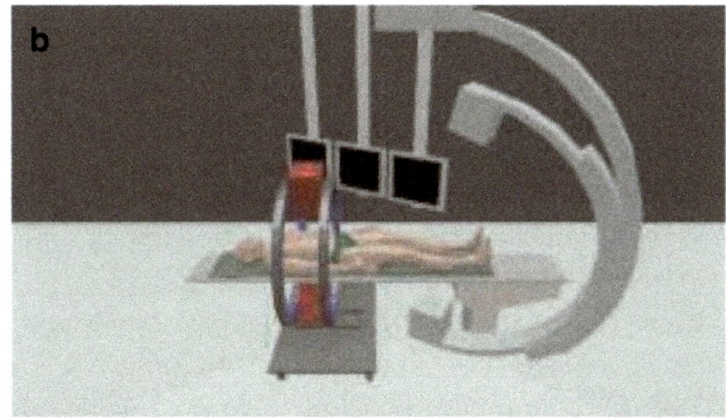

Fig. 14.6 (**a**) Monte-Carlo simulations of detected energy spectra for a ^{90}Y source in air in front of a gamma camera including a NaI crystal and equipped with a high-energy general purpose (HEGP) collimator (red curve), including a BGO crystal and equipped with a HEGP (green curve) or a high-energy pinhole (HEPH) collimator (blue curve) [37]. The curves represent the ratio of geo-metric counts to scattered counts with respect to the detected ray energy. (**b**) Illustration of a mobile dual head BGO-camera equipped with HEPH collimators to be used directly in the catheterization room to image the microspheres distribution and help the radiologist in optimizing the patient dose

bly be made in tungsten which has its fluorescence X-rays emission around 10 keV [23].

Recently Walrand et al. [37] simulated the detected energy spectra for ^{90}Y to illustrate the impact of scattered bremsstrahlung rays. Figure 14.6a represents the signal to scatter ratio, i.e. the total counts coming from the geometric X-rays to those coming from scattered X-rays, with respect to the detected X-rays energy. The signal clearly increases when the NaI crystal is replaced by a BGO crystal, and again when the high-energy parallel hole collimator is replaced by a pinhole collimator.

The simulation of the BGO-pinhole camera shows that the ratio is above 1 (geometric X-rays outnumber scattered ones) in almost all the 50–500 keV energy range. This opens the way to the development of the continuous energy tomography where the detected X-rays energy provides additional information for the image reconstruction similarly to the detector angle in conventional SPECT imaging.

This could be used to optimize the patient dose directly in the catheterization room (Fig. 14.6b). After a first injection of microspheres (^{90}Y, ^{166}Ho or ^{32}P), a BGO-pinhole camera is moved around the patient and a 2 min scan provides data that are treated by a dosimetric software. From its results the radiologist can estimate if and how much activity can still be injected in the patient. The procedure can be iterated until optimal activity has been injected.

Compton cameras are under intensive development in physics labs [27]. Similarly to PET, the purpose of Compton camera is to get free of the mechanical collimator in order to improve both the spatial resolution and the sensitivity as well. Applied to bremsstrahlung imaging, Compton camera will be free of any collimator disturbing effects. In Compton camera the photon is detected in two distant planes, i.e. the Compton and the scintillation detector. Thus, measuring the time detection sequence between these two planes will also allow discrimination between primary and backscattered photons. Lastly, sensitivity of Compton camera increases with rays energy, and acquisition with very wide energy window could be used to further increase the sensitivity.

14.8 Conclusions

With the increasing accessibility to PET systems, ^{90}Y PET imaging will likely remain the gold standard for ^{90}Y imaging. However the increasing amount of performed ^{90}Y therapies will see the continuing developments and improvements of ^{90}Y bremsstrahlung SPECT imaging, especially on the software side with better corrections to achieve imaging quality similar to PET. Moreover, bremsstrahlung SPECT will remain the only way to image ^{32}P and ^{89}Sr, two isotopes regaining interest in radiotherapy. In addition, use of a dedicated pinhole collimator could allow performing fast bremsstrahlung SPECT quantification during liver radioembolization. Soon, the emerging CZT detectors should further improve bremsstrahlung SPECT. In a distant future, Compton camera could revolutionize this imaging modality.

References

1. Simon N, Feitelberg S, Warner RRP, Greenspan EM, Edelman S, Baron MG. External scanning of internal beta-emitters. J Mt Sinai Hosp. 1966;33:365–70.
2. Simon N, Feitelberg S. Scanning Bremsstrahlung of Yttrium-90 microspheres injected intra-arterially. Radiology. 1967;88:719–24.
3. Kaplan WD, Zimmerman RE, Bloomer WD, Knapp RC, Adelstein AJ. Therapeutic intraperitoneal 32P: a clinical assessment of the dynamics of distribution. Radiology. 1981;138:683.
4. Lhommel R, Goffette P, Van den Eynde M, Jamar F, Pauwels S, Bilbao JI, Walrand S. Yttrium-90 TOF PET scan demonstrates high-resolution biodistribution after liver SIRT. Eur J Nucl Med Mol Imaging. 2009;36(10):1969.
5. Lhommel R, van Elmbt L, Goffette P, Van den Eynde M, Jamar F, Pauwels S, Walrand S. Feasibility of Yttrium-90 TOF-PET based dosimetry in liver metastasis therapy using SIR-spheres. Eur J Nucl Med Mol Imaging. 2010;37(9):1654–62.
6. Walrand S, Jamar F, van Elmbt L, Lhommel R, Bidja'a Bekonde E, Pauwels S. 4-Step renal dosimetry dependent on cortex geometry applied to 90Y peptide receptor radiotherapy: evaluation using a fillable kidney phantom imaged by 90Y PET. J Nucl Med. 2010;51:1969–73.
7. Walrand S, Flux GD, Konijnenberg MW, Valkema R, Krenning EP, Lhommel R, Pauwels S, Jamar F. Dosimetry of yttrium-labelled radiopharmaceuticals for internal therapy: (86)Y or (90)Y imaging? Eur J Nucl Med Mol Imaging. 2011;38(1):S57–68.
8. Van Holen R, Staelens S, Vandenberghe S. SPECT imaging of high energy isotopes and isotopes with high energy contaminants with rotating slat collimators. Med Phys. 2009;36:4257–67.
9. Walrand S, Hesse S, Demonceau G, Pauwels S, Jamar F. Yttrium-90 labeled microspheres tracking during liver selective internal radiotherapy by bremsstrahlung pinhole SPECT: feasibility study and evaluation in an abdominal phantom. EJNMMI Res. 2011;1:32.
10. Heard S, Flux GD, Guy MJ, Ott RJ. Monte Carlo simulation of ^{90}Y Bremsstrahlung imaging. IEEE Nucl Sci Symp Conf Rec. 2004;6:3579–83.
11. Siegel JA. Quantitative Bremsstrahlung SPECT imaging: attenuation-corrected activity determination. J Nucl Med. 1994;35(7):1213–6.
12. Minarik D, Gleisner KS, Ljungberg M. Evaluation of quantitative (90) Y SPECT based on experimental phantom studies. Phys Med Biol. 2008;53:5689–703.
13. Frey EC, Tsui BMW. A new method for modeling the spatially variant, object-dependent scatter response function in SPECT. IEEE Nucl Sci Symp. 1996;2:1082–6.
14. Minarik D, Sjögreen-Gleisner K, Linden O, Winga K, Tennvall J, Strand S-E, Ljungberg M. ^{90}Y Bremsstrahlung imaging for absorbed-dose assessment in high-dose radioimmunotherapy. J Nucl Med. 2010;51:1974–78.
15. Elschot M, Lam MGEH, van den Bosch MAAJ, Viergever MA, de Jong HWAM. Quantitative Monte Carlo-based ^{90}Y SPECT reconstruction. J Nucl Med. 2013;54:1557–63.
16. Ronga X, Du Y, Ljungberg M, Rault E, Vandenberghe S, Frey EC. Development and evaluation of an improved quantitative ^{90}Y bremsstrahlung SPECT method. Med Phys. 2012;39:2346–58.
17. Siman W, Mikell JK, Kappadath SC. Practical reconstruction protocol for quantitative ^{90}Y bremsstrahlung SPECT/CT. Med Phys. 2016;43:5093–103.
18. Dewaraja YK, Chun SY, Srinivasa RN, Kaza RK, Cuneo KC, Majdalany BS, Novelli PM, Ljungberg M, Fessler JA. Improved quantitative 90Y bremsstrahlung SPECT/CT reconstruction with Monte Carlo scatter modeling. Med Phys. 2017;44:6364–75.
19. Chun SY, Nguyen P, Phan TQ, Kim H, Fessler JA, Dewaraja YK, et al. Algorithms and analyses for joint spectral proposed an interesting approach of joint spectral image reconstruction in Y-90 bremsstrahlung SPECT. IEEE Trans Med Imaging. 2020;39:1369–79.
20. Lim H, Fessler JA, Wilderman SJ, Brooks AF, Dewaraja YK. Y-90 SPECT ML image reconstruction with a new model for tissue-dependent bremsstrahlung production using CT information: a proof-of-concept study. Phys Med Biol. 2019;63:115001.
21. Xiang H, Lim H, Fessler JA, Dewaraja YK. A deep neural network for fast and accurate scatter estimation in quantitative SPECT/CT under challenging scatter conditions. EJNMMI. 2020;47:2956–67.
22. Walrand SH, van Elmbt LR, Pauwels S. Quantitation in SPECT using an effective model of the scattering. Phys Med Biol. 1994;39(4):719–34.
23. X-ray Department. X-ray wavelengths for spectrometer. 4th ed. Boston, MA: General Electric Company; 1966.
24. Gupta T, Virmani S, Neidt TM, Szolc-Kowalska B, Sato KT, Ryu RK, Lewandowski RJ, Gates VL, Woloschak GE, Salem R, Omary RA, Larson AC. MR tracking of iron-labeled glass radioembolization microsphres during

transcatheter delivery to rabbit VX2 livers tumors: feasibility study. Radiology. 2008;249(3):845–54.

25. Barber TW, Yap KS, Kalff V. PET/CT imaging of ^{90}Y radiation synovectomy. Eur J Nucl Med Mol Imaging. 2012;39(5):917–8.

26. Riaz A, Lewandowski RJ, Kulik LM, Mulcahy MF, Sato KT, Ryu RK, et al. Complications following radioembolization with yttrium-90 microspheres: a comprehensive literature review. J Vasc Interv Radiol. 2009;29:1121–30.

27. Ahmadzadehfar H, Muckle M, Sabet A, Wilhelm K, Kuhl C, Biermann K, Haslerud T, Biersack HJ, Ezziddin S. The significance of bremsstrahlung SPECT/CT after yttrium-90 radioembolization treatment in the prediction of extrahepatic side effects. Eur J Nucl Med Mol Imaging. 2011;39:309–15.

28. Barone R, Borson-Chazot F, Valkema R, Walrand S, Chauvin F, Gogou L, Kvols LK, Krenning EP, Jamar F, Pauwels S. Patient-specific dosimetry in predicting renal toxicity with (90)Y-DOTATOC: relevance of kidney volume and dose rate in finding a dose-effect relationship. J Nucl Med. 2005;46:99S–106S.

29. Fabbri C, Sarti G, Agostini M, Di Dia A, Paganelli G. SPECT/CT 90Y-Bremsstrahlung images for dosimetry during therapy. Ecancermedicalscience. 2008;2:106.

30. Fabbri C, Sarti G, Cremonesi M, Ferrari M, Di Dia A, Agostini M, Botta F, Paganelli G. Quantitative analysis of 90Y Bremsstrahlung SPECT-CT images for application to 3D patient-specific dosimetry. Cancer Biother Radiopharm. 2009;24(1):145–54.

31. Shiba H, Takahashi A, Baba S, Himuro K, Yamashita Y, Sasaki M. Analysis of the influence of ^{111}In on ^{90}Y-bremsstrahlung SPECT based on Monte Carlo simulation. Ann Nucl Med. 2016;30:675–81.

32. Kappadath SC, Mikell J, Balagopal A, Baladandayuthapani V, Kaseb A, Mahvash A. Hepatocellular carcinoma tumor dose response after ^{90}Y-radioembolization with glass microspheres using ^{90}Y-SPECT/CT-based voxel dosimetry. Int J Radiat Oncol Biol Phys. 2018;102:451–61.

33. Piasecki P, Narloch J, Brzozowski K, Ziecina P, Mazurek A, Budzynska A, Korniluk J, Dziuk M. The predictive value of SPECT/CT imaging in colorectal liver metastases response after ^{90}Y-radioembolization. PLoS One. 2018;13:e0200488. https://doi.org/10.1371/journal.pone.0200488.

34. Schobert I, Chapiro J, Nezami N, Hamm CA, Gebauer B, Lin M, Pollak J, Saperstein L, Schlachter T, Savic LJ. Quantitative imaging biomarkers for Yttrium-90 distribution on bremsstrahlung single photon emission computed tomography after resin-based radioembolization. J Nucl Med. 2019;60:1066–72.

35. Slomka PJ, Patton JA, Berman DS, Germano G. Advances in technical aspects of myocardial perfusion SPECT imaging. J Nucl Cardiol. 2009;16(2):255–76.

36. Walrand S, Jamar F. Imaging in nuclear medicine. In: Giussani A, editor. Perspectives in nuclear medicine tomography: a physicist's point of view. Berlin: Springer; 2013.

37. Walrand S, Hesse M, Wojcik R, Lhommel R, Jamar F. Optimal design of Anger camera for bremsstrahlung imaging: Monte Carlo evaluation. Front Oncol. 2014;4:149.

Miscellaneous: SPECT and SPECT/CT for Brain and Inflammation Imaging and Radiation Planning

15

Sanaz Katal and Ali Gholamrezanezhad

15.1 Introduction

Combination of SPECT (single-photon emission computed tomography) with CT (computed tomography) provides the opportunity for a direct correlation of anatomic information and functional data and leads to a better localization and definition of scintigraphic findings. Besides anatomic referencing, the other advantage of CT co-registration is the attenuation correction capabilities of CT. These advantages together result in a higher specificity of imaging and a significant reduction in indeterminate findings. This chapter highlights the potential clinical applications of integrated SPECT/CT in neurology, inflammation imaging, and radiation planning and summarizes future directions for SPECT/CT in these fields.

15.2 SPECT/CT for Inflammation Imaging

Depending on the type of suspected disease and the clinical presentation, diagnosis of inflammatory diseases usually requires laboratory and imaging procedures to confirm clinical diagnosis. Therefore, the context in which specific imaging procedures are needed should be selected as in a case-by-case approach. Cross-sectional imaging modalities, mainly CT and MRI, provide high-quality anatomical details, but structural changes that are developed due to inflammatory processes are usually nonspecific.

The role of nuclear medicine imaging procedures, including SPECT/CT and PET (positron emission tomography) imaging using different radiopharmaceuticals, has been specifically appreciated in the diagnosis of infection of joint prostheses, infected vascular grafts, and a number of other inflammatory processes. [67]Gallium citrate, [111]Indium, [99m]Technetium HMPAO-labeled white blood cell (WBC) and bone scintigraphies are widely used in the assessment of suspected infection/inflammation. These scintigraphies suffer from poor spatial resolution and still somewhat low specificity, because of the absence or paucity of anatomical landmarks, a shortcoming which has been partly overcome by the co-registration to CT images. It has been confirmed that combined functional/anatomical imaging techniques, such as SPECT/CT, facili-

S. Katal
Department of Nuclear Medicine, Shiraz Kowsar Hospital, Shiraz, Iran

A. Gholamrezanezhad (✉)
Diagnostic Radiology, Keck School of Medicine, University of Southern California (USC), Los Angles, CA, USA
e-mail: ali.gholamrezanezhad@med.usc.edu

tate more precise localization and accurate characterization of inflammatory lesions and improve the specificity of the test. SPECT provides unique abilities in some disorders, and therefore, in spite of recent advances (specifically PET), this traditionally imaging mode will continue to survive [1]. Here we describe in brief, the application of SPECT/CT in such cases.

15.2.1 Infection of Joint Prostheses

More than 700,000 hip and knee arthroplasties are performed annually in the USA, and this number may exceed 700,000 by the year 2030 [2–5]. Aseptic loosening, dislocation, fracture, and infection are the most important complications of these procedures. As the clinical presentations and histopathologic changes of infection and aseptic loosening are remarkably similar, differentiation of these entities is sometimes problematic and needs appropriate and often multimodality imaging [3, 4].

Although conventional radiography is usually the first imaging test requested, bone scintigraphy with bone-seeking agents (like ^{99m}Tc-MDP), as a widely available, inexpensive, and exquisitely sensitive modality (sensitivity exceeding 80%), has been frequently employed as the second line of diagnosis. A normal bone scintigram has been defined as a scan in which periprosthetic uptake is indistinguishable from that of surrounding nonarticular bone. Regarding the high sensitivity of the test, such a scan is strongly against a prosthetic abnormality [3]. However, the specificity of the test is not optimal (a limited specificity reaching up to 50%), so the clinical significance of an abnormal scan, as increased periprosthetic uptake, is less certain. Any cause of increased osteoblastic activity, including infection and aseptic loosening secondary to sterile inflammation, may result in increased periprosthetic activity on bone scintigraphy, so these entities might be indistinguishable at scintigraphy. To overcome the shortcomings of bone scintigraphy, other radiopharmaceuticals—such as gallium or ^{99m}Tc-labeled WBC, labeled nanocolloids,

and ^{99m}Tc- or ^{111}In-labeled proteins, such as IgG or albumin—have been used.

As the anatomic details of bones are not as clear of bone scintigraphy, in such scintigraphies co-registration of the images with an anatomic modality like CT is more required and, in some cases, is critical in discriminating between pathologic and physiologic uptake. Several studies have shown the benefit of hybrid imaging of infection and have confirmed that SPECT/CT may significantly affect disease management by increasing specificity. By combined SPECT/CT, the specificity increases considerably to above 80%. However, still it should be confessed that none of these radiotracers are optimally specific for infection, and none offers the possibility of optimally differentiating sterile from septic inflammation. The main reason for limited specificity is that the main mechanism of action for most of these radiotracers is nonspecific accumulation at the site of inflammation secondary to increased blood flow and vascular permeability.

For the case of WBC scintigraphy, it is the physiologic uptake into bone marrow that impairs both sensitivity and specificity. Therefore, dual imaging of inflammation with WBC and nanocolloids for bone marrow has been suggested. The rationale for the dual imaging is that in infectious etiologies, bone marrow is replaced by the infectious process, so bone marrow imaging will be negative, whereas WBC scanning in the same location is still positive. This combined imaging approach has resulted in an excellent sensitivity and specificity above 90%. It appears that combined in vitro labeled leucocyte/bone marrow scintigraphy (LS/BMS) has overall diagnostic accuracy of >90% and is the imaging modality of choice for diagnosing PJI. Of note, semiquantitative analysis of the target-to-background (T/B) ratio, particularly if performed with dual-time imaging (both at 3–4 and 20 h), has been offered to improve the diagnostic accuracy of WBC imaging. Moreover, SPECT/CT could offer an added value to the dual imaging of WBC/nanocolloid scintigraphy, as it provides more accurate comparison of uptake of radiotracers in different parts of the bony structures (Fig. 15.1).

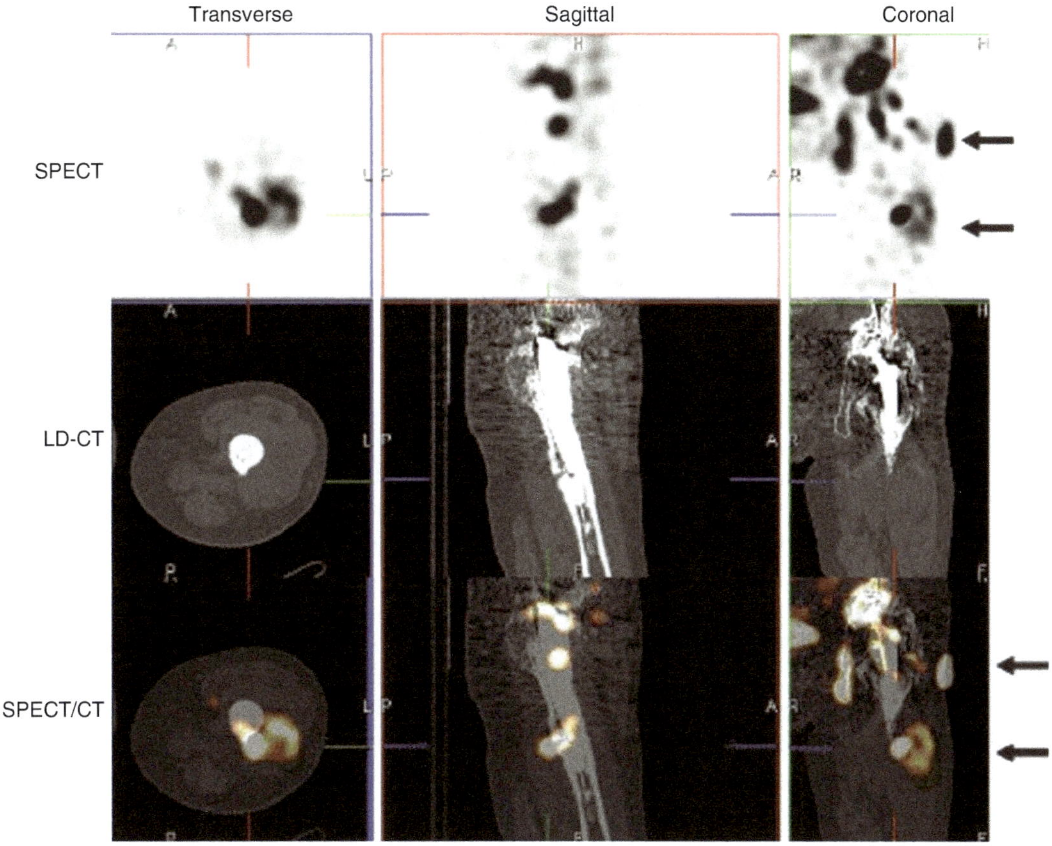

Fig. 15.1 Leukocyte SPECT/CT, performed at 4 h p.i., shows pathologic activity at the prosthesis proximal part, the presence of a chronic fistulization in the upper thigh (*arrow*), and an abscess collection near the distal part of the femoral shaft (*dashed arrow*), indicating a chronic infected hip prosthesis. Combining SPECT/CT fusion images enhances the exact localization and, in particular in this case, the extent of the inflamed tissues, probably more accurately than SPECT alone. Subsequently, the orthopedic surgeon can be prepared for an extended treatment strategy. Finally, note the presence of metal artifacts, generated on the low-dose CT. (With kind permission from Springer Science + Business Media. Gemmel et al. [6] Fig. 10)

Despite its high accuracy, radiolabeled WBC suffers from several limitations, such as potential radiation exposure to staff and its time-demanding preparation. As an alternative for WBC imaging, antigranulocyte scintigraphy has been investigated with the same sensitivity and specificity, and the advantage of in vivo labeling. In two meta-analyses by Pakos et al. [7] and Xing et al. [8], the overall sensitivity and specificity of anti-granulocyte antibodies in prosthetic joint infections (83% and 79–80%, respectively) were comparable to radiolabeled white blood, except for a slightly lower specificity for antibodies. Albeit, in vivo labeling of leukocytes using anti-granulocyte antibodies has not gained full accep-

tance in the diagnostic approach of imaging of prosthetic infectious complication. Most recently, a promising role for FDG PET has been suggested in screening for suspected infection after arthroplasty, with at least the same diagnostic accuracy compared to WBC scintigraphy [9].

15.2.2 Infectious Endocarditis (IE)

The diagnosis of infectious endocarditis poses a real challenge to clinicians, as there is still no diagnostic gold standard. Its diagnosis is mainly based on a combination of clinical assessment, microbiological cultures, and echocardiography findings. However, even with all these techniques, several cases might be missed, especially the negative-culture ones. Moreover, these measures might underestimate the extent of disease burden. Nuclear medicine methods might offer a great value in the diagnostic assessment of endocarditis, particularly when clinical suspicion is high but echocardiographic data are undetermined (such as mechanical device artifacts or marantic vegetation), or when the clinical and echocardiography findings are contradictory or inconclusive. Several studies have shown the value of ^{99m}Tc-HMPAO WBC SPECT/CT to allow detection of cardiac and additional unexpected extra-cardiac sites of inflammation in up to 41% of IE cases, which will potentially alter their clinical management in this setting [10].

15.2.3 Infected Vascular Graft

The reported rate of vascular graft infections ranges from 0.5% to 5% and is associated with a high risk of mortality and morbidity (such as limb loss); so early diagnosis of these infections is of the utmost importance for the optimal timely management, which usually necessitates surgical intervention. In view of the remarkable consequences of a false-positive diagnosis, for the diagnosis of vascular graft infection, not only a high sensitivity but also a high specificity is needed. Imaging of vascular graft infection by labeled WBC SPECT has been tested previously, but the results were discouraging, as the test suffers from a chance of false-positive results caused by the inability to exactly localize the site of inflammation. Adding CT to SPECT imaging increases the diagnostic accuracy: on CT scans, air bubbles could be found around the infected graft in almost half of the cases; however, this finding is also highly nonspecific, because in 50% of grafts these bubbles are present for weeks to months after graft implantation [11]. Also, CT is often false-negative in chronic low-grade infections, and it is challenging to differentiate between acute infection, hematoma, and lymphocele on CT scans. Based on these limitations, PET/CT with a sensitivity exceeding 90%, the

specificity of 64%, positive and negative predictive values of 88% and 96%, has been preferred over SPECT, CT, or combined SPECT/CT imaging.

15.3 Imaging of Noninfectious Inflammatory Disease

15.3.1 Rheumatoid Arthritis

Rheumatoid arthritis is an inflammatory arthropathy, for which a remarkable number of new therapeutic strategies, including biological agents such as anti-TNF antibodies, have emerged. Regarding the importance of the individualized use of disease-modifying antirheumatic drugs, such as methotrexate and biological agents, monitoring of response to treatment is one of the most challenging issues in front of rheumatologists, a measurement which cannot always be easily done by clinical criteria [12]. Another aspect of the diagnostic approach to RA is also the need to stratify patients into groups with a low risk or a high risk of rapid disease progression and severe destructive arthropathy. Imaging approaches have been employed to address these issues. Ultrasonography, MRI, and a number of scintigraphic approaches (including nanocolloids and 3-phase bone scintigraphy and ^{18}F-FDG PET) have been used to detect synovitis, as well as increased synovial blood flow in affected joints. Selection of the best imaging approach to address the clinical question depends on different factors: ultrasonography is widely available, sensitive, inexpensive, convenient, and with no ionizing radiation, so it is increasingly becoming the first-line modality of screening for suspected RA or other inflammatory arthropathy patients. It may also show bone erosions in small joints (finger and toe joints) with high sensitivity [13]. MRI, although is the gold standard imaging modality for the detection of synovitis and sensitive in the detection of bone erosions, is expensive and less convenient for patients. Plain radiography is not sensitive enough to detect early lesions in RA.

Bone scintigraphy has been employed to image disease activity with planar imaging clearly less sensitive than SPECT, so minimal changes in bone metabolism may be missed [14]. For example, multipinhole SPECT of the hands has been employed to detect early stages of the rheumatoid disease with the sensitivity equal to or even more than MRI in some cases [15]. ^{99m}Tc-nanocolloids scintigraphy has also shown high diagnostic accuracy, but with limited clinical application due to advantages of competing modalities (ultrasound, MRI, and bone scintigraphy), mainly their broad availability. PET with ^{18}F-FDG or ^{11}C-choline has been studied for imaging of synovial inflammation and measurement of cell proliferation and has been proved to have high diagnostic accuracy [16]. Although scintigraphy with either ^{99m}Tc-nanocolloids or bisphosphonates could be employed in the diagnosis of RA at its early stages, its role in the evaluation of response to treatment requires repeated imaging as often as every 6–12 weeks. However, radiation exposure associated with nuclear medicine techniques puts ultrasonography and MRI at an advantage [17].

15.3.2 Sarcoidosis

SPECT/CT with ^{67}Ga-citrate has been used for imaging of sarcoidosis, in fact for determination of disease activity, monitoring of response to treatment, detection of sites of disease previously unknown, and unsuspected metabolically active disease [18–26]. However, recent studies have shown that ^{67}Ga offers no advantages over ^{18}F-FDG PET/CT for imaging of inflammatory diseases; therefore, Ga scintigraphy has been largely replaced by PET/CT for such a purpose [27]. Similarly, in the management of the cardiac sarcoidosis, FDG PET is now preferred over ^{67}Ga and myocardial perfusion scintigraphy, for both diagnosis, and to prognosis evaluation [18].

In the diagnosis of primary sarcoidosis, high ^{67}Ga uptake could be seen in lymph nodes and other involved organs [19–24]. The *lambda sign* is seen on ^{67}Ga scans in the setting of thoracic sarcoidosis. Bilateral hilar and right paratracheal lymph nodes are typically involved which can resemble the lambda symbol. The panda sign is seen as a result of ^{67}Ga citrate accumulation in both regions of chronic and regions of acute inflammation. When the normal accumulation of the radionuclide in the nasopharynx is combined with increased symmetric accumulation in the parotid and lacrimal glands, the image shows a striking similarity to the mottled coloring of the giant panda. In response to treatment, uptake of ^{67}Ga decreases, allowing for assessment of treatment effects and for early adaptation of therapy if no response is seen (Fig. 15.2).

15.3.3 Inflammatory Bowel Disease (IBD)

Ulcerative colitis and Crohn's disease are the two main subtypes of IBD, the diagnosis of which depends on direct endoscopic visualization of the GI mucosa and the histological evaluation of the tissue samples. Radiological and scintigraphic methods are mainly employed as an adjunct to endoscopy [15]. Although disease activity is usually measured clinically by clinical activity scores, endoscopy, or barium enteroclysis, this diagnostic approach has major disadvantages, as clinical activity scores are indirect and endoscopy and barium enteroclysis are both invasive techniques, which in case of severe disease predispose the patient to procedure-related complications, like colon perforation. Similarly, barium may be contraindicated in cases of severe inflammation because of the risk of perforation and subsequent peritonitis. Therefore, noninvasive imaging procedures are needed to adequately follow patients with IBD [15, 25].

Labeled leukocyte imaging (preferably with ^{99m}Tc instead of ^{111}In due to better image quality) has been extensively employed for evaluation of IBD, mainly to detect involved bowel segments and localization of the disease as well as early diagnosis of resistance to therapy. WBC scan is unlikely to miss severe inflammation, and the sensitivity and specificity of labeled WBC scanning for the correct detection of involved bowel segment have been reported to be between 80% and 90% in adults and children [25, 26, 29–31]. WBC scanning may also help to diagnose ther-

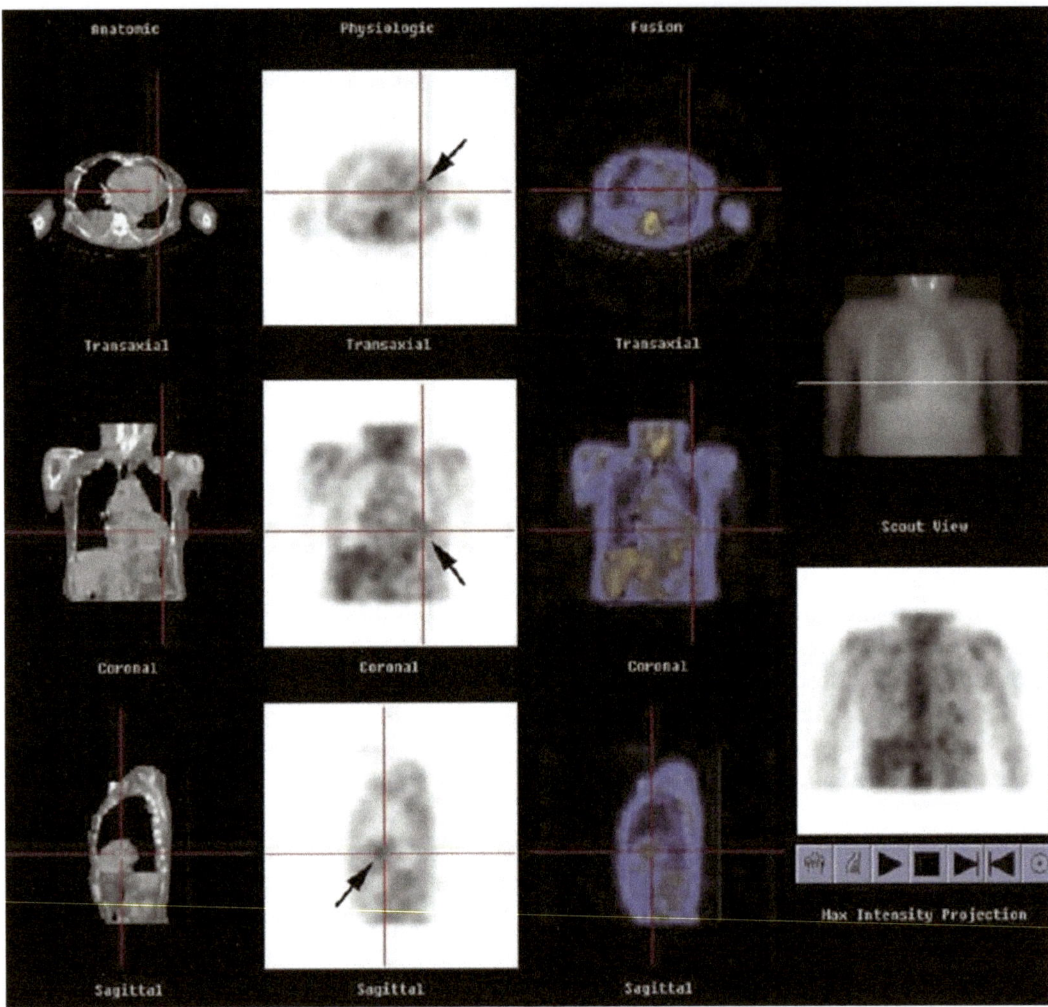

Fig. 15.2 A 60-year-old female patient with cardiac sarcoidosis. Single-photon emission computed tomography (SPECT)/CT (low-dose CT, SPECT, and fusion image) showing an abnormal uptake (*arrows*) near cardiac apex. (With kind permission from Springer Science + Business Media. Momose et al. [28])

apy resistance within days after the onset of therapy [32]. WBC scanning requires no bowel preparation, causes no patient discomfort and offers less radiation as compared to the competitive imaging modalities: the effective radiation dose for ^{99m}Tc-HMPAO WBC imaging is 3 mSv, for barium small bowel follow-through is 6 mSv, and for barium enema is 8.5 mSv [33].

Horsthuis et al. have demonstrated that WBC scanning is more sensitive than CT, but equivalent to ultrasonography and MRI in IBD imaging, with sensitivities ranging from 84% to 93% and specificities ranging from 84% to 95% [25]. Mainly based on the absence of radiation exposure, ultrasonography and MRI have been suggested as primary imaging modalities for IBD; however, it has been emphasized that ultrasonography is operator dependent, and usually not all bowel segments can be imaged by ultrasound technique [15]. For labeled leukocyte imaging, SPECT/CT should be performed for the correct localization of involved bowel segments. Controversy still exists about the optimal imaging time after infusion of labeled WBCs to the patient. Early scanning (30–60 min) has been recommended by some authors in order to avoid false-positive results caused by intestinal migration of the radionuclide, whereas late scanning (3 h) has been favored by others because of higher sensitivity [34]. Slightly lower specificity but higher sensitivity (85% vs. 100%) and accuracy (85% vs. 95%) of late scanning as compared to early scanning has been reported [32].

[99mTc]-Pentavalent dimercaptosuccinic acid [DMSA (V)] has been reported to be an accurate scintigraphic modality and has been suggested as a complementary technique to colonoscopy for the follow-up of patients and assessment of IBD activity [33, 35, 36]. Scintigraphic imaging of IBD with [111In]-anti E-selectin monoclonal antibodies and [99mTc]-labeled antigranulocyte monoclonal antibodies has been insufficiently studied and warrants further investigation [33].

15.3.4 Other Abdominal Disorders

[111In] WBC is found to accurately diagnose abdominal or pelvic abscesses with high sensitivity and specificity (90% and 95%, respectively) [37]. Comparing to [67Ga], [111In] WBC does not accumulate within the colon or sterile healing abdominal wounds, and therefore constitutes the preferred agent in assessing the patients with suspected abdominal infections.

The potential added value of SPECT/CT in the routine hepatobiliary [99mTc]-iminodiacetic acid studies has also been investigated by some studies. Although planar hepatobiliary scintigraphies usually present sufficient sensitive and specific data, Arabi et al. [38] demonstrated that SPECT/CT can alter the interpretation in 41–43% of studies, either from abnormal to normal (30%), or from normal to abnormal scan findings (13%).

The value of SPECT/CT has also been explored for the detection of liver hemangioma and splenosis [39]. In patients who have been undergone splenectomy, SPECT/CT can detect and localize active splenic tissue due to splenosis, particularly in the intrahepatic, intrapulmonary,

and pleural implants. Similarly, the usefulness of RBC SPECT/CT in detecting hepatic hemangiomas has been shown [40], especially the small ones, or those suited adjacent to the heart or vascular structures, where planar RBC imaging has major limitations.

15.4 Fever of Unknown Origin (FUO)

Although a number of definitions are found for FUO, the most commonly acceptable definition is a temperature of at least 38.3 °C (101 °F) for more than 3 weeks, with the underlying cause being uncertain after 1 week of inpatient work-up. The potential causes of FUO include a broad spectrum of diseases, mostly infectious diseases and autoimmune disorders. One third of the cases are due to an occult malignancy.

Although usually anatomic imaging is the first diagnostic approach to the patient with FUO, it suffers from remarkable limitations:

It covers just a limited area of the body, which is already selected by the referring physician, and always there is a risk that the source of fever is not included in the imaged field. Such a limitation is not present in most of nuclear medicine imaging techniques that are used for this purpose (e.g., [67Ga] scintigraphy, [18F]-FDG PET), as they are performed as whole body imaging examinations. However, SPECT/CT has the same limitation, which is mostly due to the CT component. On the other hand, anatomic imaging modalities detect anatomic changes in tissues. These changes usually are not developed, unless the underlying disease progresses beyond a specific level of tissue distortion and derangement. Functional imaging of nuclear medicine does not suffer from such a limitation and is able to detect the disease processes in an earlier stage. In addition, changes caused by previous cured diseases, radiation, or surgical interventions (scars, fibrosis) may result in false-positive interpretation of the anatomical images, a problem which is significantly less common in functional imaging (like SPECT/CT).

^{67}Ga-citrate is one of the most common agents used for the scintigraphic imaging of FUO. Whole body imaging is a great advantage of the technique, which is added to the ability of spot imaging of the areas of interest with SPECT acquisition. These areas of interest are chosen by the nuclear physician, based on the history and findings of the whole body scan. The proven efficiency of ^{67}Ga-citrate scintigraphy in the detection of inflammation is the avidity of ^{67}Ga-citrate for inflammatory molecules in the inflamed tissues. However, ^{67}Ga-citrate scintigraphy suffers from some limitations such as delayed clearance of radiotracer from the background, which requires delayed image acquisition to achieve acceptable target-to-background ratio. High γ-energy emitted by ^{67}Ga also impairs image quality by lower resolution resulting from the use of high-energy collimators. On the other hand, ^{67}Ga-citrate scintigraphy is time consuming and has a relatively high radiation burden. Meller et al. have shown that ^{67}Ga scintigraphy has a diagnostic yield nearly equivalent to that of ^{18}F-FDG coincidence PET [11, 41–43]. The alternative scintigraphic modality is labeled WBC scan, which may be used to identify infectious foci in patients with FUO. However, WBCs accumulate mainly in the foci of bacterial infections, and the scan usually has a low sensitivity in the detection of the other potential causes of FUO, such malignancies and autoimmune diseases, with a remarkable number of false-negative scans in FUO. Therefore, the clinical value of labeled WBCs for detection of the underlying etiology of FUO is limited. Considering the limitations of ^{67}Ga scintigraphy and labeled WBC scan, ^{18}F-FDG PET is the procedure of choice for the imaging evaluation of FUO, as main underlying causes of FUO (infection, autoimmune disease, and malignancy) can be detected with a high sensitivity by a single imaging. Different radiopharmaceuticals used for inflammation imaging have been listed on Table 15.1.

Table 15.1 Radiopharmaceuticals used for inflammation imaging

Radiopharmaceutical	Mechanism of action
^{99m}Tc/^{111}In-labeled autologous WBCs (white blood cells)	Active migration of WBCs to the sites of infection/inflammation
^{67}Ga-citrate	Increased perfusion of the inflamed tissues, local binding to lactoferrin, extravasation due to increased vascular permeability
^{99m}Tc-labeled bisphosphonates	Increased delivery and diffusion to the sites of infection/inflammation due to increased perfusion and extravasation (early angiographic and blood pool phases) and increased bone uptake due to higher osteoblastic activity (late phase)
^{99m}Tc-labeled nanocolloids	Uptake in macrophages (inflammation, bone marrow, liver, spleen), increased extravasation
^{99m}Tc/^{111}In-labeled proteins (IgG, albumin)	Extravasation (increased perfusion and vessel permeability)

15.5 Brain Imaging

Although functional imaging provides invaluable diagnostic information in many patients with neurological disorders [44–46], currently CT and MRI have substituted functional imaging. The most important indications of functional imaging with brain SPECT/CT are assessment of brain tumors, particularly for differentiation of postradiation necrosis versus residual/recurrent tumor, differential diagnosis of Parkinson's disease and dementia, detection of seizure focus, detection of brain death, and evaluation of substance abuse.

15.5.1 Parkinson's Disease

Parkinson's disease is one of the best examples in which functional imaging has been shown to be superior to anatomic imaging regarding clinical diagnostic efficacy. It provides invaluable information not obtainable by the other imaging modalities, which significantly influence decision making and can potentially change the therapeutic plan. ^{123}I-ioflupane with commercial name of DAT is the most commonly used and the most widely studied radiopharmaceutical for the assessment patients suspected for Parkinson's disease. It is actually one of the best radiotracers to visualize the striatum using SPECT, showing the distribution of the dopamine transporters in the striatum. After reorientation of head to avoid false impressions of asymmetry due to head tilting, images are visually interpreted [47–49].

In a normal scan the striatum is seen as symmetric, comma-shaped regions, with both caudate and putamen showing high uptake compared to background activity. With increasing age, a reduction in the target-to-background ratio is seen (5–8% decrease in ratio per decade). In early Parkinson's disease, there is usually an asymmetrical pattern of reduced DaT binding initially in the dorsal putamen contralateral to the clinically most symptomatic body side. The radiotracer binding gradually progresses anteriorly and ipsilaterally as the disease progresses. Although the activity in the caudate nucleus declines with advancing disease, it is relatively preserved in early disease. In the atypical parkinsonian syndromes, there usually is a more symmetrical decrease in DaT binding, and more involvement of caudate is detected. However, the overlap between scintigraphic features is sufficiently high not to reliably differentiate between different parkinsonian syndromes. In Lewy body dementia, DaT binding is reduced bilaterally, mainly in the putamen but also in the caudate. The reduction of radiotracer binding is generally with less asymmetry than seen in Parkinson's disease.

Moreover, other tracers have also been used for SPECT imaging in patients with Parkinson's disease. As an example, several studies have explored the ability of ^{123}I-FP-CIT SPECT for defining the reduced striatal dopamine transporters in Parkinson's disease. By defining the nigrostriatal changes in Parkinson's disease, ^{123}I-FP-CIT

SPECT also provides a robust measure of disease severity and duration of disease [50].

15.5.2 Stroke

Flow imaging with radiopharmaceuticals, which reflect regional cerebral blood flow (rCBF), has been used for early detection of stroke. Two ^{99m}Tc-labeled radiopharmaceuticals for brain flow imaging are available: hexamethylpropyleneamineoxime ([^{99m}Tc-HMPAO] Ceretec) and ethylcysteinate dimer ([^{99m}Tc-ECD] bicisate, Neurolite). Although absolute rCBF measurement using Xenon as the radiotracer is possible, such a measurement with Technetium agents has not been fully implemented, and the region of interest (ROI) analysis of rCBF has become the preferred method of quantification with these radiopharmaceuticals [51–57].

In the very early hours of stroke, rCBF is reduced, while tissue oxygen metabolism is maintained. This flow-metabolism mismatch is called "misery perfusion." In later stages, ischemia progresses and damage to blood vessels might lead to excessive or "luxury perfusion." This sequence of scintigraphic findings has been used to determine which patients may benefit from thrombolytic therapy. Some studies have shown that SPECT is able to detect the ischemic events even before MRI and the ischemic area is larger in SPECT images as compared to MRI. Such a difference is partly explained by the higher sensitivity of SPECT in detecting the penumbra area, the area that benefits from early reperfusion interventions and is at the highest risk for expansion of irreversible injury. The best candidates for fibrinolytic therapy would be those patients presenting immediately after the onset of clinical symptoms and showing an area of reduced tracer uptake (hypoperfusion) on the SPECT images. In fact, a normal brain SPECT image or just an area of hypoperfusion implies a favorable prognosis as a result of effective collateral circulation. By contrast, an area of no radiopharmaceutical uptake (cold area or absent perfusion) is more likely to be associated with hemorrhagic complications if fibrinolysis is employed. For SPECT-driven decision making, brain SPECT should be done between the first 3 and 6 h after the onset of stroke symptoms, which is usually not possible in routine clinical practice.

SPECT also has been shown to be effective in the study of transient ischemic attacks (TIA). A pharmacologic stress using acetazolamide (Diamox) injection has been employed to unmask the underlying vasculopathies limiting the vasodilatory response to Diamox. In fact, abnormal vessels do not show dilatory response to Diamox, and the blood flow is shunted away from them, leading to a kind of steal phenomenon. The final outcome in scintigraphic imaging is a significant reduction in radiotracer uptake of the cerebral regions being fed by the affected blood vessels. The rationale for the imaging is comparable to what is employed in myocardial perfusion imaging using dipyridamole.

15.5.3 Epilepsy

SPECT has been shown to be an effective modality in the detection of epileptic foci in patients with complex partial seizures refractory to medical treatment [58–65]. If the radiotracer is injected during the seizure activity, i.e., ictal SPECT, the sensitivity and specificity of the imaging, is as high as 95%. This is why ictal imaging has been considered as the gold standard for the presurgical detection of epileptic foci. In ictal imaging, ictal foci are found as areas of hyperactivity. Although the negative predictive value of an early postictal SPECT (injecting the radiopharmaceutical immediately after the seizure) is low and therefore a negative scan is not clinically useful, the positive predictive value in localizing a unilateral focus is as high as 97%. By contrast, interictal SPECT, in which the radiotracer is injected when the patient is seizure-free, provides a significantly lower diagnostic accuracy of 60–70%. Interictal images usually show hypoactivity in the epileptic focus, if they can detect any abnormality.

15.5.4 Dementia

Precise classification of dementias is crucially important in choosing the best treatment plan and for optimal prognostic evaluation of patients. Different cerebral perfusion patterns have been found to be associated with different types of dementia. Therefore, SPECT has an effective impact on therapeutic decision making by differentiating dementia of Alzheimer's type from other causes of impaired cognitive status, such as pseudodementia (depression), multi-infarct dementia, and Pick's disease [66–73].

Pseudodementia is a depressive syndrome, which manifests as an impaired cognitive status and memory loss and can be effectively managed by antidepressant medications. Pseudodementia presents with prefrontal perfusion impairment in brain SPECT imaging. The severity of the perfusion abnormality may evolve with increasing clinical impairment, providing an additional role for brain SPECT imaging in disease staging. A decreased perfusion in frontal or frontotemporal regions of the brain suggests frontal lobe dementia, such as Pick's disease, whereas decreased perfusion in the temporoparietal regions is associated with posterior dementia, such as Alzheimer's type.

In Lewy body dementia, ^{23}I-FP-CIT SPECT has also been tested, which revealed high diagnostic accuracy, and thus is included as an indicative biomarker in its diagnostic criterion [74]. ^{123}I-FP-CIT SPECT is able to differentiate between Alzheimer's Disease and Lewy body dementia [75]. Most recently, ^{99m}Tc-peptide targeting Aβ plaques has also been introduced as a potential agent for SPECT imaging in Alzheimer disease, which has shown promising results in the non-human models [76]. They found the ability of ^{99m}Tc-labeled agents for early imaging of Aβ plaques in the brain [77].

15.5.5 Restless Legs Syndrome (RLS)

Pharmacologic evidence suggests that restless legs syndrome might be associated with central dopaminergic dysfunction. Neurofunctioning

SPECT imaging of the dopaminergic alteration in patients with restless legs syndrome has been previously investigated, both at presynaptic (using ^{123}I-IPT, ^{123}I-βCIT, ^{99m}Tc-TRODAT-1) and postsynaptic ([23]I-IBZM) levels. However, the earlier studies found some controversial results [78], which might be linked to some methodological limitations. A recent study [79] on ^{99m}Tc-TRODAT-1 SPECT in 34 patients with RLS found reduced uptake in the striatum. This suggests significantly impaired striatal dopamine transporter density and activity in RLS patients, compared to healthy subjects. Moreover, in patients with RLS and end-stage renal disease (ESRD), Tc-99m TRODAT SPECT might play as a potential biomarker [80]. TRODAT uptake ratio was lower in patients with RLS and ESRD. In addition, the uptake was correlated with serum parathyroid hormone, dysregulated hemoglobin, and serum ferritin concentrations.

15.5.6 Psychiatric Disorders, and Traumatic Brain Injury

SPECT neuroimaging with perfusion and receptor agents disclose complementary aspects of the major functional changes in a wide range of psychiatric diseases. This imaging tool holds great value in diagnosis, risk stratification, prognosis assessment, and monitoring therapy response. The role of brain SPECT in major psychiatric disorders, including obsessive-compulsive disorder (OCD), Tourette's syndrome, schizophrenia, depression, panic disorder, and drug abuse, have been previously debated [81, 82]. However, only a few psychiatrists have adopted functional neuroimaging methods such as brain SPECT in routine clinical practice.

Similarly, brain SPECT imaging can be utilized in the diagnosis, prognosis, and treatment of patients who have sustained brain trauma [83]. It acts as a powerful second test when CT or MRI is inconclusive or negative after a head injury with post-injury neurological or neuropsychiatric symptoms. Not only detects the early changes before CT or MRI, but also predicts the neurological outcomes, and guides the clinicians for the optimal treatment strategy. A positive initial brain SPECT after a closed head injury might prompt aggressive treatment intervention, even in the absence of clinical symptoms. On the other hand, given its 100% negative predictive value, brain SPECT can be reliably applied to exclude clinically significant sequels shortly after a closed head injury.

15.6 SPECT/CT for Radiation Planning

An optimal radiation therapy allows delivery of high radiation doses to the tumor, while avoiding radiation to nearby non-tumoral tissues. Achieving this goal requires the exact delineation of tumor, which is provided by didactic imaging techniques [84]. Although CT and MRI have been extensively used to delineate tumor margins, they are not tumor specific. For example, gadolinium enhancement could be seen merely as a result of blood–brain barrier (BBB) breakdown, which can lead to pseudo-progression and pseudo-response findings by MRI. To overcome the limitations of anatomic imaging, functional-physiologic-metabolic imaging by SPECT and PET has been introduced, which itself suffers from limited spatial/anatomic resolution. The current state-of-the-art techniques of clinical imaging, SPECT/CT and PET/CT, in which metabolic imaging is combined with anatomical imaging, seem to be superior to both techniques and have the advantages of higher spatial resolution than SPECT and tumor specificity inherent to metabolic imaging. SPECT/CT has the potential to change the diagnostic information in 20–25% of cases compared to SPECT or to CT alone, so influencing the treatment strategy, for instance, by better defining the target volume for external beam radiotherapy planning.

15.6.1 Brain Tumors

SPECT and SPECT/CT have been employed to determine functional areas of the brain and to optimize radiation planning by sparing "functional" areas of the brain in the treatment of brain malignant neoplasms [85]. The silent areas of the brain, however, might not be totally nonfunctional, and caution is still crucial in delivering higher doses of radiation to less "functional" areas on SPECT. Although a number of radiotracers have been employed for radiation planning by SPECT and SPECT/CT, Iodine-123-alpha-methyl-L-tyrosine (IMT) is one of the most widely used tracers. It is an amino acid, which is actively accumulated in brain tumors, but not in normal brain parenchyma. It has been shown that 23% of patients with non-resected glioma have IMT tumor uptake 2 cm outside of gross tumor volume defined by a T2-weighted MRI study [86]. In another study, 29% of patients showed IMT uptake located outside the MRI postoperative changes, which leads to an increase of 20% more tissue in the boost volume [87]. Therefore, it has been generally accepted that findings on IMT-SPECT might modify target volumes for gliomas planned with MRI imaging alone.

15.6.2 Lung Cancers

SPECT lung perfusion scans provide information regarding the functionality of lung tissue and designing radiotherapy fields. SPECT/CT detects 48% of patients with hypoperfused regions of the lung, so in 11% of patients, the radiation field angles are altered to avoid highly functional lung tissue [88]. Using SPECT/CT for radiation planning has been shown to lead to a 6% gain in lung perfusion as compared with geometrically optimized CT planning in patients with one hypoperfused hemithorax [89]. For patients with smaller perfusion defects, SPECT/CT perfusion-weighted optimization resulted in the same planning as the CT-only geometrically designed planning. A recent meta-analysis by Bucknell et al. on 114 publications [90] demonstrated that functional lung imaging (mostly using SPECT) offered a greater ability for predicting postradiation pneumonitis, compared to anatomic methods. They also found a reduction of the mean lung dose by 2.2 Gy, which holds a potential dosimetry benefit for functional imaging methods, in order to spare lung functioning tissue [91].

15.6.3 Breast Cancers

In women with early breast cancer, SPECT-CT visualization of SLNs is a potentially valuable method for radiotherapy planning, especially when no surgical sampling of axillary SLNs is planned. By imagining different variants of SLN locations in the axillary fossa, SPECT-CT offers a great opportunity for SLN tumoricidal-dose irradiation using different modifications of tangential fields [92], while sparing the critical non-tumoral nodes. The addition of SPECT-CT scintigraphy into breast cancer radiation treatment planning reduces the unnecessary radiation exposure to the arm-draining lymph nodes and therefore lessens the risk of developing lymphedema [93].

References

1. Gholamrezanejhad A, Mirpour S, Mariani G. Future of nuclear medicine: SPECT versus PET. J Nucl Med. 2009;50(7):16N–8N.
2. Love C, Marwin SE, Palestro CJ. Nuclear medicine and the infected joint replacement. Semin Nucl Med. 2009;39:66–78.
3. Love C, Tomas MB, Marwin SE, Pugliese PV, Palestro CJ. Role of nuclear medicine in diagnosis of the infected joint replacement. Radiographics. 2001;21:1229–38.
4. Segura AB, Muñoz A, Brulles YR, Hermoso JA, Díaz MC, Lazaro MT, Martín-Comín J. What is the role of bone scintigraphy in the diagnosis of infected joint prostheses? Nucl Med Commun. 2004;25(5):527–32.
5. Tahmasebi MN, Saghari M, Moslehi M, Gholamrezanezhad A. Comparison of SPECT bone scintigraphy with MRI for diagnosis of meniscal tears. BMC Nucl Med. 2005;5:2. https://doi.org/10.1186/1471-2385-5-2. PMID: 15831098; PMCID: PMC1090590.
6. Gemmel F, et al. Prosthetic joint infections: radionuclide state-of-the-art imaging. Eur J Nucl Med Mol Imaging. 2012;39(5):892–909.
7. Pakos EE, Trikalinos TA, Fotopoulos AD, Ioannidis JP. Prosthesis infection: diagnosis after total joint arthroplasty with antigranulocyte scintigraphy with 99mTc-labeled monoclonal antibodies—a meta-analysis. Radiology. 2007;242(1):101–8.

8. Xing D, Ma X, Ma J, et al. Use of anti-granulocyte scintigraphy with 99mTc-labeled monoclonal antibodies for the diagnosis of periprosthetic infection in patients after total joint arthroplasty: a diagnostic meta-analysis. PLoS One. 2013;8(7):e69857.

9. Basu S, Kwee TC, Saboury B, et al. FDG-PET for diagnosing infection in hip and knee prostheses: prospective study in 221 prostheses and subgroup comparison with combined 111In-labeled leukocyte/99mTc-sulfur colloid bone marrow imaging in 88 prostheses. Clin Nucl Med. 2014;39(7):609.

10. Erba PA, Israel O. SPECT/CT in infection and inflammation. Clin Transl Imaging. 2014;2(6):519–35.

11. Meller J, Sahlmann CO, Gurocak O, Liersch T, Meller B. FDG-PET in patients with fever of unknown origin: the importance of diagnosing large vessel vasculitis. Q J Nucl Med Mol Imaging. 2009;53:51–63.

12. Harris ED Jr. Rheumatoid arthritis: pathophysiology and implications for therapy. N Engl J Med. 1990;322(18):1277–89.

13. Szkudlarek M, Narvestad E, Klarlund M, Court-Payen M, Thomsen HS, Ostergaard M. Ultrasonography of the metatarsophalangeal joints in rheumatoid arthritis: comparison with magnetic resonance imaging, conventional radiography, and clinical examination. Arthritis Rheum. 2004;50:2103–12.

14. Gotthardt M, Bleeker-Rovers CP, Boerman OC, Oyen WJG. Imaging of inflammation by PET, conventional scintigraphy, and other imaging techniques. J Nucl Med. 2010;51:1937–49.

15. Ostendorf B, Mattes-Gyorgy K, Reichelt DC, Blondin D, Wirrwar A, Lanzman R, et al. Early detection of bony alterations in rheumatoid and erosive arthritis of finger joints with high-resolution single photon emission computed tomography, and differentiation between them. Skelet Radiol. 2010;39:55–61.

16. Roivainen A, Parkkola R, Yli-Kerttula T, Lehikoinen P, Viljanen T, Mottonen T, et al. Use of positron emission tomography with methyl-11C-choline and 2-18F-fluoro-2-deoxy-D-glucose in comparison with magnetic resonance imaging for the assessment of inflammatory proliferation of synovium. Arthritis Rheum. 2003;48:3077–84.

17. Buchbender C, Ostendorf B, Mattes-Gyorgy K, Miese F, Wittsack H-J, Quentin M, et al. Synovitis and bone inflammation in early rheumatoid arthritis: high-resolution multi-pinhole SPECT versus MRI. Diagn Interv Radiol. 2013;19:20–4.

18. Kouranos V, Wells AU, Sharma R, Underwood SR, Wechalekar K. Advances in radionuclide imaging of cardiac sarcoidosis. Br Med Bull. 2015;115(1):151–63.

19. Homonnai A, Kontz K, Tombacz A. The role of gallium scintigraphy in the diagnosis of sarcoidosis and in monitoring treatment effectiveness. Orv Hetil. 2006;147:1229–32.

20. Jin S, Wang G, He B, Zhu M. Gallium-67 scanning for detection of alveolitis in idiopathic pulmonary fibrosis and sarcoidosis. Chin Med J. 1996;109:519–21.

21. Lebtahi R, Crestani B, Belmatoug N, Daou D, Genin R, Dombret MC, et al. Somatostatin receptor scintigraphy and gallium scintigraphy in patients with sarcoidosis. J Nucl Med. 2001;42:21–6.

22. Okayama K, Kurata C, Tawarahara K, Wakabayashi Y, Chida K, Sato A. Diagnostic and prognostic value of myocardial scintigraphy with thallium-201 and gallium-67 in cardiac sarcoidosis. Chest. 1995;107:330–4.

23. Sy WM, Seo IS, Homs CJ, Gulrajani R, Sze P, Smith KF, et al. The evolutional stage changes in sarcoidosis on gallium-67 scintigraphy. Ann Nucl Med. 1998;12:77–82.

24. Tawarahara K, Kurata C, Okayama K, Kobayashi A, Yamazaki N. Thallium-201 and gallium 67 single photon emission computed tomographic imaging in cardiac sarcoidosis. Am Heart J. 1992;124:1383–4.

25. Spier BJ, Perlman SB, Reichelderfer M. FDG-PET in inflammatory bowel disease. Q J Nucl Med Mol Imaging. 2009;53:64–71.

26. Charron M, del Rosario FJ, Kocoshis SA. Pediatric inflammatory bowel disease: assessment with scintigraphy with 99mTc white blood cells. Radiology. 1999;212:507–13.

27. Xiu Y, Yu JQ, Cheng E, Kumar R, Alavi A, Zhuang H. Sarcoidosis demonstrated by FDG PET imaging with negative findings on gallium scintigraphy. Clin Nucl Med. 2005;30:193–5.

28. Momose M, et al. Usefulness of 67Ga SPECT and integrated low-dose CT scanning (SPECT/CT) in the diagnosis of cardiac sarcoidosis. Ann Nucl Med. 2007;21(10):545–51.

29. Horsthuis K, Bipat S, Bennink RJ, Stoker J. Inflammatory bowel disease diagnosed with US, MR, scintigraphy, and CT: meta-analysis of prospective studies. Radiology. 2008;247:64–79. https://doi.org/10.1148/radiol.2471070611.

30. Rispo A, Imbriaco M, Celentano L, et al. Noninvasive diagnosis of small bowel Crohn's disease: combined use of bowel sonography and Tc-99m-HMPAO leukocyte scintigraphy. Inflamm Bowel Dis. 2005;11(3):76–82.

31. Stathaki MI, Koukouraki SI, Karkavitsas NS, Koutroubakis IE. Role of scintigraphy in inflammatory bowel disease. World J Gastroenterol. 2009;15:2693–700.

32. Sans M, Fuster D, Llach J, Lomena F, Bordas JM, Herranz R, et al. Optimization of technetium-99m-HMPAO leukocyte scintigraphy in evaluation of active inflammatory bowel disease. Dig Dis Sci. 2000;45:1828–35.

33. Lee BF, Chiu NT, Wu DC, Tsai KB, Liu GC, Yu HS, et al. Use of 99mTc (V) DMSA scintigraphy in the detection and localization of intestinal inflammation: comparison of findings and colonoscopy and biopsy. Radiology. 2001;220:381–5.

34. Rothstein RD. The role of scintigraphy in the management of inflammatory bowel disease. J Nucl Med. 1991;32:856–9.

35. Koutroubakis IE, Koukouraki SI, Dimoulios PD, Velidaki AA, Karkavitsas NS, Kouroumalis

EA. Active inflammatory bowel disease: evaluation with 99mTc (V) DMSA scintigraphy. Radiology. 2003;229:70–4.

36. Stathaki MI, Koutroubakis IE, Koukouraki SI, Karmiris KP, Moschandreas JA, Kouroumalis EA, et al. Active inflammatory bowel disease: head-to-head comparison between 99mTc-hexamethylpropylene amine oxime white blood cells and 99mTc(V)-dimercaptosuccinic acid scintigraphy. Nucl Med Commun. 2008;29:27–32.

37. Coleman RE, Datz FL. Detection of inflammatory disease with radiolabeled cells. In: Diagnostic nuclear medicine. 4th ed. Philadelphia, PA: Lippincott Williams & Wilkins; 2003. p. 1219–34.

38. Arabi M, Brown RK, Dwamena BA, Jakubowski E, Kim K, Alvarez R, Piert M, Frey K. Single-photon emission computed tomography/computed tomography as a problem-solving tool in patients with suspected acute cholecystitis. J Comput Assist Tomogr. 2013;37(6):844–8.

39. Schillaci O, Filippi L, Danieli R, Simonetti G. Single-photon emission computed tomography/computed tomography in abdominal diseases. Semin Nucl Med. 2007;37(1):48–6.

40. Zheng JG, Yao ZM, Shu CY, Zhang Y, Zhang X. Role of SPECT/CT in diagnosis of hepatic hemangiomas. World J Gastroenterol. 2005;11(34):5336.

41. Meller J, Altenvoerde G, Munzel U, Jauho A, Behe M, Gratz S, et al. Fever of unknown origin: prospective comparison of [18F] FDG imaging with a double-head coincidence camera and gallium-67 citrate SPET. Eur J Nucl Med. 2000;27:1617–25.

42. Meller J, Becker W. Nuclear medicine diagnosis of patients with fever of unknown origin (FUO). Nuklearmedizin. 2001;40:59–70.

43. Meller J, Sahlmann C-O, Scheel AK. 18F-FDG PET and PET/CT in fever of unknown origin. J Nucl Med. 2007;48:35–45.

44. Shooli H, Nemati R, Chabi N, Larvie M, Jokar N, Dadgar H, Gholamrezanezhad A, Assadi M. Multimodal assessment of regional gray matter integrity in early relapsing-remitting multiple sclerosis patients with normal cognition: a voxel-based structural and perfusion approach. Br J Radiol. 2021;94(1127):20210308. https://doi.org/10.1259/bjr.20210308. Epub 2021 Sep 7. PMID: 34491820.

45. Walker L, Gholamrezanezhad A, Bucklan D, Faulhaber PF, O'Donnell JK. SPECT/CT detection of a communicating arachnoid cyst in a patient with normal pressure hydrocephalus. Clin Nucl Med. 2017;42(7):555–7. https://doi.org/10.1097/RLU.0000000000001685. PMID: 28481794.

46. Eftekhari M, Assadi M, Kazemi M, Saghari M, Esfahani AF, Sichani BF, Gholamrezanezhad A, Beiki D. A preliminary study of neuroSPECT evaluation of patients with post-traumatic smell impairment. BMC Nucl Med. 2005;5:6. https://doi.org/10.1186/1471-2385-5-6. PMID: 16313675; PMCID: PMC1314885.

47. Garibotto V, Montandon ML, Viaud CT, Allaoua M, Assal F, Burkhard PR, et al. Regions of interest-based discriminant analysis of DaTSCAN SPECT and FDG-PET for the classification of dementia. Clin Nucl Med. 2013;38:112–7.

48. Ravina B, Marek K, Eberly S, Oakes D, Kurlan R, Ascherio A, et al. Dopamine transporter imaging is associated with long-term outcomes in Parkinson's disease. Mov Disord. 2012;27:1392–7.

49. Depboylu C, Maurer L, Matusch A, Hermanns G, Windolph A, Behe M, et al. Effect of long-term treatment with pramipexole or levodopa on presynaptic markers assessed by longitudinal [(123) I] FP-CIT SPECT and histochemistry. NeuroImage. 2013;79:191–200.

50. Benamer HT, Patterson J, Wyper DJ, et al. Correlation of Parkinson's disease severity and duration with 123I-FP-CIT SPECT striatal uptake. Mov Disord. 2000;15(4):692–8.

51. Hirano T, Yonehara T, Inatomi Y, Hashimoto Y, Uchino M. Presence of early ischemic changes on computed tomography depends on severity and the duration of hypoperfusion: a single photon emission-computed tomographic study. Stroke. 2005;36:2601–8.

52. Eicker SO, Turowski B, Heiroth HJ, Steiger HJ, Hanggi D. A comparative study of perfusion CT and 99m Tc-HMPAO SPECT measurement to assess cerebrovascular reserve capacity in patients with internal carotid artery occlusion. Eur J Med Res. 2011;16:484–90.

53. Krishnananthan R, Minoshima S, Lewis D. Tc-99m ECD neuro-SPECT and diffusion weighted MRI in the detection of the anatomical extent of subacute stroke: a cautionary note regarding reperfusion hyperemia. Clin Nucl Med. 2007;32:700–2.

54. Song H-C, Bom H-S, Cho KH, Kim BC, Seo J-J, Kim C-G, et al. Prognostication of recovery in patients with acute ischemic stroke through the use of brain SPECT with technetium-99m–labeled metronidazole. Stroke. 2003;34:982–6.

55. Uruma G, Kakuda W, Abo M. Changes in regional cerebral blood flow in the right cortex homologous to left language areas are directly affected by left hemispheric damage in aphasic stroke patients: evaluation by Tc-ECD SPECT and novel analytic software. Eur J Neurol. 2010;17:461–9.

56. Ogasawara K, Ogawa A, Ezura M, Konno H, Doi M, Kuroda K, et al. Dynamic and static 99mTc-ECD SPECT imaging of subacute cerebral infarction: comparison with 133Xe SPECT. J Nucl Med. 2001;42:543–7.

57. Ogasawara K, Ogawa A, Ezura M, Konno H, Suzuki M, Yoshimoto T. Brain single-photon emission CT studies using 99mTc-HMPAO and 99mTc-ECD early after recanalization by local intraarterial thrombolysis in patients with acute embolic middle cerebral artery occlusion. AJNR Am J Neuroradiol. 2001;22:48–53.

58. Henry TR, Van Heertum RL. Positron emission tomography and single photon emission computed

tomography in epilepsy care. Semin Nucl Med. 2003;33:88–8104.
59. Brinkmann BH, O'Brien TJ, Mullan BP, O'Connor MK, Robb RA, So EL. Subtraction ictal SPECT coregistered to MRI for seizure focus localization in partial epilepsy. Mayo Clin Proc. 2000;75:615–24.
60. Hong SB, Joo EY, Tae WS, Cho J-W, Lee J-H, Seo DW, et al. Preictal versus ictal injection of radiotracer for SPECT study in partial epilepsy: SISCOM. Seizure. 2008;17:383–6.
61. Kazemi NJ, Worrell GA, Stead SM, Brinkmann BH, Mullan BP, O'Brien TJ, et al. Ictal SPECT statistical parametric mapping in temporal lobe epilepsy surgery. Neurology. 2010;74:70–6.
62. Kim JH, Im KC, Kim JS, Lee S-A, Lee JK, Khang SK, et al. Ictal hyperperfusion patterns in relation to ictal scalp EEG patterns in patients with unilateral hippocampal sclerosis: a SPECT study. Epilepsia. 2007;48:270–7.
63. Turpin S, Lambert R, Dubois J, Diadori P. F-18 FDG brain PET and Tc-99m ECD brain SPECT in a patient with multiple recurrent epileptic seizures. Clin Nucl Med. 2010;35:123–5.
64. Van Paesschen W. Ictal SPECT. Epilepsia. 2004;45(Suppl 4):35–40. https://doi.org/10.1111/j.0013-9580.2004.04008.
65. Wichert-Ana L, de Azevedo-Marques PM, Oliveira LF, Fernandes RMF, Velasco TR, Santos AC, et al. Ictal technetium-99 m ethyl cysteinate dimer single-photon emission tomographic findings in epileptic patients with polymicrogyria syndromes: a subtraction of ictal-interictal SPECT coregistered to MRI study. Eur J Nucl Med Mol Imaging. 2008;35:1159–70.
66. Devanand DP, Van Heertum RL, Kegeles LS, Liu X, Jin ZH, Pradhaban G, et al. (99m) Tc hexamethyl-propylene-aminoxime single-photon emission computed tomography prediction of conversion from mild cognitive impairment to Alzheimer disease. Am J Geriatr Psychiatry. 2010;18:959–72.
67. Honda N, Machida K, Hosono M, Matsumoto T, Matsuda H, Oshima M, et al. Interobserver variation in diagnosis of dementia by brain perfusion SPECT. Radiat Med. 2002;20:281–9.
68. Nobili F, Koulibaly M, Vitali P, Migneco O, Mariani G, Ebmeier K, et al. Brain perfusion follow-up in Alzheimer's patients during treatment with acetylcholinesterase inhibitors. J Nucl Med. 2002;43:983–90.
69. Roman G, Pascual B. Contribution of neuroimaging to the diagnosis of Alzheimer's disease and vascular dementia. Arch Med Res. 2012;43:671–6.
70. Vasquez BP, Buck BH, Black SE, Leibovitch FS, Lobaugh NJ, Caldwell CB, et al. Visual attention deficits in Alzheimer's disease: relationship to HMPAO SPECT cortical hypoperfusion. Neuropsychologia. 2011;49:1741–50.
71. Borghesani PR, DeMers SM, Manchanda V, Pruthi S, Lewis DH, Borson S. Neuroimaging in the clinical diagnosis of dementia: observations from a memory disorders clinic. J Am Geriatr Soc. 2010;58:1453–8.
72. Colloby SJ, Taylor JP, Firbank MJ, McKeith IG, Williams ED, O'Brien JT. Covariance 99mTc-exametazime SPECT patterns in Alzheimer's disease and dementia with Lewy bodies: utility in differential diagnosis. J Geriatr Psychiatry Neurol. 2010;23:54–62.
73. Mitsumoto T, Ohya N, Ichimiya A, Sakaguchi Y, Kiyota A, Abe K, et al. Diagnostic performance of Tc-99m HMPAO SPECT for early and late onset Alzheimer's disease: a clinical evaluation of linearization correction. Ann Nucl Med. 2009;23: 487–95.
74. van der Zande JJ, Joling M, Happach IG, Vriend C, Scheltens P, Booij J, Lemstra AW. Serotonergic deficits in dementia with Lewy bodies with concomitant Alzheimer's disease pathology: an 123I-FP-CIT SPECT study. NeuroImage Clin. 2020;25:102062.
75. Perlaki G, Szekeres S, Janszky J, et al. The applicability of 123I-FP-CIT SPECT dopamine transporter imaging in clinical practice. Ideggyogyaszati szemle. 2019;72(11–12):381.
76. Harpstrite S, Prior J, Cairns N, Sharma V. Evaluation of a 99mTc-peptide for imaging amyloid-β (Aβ) plaques in the brain. J Nucl Med. 2014;55(Suppl 1):1117.
77. Jokar S, Behnammanesh H, Erfani M, Sharifzadeh M, et al. Synthesis, biological evaluation and preclinical study of a novel 99mTc-peptide: a targeting probe of amyloid-β plaques as a possible diagnostic agent for Alzheimer's disease. Bioorg Chem. 2020;99:103857.
78. Wetter TC, Eisensehr I, Trenkwalder C. Functional neuroimaging studies in restless legs syndrome. Sleep Med. 2004;5(4):401–6.
79. Lin CC, Fan YM, Lin GY, Yang FC, Cheng CA, Lu KC, Lin JC, Lee JT. 99mTc-TRODAT-1 SPECT as a potential neuroimaging biomarker in patients with restless legs syndrome. Clin Nucl Med. 2016;41(1):e14–7.
80. Hou YC, Fan YM, Huang YC, et al. Tc-99m TRODAT-1 SPECT is a potential biomarker for restless leg syndrome in patients with end-stage. J Clin Med. 2020;9(3):889.
81. Santra A, Kumar R. Brain perfusion single photon emission computed tomography in major psychiatric disorders: from basics to clinical practice. Ind J Nucl Med. 2014;29(4):210.
82. Camargo EE. Brain SPECT in neurology and psychiatry. J Nucl Med. 2001;42(4):611–23.
83. Raji CA, Tarzwell R, Pavel D, et al. Clinical utility of SPECT neuroimaging in the diagnosis and treatment of traumatic brain injury: a systematic review. PLoS One. 2014;9(3):e91088.
84. Gholamrezanezhad A, Sabet A, Ezziddin S, Biersack HJ, Ahmadzadehfar H. Incremental diagnostic value of SPET/CT in precise localization of extraskeletal uptake of bone-seeking agents in multiple myeloma. Hell J Nucl Med. 2010;13(3):285–6. PMID: 21193889.
85. Paulino AC, Thorstad WL, Fox T. Role of fusion in radiotherapy treatment planning. Semin Nucl Med. 2003;33:238–43.

86. Grosu AL, Weber W, Feldmann HJ, Wuttke B, Bartenstein P, Gross MW, et al. First experience with I-123-alpha-methyl-tyrosine spect in the 3-D radiation treatment planning of brain gliomas. Int J Radiat Oncol Biol Phys. 2000;47:517–26.

87. Grosu AL, Feldmann H, Dick S, Dzewas B, Nieder C, Gumprecht H, et al. Implications of IMT-SPECT for postoperative radiotherapy planning in patients with gliomas. Int J Radiat Oncol Biol Phys. 2002;54:842–54.

88. Munley MT, Marks LB, Scarfone C, Sibley GS, Patz EF, Turkington TG, et al. Multimodality nuclear medicine imaging in three-dimensional radiation treatment planning for lung cancer: challenges and prospects. Lung Cancer. 1999;23:105–14.

89. Seppenwoolde Y, Engelsman M, De Jaeger K, Muller SH, Baas P, McShan DL, et al. Optimizing radiation treatment plans for lung cancer using lung perfusion information. Radiother Oncol. 2002;63:165–77.

90. Bucknell NW, Hardcastle N, Bressel M, Hofman MS, Kron T, Ball D, Siva S. Functional lung imaging in radiation therapy for lung cancer: a systematic review and meta-analysis. Radiother Oncol. 2018;129(2):196–208.

91. Izadyar S, Saber S, Gholamrezanezhad A. Assessment of clinical impact in the application of Chang attenuation correction to lung ventilation/perfusion SPECT. J Nucl Med Technol. 2011;39(4):290-4. https://doi.org/10.2967/jnmt.110.086470. Epub 2011 Sep 19. PMID: 21930669

92. Novikov S, Krzhivitskii P, Kanaev S, Krivorotko P, Ilin N, Melnik J, Popova N. SPECT-CT localization of axillary sentinel lymph nodes for radiotherapy of early breast cancer. Rep Pract Oncol Radiother. 2019;24(6):688–94.

93. Cheville AL, Brinkmann DH, Ward SB, Durski J, Laack NN, Yan E, Schomberg PJ, Garces YI, Suman VJ, Petersen IA. The addition of SPECT/CT lymphoscintigraphy to breast cancer radiation planning spares lymph nodes critical for arm drainage. Int J Radiat Oncol Biol Phys. 2013;85(4):971–7.